D1452174

Handbook of
Clinical Geropsychology

The Plenum Series in Adult Development and Aging

SERIES EDITOR:
Jack Demick, *Suffolk University, Boston, Massachusetts*

ADULT DEVELOPMENT, THERAPY, AND CULTURE
A Postmodern Synthesis
Gerald D. Young

THE AMERICAN FATHER
Biocultural and Developmental Aspects
Wade C. Mackey

THE DEVELOPMENT OF LOGIC IN ADULTHOOD
Postformal Thought and Its Applications
Jan D. Sinnott

HANDBOOK OF AGING AND MENTAL HEALTH
An Integrative Approach
Edited by Jacob Lomranz

HANDBOOK OF CLINICAL GEROPSYCHOLOGY
Edited by Michel Hersen and Vincent B. Van Hasselt

HANDBOOK OF PAIN AND AGING
Edited by David I. Mostofsky and Jacob Lomranz

HUMAN DEVELOPMENT IN ADULTHOOD
Lewis R. Aiken

PSYCHOLOGICAL TREATMENT OF OLDER ADULTS
An Introductory Text
Edited by Michel Hersen and Vincent B. Van Hasselt

Handbook of
Clinical Geropsychology

Edited by
Michel Hersen

Pacific University
Forest Grove, Oregon

and
Vincent B. Van Hasselt

Nova Southeastern University
Fort Lauderdale, Florida

Plenum Press • New York and London

Library of Congress Cataloging-in-Publication Data

Handbook of clinical geropsychology / edited by Michel Hersen and
    Vincent B. Van Hasselt.
        p.   cm. -- (The Plenum series in adult development and aging)
    Includes bibliographical references and index.
    ISBN 0-306-45661-3
    1. Geriatric psychiatry--Handbooks, manuals, etc. 2. Aged--Mental
health--Handbooks, manuals, etc. 3. Clinical psychology--Handbooks,
manuals, etc.   I. Hersen, Michel. II. Van Hasselt, Vincent B.
III. Series.
    [DNLM: 1. Mental Disorders--in old age. 2. Mental Disorders-
-therapy. 3. Geriatric Psychiatry--methods. 4. Aged--psychology.
WT 150 H23441 1998]
RC451.4.A5H356 1998
618.97'689--dc21
DNLM/DLC
for Library of Congress   98-21527
                                                                     CIP

ISBN 0-306-45661-3

© 1998 Plenum Press, New York
A Division of Plenum Publishing Corporation
233 Spring Street, New York, N.Y. 10013

http://www.plenum.com

10 9 8 7 6 5 4 3 2 1

Printed in the United States of America

Contributors

RONALD D. ADELMAN, Division of Geriatrics and Gerontology, New York Hospital–Cornell Medical Center, New York, New York 10021

PATRICIA A. ARÉAN, Department of Psychiatry, University of California–San Francisco, San Francisco, California 94143-0984

J. GAYLE BECK, Department of Psychology, State University of New York, Buffalo, New York 14260

STEPHEN J. BARTELS, Department of Psychiatry and Community and Family Medicine, New Hampshire–Dartmouth Psychiatric Research Center, Dartmouth Medical School, Concord, New Hampshire 03301

GARY R. BIRCHLER, Department of Psychiatry, School of Medicine, University of California, San Diego, La Jolla, California 92093-0603

FRANCE C. BLAIS, École de Psychologie, Université Laval, Cité Universitaire, Québec, Canada G1K 7P4

LOUIS D. BURGIO, Center for Aging, Division of Gerontology and Geriatric Medicine, and Department of Psychology, University of Alabama at Birmingham, Birmingham, Alabama 35294-4410

TONY CELLUCCI, Department of Psychology, Francis Marion University, Florence, South Carolina 29501-0547

KATIE E. CHERRY, Department of Psychology, Louisiana State University, Baton Rouge, Louisiana 70803-5501

ANTONIA CHRONOPOLOUS, Center for Psychological Studies, Nova Southeastern University, Fort Lauderdale, Florida 33314

JOAN M. COOK, Center for Psychological Studies, Nova Southeastern University, Fort Lauderdale, Florida 33314

DAVID W. COON, Older Adult Center, Veterans Affairs Health Care System, Palo Alto, California 94304

ELLEN M. COTTER, Center for Aging, Division of Gerontology and Geriatric Medicine, and Department of Psychology, University of Alabama at Birmingham, Birmingham, Alabama 35294-4410

PATRICK H. DELEON, Administrative Assistant to U.S. Senator Daniel K. Inouye, U.S. Senate, Hart Senate Building, Washington, D.C. 20510-1102

LARRY W. DUPREE, Department of Aging and Mental Health, The Florida Mental Health Institute, University of South Florida, Tampa, Florida 33612-3899

BUNNY FALK, Center for Psychological Studies, Nova Southeastern University, Fort Lauderdale, Florida 33314

WILLIAM FALS-STEWART, Department of Psychology, Old Dominion University, Norfolk, Virginia 23529-0267

NANCY FOLDI, Division of Neurology, Winthrop–University Hospital, Mineola, New York 11501

MARY J. GAGE, Mellon Center, Cleveland Clinic, Cleveland, Ohio 44195

DOLORES GALLAGHER-THOMPSON, Older Adult Center, Veterans Affairs Health Care System, Palo Alto, California 94304 and Stanford University School of Medicine, Stanford, California

CHARLES J. GOLDEN, Center for Psychological Studies, Nova Southeastern University, Fort Lauderdale, Florida 33314

ANTHONY J. GORECZNY, Director of Clinical Training Program, Department of Psychology, University of Indianapolis, Indianapolis, Indiana 46227-3697

IGOR GRANT, Department of Psychiatry, School of Medicine, University of California, San Diego, La Jolla, California 92093-0680

CHERYL BURNS HARDISON, Program for Research on Black Americans, Institute for Social Research, University of Michigan, Ann Arbor, Michigan 48106-1248

MICHEL HERSEN, School of Professional Psychology, Pacific University, Forest Grove, Oregon 97116

JAMES S. JACKSON, Program for Research on Black Americans, Institute for Social Research, University of Michigan, Ann Arbor, Michigan 48106-1248

MICHAEL LAVIN, Department of Psychology, University of Arizona, Tucson, Arizona 85721

HOWARD D. LERNER, Department of Psychology, University of Michigan, Ann Arbor, Michigan 48104

EDITH S. LISANSKY-GOMBERG, Alcohol Research Center, Department of Psychology, University of Michigan, Ann Arbor, Michigan 48104

NATHANIEL McCONAGHY, Psychiatric Unit, Prince of Wales Hospital, Randwick 2031, New South Wales, Australia

KEITH M. MILES, Department of Psychiatry and Community and Family Medicine, New Hampshire–Dartmouth Psychiatric Research Center, Dartmouth Medical School, Concord, New Hampshire 03301

VÉRONIQUE MIMEAULT, École de Psychologie, Université Laval, Cité Universitaire, Québec, Canada G1K 7P4

CHARLES M. MORIN, École de Psychologie, Université Laval, Cité Universitaire, Québec, Canada G1K 7P4

DEBRA S. MORLEY, Department of Psychology, Boston University, Boston, Massachusetts 02215

DAVID I. MOSTOFSKY, Laboratory for Experimental Behavioral Medicine, Department of Psychology, Boston University, Boston, Massachusetts 02215

KIM T. MUESER, Department of Psychiatry and Community and Family Medicine, New Hampshire–Dartmouth Psychiatric Research Center, Dartmouth Medical School, Concord, New Hampshire 03301

TED D. NIRENBERG, Department of Psychiatry and Human Behavior, and Center for Alcohol and Addiction Studies, Brown University, and Department of Emergency Medicine, Rhode Island Hospital, Providence, Rhode Island 02908

THOMAS L. PATTERSON, Department of Psychiatry, School of Medicine, University of California, San Diego, La Jolla, California 92093-0680

DAVID POWERS, Older Adult Center, Veterans Affairs Health Care System, Palo Alto, California 94304

PETER V. RABINS, Department of Psychiatry and Behavioral Sciences, Johns Hopkins University School of Medicine, Baltimore, Maryland 21287-7279

PATRICIA RIVERA, Older Adult Center, Veterans Affairs Health Care System, Palo Alto, California 94304

BRUCE D. SALES, Department of Psychology, University of Arizona, Tucson, Arizona 85721

DEREK SATRE, Department of Psychiatry, University of California–San Francisco, San Francisco, California 94143-0984

LAWRENCE SCHONFELD, Department of Aging and Mental Health, The Florida Mental Health Institute, University of South Florida, Tampa, Florida 33612-3899

DANIEL L. SEGAL, Department of Psychology, University of Colorado at Colorado Springs, Colorado Springs, Colorado 80933-7150

SHERRILL L. SELLERS, Program for Research on Black Americans, Institute for Social Research, University of Michigan, Ann Arbor, Michigan 48106-1248

SHIRLEY SEMPLE, Department of Psychiatry, School of Medicine, University of California, San Diego, La Jolla, California 92093-0680

William S. Shaw, Department of Psychiatry, School of Medicine, University of California, San Diego, La Jolla, California 92093-0680

Henna Siddiqui, Division of Geriatrics, Winthrop–University Hospital, Mineola, New York 11501

Anderson D. Smith, School of Psychology, Georgia Institute of Technology, Atlanta, Georgia 30332-0001

Melinda A. Stanley, Department of Psychiatry and Behavioral Sciences, University of Texas Mental Sciences Institute, Health Science Center at Houston, Houston, Texas 77030

Warren W. Tryon, Department of Psychology, Fordham University, Bronx, New York 10458-5198

Heather Uncapher, Department of Psychiatry, University of California–Berkeley, Berkeley, California 94720

Vincent B. Van Hasselt, Center for Psychological Studies, Nova Southeastern University, Fort Lauderdale, Florida 33314

Gary R. VandenBos, American Psychological Association, Washington, D.C. 20002-4242

Patricia A. Wisocki, Department of Psychology, University of Massachusetts, Amherst, Massachusetts 01003

Antonette M. Zeiss, Training and Program Development, Psychology Service, and Interprofessional Team Training and Development Program, Older Adult Center, Veterans Affairs Health Care System, Palo Alto, California 94304

Preface

Clinical psychology is a relatively young profession, with its major growth spurt having occurred in the period after World War II. Clinical geropsychology, a subspecialty of clinical psychology, is of most recent vintage, with its growth spurt paralleling the dramatic increase in older adults in the United States. Indeed, in the past two decades the number of persons over 65 years of age has increased by 65%. In the year 2030, one third of the population is projected to be 55 years of age and older. In addition, the number of very old (i.e., those more than 85 years of age) is expected to increase by a factor of 6 by the middle of the next century.

Given this so-called graying of America, it should not be surprising that clinical psychologists have turned their attention to the assessment and remediation of the problems that are faced (and will continue to be faced) by our senior citizens. It is paradoxical that despite our aging population and increased longevity, the age designated as the beginning of study for geropsychology has decreased from 65 to 55, and in some instances even 50. Also of interest are the changes in terminology with respect to study of older individuals, going from the more pejorative geriatrics, to the less pejorative gerontology, to clinical geropsychology, which now reflects the work of clinical psychologists. Editors of other handbooks have used the words aging and gerontology in their titles. This is the first compendium referred to as the *Handbook of Clinical Psychology* and it, of course, highlights the contributions of *clinical* psychology.

The *Handbook of Clinical Geropsychology* contains 25 chapters divided into three parts. In Part I ("General Issues"), in addition to a historical perspective, the chapters are about clinical geropsychology and U.S. federal policy, psychodynamic issues, the values of behavioral perspectives in treating older adults, moral and ethical considerations in geropsychology, and normal memory aging.

Part II ("Psychopathology, Assessment, and Treatment") incorporates description, assessment, and treatment for dementia, substance abuse disorders, schizophrenia, depression, anxiety disorders, sexual dysfunction, sleep disturbances in late life, personality disorders, aging and mental retardation, and behavioral medicine interventions with older adults.

Finally, in Part III ("Special Issues"), nine problem areas faced by older adults and their caregivers are given consideration, including health and well-being in retirement, pain management, the experience of bereavement by older adults, marriage and divorce, family caregiving, prevention, minority issues, physical activity, and approaches to diagnosis and treatment of elder abuse and neglect.

We anticipate that this book will be of interest to professionals and students from a wide range of disciplines, including psychology, psychiatry, rehabilitation, education, social work, and nursing, especially given the explosion of new data in this area. Not only is there academic interest in the area of clinical geropsychology, but growing media and governmental attention has focused on the shift in the age spectrum of the population in our country, with its attendant problems. Given the new data and the increasing population of older people, we believe that a *new* handbook in the field of clinical geropsychology is indeed warranted, especially one that presents coverage of issues from the perspective of clinical psychology.

As an *a priori* apologia, we should note that in light of the newness of clinical geropsychology, the conclusions reached in some of the chapters can only be described as tentative. In some instances, there may be greater attention focused on where the field is going. Perhaps more definitive statements will appear in future editions of this work, as necessary.

Many individuals have contributed to the genesis and fruition of this project. First, we thank our editor and friend at Plenum Press, Eliot Werner, who understood the merits of this endeavor. Second, we thank our contributors who took time out to share their expertise with us. And finally, we thank our friend, Burt G. Bolton, who graciously has provided us with his technical expertise.

Michel Hersen
Vincent B. Van Hasselt

Contents

PART I

GENERAL ISSUES

CHAPTER 1

Historical Perspectives

Joan M. Cook, Michel Hersen, and Vincent B. Van Hasselt

INTRODUCTION

A review of the historical perspectives of geropsychology reveals a remarkable progression in standpoints on aging. The development in knowledge of aging is substantial and has been rapidly increasing in recent years. This chapter provides a historical review of the growth and development of the scientific psychological study of older adults. In the first section, we examine why there is a growing interest in the psychology of older individuals. In the second section, we examine the historical antecedents of geropsychology, ranging over three time periods: 1835 to 1918, 1919 to 1946, and 1947 to the present. Although most of the historical antecedents section focuses on perspectives on psychological research on older adults, information on policy and practice in geropsychology is added where deemed necessary. The last section of this chapter focuses on future perspectives in the field of geropsychology. It is important to understand that research, policy, and practice on aging depends in part on contextual variables such as social, economic, and political influences (Riegel, 1973).

AN INCREASING INTEREST IN PSYCHOLOGY OF AGING

In the latter half of the 20th century, there are more older persons than there have been at any other time throughout history (Dychtwald & Flower, 1989). From 1900 to 1990, the percentage of older people (65 years and over) in the population grew from 4% to 13%, while the proportion of young people (under 18 years) has diminished from 40% to 26% (U.S. Department of Health and Human Services,

Joan M. Cook and Vincent B. Van Hasselt • Center for Psychological Studies, Nova Southeastern University, Fort Lauderdale, Florida 33314.   Michel Hersen • School of Professional Psychology, Pacific University, Forest Grove, Oregon 97116.

Handbook of Clinical Geropsychology, edited by Michel Hersen and Vincent B. Van Hasselt. Plenum Press, New York, 1998.

1995). The unprecedented shift in the relative age group composition of society can be explained in part by vastly improved medical technology and care.

Contrary to popular opinion and media depiction, the elderly are not a homogeneous group. Approaches to aging must take into account the heterogeneity of older adults especially with respect to physical health, cognitive functioning, and gender. Demographic projections show that our population is changing dramatically in terms of age, ethnic, and cultural composition. For example, the oldest old, persons over the age of 85 years, are the fastest-growing segment of the aged population (Suzman, Willis, & Manton, 1992). In addition, there is a coming wave of aging "baby boomers." Further, in the next 50 years, the nonwhite portion of the elderly population is anticipated to nearly double (Angel & Hogan, 1994). In particular, according to Jackson (1988), the African American population is growing at a faster rate than any other older group.

With the dramatic increase in the population surviving to old age, the number of individuals at risk for physical, social, economic, and mental problems has also increased. Indeed, aging has often been synonymous with inevitable loss: loss of spouse, friends, and relatives, loss of work and decreased income, loss of acuity in sensory modalities, and lessening of physical abilities and cognitive functioning.

Variables under study in the field of geropsychology are wide-ranging. Psychological theories of aging address broad areas such as personality, intelligence, problem solving, sensation, perception, memory, and life satisfaction. The study of emotional well-being and social and independent functioning in older adults provides an objective basis for establishing the general experiences of older adults. Psychologists studying aging also concentrate on specific areas such as pain, insomnia, and incontinence. The behavioral functioning of an aging population includes normative aspects and deviations in the aging process.

Mental health disorders in the elderly have also received attention in the literature. As the population over 65 increases, psychological stress and mental disorders will become an increasingly important public health issue. As mentally ill persons continue to "age in place," it is imperative to assess and meet their service needs (Holhouser, 1988). Compounding the impact of mental illness are medical and social comorbidities: As the severely mentally ill age, their comorbid medical diagnoses multiply (Kramer, 1983) and mentally ill elderly are less likely to receive needed physical and mental health services than are younger persons (German, Shapiro, & Skinner, 1985). Approximately half of the older adult population who received care for physical disorders also had at least one mental disorder. Unrecognized and untreated psychopathology in conjunction with medical illness and functional difficulties place the elderly at increased risk for hospitalization and long-term institutionalization. Further, lack of appropriate diagnosis and treatment often leads to a decline in essential self-sustaining activities that are key determinants of quality of life.

As the number of elderly persons increases, there is an escalating need for mental health care and social services. Currently, there is a shortage of persons who research and provide services to aging individuals, particularly those highly qualified in the behavioral and mental health sciences and services. Although the field of psychology of aging has a substantial number of excellent re-

searchers and clinicians examining significant problems, more educational programs and incentives are needed to train and encourage people in such careers.
Despite a strong and active field of psychology and aging, there are obvious
omissions and deficiencies. For example, research on and services for special
groups of elderly individuals who are at increased risk for experiencing psychological and psychopathologic difficulties are lacking. Groups especially at
increased risk for interpersonal and intrapersonal complications are the chronically mentally ill who survive into old age, older individuals with mental retardation, and those living below poverty levels in public housing.

HISTORICAL ANTECEDENTS

As far back as ancient times, philosophers have discussed unique features
among individuals of different ages. In fact, many philosophers have concerned
themselves with defining a good old age. In the past, individuals who survived
to old age were fairly rare.

Since few people survived to old age, myths were formulated to account for
such occurrences. Human beings who lived for long periods of time were hypothesized to be favored by the gods or were suspected of ingesting special
herbs. Fascinated with the idea of rejuvenation, Ponce de Leon searched for the
Fountain of Youth in Florida. In the hope of discovering ways to increase the
lifespan, Francis Bacon observed the aging population, speculating that improvements in hygiene would reduce germs and disease and subsequently increase chances of survival. Benjamin Franklin was another investigator of aging
who searched for the answer to the rejuvenation myth. He erroneously speculated that with use of electricity deceased humans could be resurrected.

Until the early 20th century, life expectancy was relatively short (i.e., 45
years at the beginning of this century). Disease, famine, and war are among the
variables associated with a limited life span. The study of aging has a long past,
but a short history. It was not until comparatively recent times that scientists began formally to study aging.

Years 1835 to 1918

The origin of the study of the psychology of aging is often credited to Lambert Adolphe Jacques Quetelet (Birren, 1961). Quetelet, a mathematician and
astronomer, initiated the first collection of psychological data in examining human development and aging. In his book *On Man and the Development of His
Faculties,* published in 1835, Quetelet presented his data on sensory functioning, height, weight, hand strength, and productivity across various age groups
(Riegel, 1977).

The next leading researcher interested in the scientific study of aging was
Sir Francis Galton (Birren, 1961). In the 1880s, Galton collected data from 9,337
males and females, 5 to 80 years old, who visited the London International
Health Exhibitions. In his anthropometric laboratory, he employed standardized instruments to measure the degree of association of certain variables with

aging (including sensorimotor performance). Indeed, Galton was the first scientist to conclude on an empirical basis that most human capacities tend to decline as they age. These findings, published in 1885, established Galton as the founder of the psychology of individual and developmental differences.

Simultaneously, the first psychological laboratory was founded by Wilhelm Wundt in Leipzig, Germany. Wundt's physiological experiments also increased our knowledge about geropsychology. However, his students required almost a decade to become fully aware of the discrepancies in performance between subjects of different ages (Birren, 1961).

In Russia, Ivan Pavlov was also studying the connections between physiology and psychology. His studies had further implications for an evolving psychology of aging field. In particular, Pavlov's finding that the conditioning of older animals was different from that of younger animals was pivotal in establishing the importance of developmental differences (Riegel, 1977).

Years 1919 to 1946

Although largely ignored by fellow researchers, Foster and Taylor (1920) investigated differential changes in intellectual functioning of adults, including the aged. They examined the relationship of speed, functioning, and demographic variables such as educational level and socioeconomic factors to changes in intelligence.

In 1922, G. Stanley Hall, primarily known for his work on childhood and adolescence, published a book entitled *Senescence: The Second Half of Life.* This seminal work was a review of the empirical studies of aging, including psychological, biological, behavioral, and physiological perspectives. Although his review documented the status of research on aging then current, it also indicated how sparse the geropsychology literature was compared to the child psychology literature. In addition, Hall was concerned with the relationship between religious belief and fear of death.

Contemporaries of Hall who were also publishing on aging included biologists. In 1908, Minot's *The Problems of Age, Growth and Death* and Metchnikoff's *The Prolongation of Life* were both concerned with explaining aging relative to an accumulation of bacteria in the gastrointestinal tract and its believed remedy of ingesting yogurt. In addition, Pearl's (1922) *Biology of Death* basically stated that aging was caused and affected by heredity alone. At this juncture, individuals investigating aging issues had a more experimental approach and were more physiologically than socially oriented.

Interestingly, at the beginning of the 20th century, as scholars were recognizing the need for the scientific study of the aged, most clinicians were unwilling to extend psychological treatment to older adults. In fact, in the early years of psychoanalysis, Freud was very skeptical, believing that psychological treatment of individuals over the age of 50 would be ineffective (Freud, 1904/1959). Freud offered several reasons to substantiate his beliefs: older individuals have limitations in ego or intellect; analysis would have to cover a relatively longer lifetime and thus treatment would be prolonged indefinitely; and analysis would occur at a time when it was no longer important to be psychologically healthy.

In the clinical domain, Abraham (1919/1927) was the first psychoanalyst to recognize and express optimism for the psychoanalytic treatment of older adults. He described successful analyses of four older neurotic patients. His conclusions were critical. Abraham believed that the age at which the older adult started psychoanalysis or resolution of conflict was less important than the age of patient at the time the neurosis began.

Although Freud's views on older adults was typical of clinical thinking, pioneer Dr. Lillien Martin eagerly administered psychotherapy to the aged (Martin, 1944). In 1929, Dr. Martin founded and directed the San Francisco Old Age Counseling Center. This was the first established psychotherapeutic program for the aged in the United States. Dr. Martin's therapeutic techniques centered on overcoming pessimism by adopting the "will-to-do-attitude."

Concurrently, but on the research end, Walter Miles was interested in studying the problems of older workers in industry. He expanded his interests and, in 1928, with the assistance of his colleagues at Stanford University, developed a project to analyze psychological aspects of aging. Miles's initial findings from this study, named the Stanford Later Maturity Project, were published in 1931. Although the significance of this contribution to the study of intellectual development has been questioned, it undoubtedly deserves credit as one of the first studies for breadth in approach and use of experimental methods (Riegel, 1977).

Most early psychological research on adult development and aging was devoted to the study of intelligence. For example, Jones and Conrad (1933) administered the Army Alpha Test to an adult sample to test for developmental differences in intellectual functions; cohort differences and historical changes were examined.

Importantly, at this time, the notion was spreading that disciplines interested in the scientific study of aging should not be independent and unrelated. During the 1930s, the Macy Foundation developed an interest in supporting studies of aging, with an emphasis on interdisciplinary collaboration. The foundation sponsored a conference at Woods Hole, Massachusetts, where researchers with medical, social, psychological, psychiatric, and humanistic approaches met. In fact, it was the Macy Foundation that encouraged Cowdry (1939) to include multidisciplinary perspectives in his book entitled *Problems of Aging*. Indeed, Miles published some of his data from the Stanford Later Maturity Project in the first chapter of Cowdry's book. This book was a milestone, in that it brought together the ideas of several disciplines.

Sidney Pressey (1939) was the first psychologist to publish a book on development that encompassed adulthood and aging. Pressey, who taught at the department of psychology at the University of Ohio, trained many Ph.D. candidates with a focus on aging.

Despite the previously mentioned researchers' interest in and experimentation with older adults, the field of geropsychology remained in its infancy. Beyond the individuals mentioned previously, few scholars paid attention to aging until after World War II. Relatively little scientific investigation of aging and only sporadic public concern for aging issues were evident at this time. Prior to World War II, the predominant view held by psychology was that childhood was an end product rather than part of the course of an ongoing life. The belief that adolescence represented the final stage of development was widely held. Accordingly, the belief at the time was that there was little to investigate scientifically postadolescence.

World War II interrupted and curtailed the emerging interest in geropsychology. However, several studies conducted during this time found that performance of American servicemen was greatly affected by age. In the late 1930s, the surgeon general of the U.S. Public Health Service created a gerontological unit of the National Institute of Health. In 1941, Nathan Shock became the second director of this organization, and he brought to the task a psychological as well as a biological agenda. Subsequently, James Birren became associated with this group and guided its psychological research.

After World War II, the field of psychology and aging was subjected to more systematic investigation. The number of scientists interested in studying developmental and aging processes increased dramatically. These investigators emphasized that development and aging continue throughout the adult period.

In 1942, the American Geriatrics Society was established: the society publishes a journal that bears the same name. The Gerontological Society of America (GSA), a multidisciplinary association, was founded in 1945 (Adler, 1958). This organization publishes *The Journals of Gerontology* and *The Gerontologist,* two leading journals in the field of aging. In 1946, the American Psychological Association (APA) added a new division to its structure, Division 20, Maturity and Old Age (now renamed Division on Adult Development and Aging) (Pressey, 1948). The field of geropsychology gained power and momentum as psychologists acquired section representation in a multidisciplinary organization (GSA) and an independent group status within a major psychological organization, the American Psychological Association.

Although Kaplan published *Mental Disorders of Later Life* in 1945, the study of the psychopathology of later life grew relatively slowly. One reason for the lack of emphasis in this area may be stereotypes of mental illness. Although historically the mentally ill, in general, have not been treated well by society, older adults with mental health problems appear to have fared even more poorly.

Years 1947 to the Present

The International Association of Gerontology (IAG) was established in 1950. The first meeting of the IAG was primarily focused on biological processes of aging. However, in 1953, at the second IAG meeting, a large number of research papers were presented in the area of geropsychology. To help organize the wealth of information from journal articles, books, and scientific meetings, Nathan Shock (1951, 1957, 1963) started producing *A Classified Bibliography of Gerontology and Geriatrics.*

The first book on geropsychology published by the American Psychological Association was Anderson's (1956) *Psychological Aspects of Aging.* In 1959, Birren's *Handbook of Aging and the Individual* organized the scattered literature on the psychology of aging.

Despite the new data adduced, few recognized the impact that the increasing number of older adults would have on our society. Adult development traditionally was studied with a cross-sectional method, with measurements made at approximately the same time on subjects differing in chronological age. Researchers in the field of child development were the first to recognize limitations of cross-sectional analyses, and in the early part of the 20th century initiated longitudinal studies. Nearly 30 years later, scientists involved with aging research recognized the necessity of conducting longitudinal studies in adults. Most of the resulting studies, however, emphasized physiological functions and only a few studies included behavioral or personality characteristics.

In the absence of an established comprehensive theoretical paradigm for normative aging, empirical identification of aspects of aging in community settings was warranted. Beginning in 1955 at Duke University Medical Center's department of psychiatry, under the leadership of Ewald Busse (1970), a longitudinal study was conducted to explore physical, mental, and social processes of normal aging. Community-residing males and females, 60 years and older, were subjects of the study. One area of inquiry focused on characterizing behavioral correlates of changes in the aging central nervous system. Another broad area of interest concerned the adaptive aspects of behavior studied within a social psychological framework (Siegler, 1983). A significant finding from the study was that a substantial number of participants did not show decline in intellectual function. Evidence that most older people maintained high levels of cognitive functioning confirmed the notion that intellectual decline was not an inevitable concomitant of aging. In 1968, a second longitudinal study at Duke, known as the Duke Adaptation Study, was initiated. This study focused on the short- and long-term effects of stressful life events (death of spouse, retirement). One of the most important findings under the rubric of psychological inquiry was that adult personality showed little change over the eight years of the study. A third longitudinal study of aging, entitled Mental Illness and Social Support Among the Very Old, was conducted at Duke.

Yet another longitudinal study that has had a tremendous impact on current theorizing on aging processes is the Baltimore Longitudinal Study of Aging (BLSA) (Shock et al., 1984). The Duke studies included participants 60 years or older; the BLSA examined healthy aging over the entire adult life span (17 years and above). In addition, the Duke studies consisted of three separate studies in which data collection has been completed, whereas the BLSA data collection remains in progress. Beginning in 1958, participants in the BLSA were given repeated tests and examinations over their life span, including inquiries on cognitive performance, personality, and stress and coping processes. Findings from this study stress the many individual differences in the experience of aging. There is a great range of variation in psychological indicators in community-residing adults.

In the early 1960s, the National Institutes of Health (NIH) funded several programs at universities to aid scientists in the formation of systematic studies on aging. These universities included the University of Chicago, the University of Michigan–Wayne State University Institute of Gerontology, and the Ethel Percy Andrus Gerontology Center at the University of Southern California. The gerontological institutes promoted exchange of ideas and thus contributed substantially to development of the field of geropsychology.

In particular, at the University of Chicago's Committee on Human Development, under the aegis of Robert Havighurst and Bernice Neugarten, doctoral level students were trained in the social psychology of aging. In fact, some of the most significant contributions to the social psychology of aging came from this department (Neugarten, 1968). Indeed, the Kansas City Studies of Adult Life, conducted by University of Chicago researchers, greatly advanced knowledge on normal personality development in adulthood. In particular, research on ego styles and sex-role changes in middle age and later adulthood was greatly emphasized.

In 1961, the first White House Conference on Aging (WHCoA) was convened. This represented the first national symposium, joining members of the scientific, clinical, and lay communities in a productive public exchange on the elderly. By 1965, the United States Congress established Medicare and the Older Americans Act (OAA). The OAA was the first program to focus on community-based services for older adults. Two of the objectives of this Act were that the federal, state, and local governments assist older adults in obtaining mental health care and institutional, home, and community long-term care.

During the 1960s, there was a rapid expansion in the number of publications in psychological gerontology. One landmark study conducted during this period focused on life span developmental changes in intelligence (Schaie, 1965). Data collection began in 1956 for the Seattle Longitudinal Studies (SLS); the study is still in progress (Schaie, 1993). Information from the SLS on individual variation in the life course of adult intellectual abilities has been widely disseminated and its impact on the field of psychology and gerontology has been far-reaching.

Erikson (1963) proposed a theory of psychosocial development that included eight major crises an individual faces in the course of a lifetime. This theory, an alternative to Freud's psychosexual stages of human development, was the first of its kind to include phases of adult development. Recognition of developmental tasks and conflicts older individuals face was an important precedent to the increased interest in treating older adults with psychotherapy. In the late 1960s and early 1970s, innovative psychiatric programs such as the Langley Porter Neuropsychiatric Institute and the San Francisco Geriatric Screening Project encouraged older patients in the community to take advantage of services available for the detection and treatment of mental disorders in late life (Feigenbaum, 1973; Lowenthal, Berkman, & Associates, 1967).

However, despite a handful of resourceful psychiatric programs, the overall mental health service and delivery system for older adults was deficient. In the 1960s, deinstitutionalization of state psychiatric facilities was implemented. A study of patients in public hospitals estimated that one third of these residents were 65 or older and that 27% of first admissions were also in this age group (American Psychiatric Association, 1959). After deinstitutionalization, adequate care for most of the residents was not provided, and many elderly in these facilities consequently became residents of nursing homes. Thus, progress in mental health services for older adults did not keep pace with scientific progress in this field.

The second White House Conference on Aging was held in 1971. Subsequently, results of psychological investigations that were presented at the WHCoA and recommendations made by a task force organized by the American Psychological Association were compiled in a book. This second book on geropsychology issued by the APA was Eisdorfer and Lawton's (1973) *The Psychology of Adult Development and Aging.*

During the 1960s and 1970s, substantial data in geropsychology were being adduced. In 1973, Riegel categorized nine common areas of geropsychological investigation that emphasized cognitive variables: (1) intellectual deterioration, (2) general intellectual changes, (3) vocabulary performance, (4) verbal skills, (5) psychomotor skills, (6) short-term retention, (7) dichotic listening, (8) adjustment, and (9) social variables (Poon, 1980).

Subsequently, reviews of the trends and developments in the psychology of aging became more frequent. For instance, in the late 1970s, a review of the clinical psychology of aging, a topic that previously had received little attention, was published (Storandt, Siegler, & Elias, 1979). Another prime chronicle was entitled *Annual Review of Gerontology and Geriatrics* (Eisdorfer, 1980). When the American Psychological Association's third book on geropsychology, *Aging in the 1980's: Psychological Issues,* was published, it constituted evidence that the field of geropsychology had advanced and diversified, covering a wide range of topics from neuropsychological and psychopharmacological issues to environmental and interpersonal concerns (Poon, 1980).

Again, despite advancement of geropsychological science, fragmentation of clinical services was evident. In response to underutilization of community mental health centers by older adults, the Community Mental Health Centers Act of 1963, which declared access to mental health services a civil right, was amended. In 1975, this amendment mandated special services for older mentally ill individuals. Despite such legislation, Gatz, Smyer, and Lawton (1980) concluded that there was a failure of the mental health system to adequately provide services to older adults. One reason for this gap between postulated need and service may be that throughout the 1960s to the 1980s, Medicare, the national health insurance for older adults, provided little coverage for outpatient services for older adults living in the community (Gatz & Smyer, 1992). These authors concluded that despite adjustments in federal and state funding and innovative demonstrations of service, there have been only minimal improvements in the mental health system for older adults.

Many federal agencies and departments support aging-related research. Since 1965, the Administration on Aging has developed and coordinated research and service for older adults. Research on the psychology of the aged has further been supported by the National Institute on Aging (NIA) since 1974, and the National Institute of Mental Health (NIMH) since 1960. In addition, in the 1960s, as the age characteristics of the veteran population increased, the Veterans Administration (VA) began more actively participating in research projects on aging (Coppinger, 1967). While NIA and NIMH support intramural and extramural research on aging, the VA supports only intramural research. In 1975 the VA established eight geriatric research, educational, and clinical centers (GRECCs) across the country, most of which are involved in geropsychological research. Even though allocations for behavioral and social science research on aging across all agencies have increased, the biological sciences garner the lion's share of funding.

The third White House Conference on Aging was held in 1981, with the theme "The Aging Society: Challenge and Opportunity." National aging population dilemmas discussed have included life, expectancy, health, and social isolation. One of the recommendations from this WHCoA was to increase the availability of home- and community-based health care and to develop and promote effective programs for preventive health care (White House Conference on Aging, 1981).

Approaches for studying development progressed from cross-sectional to longitudinal and time lag designs. Schaie (1988) concludes that research methodology and statistics have had a tremendous impact on theorizing about aging. With availability of new techniques in statistical analysis, in particular confirma-

Table 1-1. List of Current Journals in Geropsychology

Title	Year first published
Journals of Gerontology	1946
Journal of the American Geriatrics Society	1953
Gerontologist	1960
Experimental Gerontology	1965
Journal of Geriatric Psychiatry	1967
Age and Ageing	1972
International Journal of Aging and Human Development	1973
Experimental Aging Research	1975
Journal of Ethnogerontology	1975
Journal of Gerontological Nursing	1975
Educational Gerontology	1976
Clinical Gerontologist	1977
Death Studies	1977
Journal of Gerontological Social Work	1978
Journal of Clinical and Experimental Gerontology	1979
Research on Aging	1979
Journal of Nutrition for the Elderly	1980
Activities, Adaptation and Aging	1980
Gerontology and Geriatrics Education	1980
Physical and Occupational Therapy in Geriatrics	1980
Aging and Society	1981
Geriatric Nursing	1981
Canadian Journal of Ageing	1982
Journal of Applied Gerontology	1982
Geriatrics	1984
Alzheimer Disease and Associated Disorders	1986
American Journal of Alzheimer's Care and Related Disorders and Research	1986
International Journal of Geriatric Psychiatry	1986
Journal of Cross-Cultural Gerontology	1986
Psychology and Aging	1986
Journal of Aging Studies	1988
Journal of Geriatric Psychiatry and Neurology	1988
Archives of Gerontology and Geriatrics	1989
International Psychogeriatrics	1989
Journal of Aging and Health	1989
Behavior, Health, and Aging	1990
Dementia	1990
American Journal of Geriatric Psychiatry	1993
Journal of Adult Development	1993
Education and Aging	1994
Journal of Clinical Geropsychology	1995
Journal of Mental Health and Aging	1995

tory factor analyses, possibilities for studying various aspects of gerontology have increased considerably.

As journals in the field of gerontology have proliferated from the 1970s through the 1990s, the number of journals focusing on or including psychological aspects of aging has grown (see Table 1-1). In particular, in 1985 the American Psychological Association established the journal *Psychology and Aging*. Another timely journal, inaugurated in 1995, is the *Journal of Clinical Geropsychology* which focuses on clinical issues.

In 1995, the fourth White House Conference on Aging was held, with the theme "America Now and Into the 21st Century: Generations Aging Together with Independence, Opportunity, and Dignity." In addition to discussing the needs of older Americans, the conference provided an intergenerational perspective on aging including multigenerational relationships. Emphasis was placed on the importance of a comprehensive life span developmental psychology that, of course, includes old age. Researchers and clinicians were encouraged to evaluate the organization of behaviors of adults not only at the end of life, but across the whole life span. Further resolutions from the conference included meeting mental health care needs and increasing federal funding for research in aging (diseases of older persons, long-term care, and special populations) (White House Conference on Aging, 1995).

FUTURE PERSPECTIVES

A sketch of the history of psychology and aging as it has evolved since 1835 has been provided. A more comprehensive description of major studies in psychology and aging from 1884 through 1965 has been reported elsewhere by Riegel (1973, 1977), who indicated that psychological gerontology has, in part, recapitulated the history of psychology in general. First, geropsychological studies focused on sensation and perception. The next general area of exploration was in psychophysics and psychomotor abilities. Later, geropsychology became concerned with the concept of personality, and eventually the social psychology of aging was explored.

Since the 1800s, geropsychology has grown and diversified greatly. Its burgeoning is most evident in the organizations, associations, conferences, and journals focusing on or devoted to this field. Psychology has continuing contributions to make to the research and service fields of aging. Although it is essential to gather information on the field of geropsychology, it is equally imperative to provide directions for the future.

Despite exponential growth of research in psychology and aging, much of this research involves disparate studies on narrowly defined variables. Birren (1989) stated that the field of geropsychology is data-rich and theory-poor. He further argued that the accumulated information on geropsychology is organized by microtheories. Although previous data can serve as a guideline, at the same time such information may be viewed as a constraint. A more comprehensive understanding of the older person would greatly benefit from an integration of concepts.

Several areas of psychological inquiry warrant further investigation in older adults. One area is the standardization of assessment in older adults. In particular, the discrimination of diagnostic procedures in assessing subtypes within a mental disorder and the comorbidity of disorders require our careful scrutiny. Understanding clusters of symptoms within a mental disorder of the elderly may raise questions about the symptoms used in their nomenclature. Further, symptom correlates that are unique to each disorder may identify factors that will help improve the differential diagnosis and in turn aid in the recognition of these disorders.

Further, researchers must examine and combat reasons for the low numbers of older adults seen in the current system of mental health care services. One reason may be the reluctance of some older adults to seek psychological services. For the elderly who are unwilling or unable to receive care in traditional settings, it is crucial to learn how to better deliver mental health care. One service delivery approach is the PATCH (Psychogeriatric Assessment and Treatment in City Housing) outreach model of psychiatric assessment and treatment (Roca, Storer, Robbins, Tlasek, & Rabins, 1990). Implementation and efficacy of this and other such programs have important implications for the development of service delivery models.

Although prevention programs are not necessarily capable of averting all old-age psychopathology, their contribution is essential. Primary prevention efforts aimed at avoiding psychopathology in late life are needed as are secondary and tertiary prevention targeted toward specific disorders that affect the aged. In particular, prevention of disease may rely on changing behavior (Carstensen, 1988). Behavioral assessment and treatment in older adults can lead to cost-effective solutions, which are of utmost importance during this time of shrinking government funds. Certainly, increased understanding of the nature and distribution of mental health problems in older persons, differences between late-life and earlier-onset mental disorders, and identification of etiologic and maintaining factors will facilitate developing prevention and treatment interventions.

Another area that warrants further investigation is the efficacy of psychotherapeutic intervention methods with older adults. Lebowitz and Niederehe (1992) noted that, over the past decade, clinical trials of pharmacologic, psychotherapeutic, and combined treatments have resulted in validated therapies for some disorders. For example, although limited, the data on treatment of depression in late life are strong and come from a number of clinical trials (Niederehe, 1994). However, more psychotherapeutic treatment data for the elderly are sorely needed.

With increasing numbers of individuals living considerably longer, efforts should be made not to prolong the years of life per se, but to prolong the years of healthy living. The issue, of course, is one of improving quality of life. Clearer delineations of the behavioral capabilities of older adults and of ways to make better use of their potential are topics worthy of investigation.

Recently, the U.S. Department of Health and Human Services' Task Force on Aging Research (1995) formulated future directions for research. Several key areas were proposed for evaluation, including prevalence of alcohol-related problems, treatment of depression and anxiety, and behavioral symptoms and functional disability in Alzheimer's disease patients.

With the benefit of hindsight, it is easy to be critical. Prior to the 1970s, research on aging was deficient methodologically. Replication of research on different age cohorts in the same society and on aging populations in different societies is warranted. The search for more comprehensive explanations of variations in aging continues. A complex interactional model is needed. Geropsychology should continue to benefit from multidisciplinary interaction. Our current viewpoint should emphasize how multiple factors interact to produce normal and pathological aging.

ACKNOWLEDGMENT.   We thank George Neiderehe for his comments on an earlier draft of this chapter.

REFERENCES

Abraham, K. (1927). The applicability of psycho-analytic treatment to patients at an advanced age. In D. Bryan & A. Strachey, Trans., *Selected papers on psychoanalysis* (pp. 312–317). New York: Brunner/Mazel. (Original work published 1919.)

Adler, M. (1958). History of the gerontological society. *Journal of Gerontology, 13,* 94–100.

American Psychiatric Association. (1959). Report on patients over 65 in public mental hospitals. Washington, DC: Author.

Anderson, J. E. (1956). *Psychological aspects of aging.* Washington, DC: American Psychological Association.

Angel, J. L., & Hogan, D. P. (1994). The demography of minority aging populations. In *Minority elders: Five goals toward building a public policy base.* Washington, DC: Gerontological Society of America.

Birren, J. E. (Ed.). (1959). *Handbook of aging and the individual: Psychological and biological aspects.* Chicago: University of Chicago Press.

Birren, J. E. (1961). A brief history of the psychology of aging. *Gerontologist, 1,* 69–77, 127–134.

Birren, J. E. (1989). My perspectives on research on aging. In V. L. Bengston & K. W. Schaie (Eds.), *The course of later life: Research and reflections* (pp. 135–149). New York: Springer.

Busse, E. W. (1970). A physiological, psychological and sociological study of aging. In E. Palmore (Ed.), *Normal aging.* Durham, NC: Duke University Press.

Carstensen, L. L. (1988). The emerging field of behavioral gerontology. *Behavior Therapy, 19,* 259–281.

Coppinger, N. W. (1967). Introduction. *Gerontologist, 7* (2), 1–2.

Cowdry, E. V. (Ed.). (1939). *Problems of ageing.* Baltimore: Williams & Wilkins.

Dychtwald, K., & Flower, J. (1989). *Age wave: The challenges and opportunities of an aging America.* Los Angeles: Tarcher.

Eisdorfer, C. (1980). *Annual review of gerontology and geriatrics.* New York: Springer.

Eisdorfer, C., & Lawton, M. P. (1973). *The psychology of adult development and aging.* Washington, DC: American Psychological Association.

Erikson, E. H. (1963). *Childhood and society.* New York: Norton.

Feigenbaum, E. (1973). Ambulatory treatment of the elderly. In E. W. Busse & E. Pfeiffer (Eds.), *Mental illness in later life* (pp. 153–166). Washington, DC: American Psychiatric Press.

Foster, J. C., & Taylor, G. A. (1920). The application of mental tests to persons over 50. *Journal of Applied Psychology, 4,* 29–38.

Freud, S. (1959). On psychotherapy. In J. Riviere (Trans.), *Collected papers: Volume 1. Early papers on the history of the psycho-analytic movement* (pp. 249–263). New York: Basic Books. (Original work published 1904)

Gatz, M., & Smyer, M. A. (1992). The mental health system and older adults in the 1990's. *American Psychologist, 47* (6), 741–751.

Gatz, M., Smyer, M. A., & Lawton, M. P. (1980). The mental health system and the older adult. In L. Poon (Ed.), *Aging in the 1980's: Psychological issues* (pp. 5–18). Washington, DC: American Psychological Association.

German, P. S., Shapiro, S., & Skinner, E. A. (1985). Mental health of the elderly: Use of health and mental health services. *Journal of the American Geriatrics Society, 33,* 246–252.

Hall, G. S. (1922). *Senescence: The second half of life.* New York: Appleton.

Holhouser, W. L. (1988). Aging in place: The demographics and service needs of elderly in urban public housing. *Citizens' housing and planning association.*

Jackson, J. S. (1988). *The Black American elderly: Research on physical and psychological health.* New York: Springer.

Kaplan, O. J. (1945). *Mental disorders in later life.* Stanford, CA: Stanford University Press.

Kramer, M. (1983). The continuing challenger: The rising prevalence of mental disorders, associated chronic diseases and disabling conditions. *American Journal of Social Psychiatry, 3,* 13–24.

Lebowit, B., & Niederehe, G. (1992). Concepts and issues in mental health and aging. In J. E. Birren & R. B. Sloane (Eds.), *Handbook of mental health and aging* (2nd ed., pp. 3–26). San Diego, CA: Academic.

Lowenthal, M. F., Berkman, P., & Associates. (1967). Aging *and mental disorder in San Francisco.* San Francisco: Jossey-Bass.

Martin, L. J. (1944). *A handbook for old age counselors.* San Francisco: Geertz.

Metchnikoff, E. (1908). *The prolongation of life.* New York: Putnam.

Miles, W. R. (1931). Measures of certain abilities throughout the life span. *Proceedings of the National Academy of Sciences U.S.A. 17,* 627–633.

Minot, C. (1908). *The problems of age, growth, and death.* New York: Putnam.

Neugarten, B. L. (1968). *Middle age and aging.* Chicago: University of Chicago Press.

Niederehe, G. T. (1994). Psychosocial therapies with depressed older adults. In L. S. Schneider, C. F. Reynolds, B. D. Lebowitz, & A. J. Friedhoff (Eds.), *Diagnosis and treatment of depression in late life: Results of the NIH consensus development conference.* Washington, DC: American Psychiatric Press.

Poon, L. W. (1980): *Aging in the 1980's: Psychological issues.* Washington, DC: American Psychological Association.

Pressey, S. L. (1939). *Life: A psychological survey.* New York: Harper.

Pressey, S. L. (1948). The new division on maturity and old age: Its history and potential services. *American Psychologist, 3,* 107–109.

Riegel, K. F. (1973). On the history of psychological gerontology. In C. Eisdorfer & M. P. Lawton (Eds.), *The psychology of adult development and aging* (pp. 37–68). Washington, DC: American Psychological Association.

Riegel, K. F. (1977). History of psychological gerontology. In J. E. Birren & K. W. Schaie (Eds.), *Handbook of the psychology and aging* (1st ed., pp. 70–102). New York: Van Nostrand Reinhold.

Roca, R. P., Storer, D. J., Robbins, B. M., Tlasek, M. E., & Rabins, P. V. (1990). Psychogeriatric assessment and treatment in urban public housing. *Hospital and Community Psychiatry, 8,* 916–920.

Schaie, K. W. (1965). A general model for the study of developmental problems. *Psychological Bulletin, 64,* 92–107.

Schaie, K. W. (1988). The impact of research methodology on theory building in the developmental sciences. In J. E. Birren & V. L. Bengston (Eds.), *Emergent theories of aging* (pp. 41–57). New York: Springer.

Schaie, K. W. (1993). The Seattle longitudinal studies of adult intelligence. *Psychological Science, 2* (6), 171–175.

Shock, N. W. (1951). *A classified bibliography of gerontology and geriatrics.* Stanford, CA: Stanford University Press.

Shock, N. W. (1957). *A classified bibliography of gerontology and geriatrics.* Stanford, CA: Stanford University Press.

Shock, N. W. (1963). *A classified bibliography of gerontology and geriatrics.* Stanford, CA: Stanford University Press.

Shock, N. W., Greulich, R. C., Costa P. T., Jr., Andres, R., Lakatta, E. G., Arenberg, D., & Tobin, J. D. (1984). *Normal human aging: The Baltimore longitudinal study of aging.* Washington, DC : U.S. Government Printing Office.

Siegler, I. C. (1983). Psychological aspects of the Duke Longitudinal Studies. In K. W. Schaie (Ed.), *Longitudinal studies of psychological development in adulthood* (pp. 136–190). New York: Guilford.

Storandt, M., Siegler, I. C., & Elias, M. F. (1979). *The clinical psychology of aging.* New York: Plenum.

Suzman, R. W., Willis, D. P., & Manton, K. G. (1992). *The oldest old.* New York: Oxford University Press.

U.S. Department of Health and Human Services. (1995). *The threshold of discovery: Future directions for research on aging* [Report]. Washington, DC: Task Force on Aging Research.

White House Conference on Aging. (1981). *Final report, the 1981 White House Conference on Aging: Vol. 1. A national policy on aging.* Washington, DC: Author.

White House Conference on Aging. (1995). *Proposed report: From resolutions to results, the 1995 White House Conference on Aging.* Washington, DC: Author.

CHAPTER 2

Clinical Geropsychology and U.S. Federal Policy

GARY R. VANDENBOS AND PATRICK H. DELEON

INTRODUCTION

The age distribution in American society has changed drastically since 1900 when only one in 25 Americans was age 65 or older, and the average life span was 47 years. In the year 2000 one in six Americans will be age 65 or older, and the average life span will exceed 80 (Neugarten & Neugarten, 1989).

Modern clinical psychology emerged shortly after World War II, in large part in response to initiatives of the federal government growing out of shortage of mental health professional during the war (Cummings & VandenBos, 1983). In 1950, only one out of 12 Americans was age 65 or older and the life expectancy at birth was 68.2 (Bureau of the Census, 1980, pp. 42, 96). Thus, it is not surprising that clinical geropsychology was not a significant component of training in clinical psychology in 1950, even though the American Psychological Association (APA) Division on Adult Development and Aging (Division 20) was one of the initial founding divisions of the modem APA in 1946. Clinical geropsychology has had to establish itself within clinical psychology over the last 50 years, just as aging-related policy issues have needed to seek out their own unique status within federal policy and federal legislation.

The two most significant federal legislative issues related to interests and needs of older persons are general income maintenance (e.g., retirement pensions and disability payments) and reimbursement for health care costs. The latter, which include cognitive evaluations, neuropsychological evaluations, and psychotherapeutic interventions, are obviously relevant to clinical geropsychology. The federal coordination of both programs is the responsibility of the Social Security Administration (SSA).

GARY R. VANDENBOS • American Psychological Association, Washington, D.C. 20002-4242
PATRICK H. DELEON • Administrative Assistant to U.S. Senator Daniel K. Inouye, U.S. Senate, Hart Senate Building, Washington, D.C. 20510-1102.

Handbook of Clinical Geropsychology, edited by Michel Hersen and Vincent B. Van Hasselt. Plenum Press, New York, 1998.

SOCIAL SECURITY:
A SIXTY-YEAR OVERVIEW

In 1900, most people in the United States lived and worked on farms, and economic security for the elderly was provided by the extended family. However, issues of the economic security for the young and the old changed as America became more industrialized and more people moved to urban settings. The Great Depression eventually triggered a crisis in the nation's economic life that influenced the financial security of the aged. Against this backdrop, the Social Security Act was created over 60 years ago.

In June of 1934, President Franklin Roosevelt, in a message to the Congress, announced his intention to provide a program for social security. Subsequently, the president created, by executive order, the Committee on Economic Security. The committee was instructed to study the problem of economic insecurity and to make recommendations that would serve as the basis for legislation. Within six months the committee made its report to the president. On January 17, 1935, President Roosevelt introduced the report to both houses of Congress for simultaneous consideration. Each house eventually passed its own version, but in the end the differences were resolved, and the Social Security Act was signed into law on August 14, 1935. The new Act created a social insurance program designed to pay retired workers age 65 or older a continuing income after retirement. More than 35 million Social Security cards were issued over the next two years.

The first Federal Insurance Contributions Act (FICA) taxes were collected in January of 1937. Special trust funds were created for these dedicated revenues. Benefits were then paid from the monies in the Social Security trust funds. Over the years, more than $4.5 trillion has been paid into the trust funds, and more than $4.1 trillion has been paid out in benefits (Social Security Administration, n.d.). The remainder is currently on reserve in the trust funds, and these funds will be used to pay future benefits. From 1937 until 1940, Social Security paid benefits in the form of a single, lump-sum payment. Payments of monthly benefits began in January 1940, and such payments were authorized not only for aged retired workers but for their aged wives or widows, children under age 18, and surviving aged parents.

While the Social Security System was being established in 1935, parallel efforts were also being undertaken to establish a national health insurance program. A universal, government-sponsored U.S. health system has been under discussion for many decades. The idea of government provision of health services, often referred to at that time as "socialized medicine," was particularly intriguing to proponents of the New Deal during the 1930s. Socialized medicine was only one of several ideological proposals that emerged in the first two Roosevelt administrations, but it was what organized medicine, primarily the American Medical Association (AMA), targeted for attack during the next three decades. It was ultimately defeated through AMA's intense lobbying. Socialized medicine acquired a negative connotation because of the AMA campaign, and the term was eventually replaced in the lexicon by "national health insurance" (Cummings, 1979). The initiative resurfaced under the Truman administration, but it did not really reemerge until the Great Society years of the Kennedy and Johnson administrations, when Medicare and Medicaid were established.

After 20 years, the concept behind basic Social Security began to change, and the idea of assuring economic security for disabled (younger) workers attracted greater attention. The Social Security Amendments of 1954 initiated a disability insurance program which provided Americans with additional coverage against economic insecurity. At first, federal law merely allowed a disability "freeze" of a worker's Social Security record during the years when he or she was unable to work. Although this measure offered no cash benefits, it did prevent such periods of disability from reducing or wiping out retirement and survivor benefits. The 1956 Social Security amendments provided benefits to disabled workers aged 50 to 65 and disabled adult children. Over the next 2 years, Congress broadened the scope of the program, permitting disabled workers under age 50 and their dependents to qualify for benefits. By 1960, 559,000 people were receiving disability benefits, with the average benefit amount being approximately $80 per month. The number of people receiving disability benefits more than doubled from 1961 to 1969, increasing from 742,000 to 1.7 million.

The decade of the 1960s brought major changes to the Social Security program. Under the Amendments of 1961, the age at which men were first eligible for old-age retirement benefits was lowered to 62, with benefits actuarially reduced (women previously were given this option starting in 1956). The most significant change involved the signing of the Medicare bill on July 30, 1965, by President Lyndon Johnson. With the signing of this bill, SSA became responsible for administering a new health insurance program that extended health coverage to almost all Americans aged 65 or older.

Medicare and Medicaid were enacted into public law in 1965, and nearly 20 million beneficiaries enrolled in Medicare in the first three years of the program. In fiscal year 1996, Medicare covered approximately 37.5 million aged and disabled persons (O'Sullivan & Price, 1996), and Medicaid had about 38.4 million recipients (Ford, 1996).

Medicare is a nationwide health *insurance* program of an entitlement nature in which the primary beneficiaries are those eligible for Social Security disability benefits, various railroad retirees, and, most important, nearly every senior citizen 65 years or older. Benefits under the program are uniform across the nation, and one's eligibility does not depend upon income or financial assets. Medicare is 100% federally financed.

Medicaid, on the other hand, is a medical *assistance* program (rather than health insurance program) targeted for certain needy and low-income persons. It is a state-operated and state- administered program, and each state has the authority to create its own range of programmatic benefits within broad federal guidelines. Medicaid is funded at various ratios, which can vary depending upon a number of factors. The federal government will generally pay 50% of the medical assistance costs incurred by a state. Physicians' services are a mandated benefit, but mental health services are generally optional or supplemental benefits. Accordingly, the actual provisions of the mental health components differ drastically from state to state depending upon local priorities, which can change at any given time (DeLeon & VandenBos, 1980, pp. 258–59).

The initial Medicare mental health benefit package was considerably less comprehensive than that for physical/organic illnesses. For example, inpatient care in psychiatric hospitals was limited to less than 200 days over a person's entire life, in sharp contrast to inpatient services for nonpsychiatric care. Further, when an individual had a physical illness, he or she was required to pay only 20% copayment of the cost of outpatient care. Yet, if the diagnosis was mental illness, the patient had a 50% copayment, with a $250 overall annual limit or "cap" on reimbursement. No such comparable overall limit on outpatient physical health care services existed; instead a "usual and customary" fee schedule was utilized. Psychologists were *not* expressly included as eligible providers under Medicare; this exclusion set the stage for what would become a 25-year legislative struggle for the direct recognition of psychologists under Medicare.

Of considerable historical significance to psychology is the fact that the Senate report accompanying the original bill (the Social Security Amendments of 1965, Public Law 89-97) set the tone of the orientation of Medicare as to the role of physician-provided care when it expressly stated that "the committee's bill provides that the physician is to be the key figure in determining utilization of health services" (U.S. Senate, Committee on Finance, 1965, p. 46). In response to subsequent efforts by various nonphysician health care providers to broaden the basic orientation of the programs, Congress directed the Department of Health, Education, and Welfare to conduct a formal study of the possibility of expanding the availability of various types of health services (Public Law 90-248). In December 1968 the department submitted its Independent Practitioners Study (Cohen, 1968) to Congress. While the report specifically stated that the services of clinical psychologists should be reimbursed, it recommended that such services be reimbursed only when they are provided in an organized setting and when there had been initial physician referral. Further, the report recommended that a physician should establish a plan for the patient's total care and also retain overall responsibility for patient management (DeLeon, VandenBos, & Kraut, 1986). Thus, efforts had to be made to continue to develop mechanisms for elderly patients to have easier and direct access to psychological services. Based on a 1972 amendment (Public Law 92-603) the Colorado Medicare Study (Bent, Willens, & Lassen, 1983; McCall & Rice, 1983) was conducted to test two alterations in the Medicare program, namely, a larger proportion of allowable charges for outpatient mental health services, and direct Medicare reimbursement to psychologists for providing mental health services.

In the 1970s, SSA became responsible for a new disabilities-related program, Supplemental Security Income (SSI). In the original 1935 Social Security Act, programs were introduced for needy aged and blind individuals and, in 1950, needy disabled individuals were added. These three programs were known as the "adult categories," and they were administered by state and local governments with partial federal funding. Over the years, the state programs became more complex and inconsistent, with many administrative agencies involved, and payments varying more than 300% from state to state.

In 1969, President Nixon identified a need to reform these and related welfare programs. In 1971, Secretary of Health, Education and Welfare Elliott Richardson proposed that SSA assume responsibility for the adult categories. In the Social Security Amendments of 1972, Congress federalized the adult categories by creating the SSI program and assigning responsibility for it to SSA.

More than 3 million people were transferred from state welfare programs to SSI. Some feared that redirecting a significant proportion of effort away from a focus on income security and health care access needs of the elderly would cause administrative inefficiencies and otherwise be detrimental to the integrity of the basic purpose of Social Security. The 1980 Social Security Amendments required SSA to conduct periodic reviews of current disability beneficiaries to certify their continuing eligibility. By 1983, the reviews had been halted, and in 1984, Congress passed the Disability Benefits Reform Act modifying several aspects of the disability program, with a goal of reducing paperwork.

In the early 1980s the Social Security program faced a serious long-term financing crisis. President Reagan appointed a blue-ribbon panel, known as the Greenspan Commission, to study the financing issues and make recommendations for legislative changes. The final bill, signed into law in 1983, made numerous changes in the Social Security and Medicare programs, including the taxation of Social Security benefits, the first coverage of federal employees under Social Security, and an increase in the retirement age in the next century.

Changes also continued to be made in the 1980s in terms of mental health care. In 1980, psychological services and psychotherapy were expressly enumerated under several Medicare provisions (Public Law 96-499) authorizing payment for rehabilitation services. In 1984, the first significant Medicare success directly benefitting psychologists was the inclusion of language in the Deficit Reduction Act of 1984 (Public Law 98-369) that authorized coverage for psychologists as autonomous providers under the risk-sharing health maintenance organization (HMO) provisions of the Act. Public Law 98-369 also allowed nonphysicians to head a Medicaid clinic. The Mental Health Organizational Amendments of 1986 (Public Law 99-660) explicitly listed psychologists among the authorized HMO professions, whereas prior to this modification, psychologists' services were actually recognized only under the broad heading of "other health care providers."

In 1989, during the 101st Congress, professional psychologists finally obtained direct and autonomous recognition under Medicare, as a provision of the Omnibus Budget Reconciliation Act of 1989 (Public Law 101-239) (VandenBos, Cummings, & DeLeon, 1992). On November 22, 1989, Congress passed a large package of bills, an omnibus budget reconciliation act, that included, among others, direct reimbursement of psychologists for services provided to the elderly and the disabled under Medicare; on December 19, 1989, President Bush signed the bill into law, effective on July 1, 1990. This landmark legislation marked the end of the exclusion of psychologists as reimbursable providers of services within the Medicare program, the only federal program that had excluded psychologists (Buie, 1990; Youngstrom, 1990). This legislation allowed elderly patients access to the services of psychologists. In addition, the new law removed many of the limits and arbitrarily low reimbursement ceilings from both inpatient and outpatient mental health care, although mental health services were still eligible for only 50% reimbursement (in contrast to 80% reimbursement for physical health services).

Throughout the 1980s and 1990s, there was growing bipartisan support for removing SSA from under its departmental umbrella and establishing it as an independent agency. Finally, in 1994 the Social Security Independence and

Program Improvements Act of 1994 (Public Law 103-296) was passed unanimously by Congress and, in a ceremony in the Rose Garden of the White House, President Clinton signed the act into law on August 15, 1994.

From its modest beginnings, Social Security has grown to become an essential facet of modern life, and one of particular importance to the economic security and health care of older Americans. One in seven Americans receives a Social Security benefit, and more than 90% of all workers are in jobs covered by Social Security. From 1940, when slightly more than 222,000 people received monthly Social Security benefits, until today, when more than 42 million people receive such benefits, Social Security has grown steadily. Thus, the basic Social Security System (that is, the retirement pension portion) has been in place for over 60 years and provides a base of financial income for almost everyone over 65. This program has been successful in minimizing the number of American elderly living in abject poverty. Although other retirement funds are necessary for most elderly Americans to maintain the lifestyle of their adult years, Social Security, when combined with other benefit programs and social services, provides most elderly Americans with the means to meet their basic needs with some degree of flexibility. In a parallel manner, Medicare provides aged Americans with a guaranteed basic level of health care, although mental health care still has somewhat inferior reimbursement provisions in comparison to physical health care.

CONTINUING POLICY AND
CLINICAL ISSUES

The sad fact is that the elderly are underserved by all current mental health service delivery systems and all current health care funding mechanisms. The mental health needs of the elderly simply are not being adequately met. In the mid-1980s, there were approximately 26 million individuals aged 65 or older, representing about 12% of the total U.S. population. Rough estimates suggested that between 2.5 and 7.5 million individuals out of this elderly population had emotional and behavioral problems that were serious enough to warrant professional intervention, with federal estimates suggesting a target number of 5 million individuals.

Several factors seem to contribute to the underutilization of mental health services among the elderly. It has been fashionable to talk about the anti-mental health bias within the current elderly population. There is no question that today's elderly are less psychologically sophisticated and less psychologically oriented than younger age groups. Public information campaigns about the nature of psychological and memory problems, and psychological and behavioral interventions with them, would be useful activities for government, associations, and individual psychologists. However, the level of knowledge about psychological issues and psychotherapeutic interventions is likely to increase as a more highly educated and psychologically oriented middle-aged cohort enters their retirement years.

Other reasons for the low utilization of mental health services by the elderly include misinformation about the nature and value of psychological care; lack of knowledge about the availability of services; inaccessibility due to a general lack of integrated support services (e.g., outreach, home visits, and transportation); the intimidating regulations and paperwork required for mental health insurance benefits; bias among mental health providers regarding the elderly; and financial, language, and cultural barriers in the case of elderly minorities.

Until very recently, major biases in the funding mechanisms have made it difficult for the elderly to seek psychological help. These include the artificial cap on mental health services funding under Medicare and the ineligibility for reimbursement of psychologists and other nonphysician mental health professionals by this program. As noted, these regulations were amended in 1990, so the pattern of underutilization by the elderly will soon change. Thus, it is critical for clinical geropsychology to expand and evolve rapidly so that more professional psychologists are prepared for and experienced in working with older patients.

Psychological and behavioral issues related to the elderly have been relatively neglected in psychology training programs for a long time (Storandt, 1982). Surveys in the mid-1970s revealed that as few as 100 psychologists had specialized training concentrated on serving older populations and that only a handful of programs had some type of clinical track that might be referred to as clinical geropsychology. Later, geropsychology training conferences (Knight, Teri, Wohlford, & Santos, 1995) found improvements in the availability of predoctoral course work and practicum, although such availability is still far from widespread. Moreover, aging-related knowledge is often presented to students across several courses, such as psychopathology, neuropsychology, health psychology, psychopharmacology, and so forth. Without a core course that serves as a coordinating point for such scholarly knowledge, it may be difficult to integrate all of the separate pieces with the normal developmental tasks and functions of older adults. It may be necessary, in the short term, for the federal government to target training support for clinical geropsychology, whether from Social Security funds, General Medical Education (GME) support, or National Institutes of Mental Health (NIMH) training grants. It will take active advocacy efforts by psychologists for this to occur.

In many ways, clinical problems for which older individuals see psychologists are similar to those of other age groups in the general U.S. population. This means that many skills learned and refined with other age groups can be transferred to clinical work with the elderly, once appropriate supplemental knowledge is acquired. The elderly, as a group, are generally found to have slightly fewer mental health problems of all types, with the exception of dementia. The major mental health problems among the elderly include depression and other mood disorders; dementia and severe cognitive impairment; suicide (particularly among men over 75); alcohol abuse; polydrug use and misuse of prescription medications; and chronic mental disability. Such problems frequently involve difficult behavior, memory problems, and strained family and social relations (VandenBos, 1993). Fortunately, new books and other resources are becoming available for use by practicing professionals, continuing education (CE) trainers, and predoctoral education. Such resources include *A Guide to Psychotherapy and Aging: Effective Clinical Intervention in a Life-Stage Context* (Zarit & Knight, 1996) and *Neuropsychological Assessment of Dementia and Depression in Older Adults: A Clinical Guide* (Storandt & VandenBos, 1994).

The financing of long-term nursing home care is a continuing unresolved policy issue relevant to older populations. Older Americans are generally living on fixed incomes with little potential for increases from year to year. The hall-mark of federal initiatives related to the elderly over the last 60 years has been the protection from unexpected and sudden catastrophic financial ruin. Basic Social Security provided a guaranteed income in old age. Medicare and Medic-aid provided protection from catastrophic health care costs. Perhaps the last catastrophic financial risk for the elderly yet to be addressed relates to long-term care. Twenty-four-hour day care in a residential facility is expensive and can wipe out an individual's lifetime savings in a short period of time. Although, at any given moment, only 5% of persons over 65 reside in a nursing home, the chance that people who survive to age 65 will enter a nursing home for some period of time before their death is better than one in four (Berkman & Kane, 1993).

However, for every nursing home resident, two equally impaired individuals are living in a community. Thus, availability of community-based home health care is vital. Impaired community-based elders sometimes struggle along caring for themselves under great hardship, and in other cases they survive with occasional help from family members or nearby neighbors. Availability and quality of home care services vary greatly from community to community, and the funding is often precarious. Despite the fact that home care services can be highly cost effective by both preventing institutionalization and encouraging self-reliance and independent functioning, such services often lack a firm legislative base. It is vital that, at both federal and state levels, legislative initiatives for provision of long-term care or preventive home care be supported by clinical geropsychologists.

Nursing homes and home care programs also offer the potential for clinical geropsychologists to have an important clinical impact and to gain employment. Clinically significant depression and anxiety are generally apparent in large percentages of the resident population of nursing homes. Clinical geropsychologists are needed in such settings for screening, short-term clinical interventions, and family work, and clinical opportunities exist for geropsychologists in home health care programs. Many individuals recuperating at home from physical problems and those coping with long-term chronic conditions often have elevated levels of depressive symptomatology. Social support, presence versus absence of psychopathology, and access to psycho-educational information are correlated with speed of recovery and return to self-care functional levels among those receiving home health care services. Clinical geropsychologists can aid in such programming as clinical supervisors, program managers, and direct services providers to more severely impaired individuals. However, advocacy is needed to assure that such conceptualizations (and clinical positions) are built into the legislation authorizing such service programs.

One message that is important for geropsychologists to introduce into legislative and policy discussions is the concept of individual differences. Far too often legislators working on one issue or another conceptualize older individuals in some overly simplified manner. It might be that the image of the nursing home resident momentarily stands as the image for all older adults, when at another moment the image of a frail 80-year-old man timidly driving a large car through busy traffic may stand as the image for all older drivers. Geropsychologists, likewise, need to remind legislators that there may be vast differences in physical health and psychological functioning between two 74-year-old individuals. Just as individual differences exist and are important among children, teenagers, and middle-aged adults, such differences exist in elderly populations, but may be momentarily forgotten as policy officials address a particular social issue related to a particular subset of the elderly. Legislative solutions to particular social problems must be crafted and applied with an awareness of such individual differences so as not to unintentionally hamper the functioning of other older individuals with different abilities and functional capacities.

SUMMARY

American society is aging. Older individuals will increasingly present clinical challenges to professional psychologists. Our training systems must continue to evolve so that all practitioners are appropriately trained and experienced to serve the psychological needs of older individuals. And psychology must also work to ensure that appropriate, fair, and equitable funding mechanisms are in place, so as to permit older individuals direct access to needed psychological care.

REFERENCES

Bent, R. J., Willens, J. G., & Lassen, C. L. (1983). The Colorado Clinical Psychology/Expanded Mental Health Benefits Experiment: An introductory commentary. *American Psychologist, 38,* 1274–1278.

Berkman, B., & Kane, R. A. (1993). Social work services for older people in acute or long-term care. In F. Lieberman & M. F. Collen (Eds.), *Aging in good health: A quality lifestyle for the later years* (pp. 279–294). New York: Plenum.

Buie, J. (1990, January). President signs Medicare bill. Victory caps uphill trek. *APA Monitor, 21,* pp. 1, 17–19.

Bureau of the Census, U.S. Department of Commerce. (1980, December). *Social indicators III. Selected data on social conditions and trends in the United States.* Washington, DC: Federal Statistical System.

Cohen, W. J. (1968). *Independent practitioners under Medicare: A report to the Congress.* Washington, DC: Department of Health, Education, and Welfare.

Cummings, N. A. (1979). Mental health and national health insurance: A case history of the struggle for professional autonomy. In C. A. Kiesler, N. A. Cummings, & G. R. VandenBos (Eds.), *Psychology and national health insurance* (pp. 5–16). Washington, DC: American Psychological Association.

Cummings, N. A., & VandenBos, G. R. (1983). Relations with other professions. In C. E. Walker (Ed.), *Handbook of clinical psychology* (pp. 1301–1327). Homewood, IL: Dow-Jones.

DeLeon, P. H., & VandenBos, G. R. (1980). Psychotherapy reimbursement in federal programs: Political factors. In G. R. VandenBos (Ed.), *Psychotherapy: Practice, research, policy* (pp. 247–284). Sage studies in community mental health #1. Beverly Hills, CA: Sage.

DeLeon, P. H., VandenBos, G. R., & Kraut, A. G. (1986). Federal recognition of psychology as a profession. In H. Dorken & Associates (Eds.), *Professional psychology in transition: Meeting today's challenges* (pp. 99–117). San Francisco, CA: Jossey-Bass.

Ford, M. (1996, March 26). Medicaid reform. *CRS issue brief.* Washington, DC: Congressional Research Service, Education and Public Welfare Division, Library of Congress.

Knight, B. G., Teri, L., Wohlford, P., & Santos, J. (Eds.). (1995). *Mental health services for older adults: Implications for training and practice in geropsychology.* Washington, DC: American Psychological Association.

McCall, N., & Rice, T. (1983). A summary of the Colorado Clinical Psychology/Expanded Mental Health Benefits Experiment. *American Psychologist, 38,* 1279–1291.

Neugarten, B. L., & Neugarten, D. A. (1989). Policy issues in an aging society. In M. Storandt & G. R. VandenBos (Eds.), *The adult years: Continuity and change* (pp. 147–167). Washington, DC: American Psychological Association.

O'Sullivan, J., & Price, R. (1996, May 31). Medicare. *CRS issue brief.* Washington, DC: Congressional Research Service, Education and Public Welfare Division, Library of Congress.

Social Security Administration. (n.d.). *Social security—A brief history.* Retrieved from World Wide Web: http//www.ssa.gov/history/history.html.

Storandt, M. (1982). Where have we been? Where are we going? In J. F. Santos & G. R. VandenBos (Eds.), *Psychology and the older adult: Challenges for training in the 1980s* (pp. 11–17). Washington, DC: American Psychological Association.

Storandt, M., & VandenBos, G. R. (Eds.). (1994). *Neuropsychological assessment of dementia and depression in older adults: A clinician's guide.* Washington, DC: American Psychological Association.

U.S. Senate, Committee on Finance. (1965). *Social Security Amendments of 1965* (U.S. Senate report No. 389-404, Part 1, to accompany H.R. 6675). Washington, DC: U.S. Government Printing Office.

VandenBos, G. R. (1993). Psychology and the mental health needs of the elderly. In F. Lieberman & M. F. Collen (Eds.), *Aging in good health: A quality lifestyle for the later years* (pp. 189–202). New York: Plenum.

VandenBos, G. R., Cummings, N. A., & DeLeon, P. H. (1992). A century of psychotherapy: Economic and environmental influences. In D. K. Freedheim (Ed.), *History of psychotherapy: A century of change* (pp. 65–102). Washington, DC: American Psychological Association.

Youngstrom, N. (1990, July). Register with carrier for Medicare payment. *APA Monitor, 21,* p. 23.

Zarit, S. H., & Knight, B. G. (Eds.). (1996). *A guide to psychotherapy and aging: Effective clinical interventions in a life-stage context.* Washington, DC: American Psychological Association.

CHAPTER 3

Psychodynamic Issues

Howard D. Lerner

INTRODUCTION

Psychoanalytic theory does not offer a single, coherent account of the aging process across the life cycle. First, psychoanalysis does not represent one unified, tightly knit theory. As explored in the first section of this chapter, psychoanalysis can be represented by four internally consistent theoretical models that, to a large extent, intersect and overlap but that cannot be unified into a single theory. Each model offers its own perspective on geropsychology. Second, from the perspective of psychoanalytic theorists and clinicians, issues involving geropsychology are far too complex and multidetermined to elaborate in terms of a single thread or dimension. In this chapter, therefore, aging will be examined in terms of eight "dimensions of development." These dimensions, as will be articulated, interdigitate with one another in complex ways. However, for heuristic reasons, each will be considered separately in order to offer some idea of the rich tapestry that comprises geriatric psychology from the perspective of psychoanalytic theory.

Psychoanalysis has traditionally focused little attention on aging. Its focus has been on internal, intrapsychic development during the first five or so years of life and the impact that this early development exerts on all ensuing development. In recent years, however, psychoanalytic theorists have paid increasing attention to the vicissitudes of development at all stages through the life cycle and have considered the ongoing influence that real-life experiences such as trauma, aging, and close relationships exert on the individual's inner world. The aim of this chapter is to integrate the central emphasis within psychoanalysis on internal experience with its increased attention to the formative impact of ongoing processes of maturation and real-life experience. In the first section of this chapter, the four dominant conceptual paradigms of psychoanalysis will be examined as a general introduction to contemporary

Howard D. Lerner • Department of Psychiatry, University of Michigan, Ann Arbor, Michigan 48104.

Handbook of Clinical Geropsychology, edited by Michel Hersen and Vincent B. Van Hasselt. Plenum Press, New York, 1998.

psychoanalytic thought and to establish a conceptual framework for the discussion that follows. Specific issues in aging will then be examined to demonstrate how psychoanalysis has come to incorporate the role of ongoing life experience into a predominantly internal, intrapsychic framework. In the third section, eight dimensions of development will be examined in order to shed light on the question of what, in fact, develops in aging and what the nature of this development is. In the final section, to add specificity to the discussion, the issue of aging and the mourning process will be examined.

PSYCHOANALYTIC MODELS

In formulating a psychoanalytic approach to geropsychology, it is important to recognize that psychoanalysis is not one closed, totally coherent theory of personality. Rather, it consists of a loose-fitting composite of four complementary, internally consistent models. Each model furnishes formulations for observing and understanding crucial dimensions of personality development.

Through the course of Freud's writings, he developed a wide range of formulations concerning psychological functioning and accordingly created various conceptualizations of the mind and how it works. He changed from one theory to another theory whenever prior concepts failed to explain newly observed phenomena. However, the transition from one set of formulations to another did not indicate that one superseded the other. That is, Freud did not intend to dispense with older concepts as he proposed newer ones. He assumed that a given set of clinical phenomena might be understood most clearly by using one frame of reference, whereas another set of data required a different set of concepts to explain the data. The principle of several concurrent and valid avenues for organizing the data of observation has been termed *theoretical complementarity* (Gedo & Goldberg, 1973). This is consistent with Waelder's (1930) notion of the principle of multiple functioning of the psychic apparatus that recognizes that the "final pathway" in behavior is a compromise that serves many masters or psychic agencies. No single motive or significant factor can ever be isolated.

Psychology of the Self

Heinz Kohut (1971, 1977), in a series of influential publications, laid the theoretical foundation for a systematic psychoanalytic psychology of the self. Self psychology may be characterized by its emphasis on the vicissitudes of the structure of the self, the associated subjective, conscious, preconscious, and unconscious experience of selfhood, and the self in relation to sustaining "selfobjects." The "selfobject" is one's subjective experience of another person who provides a sustaining function to the self within a relationship, evoking and maintaining the self and the experience of selfhood by his or her presence or activity. Kohut (1977) suggests that individuals need significant others who can assume selfobject functions throughout the life cycle. Self psychology recognizes as the most significant need of the individual to organize his or her internal world into a cohesive configuration, the self, and to establish self-sustaining relationships between this self and its surroundings: that is, relationships that evoke, maintain, and strengthen one's sense of coherence, vigor, and balanced harmony among the constituents of the self. In psychoanalytic treatment, from this perspective, *empathy* is considered to be the cardinal means of data collection and the primary therapeutic instrument.

Utilizing a self psychology approach, Muslin (1992) has offered the following definition of the "elderly self":

> The elderly self is the self of aging people that has become altered in all or many of its structures and functions in reaction to a constellation of societal and biological influences that reflect a particular society's views of an aging person, as well as the individual's biological givens. An "elderly self" is a self that has passed through specific alterations in its self structures that have evolved in reaction to the specific internal and external milieus. A cohesive elderly self is one in which the self-alterations have resulted in an adaptive self without the symptoms and signs of excessive reactions to the external world in the form of loss of worth or self-fragmentation and its vicissitudes as evidenced in neurosis or psychosis. (p. 5)

Object Relations Theory

A second major advance within psychoanalytic theory is modern object relations theory. Object relations theory, or "object-relational thinking" (Guntrip, 1974), does not constitute a singular organized set of concepts, principles, formulations, or a systematized theory. Rather, it represents a broad spectrum of thought that historically and collectively has taken the form of a significant movement within psychoanalysis. Within object relations theory, the concept of object representation has served as a superordinate construct. Defined broadly, object representation refers to the conscious and unconscious mental schemata, including cognitive, affective, and experiential dimensions of others, termed "objects," encountered in reality (Blatt, 1974). From a developmental perspective, beginning within an interpersonal matrix as vague and variable sensorimotor experience of pleasure and unpleasure, these schemata develop into increasingly differentiated, consistent, and relatively realistic representations of the self and the world of others. Developmentally, earlier forms of representations are based more on action sequences associated with gratification of basic needs; intermediate forms are based on specific perceptual features; and higher forms are thought to be more symbolic and conceptual. Whereas these schemata evolve from and are intertwined with the developmental internalization of object relations and ego functions, the developing representations provide a new organization or template throughout the life span for experiencing ongoing interpersonal relationships internally. From this perspective, psychoanalytic treatment attempts to help elucidate, articulate, and, it is hoped, modify one's internal representation of one's self and one's self in relationship to other people. Recently, some proponents of both self psychology and object relations theory have defined themselves as "relational theorists," and have moved from what they term a "one person psychology," which they link to classical Freudian thinking, to what they term a "two person psychology."

Modern Structural Theory

A third major dimension in psychoanalysis has been *modern structural theory.* Taking as its point of departure S. Freud's (1923/1957) tripartite model of id, ego, and superego, and dispensing with older concepts of psychic energy such as libido, modern structural theory, despite challenges from other perspectives, remains the "mainstream hypothesis of modern psychoanalysis" (Boesky, 1989).

Modern structural theory takes as its fundamental assumption the ubiquitous nature of internal conflict throughout the life cycle and the view that this conflict can be conceptualized broadly through the interaction of the id, ego, and superego. Charles Brenner has been one of the most articulate spokesmen for this point of view. According to Brenner, internal conflict is at the heart of psychoanalytic theory and treatment, the components and interactions of which result in "compromise formations." All thoughts, actions, plans, fantasies, and symptoms are thought of as compromise formations, which are understood to be multidetermined by the components of conflict. All compromise formations represent a combination of a drive derivative (a specific personal and unique wish of an individual, originating in childhood, for gratification); unpleasure in the form of anxiety or depressive affect and their ideational contents of either object loss, loss of other, or bodily damage associated with the drive derivative; defense that functions to minimize unpleasure; and various manifestations of superego or moral functioning such as guilt, self punishment, remorse, and atonement.

According to Brenner (1986), compromise formations are the observational database for the study of all psychic functioning; that is, they are the data of observation when one applies the psychoanalytic method to observe all psychological phenomena.

> To say everything is a compromise formation, means everything. Not just symptoms, not just neurotic character traits, not just the slips and errors of daily living, but everything, the normal as well as the pathological. Just as nothing is ever just defense or only wish-fulfillment, so nothing is ever only "realistic" as opposed to "neurotic." One of the principal contributions of psychoanalysis to human psychology is precisely this. The various components of conflict over wishes of childhood origin play as important a part in normal psychic functioning as they do in pathological psychic functioning. (p. 41)

From the perspective of modern structural theory, important questions asked for understanding all psychological phenomena, including those of aging, are, What wishes of childhood are being gratified? What unpleasure or pain (anxiety and depressive affect) are they arousing? What are the defensive and superego aspects? According to Brenner, the answers to these questions provide a distinctive psychoanalytic understanding of all psychological phenomena and in the treatment situation guide the timing and nature of interactions.

Developmental Theory

A fourth and increasingly popular major model in psychoanalysis is a dynamically based, developmental theory. Several contemporary clinicians, theorists, and researchers have concluded independently that developmentally salient aspects of psychological structure and functioning are initiated in and stem from the early mother–child relationship. The developmental perspective provides an assimilative and unifying focus within which multiple approaches can be organized to understand the vicissitudes of aging. The developmental perspective is rooted deeply in the psychoanalytic tradition and embraces all aspects of psychological functioning, especially the relationship between past experience and present functioning (temporal progression), between early trauma and present symptoms (phase-specific deficits), and between historical actualities and psychic realities. In addition, a developmental focus provides a framework for discerning the relative ideological weight of constitutional and experiential factors throughout the life cycle.

The developmental approach within psychoanalysis, especially as it has been built upon the systematic, naturalistic, and longitudinal study of infants and children, provides a methodological link between psychoanalysis and the social sciences and a bridge between clinical and research approaches to the individual. Mahler and her colleagues (Mahler, Pine, & Bergman, 1975) have carefully observed children and their caregivers and have described the steps in what they term the separation-individuation process. Beginning with the earliest signs of the infant's differentiation or "hatching" from a symbiotic fusion with the mother, the infant proceeds through the period of his or her absorption in his or her own autonomous functioning to the near exclusion of the mother (practicing subphase), then through the all-important period of rapprochement in which the child, precisely because of a more clearly perceived state of separateness from mother, is prompted to redirect attention back to the mother, often in provocative ways, and finally to a feeling of a primitive sense of individual identity and of object constancy. Several authors, including Behrends and Blatt (1985), have conceptualized the major task throughout the course of the life cycle as a continuation of this separation-individuation process, which is accomplished through progressive internalization of need gratifying aspects of relationships with significant others.

In his seminal work based on empirical data, Erik Erikson (1976) described stages in ego or self development at eight different stages of life. Each stage was thought to present its own psychosocial crisis. If the crisis is satisfactorily resolved, a positive quality is added to development. If it is unsatisfactorily resolved, a negative factor is added. Erikson's eight stages of the life cycle are as follows: trust versus mistrust which leads to hope; autonomy versus shame and doubt which leads to will; initiative versus guilt which leads to a sense of purpose; industry versus inferiority which gives rise to a sense of competence; the adolescent crisis of identity versus identity confusion; in young adulthood, the conflict of intimacy versus isolation; in the mature years, generativity versus self-absorption; and finally, the task of old age, which is integrity versus despair and disgust, in which a favorable outcome gives rise to wisdom.

The studies of Mahler and her colleagues, and Erikson combine many of the empirical values extant in the social sciences with the intensive, clinical study of single subjects favored by psychoanalysis. The developmental perspective and associated methodologies offer a corrective influence for both blind adherence to theoretical constructs and equally blind reliance on group data and inferential statistics. This approach thus offers a flexible balance between idiographic and nomothetic methodologies, while providing a context from which to distill theoretical formulations as they emerge from and are rooted in human experience throughout the life cycle.

ADULT DEVELOPMENT: GENERAL CONSIDERATIONS

Traditionally, psychoanalysis has viewed adulthood as the endpoint of development. An epic of relative quietude and stability, adulthood has stood within psychoanalysis as a monument to the formative developmental experiences of the early years and to the resurgence of developmental processes catalyzed at puberty that characterizes adolescence. In general, psychoanalysts have conceptualized childhood in terms of its ongoing, age-specific developmental tasks. In contrast, they have seen adulthood in terms of *already accomplished* developmental tasks.

From its inception, psychoanalysis has viewed early, infantile development as decisive for all subsequent personality development. Emphasis was on the past, in what was formative. Traditionally, psychoanalytic thinkers have emphasized the repetitive nature of human behavior, stressing the individual's drive to reenact early, formative, and unconscious experience, conflict, and fantasy throughout life.

Although the formative impact of early development remains a cornerstone of psychoanalytic theory and treatment, psychoanalysts increasingly have moved to explore the ways in which development proceeds across the life cycle. A developmental point of view implies an ongoing process, not only with a past, but also with a present and future. From this vantage point, early phases of life, not only early childhood, bring with them distinctive developmental challenges and possibilities. Further, advances in psychological structure are seen as accruing across all phases of the life cycle, including late adulthood, so that each developmental experience is thought to incorporate all development that precedes it.

Erik Erikson was the first psychoanalyst to advance an integrated psychosocial view of individual development through the course of the life cycle. Erikson has had an enormous impact in various fields throughout the social sciences and humanities. He has highlighted the interaction between the individual's internal psychological state and external social events. Central to the Eriksonian perspective on development is the "epigenetic" principal, which assumes that anything that grows has an internal "game plan." Each stage of life, including those that comprise adulthood, brings with it new challenges that the individual must master. According to this point of view, individuals who are able to meet these tasks or challenges create the opportunity to face life with renewed energy, creativity, and adaptive capacities. Each of Erikson's previously mentioned eight stages revolves around a crucial developmental task for the individual self in relation to the social world. According to Erikson, in the sixth, or young adult stage (20s and 30s), the individual deals with issues of intimacy versus self-absorption. Issues of intimacy, sexuality, and empathy in the context of a cohesive sense of self in relationship with another person are salient. In the seventh or mid-life period, the task or conflict is between generativity and stagnation. Here, generativity goes beyond the care of one's own children to guiding or mentoring the next generation through teaching, creativity, and, most importantly, participation in society. In the eighth or last stage, the conflict is between integrity and despair with integrity epitomizing an acceptance of one's life as it has been lived and letting it go with equanimity.

Settlage and his colleagues (Settlage, Curtis, Lozoff, Silbershatz, & Simburg, 1988) compare personality development in adulthood with the developmental processes of childhood and adolescence. Development, the authors suggest, is a

> process of growth, differentiation, and integration that progresses from lower and simpler to higher and more complex forms of organization and functioning . . . the functions and structures resulting from development constitute additions to or advances in the self-regulatory and adaptive capacities. (p. 35)

Psychoanalysts have traditionally conceptualized personality development as occurring at the interface between the individual's internal biological maturation and environmental forces that he or she faces. Specifically, personality formation proceeds in the context of a predetermined unfolding of stages in childhood and the biologically driven resurgence of strivings of puberty. Although biological maturation contributes to psychological development in adulthood and biological changes have a major impact on old age, the impact of biological forces are less dramatic and clear-cut than in childhood; however, easily discerned, predetermined, invariant stages of maturation characterize psychological development in the adult years.

In light of these considerations, Settlage and colleagues (1988) suggest that personality development in adulthood be conceptualized in terms of a developmental process. Within this context, the stimulus for development is a disruption in the individual's previously adequate self-regulatory and adaptive functions. Such a disruption can come in the form of biological maturation or change, environmental demand, a traumatic event such as loss, or a self-initiated pursuit of better adaptation. Examples of events or experiences that disrupt adult psychic equilibrium, particularly in the more advanced years, include loss of parents and potentially of spouse, retirement, illnesses, and loss of functions due to aging.

In response to developmental challenges, the individual experiences a conflict in which he or she must confront the need to adapt and attempt to negotiate the anxiety and conflict that any change entails. Resolution of developmental conflict potentially leads to structural change in self-regulatory and adaptive functioning. In turn this can lead to a change in the individual's self and object representations, level of separation-individuation, sense of identity, self-esteem, and compromise formations.

MULTIPLE DIMENSIONS OF DEVELOPMENT IN OLD AGE: A LIFE CYCLE PERSPECTIVE

In constructing a psychoanalytic framework for development across the life cycle, it is essential to clarify *what,* in fact, develops. Anna Freud (1965), in her deceptively simple yet sophisticated way, offered a significant conceptual framework in her discussion of "developmental lines." She described developmental lines in terms of fundamental aspects of personality that unfold in a regular sequence in the context of child and adolescent maturation. She described, as examples, one developmental line that leads from dependency to emotional self-reliance and another that leads from irresponsibility to responsibility in body management. Several authors have advanced perspectives on development that allow us to expand on Anna Freud's valuable concept of developmental lines; these perspectives are termed *dimensions of development* and they are extended across the life cycle to old age. The model of dimensions of development has been applied to adolescents (Lerner, 1987; Sugarman, Bloom-Feshbach, & Bloom-Feshbach, 1980) and social development across the life cycle (Lerner & Ehrlich, 1992).

As outlined by Lerner and Ehrlich (1992) the major task of adult development is *synthesis*—specifically, the integration of the various dimensions of development (psychosocial, cognitive, moral, etc.). The dimensions may integrate and reintegrate, at higher or lower levels of synthesis, around nodal points or tasks in development such as marriage, parenthood, retirement, and loss—what Neugarten (1979) refers to as "the normal turning points, the punctuation marks along the lifeline" (p. 889). In terms of old age, the dimensions of development may also be thought to integrate and reintegrate either toward higher or lower levels of adaptation around such crises as decline in bodily function, serious illnesses, losses, and, ultimately confronting death.

The eight dimensions of development that are examined next entail salient aspects of psychological development beginning in childhood that are transformed over time and are shaped by both maturation and life experience. Although actual development is multifaceted and exceedingly complex, these dimensions of development will be considered separately for heuristic and conceptual purposes.

As Neugarten (1979) reminds us, old age presents both old and new issues. Some of these issues are connected to renunciation such as adapting to losses, relinquishment of a position of authority, and questioning of one's former competencies; the reconciliation with significant others of one's achievements and failures; the resolution of grief over the death of important others and of one's own approaching death; the maintenance of a sense of integrity in terms of what one has been, rather than what one is, and the concern over legacy and how to leave traces of oneself.

Old age is not what many imagine. It is, in fact, becoming a longer portion of the life cycle. With improved health care, the fastest-growing segment of the population is composed of persons 85 years old and older. Individuals over 65 are becoming an increasingly powerful force in society. A larger proportion of individuals 65 and older vote than any other age group in the population. The American Association of Retired Persons, with more than 32 million members, is among the most powerful lobbying groups in Washington. There are many myths about old age that conceal the triumphs of survivorship and the recognition that one has weathered a wide range of experiences and therefore has a certain "savoir faire" in ways in which younger people cannot know. These include knowledge and strength from having lived through physical and psychological pain that can give confidence that one can recover and deal also with the contingencies that lie ahead (the sense that one is now the possessor and conservator of eternal truths, or what Erikson terms wisdom).

Psychosexual Development: Drives and Bodily Experience

There is general agreement among most psychoanalysts that many of the major psychosexual passions and conflicts of the first five years of life are rekindled and reworked not only during adolescence but also at other nodal points of adulthood. The notion of psychosexual stages was S. Freud's (1905/1951) frame of reference for conceptualizing development based on his examination of the origin and dynamics of neurotic symptoms and character traits that he connected to successive phases of the libidinal drives. He had observed that early phases of what he termed "infantile sexuality" were organized around energic investment of the oral, anal, and phallic erotogenic bodily zones, each achieving, in turn, a relative dominance over the preceding phases. Bodily activities and sensations connected with each zone are thought to be accompanied by phase-related fantasies and conflicts with the parents or other important persons in the child's environment. Despite the continuum in sensual experience (G. Klein, 1976) implied in Freud's theory of psychosexual development, few have traced the developmental line of psychosexuality into adulthood.

Colarusso and Nemiroff (1981) observed that in American society there is a tendency to associate increased age with a decrease in sexual interest and activity. This myth of diminished sexuality with age is not biologically mandated. Far-reaching and deep social and cultural changes have brought about a greater flexibility in social norms regarding sex roles and increased external freedom, despite the AIDS epidemic. For many, however, external freedom does not bring about a corresponding internal freedom from conflict. For example, the women's movement has brought new role conflict for women who simultaneously pursue occupational success and motherhood and for men who seek new freedom and new combinations of roles as worker, parent, and homemaker. As Neugarten (1979) observes, for women there is new freedom and increased energy available when children leave home, and freedom from unwanted pregnancy and, for many, new pleasures in sexual activity that accompany menopause. Nevertheless, for both sexes, there is an increased realization that, with age, the body is increasingly less predictable than earlier and there is increased attention to body monitoring. The psychological counterpart of the inevitable aging of the body is changes in the experience of time. Middle age is thought to bring with it a change in time perspective, in that time becomes restructured in terms of time left to live rather than time since birth.

Sexual behavior changes with aging (Harman, 1978; Martin, 1977). The most significant factors in determining the level of sexual activity with increased age appear to be general health and survival of the spouse. Colarusso and Nemiroff (1981), based on their review of the biological literature on aging, conclude that some degree of declining sexual function and interest appears to be an inevitable consequence of aging, but health, social, and cultural factors rather than physiological change per se seem to be responsible for most of the sexual changes seen with aging. These authors note that prevalent attitudes about brain functioning in late adulthood are just as skewed as those about sexual functioning. Mental functioning need not necessarily decline with age because of inevitable degenerative changes in the brain. Health, social factors, interpersonal relationships, and environmental stimulation, rather than a decline in brain functioning and the central nervous system, appear to be important determinants of the course of psychological development in middle and late adulthood.

Attitudes toward the body change through the life span. During adolescence and early adulthood there is a casual acceptance of the body with concerns revolving around invincibility versus vulnerability as well as the development of physical abilities and care of the body. Through the 30s and 40s there is a growing awareness of physical limitations, often signaled by baldness, gray hair, wrinkles, and changes in vision. These changes are reflected in fantasies having to do with the body of youth, a mourning process, and the emergence of a new body image, one that increasingly approximates reality with an acceptance of physical limitations and an enjoyment of the body in new ways. With advanced age, continued care or neglect of the body becomes an increasingly important psychological issue. With this come increased efforts to compensate for diminished physical energy by altering schedules, diets, and sleep patterns. These changes are also accompanied by increased fantasies of death, heart attacks, and, for many women, widowhood. With increased time, the psychological focus becomes one of remaining active despite frequent physical infirmity and with it the acceptance of permanent, irreversible physical impairment.

The Psychosocial Dimension: Striving for Ego Identity

As has been noted, most classical psychoanalytic thinkers beginning with Freud have conceptualized development from an intrapsychic perspective. Erikson, however, in a series of influential papers and books, has stressed the importance of the broader social context. It is specifically within the context of the task of integrating psychosexual and bodily changes that Erikson notes that the adolescent is confronted with the difficult task of assessing society, assimilating those values that appear sensible, and finding a place within society. To do so, according to Erikson, is to development a sense of identity, a sense of who one is as a unique individual across different situations and through historical time, a sense of self-sameness.

Formation of identity, however, does not end with adolescence. The adult phases of the life span require a continuing although less rapid and dramatic evolution, refinement, and maturation of identity for the maintenance of optimal adaptation and functioning. Michels (1980) has outlined four major themes of adult develop that can be considered in terms of their impact on ego identity: work, sex, parenthood, and aging.

One major task of adulthood involves development and integration of a work identity. During adolescence and young adulthood, the ability to make choices, to identify and develop work skills, to maintain a capacity for sustained and committed work and derive pleasure from it, as well as the experience of success and failure in the workplace are key determinants of an adult work identity. The role of a mentor relationship is often instrumental during this phase as well as during the 30s, in which there is a solidification of a work identity, the continued development of skills, increased attention to levels of achievement in terms of economic and social status, and increased internal and external pressures involving balancing of work and family life.

Through the 40s there is a transformation from student to mentor, and with it an acceptance of limitations and failure to reach certain goals. Issues of facilitation versus competitiveness and jealousy and the use of power and position come into play. With age, the successful adult must also synthesize a work identity with the aging process and must be able to diminish the role of work in his or her life as capacity progressively diminishes, and yet maintain self-esteem and a capacity for pleasure. A stable identity can insulate an individual from some of the narcissistic knocks of a decrease in work capacity. A major psychological challenge is associated with leaving the work force. No longer is the individual an accountant, a sales representative, or an electrician. The sense of self so long linked to a career is gone, and the new retiree's challenge is to find alternative ways to feel that life has purpose and meaning. Feelings of self-worth, creativity, and nurturance must be sustained. Often, mentoring or volunteer work provides opportunities for older people to pass on their expertise and wisdom. Unfortunately, some individuals leaving the work force, as they work further into old age, may withdraw and become even more self-absorbed. Conflicts involving activity versus passivity become paramount.

In terms of sexuality, according to Michels (1980), the adult has two developmental tasks: to structure a pattern of sexual behavior that incorporates biological, psychological, and social reality, and to integrate that pattern with the rest of his or her personality and to achieve maximal satisfaction from it. With age comes increased pressure to redefine relationships to the partner, to care for the partner in the face of illness and aging, to develop capacities for sharing new activities, to continue an active sexual life, and eventually the capacity to tolerate separation, loss, and death.

According to Erikson (1978), aging begins at conception but has special characteristics at each phase of the life cycle. Jacques (1965) notes that the psychological meaning of death is transformed in adult life from one of fear associated with traumatic experience to one in which death begins to be more familiar and gradually accepted. The actual loss of one's parents, friends, and loved ones, as well as the inevitability of one's own death replaces the child's unconscious fantasies as the symbolic equivalent of death. The social meaning of adulthood and of being older must be integrated into the adult identity. With development, the social impact of aging joins race, gender, and physical handicap as roles that must be redefined and reintegrated into the identity.

An example of the integrative task of identity for the elderly is offered by Erikson (1976) in his essay, "Reflections on Dr. Borg's Lifecycle," a commentary on Ingmar Bergman's film *Wild Strawberries*. The film shows the journey of Isak Borg, a 76-year-old professor driving through the Swedish countryside of his youth to attend a public ceremony in honor of his enormous accomplishments. The journey highlights poignant features of his developmental history. The countryside rekindles memories of his early years, as do hitchhikers of diverse ages and personalities who enter and leave Borg's car during the course of his journey. As Erikson points out, many of Borg's memories and thoughts revolve around the last four stages in his life-cycle model (identity versus identification, intimacy versus isolation, generativity versus stagnation, and integrity versus despair). Yet Erikson points out that Borg experiences much more than his struggle with the eighth developmental stage, the conflict between integrity and despair, out of which wisdom is cultivated. As Dr. Borg struggles with the psychological issues of this stage, he simultaneously grapples with issues from *all* the prior stages of the life cycle. As Fitzpatrick and Friedman (1983) point out, Erikson converts his life cycle model into a "life-spiral" model in which earlier developmental stages are never even partially transcended or bypassed in development. That is to say, the issues an individual struggles with in prior stages invariably reoccur alongside new issues at later stages. Development is not thought to be primarily a linear progression but rather a spiral or mosaic in which multiple interactions simultaneously link the past and the present. As each stage is negotiated, issues from prior stages are simultaneously repeated but in different terms.

The Cognitive Dimension

As with all dimensions of adult development, the cognitive dimension underlies and interdigitates with other dimensions in important and complex ways. Nevertheless, for conceptual purposes it will be considered here separately. An important cognitive transformation and development that is decisive for the remainder of the life cycle takes place during adolescence. Thought of in Piagetian theory (Inhelder & Piaget, 1958), this shift is from concrete to formal operations. As Piaget (1954) asserts, the principle of formal operations involves the real versus the possible. Formal operational thinking permits the adolescent to progress from combining the properties of objects into classes to combining classes into classes. Thus, the adolescent has access to a complete system of all possible combinations. The system can be used to solve problems, to generate hypotheses, and to integrate identifications. Reversibility of thinking frees the individual from the constraints of concrete reality. With this accomplishment, adolescents and later adults can act on representations of reality rather than on concrete reality itself. This transformation enhances adaptation in many ways. Formal operations permit enhanced freedom in dealing with wishes, affects, and interpersonal relationships, and both the real and the possible can be considered. Fantasy can become an adaptive and creative modality. Affect-laden issues such as intimacy, death, and the meaning of life can be considered: in the abstract; all possibilities and consequences can be considered; and the internal world takes on the quality of a real place. These cognitive developments permit increased freedom to experience a wider range of both internal and external issues.

Beginning with adolescence and through adulthood to old age, with the successful resolution of conflict and the struggle with crises, the individual can experience his or her internal world in a more reflective and flexible manner because an enhanced appreciation of the possible significantly reduces the fearful aspects of internal stimuli. The shift from concrete to formal operations also facilitates identity formation by affording the individual the cognitive capacities to organize and integrate representations of the past with those of the present and the future. With certain progressive neurological illnesses as well as regressions secondary to illness, depression, and psychological stresses and strains, there can be a shift back from formal to concrete operations in the elderly. In many cases, with needed stimulation, empathic responsiveness, and psychotherapy, these regressions can be reversed.

The Object Relations Dimension: Separation-Individuation and Underlying Representations

In keeping with the hypothesis advanced by Colarusso and Nemiroff (1981) that the fundamental issues of childhood continue as salient aspects of adult development but in altered forms, several writers have examined the basic process of separation-individuation through various phases of the life cycle, rather than only as a significant event of childhood. According to Mahler (1973):

> The entire life cycle constitutes a more or less successful process of distancing from an introjection of the lost symbiotic mother, and external longing for the actual or fantasized ideal state of self, with the latter standing for a symbiotic fusion with the all-good symbiotic mother who was at one time part of the self in a blissful state of well-being. (p. 138)

Colarusso and Nemiroff (1981) assert that the quest for enhanced differentiation between self and other ends only with biological death. Formative adult experiences, such as changing interpersonal relationships and investments, the recognition of interdependence with others, the experience of parenthood and grandparenthood, and the relationship with the spouse, all involve enhanced separation-individuation secondary to the gradual acceptance of real over idealized aspects of relationships and the acceptance of the aging process in both self and others.

From a life-span perspective, there are important developmental changes not only in the significance of interpersonal relationships but also in the significance of being alone and maintaining an aloneness that is satisfying. The experience of comforting aloneness becomes increasingly important during the second half of life, with the realization of the finitude of life (Jacques, 1965) to some extent replacing contact with others as a source of solace and well-being. The increased preference for solitude and aloneness must be understood as different from feelings of isolation. What may be more important in sustaining the capacity for solace and comfort in aloneness are memories of time spent together in the past which draw upon an individual's internal representations of themselves and other people. Drawing upon these representations, reminiscence replaces actual contacts with others as a major source of solace and self-soothing in later adulthood and may become increasingly adaptive as the loss of loved ones and impairment of mobility make actual contact more difficult.

The Structural Dimension: Ego Development

The structural dimension of development refers specifically to ego development; that is, a complex and multifaceted set of psychological functions based on interactions among innate constitutional givens, maturational forces, and experiential and social influences. This dimension includes the innate developmental strengths and weaknesses of underlying cognitive and representational structures and of drive-affect modulating structures such as defenses. Under optimal conditions, when these various functions operate effectively, they facilitate adaptation and further development by freeing the individual from conflict. The term "ego weakness" refers to either a diffusion or severe inhibition of drives and affects; there may be more pervasive regressions that impinge on personality structures, and the vulnerable individual faced with such threats to structural integrity may decompensate. Inhibitions include a limitation of experience, of feelings and thoughts or both, a restriction of the experience of pleasure, a tendency to externalize internal events and negative feelings, and a host of limitations of internalization necessary for the regulation of impulses, affects, and thoughts, as well as limitations in the maintenance of self-esteem. Naturally, for older people, experiences of physical illness, multiple losses, and the specter of death pose a mature stress on the integrity of the ego structure and exert a regressive pull.

Affect tolerance is considered an important aspect of the structural dimension. Although the intensity, depth, and range of affects can vary along both qualitative and quantitative continua, both between individuals and across the life span, more pathological expressions of affect tend to be less differentiated and articulated. Level of development and structural integrity of the defensive organization represents an important aspect of affect tolerance and expression.

Vaillant's (1977) longitudinal study of adaptation across the life span focused on defensive organization. Central to Vaillant's study is the assumption that for individuals to master conflict adaptively and to utilize internal resources creatively, adaptive styles, that is, defense mechanisms, must mature and develop throughout the life cycle. Ordering defenses into a theoretical hierarchy in terms of relative maturity, Vaillant found in a group of normal men over time a progressive decline in less mature defense mechanisms of fantasy and action and a concomitant increase in more mature defense mechanisms such as suppression. He noted an increase in defenses such as sublimation and altruism with age. Such changes in defensive organization provide evidence that internal structural change occurs throughout the life span.

The Moral Dimension: Superego and Ego Ideal

Both psychoanalysis and developmental-cognitive psychology have made important contributions to theories of moral development. Although traditional psychoanalytic theory related moral development to psychosexual drive states, cognitive psychology has been primarily concerned with moral judgment; hence, the scope of cognitive theory is narrower than formulations derived from psychoanalysis. Psychoanalytic inquiry has revolved around moral development in terms of the socialization process and the progressive internalization of standards that modulate potentially disruptive drives, and eventually, with the development of the ego ideal, take the form of an integrated value system. On the other hand, cognitive theorists have focused on the role of higher cognitive processes and role-taking ability in moral judgment. Nevertheless, higher levels of morality are thought to be inextricably contingent upon the achievement of formal operations.

Psychoanalysts have approached moral development from the perspective of transformations and consolidations of the superego. According to theory, during adolescence external changes in relationship with the parents are paralleled by internal changes in the superego in terms of a revival of earlier conflicts. It is thought that these changes exert a disruptive and destabilizing effect on self-regulation and self-esteem. Freud (1923/1957) thought of the superego as a precipitate of the ego, consisting of identifications with the parents and reactions against them. According to Freud, functions of the superego including judgment, prohibitions and injunctions, moral censorship, a sense of guilt and social feeling, and identifications are all subsumed under the superego rubric. According to modern structural theory, all compromise formations include a superego or moral dimension, and the superego itself is understood as a compromise formation. These formulations all suggest that the moral dimension and superego functioning in particular is a dynamic process that develops and becomes transformed throughout the life cycle.

Transitional Objects

The work of D. W. Winnicott, a British object-relations theorist, has had a major impact on psychoanalytic thought. Winnicott's formulations concerning transitional objects and self-development have important implications for understanding development through the life cycle. It is in describing the infant's experience of adapting to a shared reality through the transition from absolute to relative dependence that Winnicott's most original and creative contributions are made.

Winnicott (1951/1958) evocatively described the child's earliest experience of decentering in efforts to bridge the gap between fantasy and reality. It was through his deceptively simple and direct clinical observations that Winnicott was led to the remarkable discovery of the child's first "not-me" possession, that is, the "transitional object." Winnicott traced that transitional object (e.g., a bundle of wool, the corner of a blanket, a teddy bear) to very early forms of relating and playing. The relationship of the infant to the transitional object is marked by several qualities, including a decrease in omnipotence, a relationship in which the object is totally controlled by the infant, and in which the object becomes the target for love and hate. The transitional object takes on a reality of its own, combining the qualities of being paradoxically created and discovered:

> In the course of years it becomes not so much forgotten as relegated to limbo . . . it is not forgotten and it is not mourned, it loses meaning, and this is because the transitional phenomena have become diffused, have become spread out over the whole intermediate territory between "inner psychic reality" and the external world as perceived by two people in common, that is to say, over the whole cultural field. (p. 233)

Taking these formulations as a point of departure, Sugarman and Jaffe (1987) claim that multiple developmental transitions occur throughout the life cycle;

the transitional phenomena are psychologically called upon and used to "regain inner-outer equilibrium at each phase." In keeping with Winnicott's original formulations, transitional phenomena are conceptualized as adaptive mechanisms that are used throughout the life span. A core premise is that equilibrium between the individual and the environment is promoted through internalization of key self-regulatory functions. Transitional phenomena are seen as central aspects of this process as they foster internalization. As a consequence, the "self representation becomes increasingly differentiated and integrated through a series of internalizations" (Sugarman & Jaffe, 1987, p. 421). In essence, these authors demonstrate how the transitional object facilitates modulation of tension created by internal and external stresses throughout development.

The level of cognitive maturity and other dimensions of personality become important in determining the manifest forms of transitional phenomena. As other functions, including self and object representations, become increasingly differentiated, transitional objects are thought to become increasingly less tangible and more abstract. For example, in contrast to the transitional objects of early childhood, the transitional phenomena of adolescence such as career aspirations, music, and literature are more abstract, ideational, depersonified, and less animistic. They increasingly approximate reality. Rather than the concrete fantasy representation, it is ideas, causes, or symbolic value that become meaningful. Regardless of the manifest content of transitional objects, transitional phenomena are thought to promote the internalization of core self-regulatory functions that include narcissistic regulation such as sustaining self-esteem, drive regulation, superego integration, ego functioning, and interpersonal relationships. Through use of increasingly abstract transitional phenomena, the individual is better able to synthesize discrepant events in his or her life experience. With increased development, the function of transitional phenomena also changes from one of self-soothing to one of enriching the quality of life. For older persons, in many ways sustaining memories, reminiscence, stories, and even photos become important transitional phenomena.

Narcissism

One of the liveliest debates in contemporary psychoanalysis revolves around the concept and nature of narcissism and its role in normal development. Freud's use of the term left many areas of ambiguity that subsequent investigators have attempted to clarify. Stolorow (1975) offered a functional as well as heuristic definition of narcissism: the "structural cohesiveness, temporal stability and positive affective coloring of the self-representation" (p. 174). Psychological functioning is seen as narcissistic to the degree that it establishes and maintains cohesiveness, stability, and positive affective coloring of the self. Most authors use the term in the context of self-esteem. Normal narcissism has been distinguished from pathological narcissism (Kernberg, 1976). Normal narcissism is thought to depend on the structural integrity of the self-representation, the achievement of self and object constancy, harmony between the self and superego structures, the capacity to receive gratification from external objects, and a state of physical well-being. Pathological variants of narcissism include a defensive self-inflation with an associated lack of integration of the self-concept. Whereas normal narcissism leads to sustained, realistic self-regard and mature aspirations and ideals accompanied by the capacity for deep relationships, pathological narcissism is accompanied by grandiose views of the self, a dependency on the admiration of others, and poor object relations. It is manifested in terms of a sense of entitlement, a pursuit of perfection, and impaired capacities for concern, empathy, and love for others.

Although little has been written systematically about the vicissitudes of narcissism throughout the life cycle, it is generally agreed that narcissism is either altered or transformed as development occurs. Advances in the capacity to love another suggests advances in narcissism. According to Spruiell (1975), transformation of narcissism parallels transformations in object relations. Colarusso and Nemiroff (1981) use the term *authentic self* to characterize the mature adult, in that it describes the capacity to accept what is genuine within the self and the outer world, regardless of narcissistic injury involved. According to these authors, significant influences in later adulthood are narcissistic issues relating to the aging body, the impact of aging on the time sense, and issues related to the loss of work and significant relationships.

Normative narcissistic regressions are precipitated by developmental tasks and stresses such as the approach of mid-life, which often lead to a reemergence of elements of more infantile forms of narcissism. The reworking and reintegration of aspects of infantile narcissism can be seen as an integral part of normal development throughout the life cycle. In older persons, more infantile manifestations of narcissism can occur secondary to the loss of affirmation, calming, and soothing from significant others. Of course, these experiences are more prominent in those who depend on external reminders of their worth as a major factor in maintaining their self-esteem and equilibrium. Among the painful symptoms of "narcissistic injury" suffered by older persons are intense feelings of emptiness, hypersensitivity to insult or lack of appropriate recognition, feelings of inferiority, agitation, and exquisite feelings of vulnerability.

In each developmental phase throughout the life cycle, there are environmental situations that are experienced as narcissistic stressors. Those situations that are prone to cause more psychic pain in older persons include the loss of significant objects and self objects; illnesses both of themselves and of others; interpersonal difficulties, and a host of situations in the culture, including relocation and economic hardship. To many elderly persons, the losses of people who were important to them are the most difficult hardships to bear. Most painful are those losses that involve significant others who were the source of narcissistic supplies. It is for this reason that the experience of mourning and one's capacity to bear it is a significant developmental task for older persons.

MOURNING

Loss is a pervasive experience in the normal developmental process. That is, loss goes hand in hand with development. Pine (1985) has outlined four losses that are thought to be normative, universal, and affectively powerful during adulthood. During adulthood, in contrast to adolescence, there is a loss of omnipotentiality: an awareness of limitations and roads not taken. A second loss during adulthood is that of optimal body functioning and appearance. A third loss is the progressive loss of one's own children that begins with the birth of the child. The fourth and final loss during the adult period is the loss of peers through death and the preparation for one's own death (the final step in loss of body function and the loss of self and consciousness that goes with it).

Lerner and Lerner (1987) observed that Freud's original definition of mourning and its distinction from melancholia is still accepted by most psychoanalysts. According to S. Freud (1917/1951) the distinguishing mental features of mourning are feelings of painful dejection, loss of interest in the outside world, inability to love, and massive inhibition of all activity. Melancholia involves the identical features as well as "a lowering of the self-regarding feelings to a degree that finds utterances and self-reproaches and self-revelings and culminate in a delusional expectation of punishment" (p. 244). Freud went on to note that whereas melancholia, like mourning, may be a reaction to the loss of a loved one, it differs in that "one cannot see clearly what it is that has been lost—[the person] knows whom he has lost but not what he has lost in him" (p. 245). These observations led Freud to conclude that "in mourning it is the world which has become poor and empty; in melancholia it is the ego itself" (p. 246). If one substitutes the term "self" for "ego" these statements make phenomenological sense.

The process of mourning involves a gradual relinquishment and severing of emotional ties to the lost object and a corresponding displacement of interest or attachment onto other objects. According to Freud (1917/1951):

> [E]ach single one of the memories and situations of expectancy which demonstrate the libido's attachment to the lost object is met by the verdict of reality that the object no longer exists; and the ego, confronted as it were with the question whether it shall share this state, is persuaded by the sum of the narcissistic satisfactions it derives from being alive to sever its attachment to the object that has been abolished. (p. 237)

Melancholia also involves a withdrawal of interest or attachment from the lost object. However, rather than being displaced onto other objects, the libido, by means of regressive identification, is withdrawn back into the self. In this way the object loss is transformed into a loss of self, and the conflict between the self and the lost object is experienced as a "cleavage" within the self.

According to Lerner and Lerner (1987), the impact of loss on personality is dramatic, intense, complex, and dependent on a multitude of internal and external factors, including levels of separation-individuation, drive development, level of defense, and, most significantly, the developmental level of mental representations of self and other, as well as the availability of substitute objects and the degree to which inner psychological structures have become autonomous from supporting objects or self-objects. According to these authors, the impact of object loss on object relations and narcissism can be viewed on a developmental continuum in relation to self-object differentiation, level of mental representation, and degree of self and object constancy. When these particular lines of development are not fully structuralized or autonomous from supporting objects, the response to object loss is more likely to be one of melancholia; that is, a loss of self as opposed to mourning a loss of the other.

George Pollock, more than any other psychoanalyst, has studied the mourning process and has reported that this most poignant human experience potentially serves as an adaptation to various losses throughout the life cycle. According to Pollock, bereavement is only one dimension of mourning. Mourning can be set in motion not only after death, but also by loss, disappointment, or change, and is a normative part of development throughout life. Colarusso and Nemiroff (1981), quote Pollock (1979), who asserts:

> Mourning is a universal transformational process that allows us to accept the reality that exists which may be different from our wishes and hopes, which recognizes loss and change, both externally and internally, and which . . . can result in a happier life, fulfilled and fulfilling for ourselves and for others. For the gifted the mourning process may be part of or the end product that can result in creativity in art, music, literature, science, philosophy, religion. (p. 10)

Mourning, seen in this vein, is an adaptive process that facilitates development. According to Shabad and Dietrich (1989), death of the old gives way to the birth of the new in ways that are not always immediately apparent in the midst of grief. Loss, despite potentially pathogenic consequences, may also have other creative, constructive, long-term consequences that are not always recognizable in the immediate aftermath of death. The process of increased internalization of the representation of lost objects sets the stage for what Pollock (1979) refers to as the mourning-liberation process. The pain of working through the process of mourning can be gradually replaced by the relative psychological freedom brought about by an acceptance that loss is final. A person may then direct his or her creative capacities toward reconstituting a replacement for the lost object (Shabad and Dietrich, 1989). The relative balance between acceptance of or denial of the finality of loss and death significantly influences the individual's capacity to eventually work through and resolve the loss experience.

The lifelong experience of separation and loss is what links mourning and aging. Aging begins at conception but has unique characteristics at each phase of the life cycle (Erikson, 1978). According to Michels (1980), aging means for the first time a diminution of capacity and potential rather than the steady progressive growth associated with childhood. Michels states:

> For the adult, death begins to be more familiar and gradually accepted. Friends and loved ones die; one's own death is no longer beyond the psychologically meaningful horizon of future time; and the inevitable diseases and disabilities of middle life begin to replace the child's unconscious fantasies as the symbolic equivalent of death. (p. 33)

Compulsive attempts in middle age to remain young, hypochondriacal preoccupations with health in the parents, emergence of sexual promiscuity in order to prove oneself youthful and potent, lack of authentic enjoyment of life, and frequency of religious concern in middle age are familiar defensive patterns of coping with the inevitability of death (Jacques, 1980). The aging process, and with it, loss of physical and mental capacities, can represent an adult life crisis. It intensifies narcissistic vulnerability, recognition of mortality, and the inevitable approach of death, which demands adaptation to this most imminent threat and stress. Dealing with the issue of death itself, both for the individual approaching it, as well as survivors, involves a major shift in internal, interpersonal, and social factors and the need for psychological adaptations to new circumstances. Mourning and the aging process require a continuing evolution and maturation in order to maintain adaptation and functioning. Inevitably, the vicissitudes of life experience increasingly include separation, loss, and mourning. And no one is immune to them. Positive adaptation to these inevitable life experiences are less related to their existence than to the individual's capacity for conflict resolution and continued adaptation. These adaptations are results of the multiple dimensions or lines of development considered in this chapter.

SUMMARY

Recent contributions to psychoanalytic theory have begun to examine and refine multiple dimensions of development as they extend across the life cycle. Several authors have offered formulations as to how individuals deal with the ongoing developmental task of separation-individuation in the adult years approaching old age. In line with the approach of such contributions, this chapter, in exploring multiple dimensions of development in old age, has sought to integrate the formative, ongoing influences of intrapsychic processes with the continuous impact of maturation and life experience. Evolution of the various dimensions of development during the later years will be of increased interest to psychoanalysts as the "baby boomers" approach later stages of adulthood. Continued work will be done on the impact that specific life experiences exert on adult development. Too often, researchers and theorists formulate significant life experiences of adulthood, such as close relationships, divorce, loss, and illness, outside the context of an individual's ongoing development. This makes it easy to lose sight of the multiple dimensions of development that prestage each adult experience. Further, we fail to consider the role that each new experience of later adulthood potentially plays in the refinement and reorganization of previous dimensions of development. Individual experience thus becomes static and detached. It is important to understand how an individual's ongoing development sets the stage for a particular life event and then is transformed by it. Our understanding of critical life experiences during old age, for example, retirement, grandparenthood, illness, the loss of a spouse, and preparation for the loss of one's self, can be greatly enriched by viewing such experiences in the context of multiple dimensions of development.

REFERENCES

Behrends, R. S., & Blatt, S. J. (1985). Internalization and psychological development throughout the life cycle. *Psychoanalytic Study of the Child, 40,* 11–40.

Blatt, S. J. (1974). Levels of object representation in anaclitic and introjective depression. *Psychoanalytic Study of the Child, 29,* 107–157.

Boesky, D. (1989). A discussion of evidential criteria for therapeutic change. In A. Rothstein (Ed.), *How does treatment help: Modes of therapeutic action of psychoanalytic therapy.* Madison, CT: International Universities Press.

Brenner, C. (1986). Reflections. In A. Richards & M. S. Willock (Eds.), *Psychoanalysis: The science of mental conflict. Essays in honor of Charles Brenner.* Hillsdale, NJ: Analytic Press.

Colarusso, C. A., & Nemiroff, R. A. (1981). *Adult development.* New York: Plenum.

Erikson, E. (1976). Reflections of Dr. Borg's lifecycle. *Daedalus, 105,* 1–28.

Erikson, E. (1978). *Life history and historical moment.* New York: Norton.

Fitzpatrick, J. J., & Friedman, L. J. (1983). Adult developmental theories and Eric Erikson's lifecycle model. *Bulletin of the Menninger Clinic, 47,* 401–416.

Freud, A. (1965). *Normality and pathology in childhood.* New York: International Universities Press.

Freud, S. (1951). Mourning and melancholia. In J. Strachey (Ed. and Trans.), *The standard edition of the complete psychological works of Sigmund Freud* (Vol. XIV, pp. 237–258). London: Hogarth Press. (Original work published 1917).

Freud, S. (1951). Three essays on the theory of sexuality. In J. Strachey (Ed. and Trans.), *The standard edition of the complete psychological works of Sigmund Freud* (Vol. VII, pp. 125–243). London: Hogarth Press. (Original work published 1905).

Freud, S. (1957). The ego and the id. In J. Strachey (Ed. and Trans.). *The standard edition of the complete psychological works of Sigmund Freud* (Vol. IX, pp. 12–68). London: Hogarth Press. (Original work published 1923).

Gedo, J., & Goldberg, A. (1973). *Models of the mind.* Chicago: University of Chicago Press.

Guntrip, H. (1974). Psychoanalytic object relations theory: The Fairbairn–Guntrip approach. In S. Arieti (Ed.), *American handbook of psychiatry* (Vol. 1). New York: Basic Books.

Harman, S. W. (1978). Male menopause? The hormones flow but sex does slow. *Medical World, 20,* 11.

Inhelder, B., & Piaget, J. (1958). *The growth of logical thinking from childhood to adolescence: An essay on the construction of formal operational structures.* New York: International Universities Press.

Jacques, E. (1965). Death and the mid-life crisis. *International Journal of Psycho-Analysis, 46,* 502–514.

Jacques, E. (1980). The mid-life crisis. In S. Greenspan & G. Pollock (Eds.), *The course of the life cycle: Psychoanalytic contributions toward understanding personality development* Vol. 3, pp. 1–24). Washington, DC: National Institute of Mental Health.

Kernberg, O. (1976). *Borderline conditions and pathological narcissism.* New York: International Universities Press.

Klein, G. (1976). *Psychoanalytic theory: An exploration of essentials.* New York: International Universities Press.

Kohut, H. (1971). *The analysis of the self.* New York: International Universities Press.

Kohut, H. (1977). *The restoration of the self.* New York: International Universities Press.

Lerner, H. (1987). Psychodynamic models of adolescence. In M. Hersen & V. Van Hasselt (Eds.), *Handbook of adolescent psychology* (pp. 53–76). New York: Pergamon.

Lerner, H., & Ehrlich, J. (1992). Psychodynamic models. In V. Van Hasselt & M. Hersen (Eds.), *Handbook of social development: A lifespan perspective* (pp. 51–79). New York: Pergamon.

Lerner, H., & Lerner, P. (1987). Separation, depression, and object loss: Implications for narcissism and object relations. In J. Bloom-Feshbach & S. Bloom-Feshbach (Eds.), *The psychology of separation and loss* (pp. 375–395). San Francisco: Jossey-Bass.

Mahler, M. (1973). The experience of separation–individuation in infancy and its reverberations through the course of life: Infancy and childhood (panel report). *Journal of the American Psychoanalytic Association, 21,* 135.

Mahler, M., Pine, F., & Bergman, A. (1975). *The psychological birth of the human infant.* New York: Basic Books.

Martin, C. E. (1977). Sexual activity in the aging male. In J. Money & H. Musaph (Eds.), *Handbook of sexology.* Amsterdam: Elsevier/North Holland.

Michels, R. (1980). Adulthood. In S. Greenspan & G. Pollock (Eds.), *The course of the life cycle: Psychoanalytic contributions toward understanding personality development.* (Vol. 3, pp. 25–34). Washington, DC: National Institute of Mental Health.

Muslin, H. (1992). *The psychotherapy of the elderly self.* New York: Brunner/Mazel.

Neugarten, B. (1979). Time, age, and the life cycle. *American Journal of Psychiatry, 136,* 887–894.

Piaget, J. (1954). *The construction of reality.* New York: Basic Books.

Pine, F. (1985). *Developmental theory and clinical process.* New Haven, CT: Yale University Press.

Pollock, G. (1979). *Aging or aged: Development or pathology?* Unpublished manuscript.

Settlage, C. F., Curtis, J., Lozoff, M., Silbershatz, G., & Simburg, E. (1988). Conceptualizing adult development. *Journal of the American Psychoanalytic Association, 36,* 347–369.

Shabad, P., & Dietrich, D. (1989). Reflections on loss, mourning, and the unconscious process of regeneration. In D. Dietrich & P. Shabad (Eds.), *The problem of loss and mourning* (pp. 461–470). Madison, CT: International Universities Press.

Spruiell, V. (1975). Narcissistic transformation in adolescence. *International Journal of Psychoanalytic Psychotherapy, 4,* 518–535.

Stolorow, R. (1975). Toward a functional definition of narcissism. *International Journal of Psychoanalysis, 56,* 179–185.

Sugarman, A., & Jaffe, L. (1987). Transitional phenomena and psychological separateness in schizophrenic, borderline, and bulimic patients. In J. Bloom-Feshbach & S. Bloom-Feshbach (Eds.), *The psychology of separation and loss* (pp. 416–458). San Francisco: Jossey-Bass.

Sugarman, A., Bloom-Feshbach, J., & Bloom-Feshbach, S. (1980). The psychological dimensions of borderline adolescence. In J. Kwawer, H. Lerner, P. Lerner, & A. Sugarman (Eds.), *Borderline phenomena and the Rorschach test* (pp. 469–494). New York: International Universities Press.

Vaillant, G. E. (1977). *Adaptation of life.* Boston: Little, Brown.

Waelder, R. (1930). The principle of multiple function: Observations on overdetermination. In S. Guttman (Ed.), *Psychoanalysis: Observation, theory, application* (pp. 68–83). New York: International Universities Press.

Winnicott, D. (1958). Transitional objects and transitional phenomena. In D. Winnicott (Ed.), *Collected papers: Through pediatrics to psychoanalysis* (pp. 229–242). New York: Basic Books. (Original work published 1951)

CHAPTER 4

The Value of Behavioral Perspectives in Treating Older Adults

LARRY W. DUPREE AND LAWRENCE SCHONFELD

INTRODUCTION

Behavioral approaches used in the treatment of older adults have now been implemented and evaluated over about a 25-year period. The field of behavioral gerontology, as it is known, is noted by Wisocki (1991) to be "best defined as the application of behavioral principles and procedures to the problems of the elderly and the issues of aging" (p. 3). Interventions based on these principles have proven to be among the most effective treatments for a wide variety of behavior problems for all age groups.

In this chapter, we discuss three models for explaining behavior problems, the advantages of behavioral interventions in overcoming "ageism," and the value of the behavioral perspective at various stages of the intervention process (case finding, assessment, intervention, and outcome). In addition, we discuss the advantages for treatment staff and the problems they often encounter in using behavioral approaches.

CONCEPTUALIZING THE PROBLEMS OF OLDER ADULTS

Three common models used in conceptualizing behavior problems have important implications for the assessment and treatment of older adults. The medical, social, and behavioral models are all deterministic in that behavior is believed to be influenced by previous events.

LARRY W. DUPREE AND LAWRENCE SCHONFELD • Department of Aging and Mental Health, The Florida Mental Health Institute, University of South Florida, Tampa, Florida 33612-3899.

Handbook of Clinical Geropsychology, edited by Michel Hersen and Vincent B. Van Hasselt. Plenum Press, New York, 1998.

The medical model considers deviations from normal functioning as due to illness or disease, most notably improper physiological functioning that purportedly occurs as a natural (and expected) consequence of aging. Advocates of the medical model assume that an underlying cause such as a biologically based disease or an unobservable psychological process leads to the behavior problems or "symptoms." In this regard, Estes and Binney (1989) describe the dangers of the "biomedicalization of aging" (i.e., the powerful influence the medical field has on the process and problems of aging). This not only places treatment under the domain of biomedicine, but also leads to assumptions that behaviors are difficult to change, biologically determined, and possibly irreversible. Such assumptions easily interact with insidious ageism to markedly influence case finding, assessment, and intervention.

The social model attributes changes in behavior or differences in behavior between older and younger adults to different roles assigned to each of these age groups by the culture or society. We tend to expect less responsibility and decreased functional ability in our society's older members. Miller (1979) noted that we accept (and expect) lesser levels of functioning in these specific areas: self-care behavior, task behavior, and relationship behavior.

According to the behavioral model, behavior is the product of learning, preceded by antecedent events and followed by consequences or reinforcers. As one ages, changes in both the antecedent and the consequent events are associated with changes in behaviors (M. M. Baltes & Barton, 1977; Patterson & Jackson, 1980a, 1980b). In response to newer environmental antecedents and consequences, some appropriate behaviors are gradually lost, and other (perhaps inappropriate) behaviors appear. Within this model, behavior is assessed, evaluated, and validated through direct observation, rather than theoretically based. The approach is problem-oriented rather than age-specific and appears to be applicable to many of the well-documented problems noted in later life.

It should be noted that although behaviorists concentrate on nonmedical determinants of behavior change, behavioral gerontologists are aware that, in comparison to younger adults, older adults more frequently experience physical illness, dementia, stroke, or medication side effects, all of which may influence behavior. Older adults should have both behavioral and medical evaluations to determine the separate or combined influences of these problems. In most cases, behavioral interventions can be used concurrently with medical interventions.

ADVANTAGES OF
THE BEHAVIORAL APPROACH

Use of the behavioral approach avoids many of the stereotypes, biases, and unfounded assumptions known as "ageism" that negatively impact the delivery of mental health services to older adults. Ageism reflects a personal revulsion to, and distaste for, growing old, and a fear of powerlessness, "uselessness," and death. Older adults themselves, as well as family members and others in their community, demonstrate stereotypic beliefs which can act as barriers to asking for mental health care (Bernstein, 1990; Butler, 1980; L. W. Dupree, O'Sullivan, & Patterson, 1982). Mental health professionals may also exhibit ageism by equating aging with inevitable decline, being pessimistic about the likelihood and speed of change, believing that it is futile to invest effort in a person with limited life expectancy, or assuming that behavioral change is a one-to-one correlate of physical change (M. M. Baltes & Barton, 1977; Gatz & Pearson, 1988; Patterson & Dupree, 1994).

Because the behavior therapist usually explores the possibilities of factors other than age and physiological changes as underlying behavior, the notion of reversibility of functional age decrements and apparent cognitive impairment remains viable until proven otherwise (M. M. Baltes & Baltes, 1977; Baltes & Barton, 1977; P. B. Baltes & Willis, 1977; Hoyer, Mishara, & Reidel, 1975; Patterson & Jackson, 1980a, 1980b; Rebok & Hoyer, 1977). Almost 20 years ago, Cautela and Mansfield (1977) reported that, "even when organic dysfunction is noted it can be of practical value to assume that many behaviors can be modified somewhat by applying specific behavior therapy procedures regardless of past history or organic involvement" (p. 23). The cultural notion of behavioral inflexibility often attributed to the elderly becomes an empirical question rather than a "fact." Such an empirical approach has resulted in doubts as to the general validity of a biological decrement model (M. M. Baltes & Baltes, 1977; M. M. Baltes & Barton, 1977; P. B. Baltes & Willis, 1977). Thus, in directing the treatment specialist to consider factors other than age, the behavioral model has long permitted, and has even prompted, an optimistic attitude regarding the mental health problems of older people. Problems are defined in terms of occurring behavior, and are treated on the assumption that they can be remedied.

Cautela and Mansfield (1977) noted additional benefits of the behavioral model for the problem behavior of the elderly: (1) time is not unnecessarily spent on determining the "true" impact of all past life experience, (2) present behavior is the target for change (rather than seeking some unconscious motivator of behavior), (3) older individuals profit more from active therapists and treatment involving problem-oriented behavior rehearsal (as opposed to the more passive insight therapy), and (4) negative diagnostic labels are applied less frequently. Such labels, particularly when applied to older adults, are rarely removed, and often lead to less than enthusiastic efforts to change the unwanted behavior of the older adult.

The behavioral model is also useful in the treatment of older individuals in terms of its cost effectiveness, its replicability or consistency of treatment or both, the value of negative results as well as positive, the structure it affords staff in attending to individuals in treatment, and its potential for contributing to suitable community placement based on individual circumstances. For example, Dupree and his colleagues (L. Dupree, 1994; L. Dupree, Broskowski, & Schonfeld, 1984; Patterson *et al.,* 1982) described group "modular" approaches with monitoring that helps to ensure that today's validated program is tomorrow's. Treatment modules have defined objectives, defined and operationalized teaching techniques and materials, specific assessment techniques, and a module manual to support a high level of standardization. These characteristics permit consistency over time even with staff turnover or various levels of staff training and disciplines. Module standardization also permits replication of the modules in state psychiatric facilities and community mental health centers.

Modular activities are conducted in groups for reasons of economy and efficiency. Staff are trained to criterion (i.e., ability to lead in accord with manual standards). The daily availability of module manuals to staff greatly aids in sustaining the program-sanctioned philosophy, content, and methodology. Again, consistency and continuity (regardless of the therapist present) can be maintained for an organization in both good and bad times. Elderly clients perceive that same continuity as well. Thus, the value of structured behavior therapy to any treatment program is a sense of quality control including treatment stability over time and replicability both within and outside the program. Also, a group module can be used with other standardized units to form an integrated program (L. Dupree, 1994).

When budgets for mental health services are cut, often the first services that are reduced or eliminated are those specifically for older rather than younger adults (Kimmel, 1988). The potential value of modularized approaches for older people increases as these resources become limited.

An often overlooked value of operant-based intervention is that it requires observation on the part of those who are involved in the treatment plan. The frequent attention of staff and others is intentionally directed toward individuals' behavior. By using basic learning principles and structured interventions, such as a token economy system, treatment specialists can be "forced" to attend to targeted behaviors and then function as both providers of tokens and social reinforcers. Richards and Thorpe (1978) also report studies in which behavioral techniques were successfully applied to the behavior and attitudes of treatment staff caring for older adults in institutional settings.

The behavioral perspective assumes that human behavior is alterable, or that the problem behavior is reversible, until empirically demonstrated otherwise. Such an approach attends to concrete events (deficits and excesses, strengths and weaknesses, antecedents and consequences) as explanations for behavior rather than invoking constructs or labels. It does not overly rely on physical entities as the basis for behavior. The smallest units of analysis in relevant diagnostic interviewing of an elderly individual are the mutual and interdependent relations between the individual and his or her environment (Rebok & Hoyer, 1977). Mahoney (1975) asserts that it is more productive to examine the nature of the interdependence than to maintain that one's internal environment has greater effect on behavior than does the external environment. Even though physical changes may account for some part of any loss of environmental competence, using a strictly physical model of aging and the diagnostic process based on such an approach is not appropriate. Indeed, the physical model is biased against intervention with older adults by assuming an irreversibility of behavior (purportedly based on aging-related, irreversible physical changes).Finally, the precision or clarity of most information produced in treatment programs emphasizing the behavioral model is also valuable relative to client placement. For example, if an individual does not know what medications to take, when to take them, and, even with continued training and assessment, never significantly improves over baseline, then the community placement setting should provide enough structure and assistance to ensure that that individual is prompted to take it properly.

CATEGORIES OF BEHAVIORAL APPROACHES

There are three broad categories of behavioral approaches. The first, behavior modification or therapy, focuses on observations of overt behaviors and the application of learning and conditioning principles to modify the behavior in question (Powers & Osborne, 1976; Spiegler & Guevremont, 1993). Overt behaviors are those easily observed by the client, family member, therapist, or staff. The second category, self-management techniques, involves teaching the client to use behavior modification strategies to modify his or her own behavior (either overt or covert). The third category, cognitive-behavioral therapies, involves modification of covert behaviors or private events that only the client can observe.

BASIC BEHAVIOR MODIFICATION

Individuals who are retired, widowed, and living alone may experience significant mental health problems that are not noticed by service providers or family members. In comparison to their proportion of the general population, older adults underutilize mental health services, such as community mental health centers or psychotherapists in independent practice (Knight, 1986; Lebowitz, 1988). Lasoski (1986) suggested that this underutilization may be the result of misassumptions about irreversibility, ageism, transportation problems, lack of referral, lack of outreach, organizational barriers, or even the attitudes of the elderly about mental health services (i.e., stigma of mental illness, fears about the consequences). Assuming that someone brings the problem behavior to the attention of a mental health professional, the next task is for that professional to (1) determine whether it is a high-frequency problem behavior, and (2) define the behavior. Behavior is considered maladaptive when it is urgent, of a high frequency, and affects some quality of life of the individual, the person's family, or significant others. In extreme cases, that behavior may place the person at risk of being transferred to another living environment or becoming institutionalized.

The Assessment Process

Once the problem behavior is brought to the attention of the therapist, he or she must begin the process of assessment (i.e., to understand what events precede and follow the behavior). The older adult's adaptive behavior should be assessed relative to actual daily living tasks (DeNelsky & Boat, 1986; Goodstein, 1980; Kaszniak, 1990; Lawton, Whelihan, & Belsky, 1980). The delineation of specific behavioral and environmental deficits should demonstrate the type and degree of support needed for maintaining residence in the surroundings in which the person is assessed (Lawton, 1986; Patterson & Dupree, 1994).

What we are most often interested in understanding and measuring with regard to older clients are environmental interactions that "support' (i.e., prompt, reinforce, or otherwise help to maintain) maximally independent, organized, and generally adaptive behaviors. Consistent with our previous discussion, the focus is on person–environment interactions. This approach is quite different from more common approaches that treat the elderly person as a mere passive recipient of supports.

A comprehensive behavioral interview can generate information about deficits and supports that more directly explains behavior and that needs less specialized or "expert" interpretation (Patterson & Dupree, 1994). In contrast, psychometric data require sophisticated interpretation and interpretive comments, resulting in evaluation reports based on secondary data or norms. These norms discount the uniqueness of the older person's behavior in his or her particular context. However, this discounting can be countered by using structured behavioral interviews that guide the clinician over specified life domains.

In summary, any reasonable assessment approach relative to an elderly individual must ameliorate cultural and professional ageism (Meeks, 1990), assess diverse areas of the older person's life, and highlight both internal and external antecedents for the expressed problem behaviors. For older adults, appropriate assessment is on a broader scale than for many younger populations, and positive change is based on a broad assessment of strengths and deficits. The essential diagnostic product is an indication of the older person's capacity to do things required in his or her own environment. This incorporates the notion of "age-free" assessment, a value to older adults.

Problem Definition

The product of the assessment process is the definition of the problem behavior. A good definition is objective in that the behavior can be verified by observations of the therapist and significant others over a specified period of time with data recorded in terms of frequency, duration, magnitude, antecedents, consequences of the behavior, and so on. The principle of parsimony should be used to guide the process leading to definition of the problem. This principle suggests that whenever a therapist has a choice between a simple explanation suggested by observable events or a more complex explanation perhaps based on unobservable events, the therapist should choose the simpler explanation, leading to fewer assumptions and more conservative interpretations.

Although it is tempting to rely on a DSM-IV diagnosis (American Psychiatric Association, 1994), or to define a problem in terms of theoretical constructs such as "depression," a behavior therapist must define the problem behavior in terms of the observed behaviors (e.g., "does not participate in group activities," "client observed crying when asked to talk about family issues," "the client makes frequent negative self-statements"). Problem definition is critical to the evaluation of more immediate and future (posttreatment) success. By defining behaviors in specific, parsimonious terms that require data and objective observation, rather than speculating about underlying motives, the client's success in treatment (i.e., change in targeted problem behavior) can be evaluated. When staff are in doubt about operationally defining a problem, we suggest that they consider the question: How will you know when there is improvement in the problem? To answer this question, the staff member must consider overt, observable behaviors, rather than theoretical constructs or diagnostic categories.

After operationally defining a problem, staff observe the client's unwanted behavior to determine what events precede it (antecedents) and what events follow that behavior (consequences). Consequences reveal the potential reinforcers that maintain the behavior. Thus, the observations allow the therapist to construct a behavior chain of antecedents-behavior-consequences or "A-B-C's." Finally, after the behavior is defined, the type of data to be recorded becomes evident. In most cases, it is the frequency of a behavior: however, in other cases, it may represent magnitude or intensity (e.g., how loud a person yells when disrupting a group), or duration (the length of the behavior episode) or both. Once the measure can be determined, staff can proceed with baseline observations.

Baseline

Following identification of the problem and prior to implementing treatment, the therapist conducts baseline observations. The therapist allows sufficient time and observations to establish a baseline level (pattern) of the behavior. This is especially important for older adults who are admitted to new residences or facilities. Should a treatment plan be implemented while the person becomes oriented to the new environment, any resulting change in behavior may be falsely attributed to the treatment. Thus, determining when a "stable" baseline is reached depends on many factors: frequency of the behavior, the conditions under which it occurs, and the projected length of treatment (or length of stay in a residential treatment program). Stability in the frequency of a behavior might be considered a fluctuation of no more than a certain percentage from the average behavior of, for example, five consecutive observations of the behavior during specified periods of time.

Development of Treatment Goals

The goal of treatment is the development of alternative behaviors that are socially acceptable and adaptive, rather than simply the application of conditioning principles to reduce maladaptive behaviors (Powers & Osborne, 1976). Treatment goals should be developed as early in the process as is feasible. Short-term goals, such as those met between case reviews or treatment team meetings, are modified as progress toward the target behavior is assessed. Long-term goals remain relatively consistent and often reflect the final behavioral goal after intervention ends.

Our observations of staff from geriatric units of state psychiatric hospitals and other treatment facilities suggest that staff believe they are "required" by policy to develop goals and treatment plans to eliminate or reduce maladaptive behaviors. Consequently, they frequently ignore goals focusing on the development of new, more adaptive behaviors. For example, a client in a residential facility may be observed returning to his or her bedroom rather than participating in activities. Staff may list the goal as "decrease the number of times per day the client is observed in bedroom." In another example, the client may be observed as "yelling obscenities when asked to attend group treatment" with the goal being to decrease the yelling and obscenities. When such goals are identified, they often lead to the use of punishment techniques, such as seclusion or removal of privileges, to suppress maladaptive behaviors.

In working with such staff, we pose two key questions they should answer before developing treatment goals and plans: What positive, adaptive behavior is expected to replace the maladaptive behavior? and What skill must the client learn to improve functioning and be discharged successfully? Rather than fighting their perceptions of what the program policies should be (i.e., listing only suppression of behavior as a goal in the written treatment plan), we found that it was helpful to ask staff to develop a second goal in the client's treatment plan, identifying the new, "replacement" behavior. Thus, in the examples provided above, we might list the adaptive goal as "increase group participation" or "develop conversational skills."

Finally, the question of how the client participates in the development of the treatment goals and plan is extremely relevant given current concerns for consumer rights, licensure requirements, and accreditation policies. Traditionally, with basic behavior modification approaches, the treatment staff decided the methods of observation, treatment, or reinforcement, and so on, with little or no input by the client. Informing a client about the plan may have been perceived as awkward or even in conflict with unobtrusive observation. Today, most guidelines emphasize a more active client role by requiring a written plan and staff documentation of how the person was informed and involved in the process. This can be accomplished in day treatment and residential programs by inviting the person, guardian, and significant others into the treatment team meeting. However, if the person feels uncomfortable or "confronted" by the professionals, the therapist and the client can meet and identify problem behaviors that they believe should be high priority. The therapist, after meeting with the treatment team, can then respond to the client regarding the specifics of the plan.

Active participation by the client in the treatment planning process may make unobtrusive observation difficult. However, informing the person of the future consequences of behaviors may accelerate the modification of his or her behavior. Further, for older adults in outpatient treatment, it is essential that the therapist and client work closely together in developing goals and implementing and evaluating treatment. Providing clients with feedback as to their progress (verbal reports, graphs of their behavior) is a valuable form of positive reinforcement. The written treatment plan, which indicates who is responsible for what, will serve a similar function as a behavioral contract.

Implementing the Behavior Modification Program

Behavioral techniques have proven effective for many older clients who are deficient in activities of daily living or social skills. Patterson and colleagues (1982) describe a variety of techniques used to teach older adults adaptive behaviors, by delivery of reinforcement contingent upon the observation of the target behavior or, in the case of a shaping procedure, a reasonable approximation of the target behavior. For example, using a token economy, very simple skills, such as time conversing with other people, can be increased by providing tokens and praise after certain intervals of time in which staff observe such behavior. More complex skills (e.g., maintaining a household) may require didactic methods, modeling, prompting, and so on, to teach sequences of behavior, after which reinforcement follows.

According to the Law of Effect, response-contingent positive reinforcement increases the probability of certain behaviors (goals), whereas response contingent punishment (e.g., removal of reinforcers, time-out) decreases the probability. Our experience in training staff from geriatric treatment units in state psychiatric hospitals suggests that staff more easily identified and used aversive procedures than positive reinforcement. In conjunction with an overemphasis on suppression of behavior, this led to increased use of seclusion, restraints, or geri-chairs; overreliance on medications to control behavior; or removal of unit privileges. Referring to the earlier example, staff believed they resolved the problem of the clients' returning to their rooms during daytime hours by locking the bedrooms during those hours. As a result, instead of becoming active or involved in unit activities, some patients lay on the floor in the halls or in day area rooms, while others sat passively in chairs around the perimeter of the activity room. To address this issue, we suggested that staff use the Premack principle (Premack, 1962) to increase adaptive behaviors. This principle states that a behavior that has a high probability of occurrence (e.g., going to the bedroom) can be used as a reinforcer for a low-probability behavior. By asking the key questions noted earlier, staff easily determined that it would be desirable for the client to participate in group treatment. Using the Premack principle, the client could be informed that if he or she met a minimal criterion of group participation (e.g., 10 minutes), he or she would be free to choose to return to the bedroom later. On future trials, the amount of time required for earning reinforcement is increased and time spent in the room decreased.

One of the problems encountered by staff in geriatric units is difficulty in identification of reinforcers. For example, staff may inadvertently reinforce and maintain maladaptive behavior such as yelling or screaming by paying attention to that behavior, but paying little or no attention to the individual when he or she is calm and sociable. Staff may also assume that what is reinforcing for them is also reinforcing for everyone else. However, for some people, the administration of candy, tokens (in a token economy), or additional unit privileges may not be motivating. Determination of appropriate positive reinforcement requires interaction with and observation of each individual. Many older adults in mental health facilities have responded well to the use of praise or by being rewarded with conversation with a staff member in whom they have shown interest.

Even when appropriate reinforcers are identified, people can become satiated with reinforcement. It is helpful for staff to identify a menu of reinforcers prior to the development of a treatment plan in order to shift to another when satiation occurs. We encourage the staff to spend extra time observing how their older clients spend much of their time while on the unit, to ask them or their families about the activities they enjoy, and to experiment with the use of praise and social contact as potential reinforcers.

Evaluation of the Treatment Plan

Evaluation of the treatment plan is an ongoing process. During the assessment phase, the type of data to be recorded is determined (e.g., frequency, duration, magnitude). As treatment progresses and criteria are met, the plan can be altered to make the short-term goals more similar to the long-term goal. Relative to the earlier example, there would be an increase in group participation or other adaptive skills, with a simultaneous decrease of the maladaptive behaviors.

In the simplest form of evaluation, using single case analyses, a therapist will measure the rate or level of the target behavior during baseline ("A") and compare it to that during the treatment ("B"). Also, effectiveness of treatment can be evaluated by removing the treatment conditions (i.e., a return to the baseline condition). If the behavior returns to its former, pretreatment level, then the therapist can state that the treatment was the most likely cause of the change. However, because therapists wish to discharge the patient successfully, a typical design will be an ABAB design in which the final phase of treatment is a second implementation of treatment, or more practically, a variation of the treatment that prepares the client for discharge and appropriate behavior in his or her environment (e.g., fading the treatment over time, gradually reducing the number of reinforcers, adding new reinforcers likely to be found in the community).

Assessment of skill deficiencies that create barriers to successful community placement and independence is critical for evaluation at admission, to assess progress, and to determine discharge readiness. Staff must respond to the questions, How can we demonstrate that the individual is improving relative to the identified problem behavior as the result of this intervention? and, Is this person behaviorally capable of managing the circumstances of his or her extratreatment environment? or, Has he or she acquired necessary skills and behaviors? We encourage staff to graph data when feasible to determine changes or stability in the measured target behavior, and to demonstrate to staff and to the client that changes in behavior have or have not taken place. People often tend to believe that if they have not accomplished the final target behavior in its entirety, they have failed. To counteract this notion, it is suggested that even small improvements in behavior should be highlighted in discussions with the client to encourage further progress.

BEHAVIORAL INTERVENTIONS DEVELOPED IN FLORIDA

Thus far, we have posed several questions to help staff define target behaviors and implement the plan: (1) How do we know a problem exists? (2) How will you know when there is improvement in the problem? (3) What positive, adaptive behavior is expected to replace the maladaptive behavior? (4) What skill should the client learn to improve functioning and be discharged successfully? (5) How can we demonstrate that the individual is improving as the result of this treatment? and (6) Is this person ready to be discharged from treatment? In other words: have problem-specific skills been acquired; have unwanted behaviors been brought under control; do the more adaptive skills respond to individual person–environment interactions (do the skills fit the environment); and will intervention results generalize to the individual's likely place of residence? To address these questions, we summarize our early attempts at deinstitutionalization of older adults.

Our department's early efforts were aimed at geriatric units from state hospitals and at local psychiatric facilities (Patterson et al., 1982). Thus, the first elderly clients admitted to the gerontology program at the Florida Mental Health Institute were transferred from a state hospital. To determine what problem behaviors existed, each newly admitted client was assessed to identify his or her deficits in a variety of skills which might prevent their successful placement in community-based settings: basic and instrumental activities of daily living, communication skills, conversation, personal information training, personal effectiveness training, self-esteem, ability to manage one's medications, and leisure skills. Those clients not meeting the basic cutoff scores for any particular skill (e.g., personal grooming), entered a group training module. A module was group treatment involving a set of behavioral skills to be taught. Standardized manuals for staff to follow were also developed. These manuals included a statement of objectives, brief explanation of the behavioral principles and procedures to be used, the forms and instructions for assessing the client, descriptions of specific content (including materials and teaching aids), client objectives, and forms to graph and record data.

Teaching methods consisted of lectures and the behavioral techniques of modeling, prompting, chaining, and shaping. Clients were reassessed every four weeks to determine whether they had improved their skills adequately to "graduate" from the group and eventually to determine whether they were ready to be discharged to a community-based setting, such as independent living or an assisted-living facility. Typically, the largest change occurred within the first four weeks of treatment. However, average length of stay was approximately three months. Patterson and colleagues (1982) demonstrated that one year after discharge, the majority of individuals discharged from the Gerontology Residential Program remained in community settings, whereas the majority of a comparison group of state hospital patients remained institutionalized.

When unusual behavior, such as hallucinations, verbal outbursts, or other disruptive behaviors occurred but were not addressed in the modules, staff members were instructed to observe the behavior using a behavior analysis form (BAF) to determine what antecedents preceded the behavior and what consequences might have maintained it. An interdisciplinary treatment team reviewed the process and collected data in order to define the problem behavior and develop an individualized behavioral intervention to modify maladaptive behavior and replace it with adaptive behavior. Although a primary counselor was designated to monitor the accurate implementation of the treatment plan, all staff were informed of each older adult's treatment plan in order to implement it in a unified manner, ensuring uniform delivery of reinforcement, shaping, and so on, regardless of the staff person present, where on the unit the older adult might be, or the activity in which the client might be engaged.

PROBLEMS ENCOUNTERED IN GERIATRIC TREATMENT PROGRAMS

Based on our experience in the aging programs at the Florida Mental Health Institute and our attempts to disseminate these approaches to other programs and sites treating older adults, we have noted a number of areas that present problems for successful implementation of basic behavioral approaches. These areas include consistency of implementation of a treatment plan, generalization of new skills, working with individuals with memory problems, and working with individuals who reside in the community while attending the treatment program.

Consistency

In the early stages of disseminating our treatment approaches and modules to geriatric units at state hospitals, it appeared that the staff experienced a certain degree of frustration about the efficacy of behavioral approaches. With investigation, we often found that staff were not implementing the treatment plan in a consistent manner; we asked them, "Does the unit act like a unit?" If just one staff member or another person (e.g., family members, other clients) responds to the client in a manner inconsistent with the treatment plan, or is inappropriately reinforcing, that momentary lapse may inadvertently reinforce the unwanted behavior (i.e., a partial reinforcement effect in which occasional or intermittent reinforcement leads to behaviors that are substantially more difficult to extinguish than responses associated with consistent or continuous reinforcement procedure). Inconsistency may be influenced by poor staff training, inadequate treatment plans, or attitudes and stereotypes held by the staff. Although some staff members will try hard to implement a plan as written, others may resist because of beliefs that older adults' behaviors cannot be changed, that the client has no potential reinforcers, or that the behavior has a biological or physical cause.

In training geriatric staff to use behavioral techniques, we stress the need for all staff to act in unison and reinforce (and extinguish) behaviors identically. When this is done, behavior change is likely to occur more rapidly. This is accomplished by training staff in behavioral techniques including objective observation and recording of data, encouraging communication among staff in treatment team meetings, and developing standardized assessment and treatment programs. Similarly, family members and significant others should be informed of (1) the benefits and consequences of adhering to the plan, and (2) how to respond to maladaptive behavior.

Generalization of New Skills Outside the Therapeutic Environment

Patterson and Jackson (1980a, 1980b), point out that there is a significant difference between a *training environment* and a *therapeutic environment*. The former generates appropriate behavior that is maintained and generalized within that specific programmatic environment; the therapeutic environment does the same, but also results in generalization and maintenance of appropriate behavior in postdischarge settings. A major concern in the application of behavior modification is the generalization of the newly learned, adaptive behavior outside the therapeutic environment. A person discharged from a residential treatment program to a community placement (e.g., independent living or assisted living facility) may not demonstrate the skills learned prior to discharge unless certain predischarge intervention conditions are met.

Even with an A-B-A-B reversal design (Baseline-Treatment-Return to Baseline-Treatment), there is a possibility that the behavior will revert to pretreatment levels after the person is discharged. By planning a modified version of the second "B" (reimplementation of treatment) condition, reversion can be avoided by making that second condition more similar to the extratreatment environment. For example, prior to discharge, we might switch from using tokens (in a token economy) as rewards, to the reward of more off-unit activities or weekend visits to the new residence with participation in activities at that new site.

Treatment of Older Adults With Dementia

There are a variety of memory problems experienced by older adults. The individual may experience benign forgetfulness in which he or she may attribute memory problems to an age-related affliction. Individuals experiencing depression may also exhibit problems or pseudodementia. Behavioral techniques work well for such difficulties. However, the most challenging problems arise in addressing problems of people with dementia. Alzheimer's disease and related dementias often involve a slow, degenerative process of memory, language skills, and executive functions.

A number of basic behavioral procedures have been demonstrated to assist older people in the early and middle stages of dementia despite declining functioning. For example, Burgio and Burgio (1986) describe methods for helping older adults control urinary incontinence, including pelvic floor exercises, scheduled and prompted toileting, and delivery of positive reinforcement for controlled voids. McEvoy (1990) summarizes techniques for enhancing orientation, improving socialization and mood, decreasing verbal aggression, or improving activities of daily living. To reduce wandering and potential risk to one's welfare, Hussian (1982) altered the color of hallways and elevators to help residents in one facility discriminate between hazardous areas and those areas where ambulation would be safe. In another example, McEvoy and Patterson (1986) describe the use of backward chaining to teach spatial orientation (i.e., dividing the task into a series of steps, then teaching the steps in reverse order). The staff member begins by teaching the sequence nearest to the final, desired, behavior. When accomplished, the task is reinforced (e.g., by praise or delivery of tokens), and the next to last sequence is prompted by the staff member. This proceeds until the client learns the route to the desired location.

Those people in the most severe stages of dementia are less likely to retain information or maintain skills between sessions. In such cases, the long-term goals will be less ambitious, focusing less on independence and more on custodial care.

Community-Based Clients

Early applications of behavior modification with older adults were conducted in residential facilities or with individuals spending considerable amounts of time in day treatment or day care programs. Treatment planning for community-residing older adults who attend treatment programs periodically for short visits (e.g., a two-hour appointment once a week) presents greater challenges as a substantial portion of their time is spent "off-unit" and away from the controlled environment of a residential unit. Again, consistency and generalization are issues for such individuals. The primary therapist or case manager must ensure that the family, significant others, or staff from the assisted living facilities are brought into the treatment planning process, and that they are provided some instruction as to how to implement behavioral methodology consistent with that used in the treatment program.

For community-based populations, self-management and cognitive-behavioral interventions are appropriate extensions of behavior modification. In fact, more recently, self-management and cognitive-behavioral interventions are complementary alternatives to more traditional behavior therapies even within residential settings.

SELF-MANAGEMENT APPROACHES

Later-life onset problems are often maladaptive responses to stress generated by the relatively rapid changes characteristic of later life. The individual's perception that he or she can no longer predict or exert reasonable control over the environment magnifies the stress effects of rapid change. The more an individual expects to be in control and to cope independently with problems, the greater the probability he or she will find a solution. Problem-solving training may be viewed as one form of training to improve the elderly individual's control over his or her own behavior and over the environment. The relationship between strategies for general problem solving and techniques for self-control of specific responses has been noted by Goldfried and Davison (1976) as follows: "The major objective in problem solving is to identify the most effective alternative, which may then be followed by other self-control operations to stimulate and maintain performance of the selected course of action. Thus, problem solving becomes a crucial initial phase in a more general self-control process" (p. 187). Goldfried and Davison suggest that additional training or therapy is often required to stimulate and maintain the behaviors necessary to follow through on a selected course of action. Our experience confirms these observations. While clients may generate an effective solution, they often have trouble trying it out. Engaging in new (or renewed) adaptive coping behaviors almost always involves increased anxiety which must be overcome if the individual is to carry out in practice a plan he or she has endorsed cognitively.

As noted by Kanfer (1975), self-management involves the use of behavioral techniques by the client to modify his or her own overt or covert behaviors. An advantage of using self-management techniques is that they allow a client to continue behavior modification outside the therapeutic environment and without constant direction by the therapist. Instead of the relatively passive participant in basic behavior modification procedures, the client becomes cotherapist by taking an active role in the identification of problems, development and implementation of the treatment plan, and evaluation of progress.

Kanfer (1975) describes three major self-control components of self-management: self-monitoring, homework and assignments, and behavior contracts. Self-monitoring includes (1) awareness that a problem behavior is occurring and (2) collecting data (e.g., frequency, magnitude, or intensity) about the behavior and its consequences. For example, we have trained older alcohol abusers to maintain a log of their urges to drink or drinking episodes (L. Dupree *et al.,* 1984). A review of their logs allows the therapist to help the client avoid a relapse following a single slip (one drink of alcohol) or to review relapse episodes to help prevent future occurrences. Another example involved an older client in our residential program. Despite taking antipsychotic medications, she reported hearing voices that were disturbing to her. Staff instructed her to log the intensity, frequency, and content of the voices she heard, as well as the antecedents to hearing the voices (e.g., where she was, what activity she was involved in, who was present). Once self-monitoring is accomplished, the client becomes aware of the circumstances under which the problem behavior occurs, and is then ready to help in the development of behavior change techniques (including self-reinforcement).

Homework or assignments by the therapist allow clients to approach their final goals. For example, older adults in day treatment mental health programs experiencing loneliness and social isolation might be assigned to visit a senior center to learn what activities the program offers and to report back to the therapist what was available. Another client who abuses alcohol might be asked to call an alcoholism hotline to determine what would happen in the event he or she experienced a slip. Such assignments can be used to diminish the stress of placement or activities that might occur posttreatment.

A behavior contract is an agreement between the client and the therapist or the client and a significant other (e.g., a spouse). The contract sets the guidelines for the expected behavior and the consequences if the behavior occurs (e.g., reinforcement) or does not occur. Thus, the therapist and client develop and agree on behavioral guidelines for the self-management treatment plan. The therapeutic aim is to provide the older individual with more effective coping skills specific to the antecedent conditions noted in his or her problem behavior chain. Also, because some behaviors (e.g., abusive drinking) have multiple antecedents and may change over time, the training of elderly clients in the analysis of problem behavior, problem solving, and self-management skills makes them better prepared for future or evolving high-risk situations. They are prepared to analyze, understand, problem solve, and respond to the factors promoting unwanted behavior. Thus, intervention placing greater emphasis on client analysis and self-intervention in order to sustain positive outcome as the older person's environment continues to change enhances community stability.

COGNITIVE-BEHAVIORAL THERAPIES

Cognitive-behavior therapies (CBT) were first developed in the 1960s and rely on the principles used in basic behavior modification and self-management to modify thoughts and feelings. Whereas behavior modification is based on the belief that overt reinforcement contingencies alter behavior, cognitive behavior therapy focuses on cognitive mechanisms to alter behavior. According to Dobson and Block (1988), "at their core, cognitive-behavior therapies share three fundamental propositions: 1) cognitive activity affects behavior, 2) cognitive activity may be monitored and altered, and 3) desired behavior change may be affected through cognitive change" (p. 4). Also, Beck (1991) notes that the psychological systems of cognition, affect, and motivation are interrelated so that changes in one system may produce changes in one or more other systems. CBT therefore teaches one to identify and modify self-defeating thoughts and beliefs (Dobson, 1988; Scott, Williams, & Beck, 1989).

Mahoney and Arnkoff (1978) categorized CBTs into three major divisions: cognitive restructuring, coping-skills therapies, and problem-solving therapies. Cognitive restructuring (CR) involves teaching the client to recognize maladaptive thoughts that are believed to be the antecedents to emotional problems. The goal of cognitive restructuring "is to establish more adaptive thought patterns" (Dobson & Block, 1988, p. 13). For example, the older client may learn to recognize his or her inaccurate thoughts or self-statements that lead to depression, and replace them with more adaptive and accurate statements.

Older clients in coping-skills therapies may learn to use new, more adaptive skills when faced with stressful events or stimulation, as evident in stress-inoculation training (Meichenbaum, 1977) and Marlatt and Gordon's (1980, 1985) Relapse Prevention (RP) model of addictive behavior. According to the RP model, when faced with high-risk situations for drinking (e.g., negative emotional states, peer pressure, conflicts with other people), individuals with inadequate coping skills experience decreased self-efficacy and increased positive expectancies about their first drink. When drinking does occur, the slip leads to an abstinence violation effect and the self-fulfilling prophecy that they might as well drink more since they did not maintain abstinence. Programs using an RP model concentrate on teaching individuals the skills necessary to cope with their high-risk situation or situations and prevent a relapse. Skills are taught using didactic approaches, cognitive-behavior therapy, modeling, behavior rehearsal, and assignments. Such approaches have been successful with regard to long-term outcome (Broskowski & Dupree, 1981; L. Dupree & West, 1990; Holder, Longabaugh, Miller, & Rubonis, 1991; Marlatt & Gordon, 1980, 1985).

In the Department of Aging and Mental Health, we have used both self-management and cognitive-behavioral techniques to help older alcohol abusers overcome their problems. Clients are taught to analyze their drinking behavior and high-risk situations into the A-B-C's described earlier. Through lecture format, behavior rehearsal, and assignments away from the program, they are taught new coping skills (e.g., refusing a drink, managing feelings of anxiety, tension, frustration, anger, grief, or depression; rebuilding a social support network; and coping with a slip or relapse). These approaches have resulted in successful outcomes one year posttreatment (L. Dupree et al., 1984; Schonfeld & Dupree, 1991). Although cognitive-behavior therapy grew out of behaviorism in its acceptance of operant and respondent components, it deviates from earlier behavior therapy in its refusal to accept the tenet that environmental factors alone determine behavior. Also, the multimodal aspect of cognitive-behavior therapy allows a variety of methods for working with clients including systematic desensitization, covert modeling, mental and emotive imagery, relaxation training, thought stopping, cognitive restructuring, biofeedback, neurolinguistic programming, and cognitive modeling. Cognitive modeling combines overt and covert strategies as the client and clinician work together to change the beliefs and attitudes of the client about a situation. The therapist acts as a role model, and the client acts out the same role while the therapist coaches and monitors.

CONCLUSION

In this chapter, we have discussed a variety of behavioral interventions used with older adults. Behavioral approaches range from very basic behavior modification to self-management approaches and to cognitive-behavioral interventions. Problems in the use of basic behavior modification procedures arise when procedures are administered inconsistently, when new behaviors do not generalize to the community, when working with individuals with memory problems, and when working with outpatient populations.

Self-management is an extension of behavior modification procedures, with the individual learning to modify his or her own behaviors and the therapist acting as a motivator and guide through the process. Cognitive-behavioral approaches involve the modification of cognitions, normally considered events unobservable by anyone but the client. All of the approaches (1) are based on principles of learning, (2) use some form of behavior analysis to identify antecedents and consequences of behavior, (3) target an increase in adaptive behaviors and a simultaneous decrease in maladaptive behaviors, and (4) often result in an improved (context-appropriate) quality of life. Behavioral applications with older adults have been effective over a broad range of presenting problems in diverse settings and appear to minimize many of the misperceptions and inaccurate assumptions resulting from ageism, as well as the overreliance on the medical model to explain behavior problems. Also, by not emphasizing intrapsychic "mysteries," and by placing less emphasis on highly degreed therapists as the sole proprietors of knowledge relative to etiology and change of behavior, the behavioral model permits greater participation in change by the client. Behavior is not explained in terms of personality theory, norms, or secondary source data. In behavioral principles, older adult behavior is understood to be a product of environmental and organismic interactions. Behavior therapies have recognized and responded to the functional context of the behavior of older adults.

Proponents of the behavioral perspective recognize the influence of physiological change, but do not overemphasize it. They assume that maladaptive behavior can be remediated or ameliorated until it can be proven otherwise. This empirical approach has been demonstrated to be successful with older populations for whom few practitioners initially held out much hope for change. Only a few years ago, major leaders of nonbehavioral therapies were speaking of the futility of treating adults over age 50 to 55. Behavior therapists have modified many assumptions and can be proud of their role in developing appropriate therapies for problems common in later life.

REFERENCES

American Psychiatric Association (1994). *Diagnostic and statistical manual of mental disorders* (4th ed.). Washington, DC: Author.

Baltes, M. M., & Baltes, P. B. (1977). The ecopsychological relativity and plasticity of psychological aging: Convergent perspectives of cohort effects and operant psychology. *Zeitschrift für Experimentelle und Angewandte Psychologie, 24,* 179–194.

Baltes, M. M., & Barton, E. M. (1977). New approaches toward aging: A case for the operant model. *Educational Gerontology, 2,* 383–405.

Baltes, P. B., & Willis, S. L. (1982). Plasticity and enhancement of intellectual functioning in old age: Penn State's Adult Development and Enrichment Project (ADEPT). In F. I. M. Craik & S. Trehub (Eds.). *Aging and cognitive processes* (pp. 353–390). New York: Plenum.

Beck, A. T. (1991). Cognitive therapy as the integrative therapy. *Journal of Psychotherapy Integration, 1,* 191–198.

Bernstein, L. O. (1990). A special service: Counseling the individual elderly client. *Generations, 14,* 35–38.

Broskowski, H., & Dupree, L. (1981). *General problem solving: An assessment and skills training manual.* Tampa: University of South Florida.

Burgio, K. L., & Burgio, L. D. (1986). Behavior therapies for urinary incontinence in the elderly. *Clinical Geriatric Medicine, 2,* 809–827.

Butler, R. N. (1980). Ageism: A foreword. *Journal of Social Issues, 36,* 8–11.

Cautela, J. R., & Mansfield, L. (1977). A behavioral approach to geriatrics. In W. D. Gentry (Ed.), *Geropsychology: A model of training and clinical service* (pp. 21–42). Cambridge, Mass.: Ballinger.

DeNelsky, G., & Boat, B. (1986). A coping skills model of psychological diagnosis and treatment. *Professional Psychology: Research and Practice, 17,* 322–330.

Dobson, K. S. (Ed.) (1988). *Handbook of cognitive-behavioral therapies.* New York: Guilford.

Dobson, K. S., & Block, L. (1988). Historical and philosophical bases of the cognitive-behavioral therapies. In K. S. Dobson (Ed.), *Handbook of cognitive-behavioral therapies* (pp. 3–38). New York: Guilford.

Dupree, L. (1994). Geropsychological modular treatment: Back to the future. *Journal of Gerontological Social Work, 22,* 211–220.

Dupree, L., & West, H. (1990). *Alcohol self-management in high risk situations: A group training manual for older adults.* FMHI Publication Series, 122. Tampa: University of South Florida.

Dupree, L., Broskowski, H., & Schonfeld, L. (1984). The Gerontology Alcohol Project: A behavioral treatment program for elderly alcohol abusers. *Gerontologist, 24,* 510–516.

Dupree, L. W., O'Sullivan, M. J., & Patterson, R. L. (1982). Problems relating to aging: Rationale for a behavioral approach. In R. L. Patterson, L. W. Dupree, D. A. Eberly, G. M. Jackson, M. J. O'Sullivan, L. A. Penner, & C. D. Kelly (Eds.), *Overcoming deficits of aging* (pp. 7–21). New York: Plenum.

Estes, C. L., & Binney, E. A. (1989). The biomedicalization of aging: Dangers and dilemmas. *Gerontologist, 29,* 587–596.

Gatz, M., & Pearson, C. (1988). Ageism revised and the provision of psychological services. *American Psychologist, 43,* 184–188.

Goldfried, M. R., & Davison, G. C. (1976). *Clinical behavior therapy.* New York: Holt, Rinehart & Winston.

Goodstein, R. K. (1980). The diagnosis and treatment of elderly patients: Some practical guidelines. *Hospital and Community Psychiatry, 31,* 19–24.

Holder, H., Longabaugh, R., Miller, W. R., & Rubonis, A. V. (1991). The cost effectiveness of treatment for alcoholism: A first approximation. *Journal of Studies on Alcohol, 52,* 517–540.

Hoyer, W. J., Mishara, B. L., & Reidel, R. G. (1975). Problem behaviors as operants: Applications with elderly individuals. *Gerontologist, 15,* 452–456.

Hussian, R. A. (1982). Stimulus control in the modification of problematic behavior in elderly institutionalized patients. *International Journal of Behavioral Geriatrics, 1,* 33–46.

Kanfer, F. (1975). Self-management methods. In F. H. Kanfer & A. P. Goldstein (Eds.), *Helping people change: A textbook of methods* (pp. 309–355). New York: Pergamon.

Kaszniak, A. W (1990). Psychological assessment of the aging individual. In J. E. Birren & K. W Schaie (Eds.), *Handbook of the psychology of aging* (pp. 427–445). San Diego, CA: Academic.

Kimmel, A. (1988). Ageism, psychology, and public policy. *American Psychologist, 45,* 175–178.

Knight, B. (1986). *Psychotherapy with older adults.* Newbury Park, CA: Sage.

Lasoski, M. C. (1986). Reasons for low utilization of mental health services by the elderly. *Clinical Gerontologist, 5,* 1–18.

Lawton, M. P. (1986). Functional assessment. In L. Teri & P. M. Lewinsohn (Eds.), *Geropsychological Assessment and Treatment* (pp. 39–84). New York: Springer.

Lawton, M. P, Whelihan, W. M., & Belsky, J. K. (1980). Personality tests and their uses with older adults. In J. Birren & R. B. Sloane (Eds.), *Handbook of mental health and aging* (pp. 537–553). Englewood Cliffs, NJ: Prentice-Hall.

Lebowitz, B. D. (1988). Correlates of success in community mental health programs for the elderly. *Hospital and Community Psychiatry, 39,* 721–722.

Mahoney, M. J. (1975). The sensitive scientists in empirical humanism. *American Psychologist, 30,* 864–867.

Mahoney, M. J., & Arnkoff, D. B. (1978). Cognitive and self-control therapies. In S. L. Garfield & A. E. Berg in (Eds.), *Handbook of psychotherapy and behavior change* (2nd ed., pp. 689–722). New York: Wiley.

Marlatt, G. A., & Gordon, J. R. (1980). Determinants of relapse: Implications for the maintenance of behavior change. In P. D. Davidson & S. M. Davidson (Eds.), *Behavioral medicine: Changing health lifestyles* (pp. 410–452). New York: Brunner/Mazel.

Marlatt, G. A., & Gordon, J. R. (1985). *Relapse prevention: Maintenance strategies in the treatment of addictive behavior.* New York: Guilford.

McEvoy, C. L. (1990). Behavioral treatment. In J. L. Cummings & B. L. Miller (Eds.), *Alzheimer's cisease: Treatment and long-term management* (pp. 207–224). New York: Dekker.

McEvoy, C. L., & Patterson, R. (1986). Behavioral treatment of deficit skills in dementia patients *Gerontologist, 26,* 475–478.

Meeks, S. (1990). Age bias in the diagnostic decision-making behavior of clinicians. *Professional Psychology: Research and Practice, 21,* 279–284.

Meichenbaum, D. (1977). *Cognitive behavior modification: An integrative approach.* New York: Plenum.

Miller, L. (1979). Toward a classification of aging behaviors. *Gerontologist, 19*(3), 282–289.

Patterson, R. L., & Dupree, L. (1994). Issues in the assessment of older adults. In M. Hersen & S. M. Turner (Eds.), *Diagnostic interviewing* (2nd ed., pp. 373–397). New York: Plenum.

Patterson, R. L., & Jackson, G. M. (1980a). Behavior modification with the elderly. In M. M. Hersen, R. M. Eisler, & P. Miller (Eds.), *Progress in behavior modification* (Vol. 9, pp. 205–239). New York: Academic.

Patterson, R. L., & Jackson, G. M. (1980b). Behavioral approaches to gerontology. In M. L. Michelson, M. Hersen, & S. M. Turner (Eds.), *Future perspectives in behavior therapy* (pp. 295–315). New York: Plenum.

Patterson, R. L., Dupree, L. W., Eberly, D. A., Jackson, G. M., O'Sullivan, M. J., Penner, L. A., & Dee-Kelly, C. (1982). *Overcoming deficits of aging: A behavioral approach*. New York: Plenum.

Powers, R. B., & Osborne, J. G. (1976). Fundamentals of behavior. New York: West.

Premack, D. (1962). Reversibility of the reinforcement relation. *Science, 136,* 235–237.

Rebok, G. W., & Hoyer, W. J. (1977). The functional context of elderly behavior. *Gerontologist, 17,* 27–34.

Richards, W., & Thorpe, G. (1978). Behavioral approaches to the problems of later life. In M. Storandt, I. Siegler, & M. Elias (Eds.). *The clinical psychology of aging* (pp. 253–267). New York: Plenum.

Schonfeld, L., & Dupree, L. (1991). Antecedents of drinking for early and late-life onset elderly alcohol abusers. *Journal of Studies on Alcohol, 52,* 587–592.

Scott, J., Williams, J. M. G., & Beck, A. (1989). *Cognitive therapy in clinical practice: An illustrative casebook*. London: Routledge.

Spiegler, M. D., & Guevremont, D. C. (1993). *Contemporary behavior therapy*. Pacific Grove, CA: Brooks/Cole.

Wisocki, P. A. (1991). *Handbook of clinical behavior therapy with the elderly client*. New York: Plenum.

CHAPTER 5

Moral and Ethical Considerations in Geropsychology

Michael Lavin and Bruce D. Sales

INTRODUCTION

Most psychologists will have acquired a working familiarity with the American Psychological Association's *Ethical Principles of Psvchologists and Code of Conduct* (1992) (hereinafter referred to as Ethics Code or Code) in the course of their professional education. They may know, for example, that the Code includes an introduction, an explanatory preamble, a set of six aspirational principles relating to competence, integrity, professional and scientific responsibility, respect for people's rights and dignity, concern for the welfare of others, and social responsibility, and that these principles are followed by eight sections of ethical standards by which members of the American Psychological Association are bound. These standards cover general issues, testing, advertising, therapy, privacy and confidentiality, teaching, research, and publication, forensics, and resolving ethical issues. Although the aspirational principles of the association are not binding, they can be used to help interpret the binding standards. If psychologists who are members of the American Psychological Association fail to abide by the standards, then an ethics complaint can be brought to the association, and the association's Ethics Committee's *Rules and Procedures* (1992) will govern the quasi-legal proceedings that follow a complaint.

If geropsychology raises any special ethical issues, it is not because geropsychologists operate with different ethical principles and standards than other psychologists. Rather, it is because of the sometimes unique challenges

Michael Lavin and Bruce D. Sales • Department of Psychology, University of Arizona, Tucson, Arizona 85721.

Handbook of Clinical Geropsychology, edited by Michel Hersen and Vincent B. Van Hasselt. Plenum Press, New York, 1998.

that their clients and patients present. This chapter explores issues that are likely to loom larger for geropsychologists than for other psychologists. No pretense is made that these are the only issues that are ethically or morally pressing for geropsychologists. Indeed, our goal is not to catalogue all issues, but to present selected problems and apply a decision framework, in order to demonstrate how geropsychologists can engage in ethical practice when confronted with such challenges. Stated another way, our focus is to explore selected issues in a way that will enhance geropsychologists' moral thinking, and thus provide a basis for analyzing other problems as they arise. In order to accomplish our goal, we first present an analysis of the benefits and limits of ethical codes for guiding professional behavior. Arguing that this approach is significantly limited, we then present relevant moral principles that geropsychologists can use to improve their decision making when confronted with difficult ethical and moral situations in practice, and apply this information to selected problems.

Our use of the words "ethical" and "moral" requires comment. Though in ordinary English these terms tend to be used interchangeably, we reserve the term "ethical" for duties, prohibitions, and permissions that are given or derived from the Ethics Code. The term "moral" is used to cover the deepest level of thought that agents engage in when thinking about what they should do. A consequence of this view is that it is conceivable that an act could be ethically forbidden (i.e., proscribed by the Code) but morally required. The analysis of the complex relations between the Ethics Code and morality is beyond the scope of this chapter.

ETHICS CODES

Benefits

There are benefits to using a profession's ethics code. First, codes set forth minimal standards of professional conduct in a public way. Second, codes may make collective wisdom available to other professionals. Third, codes give public evidence as to a profession's ethics, making professionals and nonprofessionals aware of the expectations. Fourth, codes often provide careful guidance in areas that have proven to be sources of moral difficulty for a profession.

As for the first benefit, codes provide the public with a document that informs all interested parties about a profession's minimal standards. Though psychologists, for example, have a moral obligation not to exploit clients, which exists independently of any explicit recognition in the American Psychological Association's Code, the Code articulates this obligation in a public manner. For example, because of the Code, psychologists may not plead that a sexual relationship with a client is ethical, perhaps on the ground that the sexual relation is therapeutic.

As for the second benefit, codes are often drafted by professionals who have made a career of thinking about issues that have proven morally difficult for a profession. The drafters of a code bring together a collective wisdom that is unavailable to an ordinary professional. For example, the committee developing or revising a code may have access to a history of troubling assessment cases and their resolution. The average psychologist will not have had the time to think through many of the issues connected with assessment that are explicitly addressed in the Ethics Code, and even more elaborately in the American Psychological Association's *Standards for Educational and Psychological Testing* (1985). The Code, and supplemental materials such as the Standards, thereby offers the psychologist the benefit of thoughtful, considered guidance of individuals respected for their ethical and legal knowledge.

Having a code also provides the third benefit of making ethical expectations public to professional and nonprofessionals alike. Even if, as part of their professional training, all psychologists came to have the same ethical principles and standards, the public, independent of the Code, would have no way of knowing the specifics of those principles and standards. By making their ethical principles and standards public, organizations like the American Psychological Association make it possible for family members to reach a reasoned conclusion about whether a geropsychologist's treatment of an elderly patient conforms to the association's Code or to determine in advance what kind of treatment they have a right to expect from a geropsychologist.

The final benefit of the Code is that it alerts professionals to areas that have proven to be ethical puzzles for a profession. Therapy, testing, privacy and confidentiality, forensics, research, and publication have, in the past, proven to be areas where ethical and moral lapses are prone to occur. By reading and understanding their Code, psychologists can become sensitive to areas where they are likely to encounter difficulty if they fail to proceed with suitable caution and conformity.

Limitations

Despite the above noted benefits, codes have numerous potential limitations. First, codes are conservative. Second, codes have a necessary limitation in their moral authority. Third, codes are often vague. Fourth, codes often omit mention of important topics and factors. Fifth, it is often difficult to determine what guidance codes provide in complex cases, especially in cases where the guidance is inconsistent (Sales and Schuman, 1993).

The conservative nature of codes is a consequence of their being political documents. When the American Psychological Association "wrote and revised its *Ethical Principles and Code of Conduct* (1992), it created a committee to produce the document. The committee, in turn, had to reach an internal consensus on what the code should say, while simultaneously trying to produce a document that could attain the support of the majority of American Psychological Association members.

Given the nature of the process, no attempt is made to derive specific principles and standards from widely accepted moral principles. At most, codes seek to avoid manifest conflict with these principles. Professionals might therefore wonder how much authority the Code should have. For example, a central feature of moral life is a respect for one's own conscience. lt does not seem reasonable that a code could overrule conscience, especially when the dictates of a psychologist's conscience conform to the widely accepted moral principles. For many psychologists, however, the decision-making process is far simpler. The moral authority of the American Psychological Association's Code is based in their membership in the Association, which mandates each member's compliance with the Code's standards. Obviously this contractual constraint does not apply to nonmember psychologists and nonpsychologists.

A third limit of ethics codes is that they tend to be vague, but for good reason. First, it is often only possible to attain political agreements when a code's provisions are vague enough to finesse disputed issues. It is easy to achieve a consensus that individuals should respect one another, not exploit persons over whom they have professional authority, not harass clients, and not plagiarize—all provisions of the American Psychological Association's *Ethical Principles and Code of Conduct*—but it is difficult to reach a consensus on how to operationalize these requirements. For example, at what point does a supervisor's requests for a subordinate's services become exploitive? Second, even if psychologists are conscientious in observing or trying to observe the Code, it may be difficult to document this empirically. Psychologists making a sincere attempt to avoid objectionable multiple relationships, as required by the American Psychological Association's Code, may have great difficulty determining when they have entered into an objectionable multiple role. No amount of scrutinizing of the Code will necessarily resolve the issue for them. For example, using the services of a patient to resolve a plumbing problem may be necessary for the psychologist in a rural community. Moreover, this multiple relationship may be neither exploitive nor harmful to the patient.

Because codes do not attempt to replace legal codes, they are never comprehensive. Moreover, to be of use to the average professional, codes must be of manageable length. These two facts about codes guarantee that codes will omit important topics. Geropsychologists turning to the American Psychological Association's Code may well discover that matters of pressing concern to them are not addressed. For example, although a geropsychologist might very much like to have clear advice on what informed consent should consist of, and how it should be administered, ethics codes do not provide the needed information.

Finally, even if a code provides clear advice, professionals might wonder whether it is consistent with other provisions of the relevant code. For example, a geropsychologist might well believe that he has a code-given obligation to honor a commitment of confidentiality made to a patient, yet also have another code-given obligation to surrender the otherwise confidential client records to the managed care entity that is paying for services. For example, consider the situation where the elderly patient's employer has a contract with the managed care entity rerquiring it to provide the employer with access to all employee patient records as a condition of continuing the contract. Even if the geropsychologist informs the patient of this limitation in confidentiality, he might not have informed the patient of all potential risks of divulging personal information. One example of such risk is the employer firing the employee based on information contained in the geropsychological records.

MORAL THINKING

Moral thinking has at least three salient characteristics (Rachels, 1993). It is universal; it is impartial; it is reason driven. By universality, we mean that moral claims are not local. It would be odd to claim that cheating your clients is morally permissible, if only you have the good fortune to live in the right place or right time. Also, it would be morally unacceptable to acquiesce to the wish of an elderly client's son to place his cantankerous, aging parent in a residential facility, when the neuropsychological assessment suggests that the parent is fully capable of living independently. To sell one's services in such a way is partial and immoral. Finally, when we make moral claims, we have an obligation to defend the claims with reason. Unlike personal preferences (e.g., preference for one flavored tea over another), moral judgments require reasons to be morally defensible.

These three characteristic features of moral thinking do not answer substantive moral problems. To do that, one also needs the help of moral principles. Deciding what moral principles should regulate the behavior of psychologists is a controversial matter. Nevertheless, several principles have attained prominence in recent years, especially in medical ethics writing (Beauchamp & Childress, 1994; National Commission for the Protection of Human Subjects of Biomedical and Behavioral Research, 1978; President's Commission for the Study of Ethical Problems in Medicine and Biomedical and Behavioral Research, 1981, 1983). In particular, Beauchamp and Childress (1994) have been influential in articulating four principles that have gained wide allegiance: autonomy, beneficence, nonmaleficence, and justice. To this we add a fifth principle: fidelity to one's profession and client. Though the formulation, ultimate justification, and logical relationships of these five principles are certainly controversial, their relevance to moral and ethical decision making is accepted by most psychologists.

Specifically, few, if any, psychologists would assert that it is morally irrelevant whether a decision limits a person's autonomy or self-determination. Few, if any, psychologists would claim that a client's well-being is irrelevant in deciding what to do. Few, if any, psychologists would claim that whether a client is harmed is irrelevant to their deciding what to do. Few, if any, psychologists would think issues of justice are irrelevant to moral and ethical decision making. And, finally, few, if any, psychologists would argue that they should not be faithful to the ideals and goals of their standards and to meeting the clinical needs of their clients.

Many psychologists might have other principles and moral or religious ideals that help them to reach morally sound decisions, but these five principles seem to capture features that the overwhelming majority of psychologists would be willing to acknowledge. They might well represent a minimum consensus on principles that should guide psychologists in their moral decision making and the American Psychological Association in formulating its ethical principles and standards of conduct. At a minimum, ethical principles and standards that conflict with any of these moral principles should require justification. For example, it might be that regulating the sexual conduct between competent clients and therapists, as the American Psychological Association's standards do, infringes on the principle of autonomy, but is nevertheless justified, since such restriction can prevent egregious violations of the principle of nonmaleficence.

Psychologists with a sound understanding of these five moral principles are well positioned to appraise the American Psychological Association's *Ethical Principles and Code of Conduct* and to effectively respond to many issues that are not covered by the Code.

THE SPECIAL CONCERNS
OF GEROPSYCHOLOGY

Let us now apply these lessons to a sample of geropsychological problems. Though what follows is not exhaustive, it will provide the necessary introduction to the approach that geropsychologists should assume when faced with challenging situations.

Decisional Capacity and Disease

It is a familiar idea that by the time people have entered their 60s, they no longer think as fast as they once did. A healthy person taking an intelligence test at age 65 would be expected to attain approximately the same scale score he attained as a young man but his raw score will have declined. One will need fewer right answers to have an IQ of 130 at 65 than one needed to obtain the same score at 35. A good reason for this is a general slowing. Most people will not be as nimble maneuvering blocks at 65 as they were at 35.

This kind of slowing is not particularly threatening to the judgment regarding whether a person has the capacity to make ordinary decisions. The geropsychologist will not usually view the ordinary slowing of processing or the ordinary decline of raw scores with age as symptomatic of decisional incapacity. At most, the geropsychologist may take an interest in devising techniques to make efficient thinking easier for the elderly. But there are other kinds of decline, vastly more severe than ordinary slowing, that will draw the attention of the geropsychologist.

For example, Alzheimer's disease begins to appear in the population in significant percentages during the seventh decade of life (Bachman *et al.,* 1993; Evans *et al.,* 1989; Henderson & Hasegawa, 1992; Kolb & Whishaw, 1995). At 65, about one adult in 20 would be showing the debilitating effects of Alzheimer's disease. By age 70, the number of those fighting the disease rises to one in 10, and by age 80, between 40% and 50% of the population would exhibit some form of dementia, even if not related to Alzheimer's disease.

The clinical picture of increasing diagnosable dementing disease with increased age poses a challenge to geropsychologists seeking to reach morally and ethically defensible decisions about the decisional capacity of the elderly. The first and obvious challenge is that presence of a dementing disease is not, on its own, sufficient to show a lack of decisional capacity. A person's capacity to make a decision depends on the kind of decision required (Buchanan & Brock, 1989; Drane, 1985). Many simple, low-risk choices require very little decisional capacity, whereas more complicated, riskier choices may require substantial decisional capacity. Consequently, a person in the early stages of Alzheimer's disease may have the capacity to write a living will or create a durable power of attorney for medical purposes that he would not have at a later stage of the disease.

Since presence of a dementing illness does not of itself establish a person's decisional capacity, the geropsychologist must have a clear conceptualization of what functional capacities a person needs to make competent decisions. Buchanan and Brock (1989) have made an important contribution to this point. Their analysis shows that decisional capacity requires that a person be able to understand and deliberate with reference to his own values. Further, understanding and deliberation are continuous variables; nobody understands anything perfectly, while deliberation is something that people do with varying degrees of skill. Individuals even vary in the degree to which they know, can articulate, and can recognize their own values in deliberative choice. The importance of these capacities for competent decision making is intuitively obvious. When individuals do not understand the question before them, they cannot decide it well, unless lucky. If individuals cannot deliberate, they cannot use what they understand, even if they can understand a question and the information relevant to making a choice about it. And if individuals do not know their own values or if they use values alien to them, they cannot make a choice that reflects their personal beliefs and goals.

Geropsychologists assessing whether an Alzheimer's patient has the decisional capacity to make particular kinds of choices, for example, whether to remain at home or move to a nursing home, whether to accept a life-saving surgery or to reject it, must also recognize that the degree of capacity needed to make competent choices will depend on the kinds of question at hand. A grandmother may have the ability to make a decision about whether to make a small gift to a grandchild, but lack the ability to assess the risks and benefits of a medical procedure in relationship to her own goals.

Sometimes clinicians will believe that if a patient is competent to decide to accept a procedure, then he must also be competent to reject it. This is a mistaken belief. For example, accepting a low-risk procedure that will save a person's life requires far less decisional capacity than the rejection of it might. Indeed, rejecting a procedure may require that the person understand the full range of high-risk consequences that follow and also know how to assess these consequences in relation to his conception of his own good. Moreover, given that there is normally a presumption that people are competent, there will typically be no reason to question low-risk choices, but many reasons to assess a person's capacity to make a risky choice. It is not being argued that individuals, even mildly demented individuals, should never be allowed to make a risky choice. They may well have the capacity to make the choice. Rather, it is being argued that a risky choice may serve to trigger inquiries that a nonrisky choice would not.

Using a moral and ethical analysis helps us clarify the issue. In the absence of a countervailing moral consideration, the principle of autonomy commands that a person's self-determination be respected. It is only when a person appears to have made a decision that runs counter to ordinary expectations that one has grounds for assessing his competence to make a choice of that kind, and the principles of nonmaleficence and beneficence support such questioning. Therefore, although all Alzheimer's patients will eventually lose the capacity to make risky choices of any complexity, geropsychologists need to keep in mind that moral (and ethical) principles require careful professional judgment about when to conduct a competency evaluation, and how often such an evaluation needs to be considered.

As Alzheimer's disease progresses, patients progressively lose more of the functional capacities that enable them to make competent choices. At some point, a geropsychologist, after a reevaluation of the patient, might judge that the person is no longer competent, perhaps recommending to family members that they seek guardianship over that patient. This is not an easy decision, since once declared incompetent, patients may lose control over many aspects of their life. For example, they may lose the ability to decide where to live and how to spend their money. Given the severe compromise of a person's self-determination, if declared incompetent, only the principle of nonmaleficence should underwrite this infringement on the principle of autonomy. The mere observation that a person might do better in a different setting, and concomitant desire to help that person, is not enough to justify so severe a reduction in self-determination. Indeed, severe reduction of autonomy results in harm, despite the geropsychologist's best intentions. Thus, there must be some reasoned expectation that the person declared incompetent is being spared a major harm.

Given the gravity of an incompetency determination, it should not be surprising that it might place the geropsychologist at odds with a patient's family. One source of ethical and moral difficulty in incompetency determination can be ambiguity about whether the client in assessments of decisional capacity is the person being assessed or the family members seeking (and perhaps paying for) that assessment. For example, children may wish an elderly father assessed as being incapable of managing his own affairs. The children may have difficulty understanding the geropsychologist's obligation to clarify his role in relation to the children and the father. The American Psychological Association's Ethics Code and the moral principle of fidelity to one's profession and clients, require that all parties understand the nature of the geropsychologist's relationship to each of them.

Matters can become even more difficult if the family proposes actions that the geropsychologist believes will worsen the elderly client's condition. For example, people with Alzheimer's disease, even at early stages, have diminished spatial memory (Lezak, 1995). Consequently, although they can find their way about in a familiar environment, they have enormous difficulty or even find it impossible to find their way about in a novel environment. A nursing home placement can have a devastating impact on a person with an impairment of spatial memory. And even if the children are made the guardians of the elderly person, at least in theory they have an obligation to decide in their charge's best interest (Buchanan & Brock, 1989), though this duty has been disputed (Hardwig, 1990; Nelson & Nelson, 1995). Geropsychologists have an expert knowledge of the needs of elderly clients. Moreover, geropsychologists understand how different responses of family members to their elderly person's mental disorders can affect how rapidly and severely a disorder unfolds. Given a geropsychologist's special knowledge, he may have good reasons for questioning whether an elderly client's children are, in their capacity as guardians, deciding on the basis of what is best for their impaired elderly parent. These guardians may be reaching an expedient solution that is most convenient for them. Nevertheless, although respect for moral principles requires that geropsychologists be vigilant about clear violations of the patient's interests, geropsychologists must remember that a client's best interest is not a determination made by psychologists. Rather, it is a determination that the courts will make, and one that courts are less likely to need to make if geropsychologists remain cognizant of the limits of their competence. To act otherwise assumes a competency that geropsychologists do not possess in virtue of their specialist training, and violates the moral principle of fidelity.

Assessment Issues

The issues raised in connection with Alzheimer's disease and decisional capacity make reference to assessment. Both ordinary morality and the American Psychological Association's ethics code require that clients be tested appropriately. Ordinary moral thinking forbids imposition of significant harm, and unreliable tests, and testing can threaten a person with such serious consequences as misdiagnosis and loss of liberty. Unfortunately, it is often difficult for geropsychologists to determine whether they are meeting this obligation to use appropriate tests.

The situation is acute in the case of the oldest patients. For the age group over 80, few tests have been adequately normed. When such well-known scales as Wechsler's intelligence and memory scales were first normed, insufficient numbers of people lived long enough to justify the expense of establishing norms for the oldest age group. Matters have changed as improved medical and public health measures have resulted in a rapidly growing elderly population.

The nature of this population poses serious moral questions of justice for geropsychologists. One way of understanding testing is to conceive of it as action-guiding. A person's test results enable psychologists to diagnose, identify strengths and weaknesses, and establish a coherent treatment plan. However, interpretation of test results is dependent on the norms for the relevant test. As for the moral principle of justice, establishment of norms forces geropsychologist to consider, among many other factors, the moral consequences of adopting one population sample as normative, rather than another.

Since distributive justice concerns who gets what and on what basis, the testing decisions of geropsychologists serve as information backdrops for making decisions about entitlements of the elderly. A decision to include a relatively large number of impaired people in developing norms could result in a belief that diminished abilities are a normal consequence of aging, whereas a decision to develop norms from a sample that excludes people with conditions that often accompany aging could result in stigmatizing many older people. No position on the development of norms is likely to be without difficulties; perhaps the best solution is to opt for multiple norms. For example, in relation to expectations, prospective research on the elderly might wish to employ norms based on how disease-free older adults test. Such a conception of norms would make it possible to encourage the development of lifestyles that maximize health and vigor among the elderly. At the same time, these norms may be unrealistic for a significant percentage of elderly persons. Thus, it may well be appropriate to have a second set of norms that recognizes the elderly population as it is now constituted. Consequently people who might look debilitated or mildly debilitated against a high standard are not labeled as debilitated on a less exacting conception of the appropriate norm. This proposal is not without difficulties of its own. In particular, the assignment of entitlements often flows from a significant deviation from the relevant norm. A decision to use a lower-normed group could have the effect of leaving fewer people entitled to special services. Balanced against that effect is cost savings. Society now makes significant contributions to the elderly (Daniels, 1988). Employment of a high norm could result in the diversion of resources to the elderly from some other group. Space limitations preclude us from pursuing this issue further in this chapter. Our goal here is simply to make geropsychologists aware that the setting of norms, a seemingly innocuous technical exercise, is something that has consequential moral dimensions that should be considered in professional decision making.

In addition to issues of justice, testing also raises moral and ethical issues as to how to test. Psychological testing can be time consuming and demanding on the resources of the testee (Anastasi, 1988). For example, certain approaches to testing raise an often unnoticed problem. In the interest of saving time or because they are committed to an actuarial approach to test interpretation, some psychologists rely on test batteries. At the extreme, some psychologists have a psychological examiner perform an invariant pattern of tests and interpret the results.

The present state of knowledge makes this battery approach to testing older clients morally and ethically suspect (Lezak, 1995). It can be demoralizing for a patient to attempt to answer numerous questions beyond their capacity or to continue in an examination after a psychologist has noticed that the information sought has already been obtained. By administering their own examinations or at least restricting administration of examinations to those who have the training necessary to know when a portion of a battery has ceased to contribute incremental validity to a battery, psychologists spare their patients needless testing burdens.

This objection to the unrestrained use of test batteries is rooted in the principle of nonmaleficence. However, one crucial empirical claim underlies it. If the use of a battery does indeed contribute significant incremental validity to an assessment, then there is no objection to its use. The onus, though, is on the psychologist who claims that only subjecting a stressed patient to a full battery will provide the information needed for a good assessment. The current state of knowledge does not make that an easy claim. Moreover, to the extent that a patient is not distressed or is enjoying an assessment, the moral argument against invariant administration of batteries is undermined. Again, the point is not to settle the issue, but to remind geropsychologists that many clients, especially demented elderly clients, require respectful treatment in their assessment.

Suicide

Suicide poses more questions to the geropsychologist than to psychologists working with younger populations. Young people rarely have compelling reasons for killing themselves. Among the young, psychologists assume and have reason to assume that suicidality is a state that arose from a crisis and will pass in short order. Older persons are far more likely to have good reasons for wishing to die or wishing to enlist somebody else's aid in dying. Progressive diseases such as Alzheimer's disease, horrifically painful, killing diseases such as bone cancer, and many other conditions can place an older person in a position in which, at least arguably, it is rational to want to die or to kill oneself.

And yet there is a long, venerable tradition in the caregiving professions that opposes both suicide and what is often called "active euthanasia." Physicians often support the maxim, "Thou shall not kill, but need not strive too officiously to keep alive"(American Geriatrics Society, 1991; American Medical Association, 1992). Consequently, it is often allowed that there is an important difference between killing a patient (active euthanasia) and letting a patient die (passive euthanasia). Common medical practice holds that it is permissible, if patients consent, to let them die, but not permissible, even with their consent, to kill them. Geropsychologists seeking to assess an elderly person's ability to reach a reasoned decision to end his own life or to refuse to accept potentially lifesaving interventions, need to have an understanding of the moral thinking that has shaped his reasoning about these end-of-life decisions. Even though geropsychologists themselves will not perform the acts that lead to the end of a patient's life, they need to understand the moral terrain, if they are to think coherently about life-ending decisions in elderly persons.

A person with a painful, killing disease or a progressive dementing illness may have great difficulty in understanding the refusal of many caregivers to assist them in ending their life. Ordinary thinking that suicide or the refusal of lifesaving treatment is an evil may be evaluated differently when someone is faced with a set of facts that confront many elderly persons. Unlike a young person, whose depression or disease will often succumb to treatment, elderly people face a grimmer set of realities. In some cases they are going to die, and the chief question is when or how. In other cases, even though death is not imminent, the elderly person faces disintegration of himself as a dementing illness destroys ever larger portions of his brain. Few young people encounter the numbing realities of the older person who is dying a painful death or who has a dementing disease. Moreover, older persons have had a life's experience to enable them to have a clearer recognition of what their lives mean and the circumstances under which they wish to continue to live. No two people need reach the same conclusion when confronted with the same facts. For some elderly persons, the suffering that accompanies death or disease has a religious significance that perhaps enables them to bear what awaits them. Other elderly persons have beliefs that assign no positive value to pain or loss of capacity. For them, the prospect of an existence in a demented state or in constant pain may be judged as a complete evil. They may not wish to continue to live in such circumstances. The geropsychologist, in the process of exploring a desperately ill elderly person's sense of life, will learn much about the nature of the person.

The geropsychologist, if mindful of a person's right to self-determination, will recognize that in some instances, the view that it is a good thing to try to keep a person living may not be appropriate and that to continue living can even be insulting to that person.

Suppose that an elderly man has a painful bone cancer, less than three months to live, and does not wish to wait for death to arrive naturally. If a geropsychologist's assessment of him leads to the conclusion that he is competent to make a decision to end his life, should the geropsychologist declare him incompetent solely to stop the patient from seeking the means to achieve his goal? This situation is both real and disturbing because the elderly person can receive as much medication as is necessary to keep him completely free of pain. The dying man may have no wish to die in an analgesic stupor. He may have a different preference. It is stretching credibility to argue that drugging the person to an insensate state benefits him. If he is insensate, he is obviously not benefiting. Nor is it plausible to claim that the duty of nonmaleficence requires that he be encouraged to drug himself rather than kill himself. Again, in his own, competent judgment, he has reached a conclusion that his life is no longer a good to him. The clinician has no psychological basis to overrule him.

In a seminal article, Rachels (1975) has gone further and argued that there is an absence of a morally significant difference between letting die and killing, thereby suggesting that if clinicians may withdraw life-sustaining procedures, they may also actively do what ends life, with the patient's permission. Rachels's argument for the absence of a difference ran as follows: Suppose a man wished to kill a child to gain insurance money. He enters a bathroom while the child is bathing, then drowns the child. In that case, he has intentionally killed. In case two, the man again enters the room. As he does so, the child slides under the water. The man is, prepared to kill the child if need be, but instead the child dies without his assistance. He lets the child die. According to Rachels, there is no difference between the two acts, morally speaking. He is a monster in either case. If one act were morally worse than another, the first story would result in a more severe judgment than the second. Undoubtedly, killing usually occurs in *circumstances* that make it worse than letting die; however, it is the attendant circumstances, not the fact that somebody killed rather than let die, that makes the moral difference.

Geropsychologists thinking about this issue need to understand that Rachels's argument overlooks certain clinical realities facing elderly clients. Indeed, these clients also may not understand such clinical realities at the time of being assessed by the geropsychologist. Geropsychologists need to be able to explain them. Steinbock (1979) makes the case well. Competent dying and dementing clients need to understand their true situation, so that they can make a rational choice. For example, a competent patient has a moral right and a legally recognized right to refuse treatment, even though refusal of ordinary care will sometimes hasten a person's death. Moreover, although physicians have a duty to provide ordinary care to competent and incompetent patients, they have no duty to provide extraordinary care. Although failing to provide care, in either instance, may hasten a patient's death, in the case of extraordinary treatment, benefits of treatment may be sufficiently speculative so that there is no duty to provide it. Patients need to understand that while the principle of autonomy supports their right to refuse lifesaving treatment, the same principle does not entitle them to insist that others do anything for them. If it did, autonomy would include not only a right to self-determination but also a right to "other" determination. Thus, respecting a person's self-determination does not yield a right to be killed *intentionally*. Clinicians who respect a patient's treatment refusal, or who do not provide extraordinary care, are not intentionally killing him. They are working within the traditional value system of medical practice.

Geropsychologists who understand the argument between Rachels (1975) and Steinbock (1979) can at least bring their clients to an understanding of the current situation, where physicians normally resist arguments to intentionally end a desperately ill person's life. Once geropsychologists grasp these arguments, they face a difficult choice of their own. They must grapple with their own moral beliefs and what these beliefs imply about what stance they should take toward elderly clients who wish to end their life on their own or to have the assistance of others in ending it.

In the former situation, if the patient is fully competent to reach the decision, the moral principle of autonomy requires that the geropsychologist report those results to the client (e.g., the family) and not try to achieve an alternative result that satisfies the geropsychologist's or client's wishes. In the latter situation, if the person is competent, the geropsychologist may inform the person qua client that in the current state of law, persons may ask for others to stop doing things that are keeping them alive. The client should also be made to understand that it may be illegal for his caregivers to intentionally bring about his death. Further, the geropsychologist is morally obligated to report the conclusion of competency, even though a determination of incompetency could result in the person's life being saved via the continued administration of ordinary care. The duty of geropsychologists is to give thorough and honest assessments to elderly clients, even with grim diagnoses. Being old does not inoculate clients against depression and other reactions to their illnesses that could render them incompetent to make decisions about their care, but geropsychologists must remain alert to the possibility that a desire to die is not rooted in a transient psychological problem.

Finding Meaning in One's Life

If thinking about the reasons that older people may wish to die is the night of geropsychology, helping older people see meaning in their lives is the day. Although older people suffer many of the problems that younger people do—depression, sexual dysfunction, anxiety, and the like—important differences mark the two populations. The younger person is often able to achieve a meaningful life in face of psychological obstacles. A young woman with a social phobia confronts serious impediments to leading a meaningful life. The older person seeking psychotherapy for the first time perhaps comes with a different perspective and different problems. Older clients are likely to have a vivid sense of their mortality. They often have seen loved ones die. They have seen their own physical capacities decline. They may need reassurance about the extent to which the physical and psychological changes that they are undergoing are normal. They also may be seeking a way of seeing meaning in the life they have lived and in learning ways to spend well what time they have left.

Geropsychologists should keep in mind that this is not simply the delivery of a technology, as is the case if one is teaching an elderly person effective techniques for combating insomnia, depression, bereavement, or anxiety. Clinical geropsychologists are being conscripted in an attempt to help the elderly client see meaningful patterns. When geropsychologists lack a coherent philosophy of life of their own, they are going to be at a loss as to how to help such clients. But there are good reasons for questioning whether, even when geropsychologists have a coherent philosophy of life, they should offer it as part of their services as psychologists. Indeed, the task is to help the older person see what has been good, what has been bad, and how it all has come together to give them a life that means something. Since these are questions of values, geropsychologists need to seriously consider the possibility that neither their training nor acquired expertise positions them to help the older person in his quest for meaning. What the geropsychologist can do is to try to cultivate a list of contacts that may enable meaning-seeking older people to obtain the assistance they need. In some cases, they may be encouraged to discuss their life with loved ones or a spiritual adviser. Until geropsychologists have reason to believe that they have expertise in helping people find meaning, they would do well to resist the temptation to assume the mantle of competence regarding what makes a life meaningful.

In addition to the moral argument just given against geropsychologists helping elderly clients in their meaning quests, the American Psychological Association's Ethics Code lends support to this restriction on geropsychological practice. The Code enjoins psychologists not to practice beyond their competence. Since there is reason to be skeptical that psychologists have expertise in identifying what makes a life meaningful, geropsychologists should proceed with extreme caution in assisting elderly people in the quest for meaning in their lives. It may be appropriate to help with the finding of narrative themes and the like, but the question of meaning itself is not one that a geropsychologist is well trained to answer. This is not an admonition for insensitivity to the needs of meaning-seeking elderly people, but a call for humility and recognition of the limits of one's true competence as a geropsychologist. The challenge to geropsychologists who would offer guidance in an area that has traditionally been the province of religion is to give some reasoned ground for supposing that, in offering guidance in this area, they are still working as psychologists. Indeed, this requirement is supported by the moral principles of beneficence, nonmaleficence and fidelity to one's profession and patient.

SUMMARY

We have argued that geropsychology does not call for a different set of moral or ethical principles. What is distinctive about moral and ethical reasoning in geropsychology is the problems that are confronted. In particular, the age of geropsychologists' clients makes it likely that geropsychologists will encounter certain kinds of moral and ethical problems more frequently than other psychologists. We have sampled but a few of these problems. The aim of a limited sampling was to set out a context for moral and ethical reasoning about difficult problems. By engaging in such reasoning, geropsychologists place themselves in a position to achieve an intradisciplinary, and ultimately extradisciplinary, consensus about what should be done in certain kinds of circumstances. Our approach does not assume that the principles of autonomy, beneficence, nonmaleficence, justice, or fidelity will themselves survive the dialectical process unchanged or even survive at all. The purpose of moral and ethical inquiry is to evolve deeper moral and ethical understanding, not to embalm it at some instant in time. Other areas have yielded to consensus using similar procedures. There is no reason to believe that the problems now confronted by geropsychologists cannot also attain solutions by consensus.

REFERENCES

American Geriatrics Society, Public Policy Committee. (1991). Voluntary active euthanasia. *Journal of the American Geriatrics Society, 39*, 826.

American Medical Association, Council on Ethical and Judicial Affairs. (1992). Decisions near the end of life. *Journal of the American Medical Association, 267*, 2229–2233.

American Psychological Association. (1985). *Standards for educational and psychological testing.* Washington, DC: American Psychological Association.

American Psychological Association. (1992). Ethical principles of psychologists and code of conduct. *American Psychologist, 47*, 1597–1611.

Anastasi, A. (1988). *Psychological testing* (6th ed.). New York: Macmillan.

Bachman, D. L., Wolf, P. A., Linn, R. T., Knoefel, J. E., Cobb, J. L., Belanger, A. J., White, L. R., & D'Agostino, R. B. (1993). Incidence of dementia and probable Alzheimer's disease in the general population: The Framingham Study. *Neurology, 43*, 515–519.

Beauchamp, T. L., & Childress, J. F. (1994). *Principles of biomedical ethics* (4th ed.). New York: Oxford University Press.

Buchanan, A. E., & Brock, D. W. (1989). *Deciding for others: The ethics of surrogate decision making.* New York: Cambridge University Press.

Daniels, N. (1988). *Am I my parents' keeper?* New York: Oxford University Press.

Drane, J. (1985). The many faces of competency. *Hastings Center Report, 15*, 17–21.

Ethics Committee of the American Psychological Association. (1992). Rules and procedures. *American Psychologist, 47*, 1612–1628.

Evans, D. A., Funkenstein, H., Albert, M. S., Scherr, P. A., Cook, N. R., Chown, M. J., Hebert, L. E., Hennekens, C. H., & Taylor, J. O. (1989). Prevalence of Alzheimer's disease in a community population of older persons. *Journal of the American Medical Association, 262*, 2551–2556.

Hardwig, J. (1990). What about the family? *Hastings Center Report, 20*, 5–10.

Henderson, A. S., & Hasegawa, K. (1992). The epidemology of dementia and depression in later life. In M. Bergener (Ed.), *Aging and mental disorders: International perspectives.* New York: Springer.

Kolb, B., & Whishaw, I. Q. (1995). *Fundamentals of human neuropsychology* (4th ed.). New York: W. H. Freeman.

Lezak, M. D. (1995). *Neuropsychological assessment* (3rd. ed.). New York: Oxford University Press.

National Commission for the Protection of Human Subjects in Biomedical and Behavioral Research. (1978). *The Belmont report* (DHEW Publication No. 0578-0012). Washington, DC: Author.

Nelson, H. L., & Nelson, J. L. (1995). *The patient in the family: an ethics of medicine and families.* New York: Routledge.

President's Commission for the Study of Ethical Problems in Medicine and Biomedical and Behavioral Research. (1981). *Protecting human subjects*. Washington, DC: U.S. Government Printing Office.

President's Commission for the Study of Ethical Problems in Medicine and Biomedical and Behavioral Research. (1983). *Implementing human research regulations*. Washington, DC: U.S. Government Printing Office.

Rachels, J. (1975). Active and passive euthanasia. *New England Journal of Medicine, 292*, 75–80.

Rachels, J. (1993). *The elements of moral philosophy* (2nd ed.). New York: McGraw-Hill.

Sales, B. D., & Shuman, D. (1993). Reclaiming the integrity of science in expert witnessing. *Ethics and Behavior, 3*, 223–229.

Steinback, B. (1979). The intentional termination of life. *Ethics in Science and Medicine, 6*, 59–64.

CHAPTER 6

Normal Memory Aging

Katie E. Cherry and Anderson D. Smith

INTRODUCTION

Elderly people often comment that their memory is not as good as it used to be. Complaints of memory loss vary widely among older adults. Some express little concern over age-related declines in memory, but others show greater worry and concern. Older adults' concerns are understandable in light of the increased public awareness of memory impairment associated with Alzheimer's disease (Reisberg, Ferris, deLeon, Crook, & Haynes, 1987). Nonetheless, self-reported memory problems do not necessarily provide an accurate indication of older persons' performance on laboratory-based measures of memory (Dixon, 1989).

For practicing clinicians, memory concerns raise multiple interpretive issues. A variety of factors, including emotional and physiological states, may contribute to memory problems in older persons. For instance, undue memory complaint may be symptomatic of clinical depression, whereas gross performance deficits on standardized memory measures may signal a serious health condition. Accurate identification of the source of memory deficits in older adults has important implications for treatment and prognosis. Thus, understanding the developmental course of memory abilities in adulthood and the implications of these changes for older persons' daily lives is important for clinical geropsychologists.

This chapter is organized as follows: In the first section, we distinguish between *normal memory aging* due to maturational processes and *pathological memory aging* that may be attributable to disease states or other factors. In the second section, we offer five general conclusions about normal memory functioning in adulthood based on a selective review of experimental studies of memory aging. In the third section, we explore memory intervention techniques

Katie E. Cherry • Department of Psychology, Louisiana State University, Baton Rouge, Louisiana 70803-5501. Anderson D. Smith • School of Psychology, Georgia Institute of Technology, Atlanta, Georgia 30332-0001.

Handbook of Clinical Geropsychology, edited by Michel Hersen and Vincent B. Van Hasselt. Plenum Press, New York, 1998.

and evaluate the efficacy of these methods with older persons. In the fourth section, we consider broad implications of experimental findings on memory aging for clinical practice.

NORMAL VERSUS PATHOLOGICAL MEMORY AGING

Normal Memory Aging

Scope and Definition

Persons of all ages experience memory failures that may be attributable to internal states (e.g., inattention, interference, fatigue), external factors (e.g., inadequate retrieval cues, information overload), or a combination. Forgetfulness in daily life occurs more often for older than younger adults, as revealed in survey and questionnaire studies of memory (Cavanaugh, Grady, & Perlmutter, 1983; Gilewski & Zelinski, 1986). Laboratory studies of memory in healthy older adults also provide substantial evidence of age-related deficits in both immediate and long-term retention (see Craik & Jennings, 1992; Kausler, 1994; Smith, 1996; Smith & Earles, 1996, for reviews).

Behaviors such as forgetting names, dates, or where the car keys were placed are characteristic of normal memory aging (Jarvik, 1980). Ample experimental evidence supports this view. Researchers have attempted to model everyday memory behaviors using laboratory-based procedures that permit strict control over subject characteristics, task demands, and other potentially confounding factors (West, 1989). The patterns of age-related deficits in memory for everyday materials (e.g., names and faces, prose, television programs) are generally similar to those observed on traditional laboratory memory measures (see Bäckman, Mantila, & Herlitz, 1990; Salthouse, 1991, for reviews).

Descriptive Terms

Several descriptive terms have emerged in recent years to characterize declining memory abilities in older adults who show no signs of depression or dementia. For example, the National Institute of Mental Health has proposed the term *minimal memory impairment* to describe normal age-related cognitive changes (J. A. Yesavage, Lapp, & Sheikh, 1989). Similar terms include *age-associated memory impairment* (Crook *et al.,* 1986), *normal cognitive aging* (Powell, 1994), and *benign senescent forgetfulness* (Jarvik, 1980). Although efforts have been made to develop criteria to define normal memory aging (Crook & Larrabee, 1988), systematic application of these criteria by researchers and clinicians has yet to occur. Widespread endorsement of a topology of the memory problems of normal aging is a likely trend for the future; such a topology would be beneficial for research and clinical purposes (Powell, 1994).

Pathological Memory Aging

Diagnostic Issues

An important issue for practicing clinicians is to distinguish memory problems of normal aging from those that may be caused by physiological or psychopathological factors. Forgetting names of family members or close friends,
confusion in space and time, and difficulties with simple motor tasks (e.g., un-
locking a door with a key) are behaviors that could be signaling a serious health
condition. Accurate diagnosis of conditions producing problems such as these
is imperative, as cognitive deficits may be responsive to treatment in some
cases. However, deficits such as those observed in the adult dementias are irreversible (Jarvik, 1980).

Although numerous advances in the clinical assessment of memory in
older adults have been made in recent years (Poon et al., 1986; Powell, 1994),
accurate diagnosis of memory dysfunction remains difficult. This is partly because many etiologically distinct conditions have similar behavioral symptoms
(e.g., dementia, cerebral vascular accident, nutritional and metabolic disorders,
head trauma). Consequently, extensive case histories, as well as concurrent
physical, clinical, and neurological examinations, may be necessary before definitive diagnoses would be warranted (Jarvik, 1980).

Adult Dementias

Dementia syndromes are a form of organic mental disorders defined
broadly by a constellation of symptoms and features, including gross cognitive
impairment and changes in personality and affective states (American Psychiatric Association, 1994). Progressive memory dysfunction is symptomatic of
Alzheimer's disease (AD) and other dementia syndromes that affect older adults
(see Cherry & Plauche, 1996, for review). For example, *Parkinson's disease* (a
disorder involving loss of motor ability) has associated dementia in some cases,
with memory impairment and slowness of thinking, but preserved language
ability. *Multi-infarct dementia* is a vascular dementia with an abrupt onset,
stepwise deterioration, and focal neurologic signs and symptoms. *Pick's disease,* a rare dementing disorder, is clinically similar to AD but the neurochemistry and neuropathology differs by comparison *Cruetzfeldt-Jakob disease* is a
rare, infectious disorder (caused by a slow-acting virus) with pronounced mental deterioration, involuntary muscle spasms, and rapid death. Confirmation of
diagnosis of the adult dementias occurs postmortem when specific neurologic
features are revealed on autopsy (Jarvik, 1980; Raskind & Peskind, 1992).

Physiological Conditions

Certain physiologic conditions have associated memory dysfunction that
may resemble early AD (Haase, 1971). Such conditions include but are not limited to normal-pressure hydrocephalus; metabolic, endocrine, or electrolyte disturbances; and other conditions, such as dietary insufficiencies or alcoholism.

Diagnosis and treatment of these conditions are imperative, as it may be possible to reverse the cognitive deficits in some cases (Jarvik, 1980).

Pharmacological Agents

Older persons may experience multiple health problems and illnesses that are treated with different drug therapies (e.g., Ouslander, 1981; Vestal, 1978). Physician-prescribed medications, as well as over-the-counter medications, may adversely affect older adults' memory and other aspects of cognition. For example, antimicrobials have been associated with memory disturbance in older persons. Antihypertensives, analgesics, antihistamines, and cardiovascular medications have also been shown to produce confusion (among other adverse effects) in older persons (see Ouslander, 1982). Memory problems and confusional states due to drug effects, drug–drug interactions, or drug toxicity can potentially be reversed. Risks of adverse drug reactions can be minimized by careful monitoring and appropriate adjustment of therapeutic dosages (Cherry & Morton, 1989).

Psychopathologic Conditions

Memory problems may also be due to conditions such as acute grief, paranoid disorders, and depression. In fact, clinical depression may be initially mistaken for probable AD, due to the similarity of symptoms (e.g., apathy, difficulties in concentration, psychomotor slowing). Depressed older adults may complain of memory loss, but the correspondence between self-reported memory deficits and objective memory performance tends to be poor (Kahn, Zarit, Hilbert, & Niederehe, 1975; Larrabee & Levin, 1986; Popkin, Gallagher, Thompson, & Moore, 1982). In contrast, probable AD patients may overestimate their memory ability, relative to performance on objective memory tests and reports by their relatives (Gilewski & Zelinski, 1986). Recent studies also indicate that severe depression may coexist with AD in the early stages (e.g., Lamberty & Bieliauskas, 1993). Further research is needed to clarify the conceptual and methodological issues that surround dual diagnosis of depression and dementia (Terry & Wagner, 1992).

FIVE CONCLUSIONS FROM EXPERIMENTAL STUDIES OF NORMAL MEMORY AGING

Because memory problems associated with normal aging are so prevalent, they have been very popular research topics in psychology. In fact, one third of all published research studies examining psychological aging over the past two decades have dealt with memory (Smith, 1996). Based on a selective review of this literature, we offer five general conclusions: (1) the relationship between aging and memory performance is complex; (2) individual differences within age groups are often greater than differences between age groups; (3) noncognitive factors may influence the magnitude of age differences in memory performance, but these factors do not account for all the age-related variance in memory performance; (4) much of the age-related variance in memory performance can be accounted for by simple cognitive mechanisms; and (5) successful aging is not the absence of memory changes but adaptation to them.

Description of Relationship Between Age and Memory

Memory changes associated with aging are complex and no simple description is satisfactory. To illustrate, Table 6-1 presents a summary of age effects on different types of short-term and long-term memory tasks. As can be seen in Table 6-1, changes associated with some types of memory are large and reliable, while others are negligible. Even a distinction between short-term memory and long-term memory is not sufficient to capture the complexities associated with the effects of aging.

Short-Term Memory

With short-term memory, it is not the passive capacity to keep things in mind that is affected by aging (i.e., primary memory), but rather the capacity to store and process at the same time (i.e., working memory) (Dobbs & Rule, 1989). The Forward Digit Span test on the Wechsler Adult Intelligence Scale (WAIS) provides an estimate of primary memory. Age differences are typically not found on this test, unless a very large number of subjects is used making the age comparisons powerful enough to detect very small differences (Craik & Jennings, 1992). Active working memory tasks, however, do show reliable age differences. Regardless of whether the working memory tasks involve processing verbal materials (e.g., Wingfield, Stine, Lahar, & Aberdeen, 1988), arithmetic problems (e.g., Babcock & Salthouse, 1990), or spatial information (e.g., Salthouse, 1993), older adults consistently do worse when trying to store and process information at the same time.

Long-Term Memory

Age effects on long-term memory are also specific to certain types of memory. While semantic and procedural memory are relatively spared, there are deficits in episodic memory in older adults.

Semantic memory involves the ability of subjects to recall information from their accumulated world knowledge. There is some evidence that it takes longer for older adults to retrieve semantic information, but there is little evidence that this reflects a problem with the structure or quality of semantic memory storage (e.g., Light, 1992). For example, when the structure of semantic memory (i.e., the nature of the network of semantic associations) is assessed by looking at the ability of different-aged subjects to generate free associations across a variety of different types of materials, there are no age differences in the nature of the associations given (Light, 1991, 1992).

Procedural memory refers to remembering that is automatic, memory without the requirement of deliberate recollection. Procedural memory ability requires

Table 6-1. Description of Memory Types and Age Effects on Memory Tests

Type of memory	Definition	Example test	Age effects
Short-term memory Primary memory	Passive capacity to keep things in mind; the number of things one can think of at one time.	WAIS Forward Digit Span	Little age effects; age differences only detected if large number of adults tested.
Working memory	Active capacity to store information and process information at the same time; the ability to engage in on-line information processing.	Reading span; read sentences and answer questions about each sentence; when cued, recall the last word in each sentence.	Large, reliable age differences regardless of type of processing involved. Deficits seen with semantic, spatial, or computational processing.
Long-term memory Episodic memory	Ability to remember past experiences based on contextual cues associated with original learning.	Free recall task; look at a list of familiar words and later recall as many of the words as possible.	Large, reliable age differences in recall; smaller age differences if recognition used to test memory.
Semantic memory	Ability to retrieve information as world knowledge based on semantic or conceptual cues.	WAIS Vocabulary Test or General Information Test	No age differences unless large number of adults tested and then slight advantage for older adults over younger adults.
Procedural memory	Automatic skill. Can be complex skill (e.g., riding a bicycle) to simple indirect effects of memory (e.g., implicit memory).	Implicit memory test; view list of words and then later fill in stem completions with words (e.g., ST___). Words from earlier read list are filled in even though subjects are unaware of the	Little age effects in implicit memory; slight differences detected in favaor of younger adults if large numbers of subjects used to test for implicit memory.

much practice to make remembering automatic, but there is general consensus that if memories are automatic, age differences are negligible (Hasher & Sacks, 1979). Procedural memories can range from indirect effects of memory to complex skills like riding a bicycle or driving a car.

A good example of procedural knowledge is implicit memory, a measurable effect of previous experience (i.e., memory) without awareness on the part of the subject. A typical demonstration of implicit memory involves presenting a list of words without an indication that a test will follow. Following some filled time interval, subjects are asked to supply the first word that comes to mind to a stem completion (st____ or a word fragment (p_r_di_m). Subjects will give words presented in the earlier list, even though they are unaware that the words came from the other list, and even though they cannot remember the words in an explicit recall test. Evidence suggests that there are very small age differences in implicit memory, if any at all (see Howard, 1996, for review). Although some researchers have found small but significant age differences in implicit memory, many subjects are necessary to show these differences because of the small effect sizes (e.g., Hultsch, Masson, & Small, 1991).

In contrast to semantic and procedural memory, episodic memory, which reflects memory for information experienced in specific contexts, shows age differences. The size of these deficits, however, seems to be dependent on the degree of subject-initiated processing required in the task (Craik, 1986). At both encoding (learning) and retrieval (remembering), age differences in episodic memory can be lessened by reducing the processing requirements of the task. For example, in a paired-associate memory task, age differences are smaller if the stimulus and response items are related to each other and larger if they are unrelated as the subject must generate an association between them (e.g., Park, Smith, Morrell, Puglisi, & Dudley, 1990).

Research on age differences in memory for pictures also supports the view that the processing requirements inherent in the memory task determine the magnitude of age effects. Age differences are found on several tasks that use pictorial materials (e.g., memory for faces, Bartlett, Leslie, Tubbs, & Fulton, 1989; map routes, Lipman & Caplan, 1992; simple line drawings, Puglisi & Park, 1987). However, age differences are typically not found with recognition of complex pictorial scenes (e.g., Park, Puglisi, & Smith, 1986). It has been shown that older adults do as well as younger adults in remembering complex scenes because of the rich semantic and perceptual detail found in such pictures (Smith, Park, Cherry, & Berkovsky, 1990). When the pictures were made non-meaningful or abstract, or when perceptual detail was removed from the pictures, age differences emerged. Again, the rich encoding context provided by the complex scenes may minimize the processing requirements to encode and later remember the pictures.

Similarly, reducing the effort or processing requirements at retrieval can reduce age differences on episodic tasks. Craik and McDowd (1987), for example, found large age differences when episodic memory was tested by free recall, but no age differences when memory was tested by recognition (picking out the words that were presented earlier), even when the overall level of performance on recall and recognition were equated by differentially delaying the recognition test. Craik and McDowd also measured the processing effort required of the two retrieval tasks by having subjects perform a digit-monitoring task while they were remembering the words. Slowed reaction time (RT) on the digit task indicates greater effort in the word-retrieval task because subjects have to time-share their attention to the two tasks (retrieving the words and monitoring the digits). The RTs of younger subjects were similar for the recall and recognition tasks. The older adults, however, doubled their RTs when trying to recall the items as compared to recognition. This suggests that the older adults do worse on the recall task because of the greater effort required to retrieve the words.

Summary and Implications

In short, age differences in memory depend on the nature of the memory test, the information to be remembered, and the type of memory being tested. Age differences in memory are not always found, but seem to be determined by the degree of self-initiated processing required.

For the clinician, it is important to understand that memory changes associated with normal aging are selective and that only certain memory tasks and types of memory show age differences. This allows better discrimination between memory complaints of realistic perceived changes associated with normal aging, and memory complaints that reflect other problems such as depression. Use of tasks that show minimal age effects, such as implicit (procedural) or semantic memory, also may be useful in differentiating normal memory changes from cognitive pathologies associated with dementia. Making such differentiations is complex, however, because demented patients show deficits on some procedural and semantic tasks but not others (e.g., Nebes, 1992).

Furthermore, understanding that memory differences are largest when self-initiated deliberate processing is required can be used to structure environmental interventions that minimize memory problems in older adults. As examples, Park (1992) discusses how theoretical and empirical findings from the memory laboratory can be used to help with everyday problems specific to older adults, such as medication adherence or work productivity.

Individual Differences Increase with Age

General

Although mean performance on many memory tasks decreases with age, it is evident that variance in performance increases. In fact, individual differences in memory performance within an age group are often larger than mean differences between age groups. This was demonstrated by Powell (1994) in his study of the cognitive performance of 1,002 physicians ranging in age from 25 to 92 years. Twenty-two different cognitive tests from simple reaction time (RT) to analogical reasoning were administered to the physicians. Many of the tests involved measures of memory, such as word recognition, story recall, and spatial recall. There was a steady decline in overall cognitive performance across the age groups, and this overall effect was replicated with each of the separate memory measures. More striking, however, was the increase in variability of performance. Even though the performance at age 70 was 18% lower than among the 40-year-olds, variability in performance was 60% greater. Similar results have been reported by other investigators. This indicates that the rate of memory decline differs considerably among individuals.

Summary and Implications

Because of the magnitude of individual differences and the fact that individual differences tend to increase with age, it is difficult to assess memory performance without longitudinal measures (measures of individual change). In fact, because memory pathology associated with dementia is characterized by degenerative change, care must be taken to make multiple assessments across time when early signs of dementia are suggested. Only late in dementia are qualitative differences seen between normal aging and pathological aging (Nebes, 1992).

Noncognitive Influences on Age-Related Memory Differences

General

It has been popular to attribute age differences on memory tasks to factors other than aging per se (e.g., student status, self-reported health, depression). Factors that have been hypothesized to account for age differences in memory include education (e.g., Kaufman, Reynolds, & McLean, 1989), metamemory (see Light, 1991, for review), and motivation (e.g., Hartley & Walsh, 1980). Overall, however, research has failed to show that these factors can account for significant age-related variance.

One hypothesis has been that laboratory memory tasks are more similar to academic remembering required in formal school settings and less like the everyday memory requirements of older adults (e.g., Perlmutter & Mitchell, 1982). If true, many of the memory differences would be exaggerated especially because many laboratory studies compare community-dwelling older adults to younger college students. Even though some studies have found that age differences in memory tasks are reduced when student status is controlled (e.g., comparing young vs. old college students), there are many problems with such comparisons. Often, for example, older students are taking elective single courses rather than being engaged in full academic pursuits (e.g., Zivian & Darjes, 1983). Furthermore, the findings are not consistent. Other studies have found significant age differences in memory performance when student status is controlled (e.g., Cohen, Sandler, & Schroeder, 1987).

Another factor that is obviously important in determining memory is health. Because health problems increase so dramatically with aging, health has been a likely factor producing the observed age differences in memory tasks. There have been conflicting results when self-rated health is used to account for age-related variance in cognitive performance. Some researchers have found that age-related variance is reduced when health is considered (e.g., Perlmutter & Nyquist, 1990), while others show no change at all when health is controlled (e.g., Salthouse, Kausler, & Saults, 1990). Health status, at best, accounts for only a part of the age-related memory variance.

Statistics also show depression to be more prevalent in older adults (e.g., Blazer, Hughes, & George, 1987). Depression, however, is sometimes difficult to diagnose because of the symptoms that may be associated with normal aging such as complaints about memory failures. In fact, evidence suggests that memory complaint may be more predictive of a lack of memory self-efficacy and depression than of actual memory performance (Larrabee & Levin, 1986). When validating commonly used metamemory questionnaires, Hertzog, Hultsch, and Dixon (1989) found a significant relationship between memory self-efficacy as measured on these questionnaires and measures of depression and well-being. Furthermore,

West, Crook, and Barron (1992) found that age still predicted everyday memory performance, even when scores on a test of depression were statistically controlled.

Summary and Implications

Changes in memory are real. So far, research has been unable to attribute these changes solely to factors other than aging. Thus, it is important for older adults to understand that memory change is normal and not reflective of either lack of motivation or the beginnings of dementia. Although noncognitive factors such as motivation, affect, education, socioeconomic status, experiences due to birth cohort, and physical and mental health have been shown to influence cognition, no research to date has shown that any single factor is primarily responsible for age-related memory differences (see Salthouse, 1991).

Simple Cognitive Mechanisms as Predictors of Age-Related Memory Differences

General

Although noncognitive factors have proven unsuccessful in accounting for the age-related memory differences seen in normal aging, a few cognitive mechanisms are good predictors of these differences. Earlier, it was indicated that memory differences in laboratory tasks seem to be determined by the extent of effort or deliberate processing required for the task. Even though no direct measures of deliberate processing have been developed, several specific measures have proven effective.

As discussed earlier, working memory is assumed to reflect the capacity to engage in on-line information processing (see Table 6-1). Because of the fundamental importance of working memory to cognition, researchers have attempted to determine whether individual differences in working memory predict age-related variance in other cognitive tasks. Salthouse (1992), in a review of a large number of studies examining the relationship among age, working memory, and cognition, has shown that about 50% of the age-related variance in cognition across a variety of different cognitive tasks is shared with working memory capacity. Other evidence indicates that measures of working memory account for a large proportion of the age-related variance in episodic memory performance. For example, Hultsch, Hertzog, and Dixon (1990) showed that working memory capacity accounts for much of the age difference in both word recall and text recall.

Other studies have shown that even simple measures of perceptual speed can account for the large proportion of the age-related variance in memory performance. When performance on perceptual speed tasks such as the digit-symbol substitution test or even simple perceptual comparison tasks (deciding whether digit or letter strings are the same or different) is statistically controlled, very little age-related variance remains on most memory measures. Salthouse (1994), for example, found that only 1% of the age-related variance on paired-associate memory was unique to age and not shared with perceptual speed. In one recent study, Park and colleagues (1996) found that perceptual speed accounted for most of the variance in free recall, cued recall, and spatial memory (three episodic memory tasks that show reliable age differences in the literature).

Summary and Implications

Individual difference studies show that even though interactions between age and various memory tasks are complex, cognitive mechanisms such as speed and working memory capacity may be responsible for much of the age-related variance. This research supports an inviting hypothesis that a few number of simple mechanisms may be responsible for most of the memory differences experienced by older adults. As Park (1992) points out, this means that greater attention needs to be paid to the environmental conditions faced daily by older adults that require complex, rapid decision making.

Successful Aging Is Not the Absence of Change but Adaptation to It

Baltes and Baltes (1990) propose a model of psychological aging that holds that successful aging is not the absence of psychological change, but the extent to which older adults are able to handle change (see Figure 6-1). As can be seen in the model, through various adaptive processes older adults can lead effective lives in the presence of cognitive loss. As we grow older, we are capable of a great deal of adaptation. For example, training studies show that there is a great deal of plasticity in cognitive processes with age. Willis and her colleagues have shown that even fluid intelligence skills can be improved in older adults with training (see Willis, 1989, for review). Others have shown that specific cognitive losses are often compensated for by improvements in other processes that

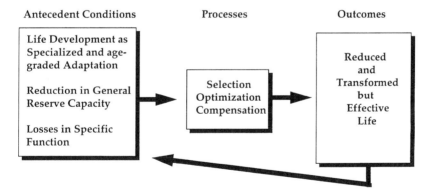

Figure 6-1. The Baltes and Baltes (1990) model of selective optimization with compensation, a model of adaptation during aging leading to successful aging. From "Psychological Perspectives on Successful Aging: The Model of Selective Optimization with Compensation," by P. B. Baltes and M. M. Baltes, 1990. In P. B. Baltes and M. M. Baltes (Eds.), *Successful Aging: Perspectives from the Social Sciences.* Cambridge: Cambridge University Press. Copyright 1990 by Cambridge University Press. Adapted with permission from P. B. Baltes.

together determine some overall cognitive behavior (Charness & Bosman, 1990). Salthouse (1984), for example, found that some expert typists will maintain their overall typing speed late into life, despite the fact that perceptual-motor speed (measured by choice RT) declines significantly. He discovered that the increases in RT were compensated for by the fact that the export typists had learned to look further ahead in the text while typing (eye-hand span).

To summarize, memory changes in normal aging are complex and individual differences tend to be large. Age-related differences in memory cannot be wholly accounted for by noncognitive variables, but can be predicted by simple cognitive mechanisms. Older adults are also capable of engaging in compensatory and optimization activities that greatly attenuate the effects of memory change on their daily lives.

MEMORY INTERVENTIONS

Researchers have attempted to offset age deficits in memory by training older adults in the use of mnemonic techniques to improve recall. Generally speaking, most mnemonic methods are efficacious for older adults, relative to baseline or appropriate control group conditions. Most studies on mnemonic methods have used visually based imagery and the classic mnemonic techniques (see Poon, Walsh-Sweeney, & Fozard, 1980, and J. A. Yesavage et al., 1989, for reviews), as described next. Interested readers arc referred to other sources where verbally based mnemonic methods are discussed (Drevenstedt & Bellezza, 1993; Hill, Allen, & McWhorter, 1991).

Classic Mnemonic Techniques

Visual Imagery

The philosophical origins of visual imagery as an aid to memory are traced back to the writings of Aristotle and other classical scholars of rhetoric (Paivio, 1971). In the commercial realm, modem-day memory professionals and authors of popular psychology books stress visually imaging the material to be remembered to promote recall (e.g., Bellezza, 1982; Bezan, 1974; Lorayne & Lucas, 1974). For example, Roth (1961) has argued that creative visualization is the sine qua non of good memory. His three cardinal principles are exaggeration, motion, and unusual association. To remember the noun pair *hen-ham,* Roth suggests visualizing "a big *ham* in the yard." "A large *hen* runs and jumps on the ham and dances a jig there" (p. 8).

In short, the popular idea has been that implausible, imaginative associations enhance recall. Experimental studies in the verbal learning tradition have documented the positive effects of visual imagery on retention (e.g., Bower, 1972). However, studies of imagery bizarreness with college students have yielded equivocal results (e.g., Kroll, Schepeler, & Angin, 1986; McDaniel & Einstein, 1986). Few studies have examined image bizarreness effects with older adults (Poon et al., 1980). Crovitz (1989) has made the point that younger adults may be comfortable with forming bizarre images of stimuli to be recalled, but older people would prefer to form plausible associations. Thus, in contrast to the popular literature, it seems more appropriate to endorse the formation of plausible rather than bizarre imagery to increase the likelihood of recall in older people.

Substantial evidence shows that imagery-based mnemonics improve recall in younger adults (e.g., word lists, Roediger, 1980; face-name associations, McCarty, 1980). For older adults, positive effects of imagery have been revealed in studies of paired-associate learning (e.g., Hulicka & Grossman, 1967) and memory for face-name associations (e.g., J. A. Yesavage & Rose, 1984a). It is clear that older adults benefit as do younger adults from visual imagery as a mediator in learning and memory. Thus, the assumption has been that older people should also profit from mnemonic techniques, such as the method of loci and pegword method, that incorporate visual imagery and other procedures that improve the organization of the material to be remembered.

Method of Loci

The method of loci is a classic mnemonic technique that was first used by ancient scholars to remember their long orations. This technique involves using a well-known sequence of spatial locations to store issues in a speech, or word lists to be remembered by imagining separate items in each location. Items are recalled in the correct sequence by visualizing each location and its contents (Bower, 1970).

Ample evidence confirms the benefit of the method of loci in word list recall for college students (e.g., Groninger, 1971; Ross & Lawrence, 1968) and older adults (e.g., Anschutz, Camp, Markley, & Kramer 1985; Hill, Yesavage, Sheikh, & Friedman, 1989; J. A. Yesavage & Rose, 1984b). The size of the memory benefit, however, tends to be smaller for older adults when compared with younger persons (Kliegl, Smith, & Baltes, 1990; Lindenberger, Kliegl, & Baltes, 1992; Robertson-Tchabo, Hausman, & Arenberg, 1976; but see Rose & Yesavage, 1983). Robertson-Tchabo and colleagues (1976) also found that older people were unlikely to use the method of loci unless experimenter-prompted. Similarly, Anschutz, Camp, Markley, and Kramer (1987) found that older adults acknowledged the efficacy of the method of loci after training, but seldom used the method in everyday life.

Pegword Method

The pegword method is similar to the method of loci in that both techniques use visual imagery to enhance serial recall of word lists. The pegword method requires subjects to first memorize a sequence of number-rhyme pairs (e.g., "one is a bun, two is a shoe . . ."). The numbers (1–10) are paired with simple concrete nouns which invoke visual images that provide a "peg" for the items to be recalled. Following training on the number-rhyme pairs, subjects are told to form a complex image where each word to be recalled interacts with its corresponding pegword (e.g., "battleship in bun," see Bugelski, Kidd, & Segmen, 1968). At recall, subjects mentally reinstate the number-rhyme sequence; successive pegwords should prompt a compound image of the pegwords' referent interacting with the word to be recalled (e.g., "one is a bun" → battleship in a bun). The mnemonic efficacy of this technique is derived from both the pegword, which serves as a retrieval cue, and the numbers, which permit serially ordered recall (Paivio, 1971).

The effectiveness of the pegword mnemonic for college students is widely recognized. For example, Bugelski and colleagues (1968) found that linking the items to be remembered with the pegwords in an interactive relationship led to greater recall relative to both rhyme and standard control group conditions. Later studies show that the benefit extends to multiple list learning (e.g., Bower & Reitman, 1972; Persensky & Senter, 1970). Studies with older adults have failed to show positive effects of the pegword mnemonic on learning and memory (Mason & Smith 1977; Wood & Pratt, 1987). Consequently, the pegword method has since received scant attention in experimental aging literature (Kausler, 1994).

Improving the Effectiveness of Mnemonic Methods

Efforts to improve the effectiveness of imagery mnemonics for older adults have been made by adding various instructional sessions to the program administered prior to training on the mnemonic method. Pretraining sessions have included both cognitive (image elaboration) and noncognitive (affective judgments, relaxation training) activities that have known or assumed beneficial effects on memory (e.g., J. A. Yesavage et al., 1989). The studies summarized next show the positive effects of stimulus elaboration and confirm that pretraining generally improves the effectiveness of the mnemonic technique for older persons.

J. A. Yesavage (1983) found that training older persons in forming visual images prior to mnemonic training improved face-name recall more than that of nonspecific pretraining on improving attitudes toward aging. In a later study, J. A. Yesavage and Rose (1984b) used a semantic orienting task (pleasantness judgment) to increase elaboration of the visually imagined associations formed during training with method of loci. They found that semantic elaboration enhanced older adults' recall of list items more than did standard mnemonic instructions (see also J. A. Yesavage, Rose, & Bower, 1983). These findings replicate other studies showing a positive effect of semantic encoding tasks on memory for visual stimuli (e.g., Bower & Karlin, 1974; Smith & Winograd, 1978).

Yesavage and his associates have also examined the effects noncognitive pretraining activities on standard free recall (J. A. Yesavage, Rose, & Spiegel, 1982) and on mnemonic training efficacy (e.g., Hill, Sheikh, & Yesavage, 1989; J. A. Yesavage & Jacob, 1984). For example, J. A. Yesavage and colleagues (1982) found that progressive muscle relaxation pretraining had no effect on overall word list recall but the two variables were positively correlated. That is, relaxation improved recall for older persons with initially high state anxiety (indicated by anxiety subscale scores on the Symptom Check List 90), but impaired recall for those low in anxiety (see Yesavage & Jacob, 1984, for similar results).

Recent studies with older adults have compared the effects of different types of pretraining activities on face-name mnemonic training. Gratzinger, Sheikh, Friedman, and Yesavage (1990) compared three pretraining activities (imagery alone, imagery plus affective judgment, relaxation) given prior to instruction on a face-name mnemonic technique. Results showed that pretraining enhanced recall, relative to baseline, but no differences occurred as a function of the type of pretraining activity (see also Hill, Sheikh, *et al.,* 1989; J. Yesavage, Sheikh, Friedman, & Tanke, 1990; but see Hill, Sheikh, & Yesavage, 1988). Moreover, Sheikh, Hill, and Yesavage (1986) found that the benefit of pretraining activities was observed at immediate testing and at 6-month posttest. Together, these studies suggest that pretraining activities improve the effectiveness of face-name mnemonics and that the benefit is temporally stable (cf. Verhaeghen, Marcoen, & Gossens, 1992).

Cautionary Note

Several limitations in the use of visual imagery to promote recall in older adults warrant brief mention. First, older adults may find the formation of complex visual images difficult. This is not surprising because the encoding processes required by imagery-based techniques may exceed the processing capabilities of older people. Second, visual imagery techniques may also be anxiety-provoking for older persons, especially in the context of testing situations (see J. A. Yesavage et al., 1989). Third, visually based mnemonic techniques are complicated and often require extensive training to master. Thus, they may not be useful for cognitively impaired, older persons or those who are unwilling to participate in multiple training sessions (J. A. Yesavage et al., 1989).

Memory Interventions with Cognitively Impaired Persons

Visual Imagery

Imagery mnemonics have been used with some success in cognitive remediation programs for adults with neurological disorders (see Poon *et al.,* 1980). There is also evidence from a single case study showing that an imagery mnemonic promoted retention of face-name associations for a probable AD patient (Hill, Evankovich, Sheikh, & Yesavage, 1987). However, Bäckman, Josephsson, Herlitz, Stigsdotter, and Viitanen (1991) later found that the same imagery mnemonic enhanced face-name retention for one AD patient, but not for seven other dementia patients, suggesting that the generalizability of mnemonic effect is limited. Group studies with older adults have also revealed that the benefit of visual mnemonic methods is positively correlated with cognitive status, as indexed by scores on the Mini-Mental State Examination (Folstein, Folstein, & McHugh, 1975; see Hill, Yesavage, *et al.,* 1989; J. Yesavage *et al.,* 1990). Thus, for older persons with mild to moderate cognitive impairment, imagery mnemonics may not be suitable, because of the limited processing resources of these persons and the complexity of the mnemonic methods (Hill, Yesavage, *et al.,* 1989).

Spaced Retrieval

The spaced retrieval technique involves successive recall attempts at expanding intervals following acquisition. The technique is based on earlier research with college students in which lengthening the amount of time between recall attempts improved performance more than that of constant repetition within fixed periods of time (cf Landauer & Bjork, 1978). The mnemonic benefit of spaced retrieval for recall of simple associations has been demonstrated for persons with neurological disorders (e.g., Schacter, Rich & Stampp, 1985) and older adults with probable AD (e.g., Camp, 1989).

Camp and his associates (1989) adapted the spaced retrieval technique for use with probable AD patients. During training trials, subjects were given specific target information to remember, such as a face-name association. Immediate recall was solicited. If recall was successful, the intertrial interval was systematically expanded (e.g., 5-, 10-, 20-, and 40-second intervals, expanding in increments of 30 seconds thereafter). Following a recall failure, the intertrial interval was reduced to that of the previous trial. Using this procedure, Camp and his associates successfully increased the duration of retention of simple associations in probable AD patients from minutes to weeks after initial acquisition (see Camp & McKitrick, 1992; Kotler-Cope & Camp, 1990, for reviews). The efficacy of spaced retrieval with demented adults has been attributed to implicit memory processes, thought to be spared until the later stages of AD (e.g., Camp *et al.*, 1993). Spaced retrieval techniques may be optimal for older adults with probable AD, who would otherwise be unlikely to profit from the more cognitively demanding imagery-based mnemonic methods.

Beyond the Laboratory: Application of Memory Interventions with Older Adults

The notion that experimental mnemonic methods could be adapted for clinical use has received a fair amount of attention (see Poon, 1985). Successful application of mnemonic methods for everyday remembering is likely to depend on careful consideration of many variables, such as individual difference and task factors that may affect the outcome of mnemonic training, as discussed next.

Subject Characteristics

Whether a person will benefit from mnemonic training is an important practical issue. Many different subject factors could limit the usefulness of visually based mnemonics applied to problems of everyday memory (e.g., age, cognitive status, motivation, state anxiety, depression). Age and cognitive status have been clearly shown to influence the success of mnemonic training (e.g., J. Yesavage et al., 1990). Less cognitively demanding techniques may be more beneficial for the oldest-old (those over 85 years) and persons with probable AD. Based on the findings of Camp and his associates (1989), spaced retrieval appears to be an optimal technique for persons with probable AD.

Duration of Effects

Whether the benefit of memory training will persist over time is another important practical issue. Studies have examined the temporal stability of both specific mnemonic methods (e.g., face-name training, Sheikh *et al.*,

1986; method of loci, Anschutz et al., 1987) and general memory skills training (Neely & Bäckman, 1993a, 1993b; Scogin & Bienias, 1988; Stigsdotter & Bäckman, 1989). Some studies indicate that the benefit of memory training is observed at 6-month follow-up (Neely & Bäckman, 1993a; Sheikh et al., 1986; Stigsdotter & Bäckman, 1989). Regarding long-term maintenance of effects, the evidence has been equivocal. Scogin and Bienias (1988) found scant evidence of overall training effectiveness at 3-year follow-up (cf. Anschutz *et al.,* 1987). In contrast, Neely and Bäckman (1993b) found that performance gains in word list recall were maintained at 3½-year follow-up. That is, older adults in the training program showed greater posttest recall (relative to pretest), whereas performance did not vary across testing sessions for the nontrained control group.

Contrasting outcomes for the durability of training effects over time may be partly due to differences in subject samples and training procedures. In the Scogin and Bienias (1988) study, those in the training program had significantly more memory complaints than did the control group at both pretest and posttest. Training was also administered via self-instruction using a memory training manual (cf. Scogin, Storandt, & Lott, 1985). In contrast, Neely and Bäckman's (1993b) program used training activities similar to those of Yesavage and his associates (e.g., interactive imagery, attention and relaxation training; see Yesavage, Lapp, & Sheikh, 1989). Interestingly, in both reports, there was no evidence of transfer of training to other cognitive measures (digit span, Benton visual retention test). Thus, extensive pretraining on *task-relevant* material may be necessary to promote long-term effectiveness of memory training programs in older adults.

Summary

Whether training programs will improve older adults' memory in daily life may ultimately depend on noncognitive subject factors, such as compliance and motivation. For example, older adults may modify the mnemonic method after training or abandon it completely (Anschutz *et al.,* 1985, 1987). Neely and Bäckman (1993a) found that only 39% of their sample reported using trained mnemonic methods in everyday life at 6-month follow-up. Scogin and Bienias (1988) reported a similar rate (28%) for self-taught memory skills at 3-year follow-up. Future research is needed to identify noncognitive factors that predict success with memory interventions (Yesavage *et al.,* 1989). In short, intervention programs applied to everyday remembering should include posttraining discussion sessions to encourage older adults to use and practice the techniques they have learned, as older persons may not use these skills on their own initiative (Flynn & Storandt, 1990; Poon *et al.,* 1980).

IMPLICATIONS FOR CLINICAL PRACTICE

Experimental studies of memory aging provide a rich source of knowledge that is potentially useful for clinicians. In closing, we consider three broad implications for clinical practice that arise from the experimental evidence presented earlier.

A Priori Beliefs About Memory Aging

People of all ages hold certain assumptions about the course of memory abilities in adulthood. Culturally shared views of memory aging, as well as everyday experience, may leave older persons with the impression that memory failures in later life are comprehensive and immutable. On the basis of experimental studies of memory aging, this assumption is largely inaccurate. There are also theoretical and practical drawbacks to viewing memory in adulthood only in terms of progressive decline.

From a theoretical viewpoint, the *universal-decrementalist perspective* is incompatible with evidence showing that age-related performance differences are smaller on some cognitive tasks and larger on others (see Table 6-1). This perspective is also antithetical to current views of cognitive plasticity in adulthood (e.g., Willis, 1989). From a practical viewpoint, a decrementalist perspective may foster the opinion that compensatory strategies and intervention techniques are of limited value, which is clearly not true. The memory intervention literature provides compelling evidence of cognitive remediation for healthy older persons, and in some cases, for those with early AD. In short, negative a priori beliefs of memory competence in adulthood may thwart efforts to improve everyday remembering, as well as limit the success to memory intervention programs that are undertaken.

Examine Practical Memory Needs

Whether laboratory-based interventions are appropriately suited for meeting the everyday memory needs of older persons has prompted some debate (West, 1989). In general, very little research has examined older adults' practical memory needs (but see Leirer, Morrow, Sheikh, & Pariante, 1990). With regard to clinical practice, defining the specific aspects of memory that an older person might want to improve may be a useful starting place. Intervention techniques could then be matched to self-expressed needs. For example, in questionnaire studies of everyday memory, older adults report difficulties in learning and remembering names (e.g., Leirer *et al.,* 1990). In response to this concern, visually based mnemonic methods could be applied, as numerous laboratory studies confirm that these techniques improve recall of face-name associations (Kausler, 1994; J. A. Yesavage *et al.,* 1989). In short, successful intervention may depend on targeting everyday memory behaviors as indicated by older persons. Specificity is especially important because there is very little evidence of transfer of broad-based memory skills training to other cognitive measures (cf. Neely & Bäckman, 1993a, 1993b).

Individual Differences and Clinical Outcomes

On the basis of the research summarized previously, it is likely that individual differences contribute to clinical outcomes with older adults. For the clinician, awareness of interindividual variability is vitally important for at least two reasons. First, differences among older people are likely to influence the choice of an appropriate treatment for memory problems. As West (1989) has pointed out, memory interventions should be tailored specifically for the individual. Some older persons may benefit from visual mnemonic methods (see J. A. Yesavage *et al.,* 1989). Others may have difficulty forming visual images and would prefer verbally based techniques, for example, those that emphasize categorical organization of material to be remembered (see Kausler, 1994). External memory aids (e.g., lists, notebooks) may also be preferable to internal mnemonic methods for some older adults (see Cavanaugh *et al.,* 1983; Crovitz, 1989). External aids could be used alone or in combination with internal mnemonic strategies to improve everyday remembering.

As a second point, individual differences are likely to affect clinical outcomes. Appropriate criteria for everyday memory performance will vary from one older person to another (J. A. Yesavage *et al.,* 1989). Moreover, positive clinical outcomes may have little to do with older adults' actual memory performance. Some studies have shown no influence of mnemonic training on memory performance, but other benefits of training were observed, such as improvements in perceived control (e.g., Lachman, Weaver, Bandura, & Lewkowicz, 1992) and reduced memory complaint (e.g., Zarit, Cole, & Guider, 1981; but see Scogin & Bienias, 1988). Thus, memory intervention training may be useful only to the extent that it reduces memory concerns and depression in some older persons (Zarit, Gallagher, & Kramer, 1981).

SUMMARY

Age-related declines in memory are well documented in experimental studies with older adults. Whether age deficits will be minimal or exaggerated depends on characteristics of the memory task, the older person, and the component mental processes involved in the act of remembering. Although normal aging is associated with reduced memory efficiency, the potential for remediation and cognitive compensation should not be overlooked. As noted previously, adaptation to cognitive changes in adulthood may be critical for successful aging (see Fig. 6-1). Practicing clinicians could apply mnemonic methods or general principles of memory from the experimental aging literature to assist older persons with adaptation to cognitive changes in later life.

REFERENCES

American Psychiatric Association. (1994). *Diagnostic and statistical manual of mental disorders* (4th ed.). Washington, DC: Author.

Anschutz, L., Camp, C. J., Markley, R P., & Kramer, J. J. (1985). Maintenance and generalization of mnemonics for grocery shopping by older adults. *Experimental Aging Research, 11,* 157–160.

Anschutz, L., Camp, C. J., Markley, R. P., & Kramer, J. J. (1987). A three-year follow-up on the effects of mnemonics training in elderly adults. *Experimental Aging Research, 13,* 141–143.

Babcock, R. L., & Salthouse, T. A. (1990). Effects of increased processing demands on age differences in working memory. *Psychology and Aging, 5,* 421–428.

Bäckman, L., Mantila, T., & Herlitz, A. (1990). The optimization of episodic remembering in old age. In P. B. Baltes & M. M. Baltes (Eds.), *Successful aging: Perspectives from the behavioral sciences* (pp. 118–163). New York: Cambridge University Press.

Bäckman, L., Josephsson, S., Herlitz, A., Stigsdotter, A., & Viitanen, M. (1991). The generalizability of training gains in dementia: Effects of an imagery-based mnemonic on face-name retention duration. *Psychology and Aging, 6,* 489–492.

Baltes, P. B., & Baltes, M. M. (1990). Psychological perspectives on successful aging: The model of selective optimization with compensation. In P. B. Baltes and M. M. Baltes (Eds.), *Successful aging: Perspectives from the behavioral sciences* (pp. 1–34). Cambridge: Cambridge University Press.

Bartlett, J. C., Leslie, J. E., Tubbs, A., & Fulton, A. (1989). Aging and memory of faces. *Psychology and Aging, 4,* 276–283.

Bellezza, F. S. (1982). *Improve your memory skills.* Englewood Cliffs, NJ: Prentice-Hall.

Bezan, T. (1974). *Use your perfect memory.* New York: Dutton.

Blazer, D., Hughes, D. C., & George, L. K. (1987). The epidemiology of depression in an elderly community sample. *Gerontologist, 27,* 281–287.

Bower, G. H. (1970). Analysis of a mnemonic device. *American Scientist, 58,* 496–510.

Bower, G. H. (1972). Mental imagery and associative learning. In L. Gregg (Ed.), *Cognition in learning and memory* (pp. 51–88). New York: Wiley.

Bower, G. H., & Karlin, M. B. (1974). Depth of processing pictures of faces and recognition memory. *Journal of Experimental Psychology, 103,* 751–757.

Bower, G. H., & Reitman, J. S. (1972). Mnemonic elaboration in multi-list learning. *Journal of Verbal Learning and Verbal Behavior, 11,* 478–485.

Bugelski, B. R., Kidd, E., & Segmen, J. (1968). Image as a mediator in one-trial paired-associate learning. *Journal of Experimental Psychology, 76,* 69–73.

Camp, C. J. (1989). Facilitation of new learning in Alzheimer's disease. In G. C. Gilmore, P. Whitehouse, & M. Wylke (Eds.), *Memory and Aging: Theory, research and practice* (pp. 212–225). New York: Springer.

Camp, C. J., & McKitrick, L. A. (1992). Memory interventions in Alzheimer's-type dementia populations: Methodological and theoretical issues. In R. L. West & J. D. Sinnott (Eds.), *Everyday memory and aging: Current research and methodology* (pp. 155–172). New York: Springer-Verlag.

Camp, C. J., Foss, J. W., Stevens, A. B., Reichard, C. C., McKitrick, L. A., & O'Hanlon, A. M. (1993). Memory training in normal and demented elderly populations: The E-I-E-I-O model. *Experimental Aging Research, 19,* 277–290.

Cavanaugh, J. C., Grady, J. G., & Perlmutter, M. (1983). Forgetting and use of memory aids in 20 to 70 year olds in everyday life. *International Journal of Aging and Human Development, 17,* 113–122.

Charness, N., & Bosman, E. A. (1990). Expertise and aging: Life in the lab. In T. M. Hess (Ed.), *Aging and cognition: Knowledge, organization, and utilization* (pp. 343–385). San Diego: Academic.

Cherry, K. E., & Morton, M. R. (1989). Drug sensitivity in older adults: The role of physiologic and pharmacokinetic factors. *International Journal of Aging and Human Development, 23,* 159–174.

Cherry, K. E., & Plauche, M. F. (1996). Memory impairment in Alzheimer's disease: Findings, interventions, and implications. *Journal of Clinical Geropsychology, 2,* 263–296.

Cohen, R. L., Sandler, S. P., & Schroeder, K. (1987). Aging and memory for words and action events: Effects of item repetition and list length. *Psychology and Aging, 2,* 280–285.

Craik, F. I. M. (1986). A functional account of age differences in memory. In F. Klix & H. Hagendorf (Eds.), *Human memory and cognitive capabilities, mechanisms, and performance* (pp. 409–422). Amsterdam: Elsevier Science.

Craik, F. I. M., & Jennings, J. M., (1992). Human memory. In F. I. M. Craik & T. A. Salthouse (Eds.), *The handbook of aging and cognition* (pp. 51–110). Hillsdale, NJ: Erlbaum.

Craik, F. I. M., & McDowd, J. M. (1987). Age differences in recall and recognition. *Journal of Experimental Psychology: Learning, Memory, and Cognition, 13,* 474–479.

Crook, T., & Larrabee, C. J. (1988). Age-associated memory impairment: Diagnostic criteria and treatment strategies. *Psychopharmacology Bulletin, 24,* 509–514.

Crook, T., Bartus, R., Ferris, S. H., Whitehouse, P., Cohen, G., & Gershon, S. (1986). Age-associated memory impairment: Proposed diagnostic criteria and measures of clinical change—Report of a National Institute of Mental Health work group. *Developmental Neuropsychology, 2,* 261–276.

Crovitz, H. F. (1989). Memory retraining: Everyday needs and future prospects. In L. W. Poon, D. C. Rubin, & B. A. Wilson (Eds.), *Everyday cognition in adulthood and late life* (pp. 681–691). New York: Cambridge University Press.

Dixon, R. A. (1989). Questionnaire research on metamemory and aging: Issues of structure and function. In L. W. Poon, D. C. Robin, & B. A. Wilson (Eds.), *Everyday cognition in adulthood and late life* (pp. 394–681). New York: Cambridge University Press.

Dobbs, A. R., & Rule, B. G. (1989). Adult age differences in working memory. *Psychology and Aging, 4,* 500–503.

Drevenstedt, J., & Bellezza, F. S. (1993). Memory for self-generated narration in the elderly. *Psychology and Aging,* 187–196.

Flynn, T. M., & Storandt, M. (1990). Supplemental group discussions in memory training for older adults. *Psychology and Aging, 5,* 178–181.

Folstein, M. F., Folstein, S. E., & McHugh, P. H. (1975). Mini-Mental State: A practical method for grading the cognitive state of patients for the clinician. *Journal of Psychiatric Research, 12,* 189–198.

Gilewski, M. J., & Zelinski, E. M. (1986). Questionnaire assessment of memory complaints. In L. W. Poon, T. Crook, K. L. Davis, C. Eisdorfer, B. J. Gurland, A. W. Kaszniak, & L. W. Thompson (Eds.), *Handbook for clinical memory assessment of older adults* (pp. 93–107). Washington, DC: American Psychological Association.

Gratzinger, P., Sheikh, J. I., Friedman, L., & Yesavage, J. A. (1990). Cognitive interventions to improve face-name recall: The role of personality differences. *Developmental Psychology, 26,* 889–893.

Groninger, L. C. (1971). Mnemonic imagery and forgetting. *Psychonomic Science, 23,* 161–163.

Haase, G. R. (1971). Diseases presenting as dementia. In C. E. Wells (Ed.), *Dementia* (pp. 163–207). Philadelphia: Davis.

Hartley, J. T., & Walsh, D. A. (1980). The effect of monetary incentive on amount and rate of free recall in older and younger adults. *Journal of Gerontology, 35,* 899–905.

Hasher, L., & Zacks, R. T. (1979). Automatic and effortful processes in memory. *Journal of Experimental Psychology: General. 108,* 356–388.

Hertzog, C., Hultsch D. F., & Dixon, R. A. (1989). Evidence for the convergent validity of two self-report metamemory questionnaires. *Developmental Psychology, 25,* 687–700.

Hill, R. D., Evankovich, K. D., Sheikh, J. I., & Yesavage, J. (1987). Imagery mnemonic training in a patient with primary degenerative dementia. *Psychology and Aging, 2,* 204–205.

Hill, R. D., Sheikh, J. I., & Yesavage, J. (1988). The effect of mnemonic training on perceived recall confidence in the elderly. *Experimental Aging Research, 13,* 185–188.

Hill, R. D., Sheikh, J. I., & Yesavage, J. (1989). Pretraining enhances mnemonic training in elderly adults. *Experimental Aging Research, 14,* 207–211.

Hill, R. D., Yesavage, J. A., Sheikh, J., & Friedman, L. (1989). Mental status as a predictor of response to memory training in older adults. *Educational Gerontology, 15,* 633–639.

Hill, R. D., Allen, C., & McWhorter, P. (1991). Stories as a mnemonic aid for older learners. *Psychology and Aging, 6,* 484–486.

Howard, D. (1996). The aging of implicit and explicit memory. In F. Blanchard-Fields & T. M. Hess (Eds.), *Perspectives on cognitive change in adulthood and aging* (pp. 221–254). New York: McGraw-Hill.

Hulicka, I. M., & Grossman, J. L. (1967). Age group comparisons for the use of mediators in paired-associate learning. *Journal of Gerontology, 22,* 46–51.

Hultsch, D. F., Hertzog, C., & Dixon, R. A. (1990). Ability correlates of memory performance in adulthood and aging. *Psychology and Aging, 5,* 356–368.

Hultsch, D. F., Masson, M., & Small, R. A. (1991). Adult age differences in direct and indirect tests of memory. *Journals of Gerontology: Psychological Sciences, 46,* P22–P30.

Jarvik, L. F. (1980). Diagnosis of dementia in the elderly: A 1980 perspective. *Annual Review of Gerontology and Geriatrics, 1,* 180–203.

Kahn, H. L., Zarit, S. H., Hilbert, N. M., & Niederehe, G. A. (1975). Memory complaint and impairment in the aged: The effect of depression and altered brain function. *Archives of General Psychiatry, 32,* 1560–1573.

Kaufman, A. S., Reynolds, C. R., & McLean, J. E. (1989). Age and WAIS-R intelligence in a national sample of adults in the 20 to 74-year age range: A cross-sectional study. *Intelligence, 13,* 235–253.

Kausler, D. H. (1994). *Learning and memory in normal aging.* San Diego, CA: Academic.

Kliegl, R., Smith, J., & Baltes, P. B. (1990). On the locus of magnification of age differences during mnemonic training. *Developmental Psychology, 26,* 894–904.

Kotler-Cope, S., & Camp, C. J. (1990). Memory interventions in aging populations. In E. A. Lovelace (Ed.), *Aging and cognition: Mental processes. self-awareness and interventions* (pp. 231–261). Amsterdam: Elsevier Science.

Kroll, N. E. A., Schepeler, E. M., & Angin, K. T. (1986). Bizarre imagery: The misremembered mnemonic. *Journal of Experimental Psychology: Learning, Memory and Cognition, 12,* 42–53.

Lachman, M. E., Weaver, S. L., Bandura, E., & Lewkowicz, C. J. (1992). Improving memory and control beliefs through cognitive restructuring and self-generated strategies. *Journal of Gerontology: Psychological Sciences, 47,* P293–299.

Lamberty, G. J., & Bieliauskas, L. A. (1993). Distinguishing between depression and dementia in the elderly: A review of neuropsychological findings. *Archives of Clinical Neuropsychology, 8,* 149–170.

Landauer, T. K., & Bjork, R. A. (1978). Optimum rehearsal patterns and name learning. In M. M. Gruneberg, P. E. Morris, & R. N. Sykes (Eds.), *Practical aspects of memory* (pp. 625–632). New York: Academic.

Larrabee, G. J., & Levin, H. S. (1986). Memory self-ratings and objective test performance in a normal elderly sample. *Journal of Clinical and Experimental, Neuropsychology, 8,* 275–284.

Leirer, V. O., Morrow, D. G., Sheikh, J. I., & Pariante, G. (1990). Memory skills elders want to improve. *Experimental Aging Research, 17,* 155–158.

Light, L. L. (1991). Memory and aging: Four hypotheses in search of data. *Annual Review of Psychology, 42,* 333–376.

Light, L. L. (1992). The organization of memory in old age. In F. I. M. Craik & T. A. Salthouse (Eds.), *The handbook of cognition and aging* (pp. 111–165). Hillsdale, NJ: Erlbaum.

Lindenberger, U., Kliegl, R., & Baltes, P. B. (1992). Professional expertise does not eliminate age differences in imagery-based memory performance during adulthood. *Psychology and Aging, 7,* 585–593.

Lipman, P. D., & Caplan, L. J. (1992). Adult age differences in memory for routes: Effects of instruction and spatial diagram. *Psychology and Aging, 7,* 435–442.

Lorayne, H., & Lucas, J. (1974). *The memory book.* New York: Stein and Day.

Mason, S. E., & Smith, A. D. (1977). Imagery in the aged. *Experimental Aging Research, 3,* 17–32.

McCarty, D. L. (1980). Investigation of a visual imagery mnemonic device for acquiring face-name associations. *Journal of Experimental Psychology: Human Learning and Memory, 6,* 145–155.

McDaniel, M. A., & Einstein, G. O. (1986). Bizarre imagery as an effective memory aid: The importance of distinctiveness. *Journal of Experimental Psychology: Learning, Memory, and Cognition, 12,* 54–65.

Nebes, R. D. (1992). Cognitive dysfunction in Alzheimer's disease. In F. I. M. Craik & T. A. Salthouse (Eds.), *The handbook of aging and cognition* (pp. 373–446). Hillsdale, NJ: Erlbaum.

Neely, A. S., & Bäckman, L. (1993a). Maintenance of gains following multifactorial and unifactorial memory training in late adulthood. *Educational Gerontology, 19,* 105–117.

Neely, A. S., & Bäckman, L. (1993b). Long-term maintenance of gains from memory training in older adults: Two $3^1/_2$ year follow-up studies. *Journal of Gerontology: Psychological Sciences, 48,* P233–P237.

Ouslander, J. G. (1981). Drug therapy in the elderly. *Annals of Internal Medicine, 95,* 711–722.

Ouslander, J. G. (1982). Illness and psychopathology in the elderly. In L. F. Jarvik & G. W. Small (Eds.), *Psychiatric clinics of North America* (pp. 145–158). Philadelphia: Saunders.

Paivio, A. (1971). *Imagery and verbal processes.* New York: Rinehart and Winston.

Park, D. C. (1992). Applied cognitive aging research. In F. I. M. Craik and T. A. Salthouse (Eds.), *The handbook of aging and cognition* (pp. 449–493). Hillsdale, NJ: Erlbaum.

Park, D. C., Puglisi, J. T., & Smith, A. D. (1986). Memory for pictures: Does an age-related decline exist? *Psychology and Aging, 1,* 11–17.

Park, D. C., Smith, A. D., Morrell, R. W., Puglisi, J. T., & Dudley, W. N. (1990). Effects of contextual integration in recall of pictures by older adults. *Journals of Gerontology: Psychological Sciences, 45,* P52–P57.

Park, D. C., Smith, A. D., Lautenschlager, G., Earles, J. L., Frieske, D., Zwahr, M., & Gaines, C. (1996). Mediators of long-term memory performance across the life span. *Psychology and Aging, 11,* 621–637.

Perlmutter, M., & Mitchell, D. B. (1982). The appearance and disappearance of age differences in adult memory. In F. I. M. Craik & S. Trehub (Eds.), *Aging and cognitive processes* (pp. 127–144). New York: Plenum.

Perlmutter, M., & Nyquist, L. (1990). Relationships between self-reported physical and mental health and intelligence performance across adulthood. *Journals of Gerontology: Psychological Sciences, 45,* P145–P155.

Persensky, J. J., & Senter, R. J. (1970). An investigation of "bizarre" imagery as a mnemonic device. *Psychological Record, 20,* 145–150.

Poon, L. W. (1985). Differences in human memory with aging: Nature, causes, and clinical implications. In J. E. Bitten & K. W. Schaie (Eds.), *Handbook of the psychology of aging* (2nd ed., pp. 427–462). New York: Van Nostrand Reinhold.

Poon, L. W., Walsh-Sweeney, L., & Fozard, J. L. (1980). Memory skill training for the elderly: Salient issues on the use of imagery mnemonics. In L. W. Poon, J. L. Fozard, L. S. Cermak, D. S. Arenberg, & L. W. Thompson (Eds.), *New directions in memory and aging: Proceedings of the George Talland memorial conference* (pp. 461–484). Hillsdale, NJ: Erlbaum.

Poon, L. W., Crook, T. Davis, K. L., Eisdorfer, C., Gurland, B. J., Kaszniak, A. W., & Thompson, L. W. (1986), *Handbook for clinical memory assessment of older adults.* Washington, DC: American Psychological Association.

Popkin, S. J., Gallagher, D., Thompson, L. W., & Moore, M. (1982). Memory complaint and performance in normal and depressed older adults. *Experimental Aging Research, 8,* 141–145.

Powell, D. H. (1994). *Profiles in cognitive aging.* Cambridge, MA: Harvard University Press.

Puglisi, J. T., & Park, D. C. (1987). Perceptual elaboration and memory in older adults. *Journal of Gerontology, 42,* 160–162.

Raskind, M. A., & Peskind, E. R. (1992). Alzheimer's disease and other dementing disorders. In J. E. Birren, R. B. Sloane, & G. D. Cohen, *Handbook of mental health and aging* (2nd ed., pp. 478–513). New York: Academic.

Reisberg, B. Ferris, S. H., deLeon, M. J., Crook, T., & Haynes, N. (1987). Senile dementia of the Alzheimer's type. In M. Bergener (Ed.), *Psychogenatrics: An international handbook* (pp. 306–334). New York: Springer.

Robertson-Tchabo, E. A., Hausman, C. P., & Arenberg, D. (1976). A classical mnemonic for older learners: A trip that works. *Educational Gerontology, 1,* 215–226.

Roediger, H. L. (1980). The effectiveness of four mnemonics in ordering recall. *Journal of Experimental Psychology: Human Learning and Memory. 6,* 558–567.

Rose, T. L., & Yesavage, J. A. (1983). Differential effects of a list-learning mnemonic in three age groups. *Gerontology, 29,* 293–293.

Ross, J., & Lawrence, K. A. (1968). Some observations on memory artifice. *Psychonomic Science, 13,* 107–108.

Roth, D. M. (1961). *Roth memory course.* New Jersey: Wehman.

Salthouse, T. A. (1984). Effect of age and skill in typing. *Journal of Experimental Psychology, General, 13,* 345–371.

Salthouse, T. A. (1991). *Theoretical perspectives on cognitive aging.* Hillsdale, NJ: Erlbaum.

Salthouse, T. A. (1992). *Mechanisms of age-cognition relations in adulthood.* Hillsdale, NJ: Erlbaum.

Salthouse, T. A. (1993). Influence of working memory on adult age differences in matrix reasoning. *British Journal of Psychology, 84,* 171–199.

Salthouse, T. A. (1994). The nature of the influence of speed on adult age differences in cognition. *Developmental Psychology, 30,* 240–259.

Salthouse, T. A., Kausler, D. H., & Saults, J. S. (1990). Age, self-assessed health status, and cognition. *Journals of Gerontology: Psychological Sciences, 45,* P156–P160.

Schacter, D. L., Rich, S. A., & Stampp, M. S. (1985). Remediation of memory disorders: Experimental evaluation of the spaced-retrieval technique. *Journal of Clinical and Experimental Neuropsychology, 7,* 79–96.

Scogin, F. R., & Bienias, J. L. (1988). A three-year follow-up of older adult participants in a memory-skills training program. *Psychology and Aging, 3,* 334–337.

Scogin, F. R., Storandt, M., & Lott, L. (1985). Memory-skills training, memory complaints, and depression in older adults. *Journal of Gerontology, 40,* 562–568.

Sheikh, J. I., Hill, R. D., & Yesavage, J. A. (1986). Long-term efficacy of cognitive training for age-associated memory impairment: A six-month follow-up study. *Developmental Neuropsychology, 2,* 413–421.

Smith, A. D. (1996). Memory. In. J. E. Birren & K. W. Schaie (Eds.), *Handbook of the psychology of aging* (4th ed., pp. 236–250). San Diego, CA: Academic.

Smith, A. D., & Earles, J. L. K. (1996). Memory changes in normal aging. In F. Blanchard-Fields & T. M. Hess (Eds.), *Perspectives on cognitive change in adulthood and aging* (pp. 192–220). New York: McGraw-Hill.

Smith, A. D., & Winograd, E. (1978). Adult age differences in remembering faces. *Developmental Psychology, 14,* 443–444.

Smith, A. D., Park, D. C., Cherry, K. E., & Berkovsky, K. (1990). Age differences in memory for concrete and abstract pictures. *Journals of Gerontology: Psychological Sciences, 45,* P205–P209.

Stigsdotter, A., & Bäckman, L., (1989). Multifactorial memory training with older adults: How to foster maintenance of improved performance. *Gerontology, 35,* 260–267.

Terry, L., & Wagner, A. (1992). Alzheimer's disease and depression. *Journal of Consulting and Clinical Psychology, 60,* 379–391.

Verhaeghen, P., Marcoen, A., & Gossens, L. (1992). Improving memory performance in the aged through mnemonic training: A meta-analytic study. *Psychology and Aging, 7,* 242–251.

Vestal, R. F. (1978). Drug use in the elderly: A review of problems and special considerations. *Drugs, 16,* 358–382.

West, R. L. (1989). Planning practical memory training for the aged. In L. W. Poon, D. C. Rubin, & B. A. Wilson (Eds.), *Everyday cognition in adulthood and late life* (pp. 573–597). New York: Cambridge University Press

West, R. L., Crook, T. H., & Barron, K. L. (1992). Everyday memory performance across the life span: Effects of age and noncognitive individual differences. *Psychology and Aging, 7,* 72–82.

Willis, S. L. (1989). Improvement with cognitive training: Which old dogs learn what tricks? In L. W. Poon, D. C. Rubin, & B. A. Wilson (Eds.), *Everyday cognition in adulthood and late life* (pp. 545–569). New York: Cambridge University Press.

Wingfield, A., Stine, E. A. L., Lahar, C. J., & Aberdeen, J. S. (1988). Does the capacity of working memory change with age? *Experimental Aging Research, 14,* 103–107.

Wood, I. E., & Pratt, J. D. (1987). Pegword mnemonic as an aid to memory in the elderly: A comparison of four age groups. *Educational Gerontology, 13,* 325–339.

Yesavage, J., Sheikh, J. I., Friedman, L., & Tanke, E. (1990). Learning mnemonics: Roles of aging and subtle cognitive impairment. *Psychology and Aging, 5,* 133–137.

Yesavage, J. A. (1983). Imagery pretraining and memory training in the elderly. *Gerontology, 29,* 271–275.

Yesavage, J. A., & Jacob, R. (1984). Effects of relaxation and mnemonics on memory attention and anxiety in the elderly. *Experimental Aging Research, 10,* 211–214.

Yesavage, J. A., & Rose, T. L. (1984a). The effects of a face-name mnemonics in young, middle-aged, and elderly adults. *Experimental Aging Research, 10,* 55–57.

Yesavage, J. A., & Rose, T. L. (1984b). Semantic elaboration and the method of loci: A new trip for older learners. *Experimental Aging Research, 10,* 155–159.

Yesavage, J. A., Rose, T. L., & Spiegel, D. (1982). Relaxation training and memory improvement in elderly normals: Correlation of anxiety ratings and recall improvement. *Experimental Aging Research, 8,* 195–198.

Yesavage, J. A., Rose, T. L., & Bower, G. H. (1983). Interactive imagery and affective judgments improve face-name learning in the elderly. *Journal of Gerontology, 38,* 197–203.

Yesavage, J. A., Lapp, D., & Sheikh, J. I. (1989). Mnemonics as modified for use by the elderly. In L. W. Poon, D. C. Rubin, & B. A. Wilson (Eds.), *Everyday cognition in adulthood and late life* (pp. 598–611). New York: Cambridge University Press.

Zarit, S. H., Cole, K. D., & Guider, R. L. (1981). Memory training strategies and subjective complaints of memory in the aged. *The Gerontologist, 21,* 158–164.

Zarit, S. H., Gallagher, D., & Kramer, N. (1981). Memory training in the community aged: Effects of depression, memory complaint, and memory performance. *Educational Gerontology, 6,* 11–27.

Zivian, M. T., & Darjes, R. W. (1983). Free recall by in-school and out-of-school adults: Performance and metamemory. *Developmental Psvchology, 19,* 513–520.

PART II

PSYCHOPATHOLOGY, ASSESSMENT, AND TREATMENT

CHAPTER 7

Dementia

CHARLES J. GOLDEN AND
ANTONIA CHRONOPOLOUS

INTRODUCTION

Dementias were first recognized as a diagnostic issue during the 1800s and have
become a major topic only within the last half century. As the population has
aged, concern over the dementias has increased because of their higher incidence and the increased sensitivity in medical and mental health circles in recognizing the symptoms of these disorders. Kraepelin (1896) saw dementia as a
disease of aging; later versions of his work recognized the writings of Alzheimer
(1898) and others who identified the presence of presenile dementias. Over
time, there has been increased attention to multiple etiologies and alternative
methods of presentation.

The dementias refer to a wide variety of disorders which are characterized
by memory problems along with at least one other cognitive problem. Dementias may vary widely in terms of severity, course, nature of the symptoms, and
etiology. Dementias may or may not be progressive, and vary in terms of treatment, although they are characterized by irreversible declines in cognitive function. Age of onset may be at any time, but most dementias occur in the second
half of the life span.

Skoog, Nilsson, Palmertz, Andreasson, and Svanborg (1993) surveyed a
sample of 494, 85-year-old Swedes to determine relative incidence of dementia
in a nonselected population. The investigators, using a wide variety of diagnostic techniques, identified dementia in nearly 30% of their sample. Slightly
more than one fourth of these subjects had mild dementia, while the remainder were divided between mild and moderate dementia.

Several classification systems of the dementias have been employed. Current classification systems recognize the dementias on the basis of the areas of

CHARLES J. GOLDEN AND ANTONIA CHRONOPOLOUS • Center for Psychological Studies, Nova Southeastern University, Fort Lauderdale, Florida 33314.

Handbook of Clinical Geropsychology, edited by Michel Hersen and Vincent B. Van Hasselt.
Plenum Press, New York, 1998.

the brain involved, or by etiology. For example, Gustafson (1992) classified dementias into frontotemporal, temporoparietal, subcortical, or other types. Gottfries (1991) separated the dementias into idiopathic dementias (in which dementia is the primary symptom of the disorder), vascular dementias, and secondary dementias (caused by trauma or substance abuse).

The Diagnostic and Statistical Manual of Mental Disorders, 4th edition (*DSM-IV*; American Psychiatric Association, 1994) classified dementias in terms of their specific etiologies: Dementia of the Alzheimer Type, Vascular Dementia, Dementia due to HIV Disease, Dementia due to Head Trauma, Dementia due to Parkinson's Disease, Dementia due to Huntington's Disease, Dementia due to Creutzfeldt–Jakob Disease, Dementia due to General Medical Conditions, Substance Induced Persisting Dementia, Dementia due to Multiple Etiologies, and Dementia Not Otherwise Specified (NOS).

Dementia-like symptoms may be seen in disorders classified as delirium. A delirium may have similar symptoms, but the disorder is generally more variable and the symptoms increase and decrease. While most cases of delirium are time limited, especially when the etiology is recognized, this is not always the case. Conversely, the symptoms in dementia are more stable or reflect deteriorating skills. However, some cases of dementia may be found to be treatable and the symptoms may remit despite the fact that one may associate the word dementia with the concept of irreversibility. Some disorders are initially classified as deliriums, but are later found to be dementias, and disorders initially seen as dementias may later be found to be cases of delirium.

DEFINITION

Regardless of etiology, all dementias are characterized by a primary loss in memory functions. Without this essential feature, no set of symptoms, regardless of severity, can be classified as a dementia. However, in addition to the symptoms of memory disturbance, there must be at least one other cognitive symptom. This may be a disorder of language, a disorder of spatial skills, a disorder of social judgment, or a disorder of executive functions of the brain.

Memory Symptoms

The most obvious of the memory symptoms is the loss of the ability to learn new material. This generally occurs early in the disorder and may be the first symptom to become evident. In individuals with extensive previous learning, this symptom may be masked as the individual may substitute previously learned knowledge for the information one wishes the person to learn. In individuals with less previous knowledge, the loss of new learning may be more evident although it may be mistaken in some cases for a generalized preexisting slowness in learning.

Other cases may report loss of long-term, preexisting memories as well, although there is some disagreement in this area; this loss is rare in mild cases. Individuals may be unable to produce specific memories on command at a specific time, but often later can relate the "forgotten" memory. In early cases, losses are rarely seen in short-term memory, in which the individual cannot retain information for several seconds or maintain a short conversation. However, losses in these areas may be quite striking in more severe cases.

Related Cognitive Disorders

Related cognitive disorders may fall into many categories. Patients may show a loss of verbal skills. These can cover a wide range of disorders: loss of naming skills, problems in grammar, loss of oral language, inability to understand language, disorders of reading, reading comprehension, writing, spelling, or arithmetic, word substitution, verbal confusion, fluent aphasias, dysfluent aphasia, and any other symptom complex seen with verbal skills.

Disorders may also be nonverbal in nature. This can include difficulty drawing simple or complex figures, difficulty with spatial relationships, problems in map reading and finding one's way around new or even familiar neighborhoods, difficulty in recognizing or maintaining sequences, problems with facial recognition, figure or background distortions, difficulties in telling time, problems in recognizing the passage of time, difficulty in recognizing nonverbal sounds (e.g., the sound of a train), and problems in expressing or recognizing emotions.

Other disorders may include inflexibility, an inability to solve problems, poor judgment, impulsivity, poor attention and concentration, inappropriateness, aggressiveness, irritability, improper social behavior, and hyper- or hypo-emotionality. Across disorders, any problem which can be caused by brain damage will be seen in some cases of dementia.

Laboratory Findings

Each type of dementia is characterized by specific laboratory findings, although there is at present only a mild to moderate relationship between the laboratory findings and the behavioral symptoms as outlined above. In many cases, absolute neuropathological identification requires an autopsy. Even with a typical autopsy exact identification of the presence of a dementing disorder or a specific dementing disorder is questionable. Alafuzoff (1992; Alafuzoff, Ronnberg, & Asikainen-Gustafsson, 1991) found a lack of correspondence between neuropathological findings and clinical findings of dementia that they blamed partially on autopsy techniques.

TYPES OF DEMENTIA

There are several systems for classifying the dementias. However, since *DSM-IV* remains the basic nomenclature in the United States, we use that classification system to structure this chapter.

Alzheimer's Disease

Alzheimer's disease (AD) represents the most common form of dementia. Skoog and colleagues (1993) identified 43% of their general dementia sample with this disorder. Precise numbers are difficult because of the problems in diagnosis without a detailed autopsy. Alzheimer's disease is characterized by severe memory disorders, loss of smell, and a wide variety of cognitive problems. Onset may be at a relatively young age (less than 50 years) or at any time thereafter. The progress of the disease may be very short or may last over a decade from the time the disorder is first diagnosed.

Alafuzoff (1992) describes the pathological changes in AD as primarily microscopic lesions in the brain including neurotic plaques and neurofibrillary changes (tangles) within clusters of nerve cells. These are accompanied by selective loss of neurons, neuronal atrophy, and the accumulations of granules between cell bodies. The plaques have a central amyloid core and other distinct neuropathological characteristics.

In his review, Edwards (1993) suggested that the most serious problems in AD are found in the temporal lobe in the hippocampus and the amygdala. Although some theorists have suggested that the problems in AD are related only to changes in cholinergic pathways, Holttum and Gershon (1992) rejected a unitary cholinergic theory. They suggested that approaches that transcend single neurotransmitter systems are necessary to explain the disorder. Some research demonstrates that AD may be related to a genetic predisposition (e.g., Jarvik, 1992).

The definitive diagnosis for AD must come from neuropathological evidence. However, such evidence is rarely available until after the death of the patient. Thus, diagnosis often comes through ruling out other causes, such as vascular dementia, rather than from a definitive constellation of symptoms that differentiates AD from other dementias. To be considered AD, there must be a gradual onset of symptoms without evidence of focal damage associated with vascular dementia or the specific features associated with other dementias. In addition, AD tends to show more symptoms over time associated with the temporoparietal areas of the brain (e.g., language problems, visual spatial difficulties, naming problems) than do other gradual dementias such as Pick's disease.

Because the presentation of AD may vary quite widely in clinical samples, there has been speculation that there may be subtypes of the disorder or even different diseases being grouped together erroneously. Although some misclassification certainly takes place because of the unavailability of a definitive diagnostic procedure, at present there is no evidence of different subtypes of AD but rather differences in presentation which depend on such factors as premorbid status, age at onset, and the overall rate of degeneration (Kurz, Haupt, Pollmann, & Romero, 1992).

Vascular Dementia

Along with Alzheimer's, this is the most common cause of dementia currently identified. Vascular dementias are characterized by the presence of cerebrovascular disease. Vascular dementia can arise from one major infarction, occlusion, cerebral hemorrhage, or from a series of vascular problems that may develop over many years. The initial symptoms vary considerably depending on the location of the vascular lesion and other related neurological factors. Unlike cases of AD, individuals with vascular dementia will often show focal neurological signs and clear areas of injury on MRI or CT scan. However, in milder cases, such tests may appear normal especially when it is the result of many small focal injuries rather than one or more larger injuries.

The wide variety of presentations possible make clear criteria difficult. Roman and colleagues (1993) developed a series of research diagnostic criteria for this disorder. They identified a series of different lesions which may be associated with the problem. Most common is multi-infarct dementia, in which there are multiple large vessel infarcts involving both cortical and subcortical areas. MRI and CT scans are typically quite abnormal in this subtype. Multi-infarct dementia may also arise from a series of small strokes that may be mistaken for Transient Ischemic Attacks (TIA) that leave no residual deficits. In these cases, the amount of damage done each time is slight and difficult to see, but the accumulating damage over time leads to dementia.

A second type of dementia arises from single infarcts which produce small, localized damage in an important part of the brain and may produce well-defined and striking forms of dementia. For example, infarcts within the left angular gyrus may produce a fluent aphasia in which the motor production of words is maintained, but their meaning or understanding may be lost. The most extreme forms of this are jargon aphasia in which the person speaks fluently but makes no sense whatsoever, or receptive aphasia in which the person is unable to understand spoken or written communications.

Infarcts of the posterior cerebral artery may present with visual field loss, visual hallucinations, agitation, confusion, and memory loss. Injuries to the anterior cerebral artery may result in a loss of initiative, inability to locate memories, agitation, irritability, and emotional liability. Middle cerebral artery infarcts can result in aphasia, irritability, spatial losses, paranoia, confusion, and impairment in all basic achievement skills. Lesions in subcortical areas may result in thalamic dementia, with severe memory loss and confusion, or disorders in which new memories are completely lost while leaving old memories intact (bilateral hippocampal lesions).

Another major subtype is small vessel disease in which blood flow is maintained within the large vessels but not within the smaller vessels. This may cause subcortical or cortical symptoms in which onset may appear to be gradual and more like AD than the more sudden or clearly stepwise deficits seen in other forms of vascular dementia. This disorder may cause small lacunar infarcts in the brain which can be detected on MRI. However, the presence of such small areas of dysfunction do not always correlate with behavioral or cognitive impairment. The deficits from this disorder may include personality change, difficulty with complex executive tasks (also as seen in Pick's disease), and diffuse memory problems. More focal and definitive cognitive signs, as seen in other forms of vascular dementia, are rare in this disorder.

Another important form of vascular dementia arises from cerebral hypoxic events. These result in a loss of oxygen to the brain secondary to the inability of the heart and lungs to provide enough oxygen to the brain, or the inability of the oxygen to reach areas of the brain due to edema or other restrictive factors. It is well known that brain damage arises quickly from a complete loss of oxygen to the brain (anoxia); partial losses of oxygen (hypoxia) can also cause damage although over longer and more indeterminate periods of time. These deficits tend to be diffuse and less focal, sometimes mimicking small vessel disease as well as dementias caused by substance abuse and poisoning.

Diagnosis of vascular dementia may be clear from CT scan or MRI studies. In addition, measures of blood flow may be used to show areas of the brain with little or no circulation even when the areas look normal on tests that show only structure. The presence of clearly abnormal findings on these tests can usually be considered diagnostic if the required memory and cognitive disorders can be demonstrated with neuropsychological tests. As noted earlier, routine neurological testing may also show clear signs of a possible disorder.

It should be noted that the various forms of vascular dementia can occur simultaneously in one person, or in conjunction with other forms of dementia.

Dementia Due to General Medical Condition

In *DSM-IV,* this diagnosis includes a wide range of subtypes in which the symptoms of a dementia can be demonstrated along with clear medical and historical information that the dementia is related to the medical condition. Each of these disorders has its own clear diagnostic requirements based on history, symptoms, and laboratory findings.

HIV

This is a relatively new and increasingly diagnosed form of dementia seen in both younger and older populations. HIV (human immunodeficiency virus) is transmitted between individuals primarily as the result of sexual contact or other forms of bodily fluid exchange including the use of contaminated needles or from contaminated blood. HIV attacks the human immune system, and is found throughout the body. Berg, Franzen, and Wedding (1994) reported that upon autopsy, pathological involvement of the brain is seen in more than 75% of all patients. In addition, the virus's attack on the immune system allows numerous opportunistic infections to attack the body, including the brain. These factors may result in a subcortical dementia characterized by memory loss, confusion, personality change, and impairment in higher cortical functions. Diagnosis depends on the demonstration of an HIV infection followed by the development of dementia-like symptoms.

Head Trauma

This is a more common cause of dementia than has been recognized in both elderly and young populations. The elderly are particularly susceptible to the effects of falls and automobile accidents because of decreased resiliency of the brain in this age group. However, this cause is often ignored because the injuries are not reported, appear not to be serious, or the symptoms are ascribed to normal aging by individuals unfamiliar with the client's premorbid status or by family in denial.

The symptoms in milder cases are difficult to identify because of the wide range of normal variation in the elderly. The most common results of mild to moderate head injury are a mild memory disorder of new memory along with mild impairment in higher-level executive functions (Golden, Zillmer, & Spiers, 1992). Emotional liability may also be seen. The memory impairment is often misdiagnosed as just normal forgetting associated with aging, and the impairment in executive function is clear only with novel stimuli or highly stressful or complex situations that are unfamiliar. In an individual who is retired, such situations may be rare. In addition, elderly clients are less likely to be in situations that they find unfamiliar. When they are, deficits are again ascribed to normal aging.

As a result, deficits may pass unnoticed for substantial periods of time until later noted during a crisis. At that time, the role of the head injury may be missed, yielding a misdiagnosis of another type of dementia (usually AD or diffuse vascular dementia) or even leading to a diagnosis of depression or schizophrenia despite the lack of premorbid history of such disorders.

Neurodiagnostic tests are rarely helpful in these cases, even when conducted immediately after the injury. Unless there is bleeding or other significant vascular events secondary to the head injury, CT and MRI may be nonsignificant and measures of blood flow will be equivocal at best in many cases. Neurological examinations may be normal. Diagnosis is most often established by a well-developed history rather than more elaborate diagnostic devices.

Parkinson's Disease

This disease, the symptoms of which have been recognized for centuries, was first embodied as a disease entity by the work of James Parkinson in 1817 (Golden et al., 1992). The disease occurs in less than 1% of the population. Parkinson's disease is a progressive disorder marked primarily by motor symptoms: tremor, rigidity, postural instability, and bradykinesia. Dementia is not always associated with the disease, but is seen in more advanced stages, with estimates of incidence ranging from 0% to 81% in different studies (Biggins *et al.,* 1992). In their own longitudinal study, Biggins and colleagues (1992) estimated an incidence of 19%. It may occur in as much as 1% of the elderly population. Parkinson's disease is considered a disorder of the basal ganglia that usually begins in middle age or later. The symptoms are related to a disturbance of dopaminergic activity in these areas.

Parkinson's disease may be idiopathic or may arise from head injury, vascular disease, or other disorders of the brain that affect the appropriate parts of the brain. Parkinson-like symptoms may develop from certain antipsychotic medications. The onset is slow in idiopathic Parkinson's disease.

Individuals with Parkinson's will initially present without any cognitive symptoms, but will show a resting tremor, rigidity, and involuntary movements. Voluntary movements may be slow. The tremors usually start distally. There may be disorders of posture, motor disturbance of speech, and motor problems with walking. Facial expression may be lost, resulting in a rigid, "masked" appearance. Repetitive movements will be slowed.

When cognitive symptoms develop, they appear more diffuse, with impairment of memory and executive functions. On many tests, however, general motor and motor speech impairment can lead to a misdiagnosis of cognitive dysfunction. For example, low performance IQs reported on the Wechsler Adult Intelligence Scale may be the result simply of motor impairment (see Marsden & Fahn, 1987). Some deficits, however, can be recognized independent of motor and speed issues but these are not clearly typical of the disease (Golden *et al.*, 1992). Diagnosis of dementia in Parkinson's arises from confirmation of the symptoms through history and neurological examination, followed by confirmation of dementia where no other likely cause is present.

Huntington's Disease

Huntington's disease is the classical prototype of a dementing disorder clearly related to genetic issues. The disease is a progressive, degenerative disorder that clearly runs in families. It is transmitted through a single autosomal dominant gene on chromosome four. The onset of symptoms is usually after age 30, but may occur at any time in the life span including well past age 60 (Golden *et al.*, 1992).

Early symptoms may reflect changes in personality: irritability, mood change, depression, anxiety, and hypersexuality. Movement disorders characterized by stereotyped atypical chorioid movements then develop. Dementing symptoms including memory problems, executive problems, and eventually problems throughout the brain accompany this degeneration. Frank psychosis may develop. The progression of the disease can be closely followed by performance on neuropsychological tests.

Diagnosis can be established through history, genetic testing, and neurological and neuropsychological examination. The disease presentation is rather clear as it progresses, and it can usually be easily distinguished from other forms of dementia.

Pick's Disease

First described by Arnold Pick in 1892, Pick's disease is a degenerative disease of the brain focused in the anterior fronto-temporal areas of the brain. The disease is progressive and irreversible. This disorder results in a wide variety of symptoms ranging from mood changes, irritability, and instability, to a lack of flexibility, planning, new memory, and judgment.

The neuropathology of the disorder is characterized by the presence of Pick's Bodies as opposed to the tangles seen in Alzheimer's disease. This is accompanied by clear atrophy of the frontal and temporal lobes which can be seen on autopsy as well as on MRI or CT scan. In summarizing the literature, Cummings and Benson (1992) described three stages for the development of the disease: loss of higher executive functions characterized by impulsivity, irritability, and loss of social skills; a second stage characterized by verbal deficits, aphasia, and deterioration of judgment; and the final third stage characterized by a disintegration of behavior across many modalities and skills.

The behavior of Pick's patients may be quite bizarre due to the loss of social skills, judgment, and social awareness. This can include roaming behavior, poor hygiene, urination in public, disinhibition, inappropriate comments, childlike behavior, hyper- or hypo-orality, hypersexuality, hyperaggressiveness, apathy, loss of initiative, echolalia, perseveration, anomia, compulsive or ritualistic behavior, lying, general criminal behavior, lack of insight, psychotic-like behavior, and mood swings (Golden, Osmon, Moses, & Berg, 1981; Jung & Solomon, 1993; Mendez, Selwood, Mastri, & Frey, 1993; Miller *et al.,* 1991).

The diagnostic dilemma in this disorder is that final diagnosis requires an autopsy as in Alzheimer's disease. In later stages, AD and Pick's may seem behaviorally similar and this can lead to misdiagnosis in the absence of a good history. In some cases, CT, MRI, and SPECT will demonstrate the clear anterior nature of the atrophy which would clearly lead to a suspicion of the disorder. This is not true in all cases, however, and autopsy may lead to reversal of the diagnosis. About 10% of all dementias are likely to be cases of Pick's disease.

Creutzfeldt–Jakob Disease

Creutzfeldt–Jakob disease is a rare degenerative disorder that is inevitably fatal and that can be transmitted from person to person. The disorder typically appears at about age 60, but can occur at any age. The disorder was first described by Creutzfeldt and Jakob in the second decade of the twentieth century (Ball, 1980; Beck & Daniel, 1987; Brown, 1989; Jones, Hedley-White, & Friedberg, 1985).

The disease follows a clear course. During the prodromal phase, the client has mild, nonspecific physical symptoms along with feelings of fatigue and concentration problems. Subsequently, a full cortical dementia develops with symptoms of aphasia, executive dysfunction, delusions, hallucinations and general intellectual deterioration. Motor symptoms and abnormalities also develop during this time. The last stage is characterized by stupor, multiple physical problems, and eventually death. The neuropathological sign of the disease is the spongiform appearance of the cerebral cortex which can be identified on autopsy.

The disease can be divided into familial and transmissible forms. There are several variants of the disease that have been identified but they all have the same fatal, rapidly degenerative course. Definitive diagnosis is difficult without biopsy, and in many cases is not even considered because the disease is so rare (1 incidence per 1 million people). Familial history or preexisting trauma or neurological disease may increase the likelihood of the disease.

Other

This category includes a wide variety of medical disorders that may have a primary or secondary effect on the function of the brain. Several of these are relatively common in elderly populations and must be considered in any case of dementia.

One of the most common of these disorders are tumors. For our purposes, tumors can roughly be divided into three categories: extrinsic, intrinsic, and metastatic (Golden *et al.,* 1992). Extrinsic tumors are those that are inside the skull but do not invade the tissue of the brain itself. Rather, these tumors cause problems by increasing in size, compressing brain tissue, and increasing intracranial pressure. The symptoms of increased intracranial pressure include headaches, nausea, incontinence, balance problems, memory problems, and difficulty with attention and concentration. More localized symptoms may occur depending on exactly which tissue in the brain is compressed (although this may not always reflect the physical location of the tumor). When extrinsic tumors are slow growing, they may show little effect. In the elderly, in whom brain atrophy is common as a result of normal aging, the tumor may have additional space in which to grow before causing any visible symptoms. Some extrinsic tumors are first discovered at autopsy without any clinical correlations before death.

Intrinsic tumors are those that invade and destroy healthy brain tissue. These tumors primarily differ (for our purposes) on the basis of speed of development from slow to very fast. The slowest tumors may cause few problems as the brain is able to adjust to the slow loss of tissue with appropriate behavioral adaptations, although problems may show after enough tissue has been compromised. Faster-growing tumors, however, may cause both highly localized effects (as seen in the localized vascular dementias) as well as more general effects from increased intracranial pressure. These disorders can develop quite quickly and may even be mistaken for a vascular disorder. All of the forms of tumors can be easily identified in most cases by MRI or CT scan.

The third form of tumors are metastatic tumors. These are usually tumors secondary to various forms of cancer, most often from lung or breast cancer although any form of cancer can metastasize to the brain. Metastatic tumors must be considered in any individual with a history of cancer who shows a quick onset of dementia-like symptoms, even years after the original cancer has been treated. The symptoms are generally highly focal and severe, and again may be mistaken in some cases for vascular dementia.

Another important disorder in the elderly is normal pressure hydrocephalus. This disorder differs from the form of hydrocephalus seen in younger individuals. In younger cases, hydrocephalus is the result of pressure within the ventricular system increasing because of blockage or a failure to reabsorb CSF fluid. In normal pressure hydrocephalus, the pressure within the ventricular system remains normal. What changes is the ability of the brain tissue to resist that pressure. Instead of "pushing back" on the ventricles, the brain tissue collapses and compresses. This results in symptoms similar to increased pressure or edema as discussed earlier.

The presence of enlarged ventricles can be easily diagnosed through CT scan or MRI, but the presence of enlarged ventricles is not diagnostic of normal pressure hydrocephalus. In many normal elderly, we see normal atrophy of the brain in which the brain shrinks on its own rather than through compression. In some of these cases, the shrinkage is due to a disease process such as AD, but in other cases it is normal. The enlargement of the ventricles is simply a "space filling" response rather than a compression of the brain tissue. In these circumstances, the ventricular enlargement has nothing to do with any symptoms shown by the patient.

Thus, normal pressure hydrocephalus can be diagnosed only in cases where the ventricular enlargement is compressing the brain. This requires both identifying the generalized symptoms of the disorder neurologically, cognitively, and behaviorally, and ruling out any other causes for the observed brain atrophy.

A third possible cause of dementia within this group are subdural hematomas. A hematoma is a "sack" of blood between layers of the meninges that occurs as a result of bleeding into the subdural space. These can occur spontaneously when a vessel breaks due to arteriosclerosis, a defect in the vessel, or as a result of a head trauma. In the elderly, such a head trauma may be very mild and may have occurred several weeks prior to the development of symptoms. Traumas such as hitting one's head on a door or a mild fall can lead to the onset of the hematoma.

The effects of the hematoma will depend on the rate at which the hematoma grows, the amount of space available in the brain, and the ability of the brain to reabsorb the hematoma. In some cases, the hematoma may pass without notice. In other cases, symptoms of a space occupying lesion will develop as is seen in extrinsic tumors and normal pressure hydrocephalus. Untreated, the dementia can become quite severe and the hematoma can become life threatening. In some cases, sustained elevations in intracranial pressure can restrict blood flow and cause a permanent dementia via sustained hypoxia. As in other space occupying lesions, the clue to diagnosis is the development, slowly or quickly, of headaches, confusion, incontinence, balance, and memory problems.

Nutritional disorders are also a common cause of dementia in the elderly. This may result from changes in smell and taste that restrict the enjoyment of food, leading to a tendency either to eat less than needed or to restrict diets to a very few foods (e.g., a patient who would only eat chocolate pudding, from a certain manufacturer, and coffee). Such restrictions may also arise from economic or physical limitations that inhibit access to a wide variety of foods, or from the presence of dental or gastrointestinal problems that interfere with consuming or absorbing foods. In all of these cases, the eventual outcome is a severe nutritional deficiency (e.g., niacin or vitamin B_{12}) that leads to generalized confusion and dementia. Such deficiencies may also be the side effects of certain medications or combinations of medications.

The elderly may also demonstrate a variety of demyelinating diseases such as multiple sclerosis (MS) or Lou Gehrig's disease. The latter are two well-known examples of a wide variety of demyelinating diseases in which the primary initial symptoms are sensory or motor in nature. As these diseases progress, however, problems with memory, attention, concentration, and executive and personality functions may develop. Dementia is by no means an inevitable outcome of these disorders, but it is seen in more severe forms of the disease. As with Parkinson's disease, it is important not to misinterpret motor and sensory problems as cognitive problems.

Infections of various kinds may also lead to dementia. These include meningitis and encephalitis, which may arise secondary to other viral and infectious diseases in individuals who are otherwise weak or have immunological impairment. In some cases, brain abscesses will develop which destroy specific areas of the brain. In the elderly, these disorders can result in permanent nonprogressive dementias characterized by memory loss, attentional loss, and disorders of executive skills. A clear history is often necessary to identify this etiology. In such cases, the onset of symptoms can usually be traced to the development of the illness, with the resolution of the illness leading to only partial remission of the symptoms. This is sometimes missed as residual symptoms are seen as signs of continuing recovery rather than as signs of permanent injury.

A final set of causes arise from treatment. These can be, for example,from the effects of general anesthesia in the elderly or the effects of chemotherapy or radiation therapy for cancer. In some cases, these disorders are correctly classified as deliriums; however, in many cases there may be residual symptoms that do not recover even after the cessation of the treatment. If the memory and cognitive symptoms are present, then these would also be properly labeled as dementias.

Substance-Induced Persisting Dementia

This class of dementia is in general less important in the elderly as onset is generally before age 50. The substance involved may be alcohol, inhalants, hypnotics, sedatives, anticonvulsants, heroin, cocaine, LSD, and so on. The most important substance issues in the elderly are the long-term effects of alcohol along with the effects of prescription medication.

Perhaps the best known of these disorders in the elderly is Korsakoff's syndrome secondary to chronic use of alcohol, the most abused substance within the elderly population. Many years of heavy drinking is necessary for the onset of this disorder, and the onset is often accompanied by other problems such as vitamin deficiencies and failure of the liver or kidneys. Berman (1990) estimated that alcoholic dementia may represent as much as 10% of all dementias although this figure is not universally accepted. This syndrome is characterized by extreme memory problems along with confabulation to fill in memory losses. Memory loss often extends back to when the person began heavy drinking although the presence of confabulation may not make this clear upon cursory examination. New memory formation is almost nonexistent (Brandt & Butters, 1986). Other symptoms may include problems with higher-level executive functions and visual spatial functions (Jacobson, Acker, & Lishman, 1990). Although improved nutrition and medical care may decrease symptoms, the likelihood of recovery remains low (Parsons & Nixon, 1993).

Another form of substance-induced dementia in the elderly is the effects of prescription medication. These medications may have relatively benign effects in younger individuals, but some elderly show significant cognitive reactions to extended pain medication, hypnotics, antipsychotics, antidepressives, anxiolitics and other medications either alone or in combination. Some of these effects may be temporary, causing delirium, but other effects may be permanent even though the length of time on medication was limited. In more chronic use, longer-lasting effects may be noted. In some cases, the effects of the medication or combination of medications is idiopathic and unexpected; others are the result of improper monitoring of the greater effects of medication in the elderly.

Other Categories of Dementia

The category of "dementia due to multiple etiologies" is used when there is more than one documented etiology for the dementia. This is commonly appropriate in the elderly as several different problems may lead to an individual presentation of dementia. The category of "Dementia NOS" is used when no cause can be established although the diagnostic symptoms of dementia are present.

DIAGNOSIS

The diagnosis of dementia takes place in several steps. First, there is a need to establish the presence of symptoms which may initially suggest the possibility of a dementia. Second, there is the need to establish that a dementia clearly exists. The third stage involves establishing a specific diagnostic type, which may in turn allow for treatment or prognostic plans. In each phase, information is gained from several specific sources: (1) history; (2) evaluation of activities of daily living; (3) screening examinations; (4) neurological, neuroradiological, and medical examinations; and (5) neuropsychological testing.

History

History is an extremely important component of any evaluation of dementia, but one which is often slighted in favor of questionnaires, screening tests, and neuroradiological findings. However, history is necessary to establish that the individual was once functioning at higher levels, as the presence of any of the disorders discussed in this chapter assumes that the person was once functioning at a higher level. Without a well-taken history, such decline may not be recognized, especially in otherwise higher-functioning individuals. Lower levels of initial function, due to education, basic IQ, or background, may be misinterpreted as signs of dementia. There is a bias to underdiagnose these disorders in highly intelligent individuals and to overdiagnose in minorities and those with lower education.

Any history should extend beyond a basic questionnaire, as families may not recognize what is important or may be in denial. They may also fail to understand the meaning of specific questions.

Histories should be oriented toward gathering basic concrete behavioral observations rather than generalities or conclusions. Thus, a complaint of memory problems should be broken down into specific acts: "he loses his key," "he can't remember the route to get to work," "he leaves the house and can't find his way home," and other such basic complaints. In addition, it is important to generate information about the frequency of the behavior, the situation that accompanies the behavior, and the frequency of the behavior in the past. If possible, it is important to identify a timeline that indicates when the behavior was absent and the speed and degree at which it developed over time. This should be done for each abnormal or changed behavior, whether this involves medical symptoms (such as headaches or nausea), cognitive changes (memory problems or problems with speech or attention), or personality change (irritability, depression, apathy, aggression. hallucinations, delusions).

History can be used as basic evidence for the existence of a dementia or an alternative diagnosis such as depression. Indeed, although the absence of a clear history does not rule out the diagnosis, a well-taken history with proper evidence clearly establishes that a problem exists and generally obviates the need for screening tests that have a high rate of misdiagnosis. In many of the dementing disorders, history (along with clear-cut evidence of a decline in functioning) is indeed the best diagnostic indicator in the absence of an autopsy.

This is especially important in such disorders as AD, Pick's disease, Korsakoff's disease, and other dementias in which there are no clear diagnostic tests that can confirm the disease process itself (although many that can identity the presence of the memory and other behavioral or personality characteristics of the disease). Vascular dementia can be recognized by its stepwise development of symptoms, as opposed to the more continuously developing disorders such as AD or Pick's disease. Korsakoff's disorder requires a clear history of alcoholism, and histories of smoking, cancer, liver disease, and others can be major markers in the diagnosis of a specific dementia.

History is important because of the overlap between the various forms of dementia in terms of symptoms and course of development. For example, some individuals with AD may have had alcohol histories simply because of the prevalence of alcoholism in our communities. It is easy to settle on alcohol as the one explanation without thoroughly investigating all of the alternative possibilities. When the differential is between two untreatable forms of dementia, this is not so serious an issue. However, when the differential involves treatable as well as untreatable alternatives, delay in getting an accurate diagnosis can be extremely dangerous to the client.

When there are alternative interpretations, histories should be gathered to indicate the possible alternatives. While this is not always definitive, good histories can clearly indicate what medical tests or further information is necessary to further refine the diagnostic procedure.

Activities of Daily Living

This is another extremely important part of the diagnosis. Many will come in with complaints that are subjective and hard to pin down, but focusing on ADLs offers both a more concrete example of the impact of the problems and an assessment of their severity in a real-life setting. This is quite important in assessing the likelihood of dementia in marginal cases and in treatment and long-term planning.

Many scales for ADL activity exist, but most are general and oriented toward acute, quick-onset disorders. These are less sensitive to the early stages of the chronic progressive disorders. Although new scales which may be more sensitive and more useful are being developed, they are as yet not well researched or ready for general use.

Thus, evaluations remain at present more subjective than objective. The focus of an evaluation should not be on the level of function of the individual in a given area (which is relatively difficult), but on change over the past year or other appropriate time period. Such investigations should obtain the report of the patient and someone close to the patient. Patient reports are often inadequate and may overestimate or underestimate the patient's actual level of function. The report of a close individual may also be biased, but separate determinations can identify areas of disagreement that may require more detailed evaluation.

ADL evaluation should cover at least the following areas:

Basic Care

Basic care includes hygiene, dressing, bathing, eating, and drinking. These areas are those most often covered in traditional ADL scales. Impairment in these areas suggests a severe disorder, an acute disorder, or a relatively progressed chronic disorder.

Social Relationships

Social relationships include the ability to interact with groups of people, handle stressful or complex relationships, act in an appropriate manner, resist impulsive behavior, act in a tactful manner, and maintain preexisting relationships. People who know the individual well at home or work can often contribute important observations.

Household Chores

Household chores include such tasks as cleaning, laundry, food preparation, gardening, and care of personal goods. These are important areas related to an individual's ability to function independently and are good markers of changes in cognitive status.

Financial Responsibilities

Financial responsibilities include paying bills, investing, budgeting, marketing, handling credit and credit cards, and other financial transactions. These areas are relatively complex and require active and continual involvement. Deficits in this area can range from simple mathematical errors, which become more common, to a loss of the ability to see the long-term consequences of specific behaviors or to understand what is being done at all.

Work Responsibilities

Work responsibilities vary depending on whether the person is employed or retired, and on the nature of the job if the client is employed. In early dementia, coworkers and superiors may notice a decrease in the quality of actions taken, a lessening of the ability to deal with stress and crisis situations, and a lessening of planning activities. Behavior may become more impulsive and less socially appropriate with coworkers as well as customers or clients. Decision making and responsible behavior will be impaired. This is often ignored or explained as temporary but needs careful investigation in identifying early onset of dementia.

Problem-Solving in Daily Life

Areas may include household repairs, responsibilities in community organizations, family obligations, and other areas where problem-solving skills are expected. Early deficits may again show up in these areas and may include withdrawal from activities to avoid making errors (although the client may not state this).

Driving Skills

This area includes the motor and perceptual act of driving as well as the more cognitive acts of planning and finding one's way in unfamiliar areas. Basic driving skills will often remain stable in early to moderate dementias, but problems will be seen in dealing with novel or complex driving situations and in spatial skills related to map reading. Motor or perceptual problems seen in some specific disorders may also appear as well.

Motor Skills

Motor skills include the necessary coordination, balance, timing, and cognitive skills for walking, running, stair climbing and other physical activities. These are common in disorders like Parkinson's disease, vascular dementias, demyelinating disorders, and other dementias that affect the motor system. Early symptoms may be reflected only in slowness. There may be a loss in the ability to continue athletic activities at the level previous to the decline.

Recreational Activities

Recreational activities include athletic activities, card games, dancing, movies, reading, hobbies and all other activities done for enjoyment. Individuals may show a loss of interest in activities without clear-cut evidence of depression. This loss of interest is usually related to an inability to perform the activities at the previous level of competence and an attempt to avoid embarrassment. Loss of interest may also arise from an inability to gain pleasure from the activity due to a recognition of the loss of skills, attentional and concentration problems, or other cognitive factors. It is important to explore this area to differentiate this change from the loss of interest that accompanies depression.

Planning and Evaluation in All Aspects of Behavior

One of the major activities which distinguishes adults from children is the ability to plan and anticipate the consequences of behavior and to learn from previous experience with a situation. This, again, may be lost early in dementing disorders with the individual becoming fixated on one approach without learning from consequences or being able to recognize what consequences are likely. Such individuals become more focused on day-to-day or hour-to-hour gains without seeing the whole picture.

Perseveration

Perseveration refers to both inflexibility and the tendency to repeat oneself. In memory disorders, this may involve forgetting that one has asked or done something, leading to repetition of the behavior. In other cases, clients may develop rituals to avoid having to make decisions or be placed at a disadvantage. In more serious cases, the client may repeat single phrases (e.g., "Kentucky Fried Chicken" or "OK. OK.").

Evaluation of these active behaviors adds a substantial amount of information to the traditional mental health or medical history. Combined with the remainder of the data, information about these behaviors adds considerably to diagnosis and treatment planning.

Screening Examinations

This is an area that has received an inordinate amount of attention in the literature. Such examinations appear to offer much to users: fast evaluation and classification of clients that can be performed even by nonprofessionals. They are often used in place of a detailed history or ADL evaluation, or as a method of justifying or not justifying ordering of neuroradiological or neuropsychological testing. They can be used for quick objective classification of clients in research studies at minimal cost.

Such tests have significant disadvantages in the diagnosis of an individual when used alone. First, all have significant error rates especially in the mild or early dementias. They do best in identifying the presence of moderate to severe dementia. The difficulty here is that moderate to advanced dementia is fairly easy to recognize without such testing. In clinical work, it is the mild cases or beginning cases that present problems. When one considers issues of base rates, false positives, and false negatives within the mild population, many individual diagnostic errors will be made that have potentially significant impact on the individual client.

The second problem is that these tests sample only a small number of the areas that can be affected in dementia, and none effectively sample such functions as personality changes, impulsivity, and loss of social skills. Even if one assumes that the tests detect everything in the areas they measure, many other areas are ignored. Thus, a given test might adequately sample for a given form of dementia, but not for others. Unfortunately, these tests are interpreted as measuring for all forms of dementia.

Despite these limitations, researchers and clinicians have focused on their use. Probably the most frequently used of these examinations has been the Mini-Mental State Examination (MMSE) (Folstein, Folstein, & McHugh, 1975).

Some studies have reported excellent results in general and patient populations between normal and demented subjects (Anthony, LeResche, Niaz, von Korff, & Folstein, 1982; Ashford et al., 1992; Van der Cammen, Van Harskamp, Stronks, Passchier, & Schudel, 1992; Galasko et al., 1990; Kay et al., 1985). However, accuracy rates generally remain under 90% and substantially less in some populations.

Fratiglioni, Grut, Forsell, Viitanen, and Winblad (1992) found that while significant results could be found for the MMSE, significant and serious errors were still made. Sabe, Jason, Juejati, Leiguarda, and Starkstein (1993) found that when normals were compared to mild (but already identified) dementia cases, no normals were misidentified; however, only 55% of the demented subjects were correctly identified. Fields, Fulop, Sachs, Strain and Fillit (1992) found the MMSE better than the Neurobehavioral Cognitive Status Examination (NCSE), but again found accuracy rates (as measured against a psychiatric opinion) to be low.

Many other tests have been suggested in the literature but none has been proven reliably superior to the MMSE or researched as well (e.g., Copeland, Kelleher, Kellett, Gourlay, & Gurland, 1976; Everhuis, 1992; Gurland, Kuriansky, Sharpe, Simon, & Stiller, 1977; Overall & Schaltenbrand, 1992; Roth, Tym, Mountjoy, Huppert, & Hendrie, 1986; Zaudig, 1992; Zaudig, Mittelhammer, Hiller, Pauls, & Thora, 1991).

Overall, these results suggest that screening tests can be used, but not as the only or most important criteria for determining the presence of dementia. They must be regarded within their individual limitations as only one source of information along with other detailed information from the other domains identified in this section These tests may also be useful as longitudinal indicators in changes in status over time rather than diagnosis per se.

Radiological and Medical Evaluations

These are essential aspects of any evaluation of dementia. Behavioral and cognitive symptoms, along with historical and ADL information, may be used to define the presence of dementia, but they can only suggest the etiology of the disorder. While establishing the absolute cause of a dementia is not always possible without an autopsy, it is absolutely necessary that medical examinations rule out the many fully or partially treatable forms of dementia in order to ensure the best possible medical care or the longest maintenance of the client's level of function.

This area includes a complete medical examination including appropriate tests for diabetes, thyroid disorders, kidney disorders, liver disorders, heart disorders, lung disorders, cancers of all kinds, blood disorders, endocrine disorders, poisoning, and other medical correlates of dementia. The specific tests conducted depend on the patient's symptom presentation, history, and other relevant factors. Such an examination needs to be thorough and complete before concluding that none of these factors are relevant to the patient's symptoms.

A complete neurological examination is useful for detecting gross distortions in mental status and the presence of any localized or diffuse neurological signs. Particular care is necessary for the identification of signs of increased intracerebral pressure, which may suggest tumors, edema, hydrocephalus, hematoma, and other disorders, and strong localizing signs, which may suggest vascular lesions, certain localized tumors, or focal areas of confusion. Neither a normal neurological examination nor a normal medical examination will rule out the presence of dementia, however.

The final aspect of the examinations is the use of neurological and neuroradiological devices. These include measures of electrical activity in the brain (EEG, evoked potential), measures of brain structure (CT scan, MRI), measures of cerebral blood flow (rCBF, SPECT, PETT), and measures of intracranial pressure (spinal tap). Each of these types of devices is useful in identifying specific disorders but none are absolute: normal results again do not predict the absence of dementia.

EEG measures have long been used in cases of dementia. In AD, many studies have shown slowing in EEG activity in more moderate to advanced cases (e.g., Brenner, Ulrich, Spiker, Sclabassi, & Reynolds, 1986; Breslau, Starr, Sicotte, Higa, & Buchsbaum, 1989; Israel, Kozarevic, & Sarorius, 1984; Saletu & Anderer, 1988). Gunther *et al.,* (1993) suggested that EEG could be effective in detecting changes at rest as well as when the client was involved in active perceptual or cognitive processing. Miyauchi and colleagues (1994) reported useful but not individually diagnostic findings using Quantitative EEG (QEEG) methods, as have Onofri and colleagues (1991) using event related potential in AD and individuals with MS dementia.

EEG can be useful in documenting cerebral dysfunction and in identifying subcortical lesions in diseases like MS. EEGs can also be utilized for the identification of certain types of seizures which may be seen secondarily in cases of dementia. In some cases treatment of the seizures will markedly improve cognitive as well as behavioral symptoms. The elimination of active seizures can improve memory concentration, and general cognitive skills, and eliminate behavioral and psychological effects of partial complex seizures which can include depression, anxiety, panic, anger, aggression, and acting-out behavior.

More extended use has been made of devices that measure structural changes in the brain. These have been used to identify general and specific brain atrophy, identify focal points of damage, and identify space occupying lesions such as hematomas and tumors. Ventricular enlargement is also easily seen by these tests. Differentiating normal and abnormal ventricular enlargement and atrophy, however, becomes increasingly difficult as the client grows older. As noted earlier, there are benign and pathological causes of atrophy that cannot be easily identified except through clinical correlation. In cases in which atrophy is present, it is not always correct or advisable to assume immediately that the atrophy is related to the dementia.

For example, Powell Mezrich, Coyne, Loesberg, and Keller (1993) found that demented subjects were more likely to show third ventricle enlargement, but that the sign was not diagnostic in individual cases. In other cases, substantial dementia may exist without any abnormal changes to the structure of the brain. These tests are more useful when finding hematomas, tumors, or other space occupying disorders. The tests are also useful in longitudinal evaluation of changes (DeCarli *et al.,* 1992).

Regional cerebral blood flow measures have opened another possible method for analyzing brain function. Since these measures depend on brain metabolism, they can remain normal despite apparent atrophy and show impairment despite apparent intact structure. These measures can also differentiate blood flow when the client is at rest and during active tasks, possibly showing abnormalities in how the brain executes a task. With the introduction of SPECT scans over the past decade, and the imminent introduction of an MRI capable of measuring blood flow, these are becoming increasingly available and cost-effective methods of evaluation.

As might be expected, blood flow is clearly reduced in AD (Bonte, Ross, Chehabi, & Devous, 1986; Burns, Philpot, Costa, Ell, & Levy, 1989; Eberling, Jagust, Reed, & Baker, 1992; Kumar *et al.,* 1991) Sawada and colleagues (1992) found cerebral blood flow useful in predicting the presence of dementia in Parkinson's disease.

As with the other measures, cerebral blood flow appears a useful adjunct in general to the study of the demented patient, but cannot differentiate reliably the presence or type of dementia. However it may provide very useful clues in certain cases in which other measures are normal or equivocal. More research needs to be done on this and the other measures, and clinical use is recommended as long as clear clinical correlations and historical issues are considered as well.

Neuropsychological Testing

Neuropsychological testing has been widely used in the diagnosis of dementia. However, such testing also has significant limitations. One of the major limitations is a tendency for norms to become much more variable with older normal populations. As a result, many tests of memory, motor speed and problem solving show considerable overlap between the performance of persons with mild dementia and normal individuals. Although there are unquestionably group differences on these measures between identified groups with dementia and normal controls, the overlap between the groups makes individual diagnosis difficult and unreliable.

Another problem has been the issue of differentiating types of dementia. Some clear-cut distinctions can be made, but they do not apply to all patients. For example vascular dementias are much more likely to be accompanied by lateralized sensory or motor symptoms or focal cognitive signs, but this is not always the case. Frontal lobe signs are prominent in Pick's disease, but may be seen in many other disorders as well.

The third problem is one of clinical correlation. Because of the overlap of patient and normal groups on many neuropsychological tests, the correlations with ADLs and practical symptoms of dementia can range between slight and moderate. The novelty of these tests can lead to overestimates of the functional disorder, which in turn can lead to suggestions for institutionalization that is unnecessary.

A good neuropsychological examination should also include a thorough personality evaluation which should consist of both objective and projective tests if at all possible. Reliance should not be placed entirely on patient self-report in this or any area of evaluation.

With these caveats, neuropsychological tests are still quite useful in identifying disorders that may be at the heart of the client's problem, an aid in differential diagnosis both of type of dementia and the presence of dementia. Again, however, they should not be used alone, but only in conjunction with other sources of data.

The Diagnostic Process

The diagnostic process is, thus, a multilevel process aimed at determining the presence of dementia and its etiology. To determine that dementia is present, there is only a need to demonstrate the presence of (1) memory problems, and (2) other cognitive problems which, in turn, lead to impairment in occupational and/or social functioning. The remainder of the differential lies in establishing the etiology of the disorder according to the criteria discussed in each area. This latter task requires the full range of diagnostic approaches, with different strategies having a more significant role in different types of cases. In general, a complete evaluation will lead to a satisfactory explanation for the disorder, although final confirmation may not be available after the death of the client given the current state of our diagnostic skills.

Differential Diagnosis

There are several major disorders for differential diagnosis. The most obvious are the deliriums. The symptoms in delirium are generally less stable and much more variable over time. Delirium and dementia may coexist, making diagnosis difficult. History may also be useful in making the discrimination and establishing a clear etiology.

Amnestic disorders are differentiated from dementias by the absence of an associated cognitive disorder. However, some systems would consider these dementias, along with cases of cognitive disorder without memory disorder, which is classified under *DSM-IV* as Cognitive Disorder NOS. Mental retardation is defined by its onset in childhood, and both disorders may be diagnosed if the individual has symptoms of both.

Schizophrenia shows overlapping symptoms, but generally has an earlier age of onset. In the elderly without a history of schizophrenia, the dementias or delirium must be considered the more likely diagnosis. However, an individual with life-long schizophrenia can develop dementia in later life; this would be marked by lower functioning, memory, and cognitive skills than they demonstrated throughout their lives.

Perhaps the diagnosis most often confused with dementia is depression. In cases where the client is not depressed, this is not a problem. In cases without a history of major depression and without a clear etiology for the depression (such as a loss of a mate), delirium or dementia again become more likely. A thorough history is absolutely necessary to see whether the course of cognitive decline is consistent with a specific form of dementia. If so, appropriate medical and neuropsychological tests can be used to confirm or disconfirm the diagnosis. If the history suggests depression, then medical and neuropsychological tests can also confirm this or suggest the concurrent existence of dementia. A thorough examination at all levels discussed here will generally lead to a reasonable discrimination (Golden *et al.,* 1992; Lamberty & Bieliaukas, 1993).

A final category which should be considered is malingering. Such a disorder generally requires some secondary motivation, which is rare in cases of dementia. In general, however, a thorough examination will reveal glaring inconsistencies in findings across and within methods. However, such evaluations must be made with the awareness that there is only a moderate correlation between different methods of evaluation.

TREATMENT

There is no definitive general treatment for the dementias. Some of these disorders are irreversible, while others may respond to timely and appropriate treatment with partial or full remission. Most can respond to behavioral and chemical interventions, as well as manipulation of the environment. We will discuss each of these alternatives.

Treatable Disorders

Many of the disorders that cause dementia have medical treatments that can fully or partially alleviate the disorder and the resultant cognitive symptoms. These disorders include diabetes, liver and kidney failure, tumors, cancers, endocrine disorders, nutritional disorders, heart disorders, lung disorders, blood disorders, hematomas, normal pressure hydrocephalus, and other related problems. The specific treatments for these disorders are not within the scope of this chapter, but their identification and treatment is a key in any initial medical "workup" of the demented client.

Pharmaceutical Intervention

Pharmaceutical intervention falls into several classes. The first of these involve medication specific to one disorder that generally addresses motor symptoms in such disorders as Parkinson's disease or MS. Since these medications do not address the symptoms of dementia per se, they are not covered in this chapter. The second class of medications attempts to limit or reverse the direct cognitive effects of dementing disorders. The final class of medication addresses the behavioral effects of dementia. We examine the effects of the latter two classes of medications.

Antidementia Medications

Medications attempt to reverse the cognitive effects of AD and other dementias are relatively new, although the investigation of substances that might reverse dementia has been popular since it was discovered that some forms of dementia were due to diseases like syphilis and others were due to vitamin and nutritional deficiencies. Medications like folate and vitamin B_{12} have been popular although results have been disappointing (e.g., Chanarin, Deacon, Lumb, and Perry, 1989; Goodwin, Goodwin, & Garry, 1983; Levitt & Karlinsky, 1992; Shorvon, Carney, Chanarin, & Reynolds, 1980; Shulman, 1967; Sneath, Chanarin, Hodkinson, McPherson, & Reynolds, 1973). Some dementias are clearly caused by deficiencies in such substances, but they comprise a very small part of the dementia population overall.

More promising medications attempt to increase levels of acetylcholine in the brain, based on the theory that AD and perhaps other disorders are related to a deficiency in this neurotransmitter. Others use different pathways but with similar goals. Although none of these drugs have been studied sufficiently to be considered "proven," they are all of interest at the time this chapter was written. Nearly all of this research has been conducted within the past 20 years, with beliefs about the efficacy of the drugs ranging from negative to more optimistic. The hope is that within the next decade a set of medications will be identified that can improve or retard degeneration in cognitive and memory performance in some cases of dementia.

These medications include such substances as oxiracetam, nicergoline, milacemide, nebracetam fumurate, denbufylline, pyritinol, and piracetam. Studies have shown cognitive improvement in animals (Artola & Singer, 1987; Banfi & Dorigotti, 1986; Giurgea, 1972; Johnson & Asher, 1987; Kuhn et al., 1988; Mondadori & Classen, 1984; Ohno, Yamamoto, Kitajima, & Ueki, 1990; Spignoli et al., 1986) and humans (e.g., Bottini et al., 1992; Cutler et al., 1993; Fischhof et al., 1992; Herrmann & Stephan, 1992; Saletu et al., 1992; Urakami et al., 1993; Zappoli et al., 1991). Improvements have been shown in a wide variety of memory areas, cognitive function, brain metabolism, brain electrical activity, and behavior.

The patients who took medication generally did better than patients who received placebo. Not all patients who responded to the medications showed improvement. Some of the patients on the medication, however, did show dramatic improvements. In well-constructed double-blind studies, the edge, or the treated group as a whole, was clearly significant. The development of these substances is still in its infancy. We will likely see better drugs developed in the future. We are also likely to find that certain symptom constellations and certain etiological actors play a major role in determining who responds and who does not respond to these medications. The research in this area is quite exciting, and it is likely that these "antidementia" medications will be a major part of the treatment of persons with dementia over the next decade and beyond.

Behavioral Control

The other use of medication is aimed at the behavioral and psychiatric symptoms which may accompany dementia. These include aggressiveness, agitation, screaming, hostility, hallucinations, dementia, eating disorders, sleep disturbance, inappropriate sexual behavior, and excessive wandering behavior. These behaviors are extremely disruptive to caregivers and may make adequate care impossible in some cases. These behaviors can be treated behaviorally or using a pharmaceutical approach.

Despite over three decades of using psychoactive medications for treating the elderly demented, well-run studies or clear results have largely been lacking and physicians have been more dependent on "feel" than fact. A metanalysis of prior studies by Schneider, Pollock, and Lyness (1990) found that the medications were better than placebo, but only by a small amount, regardless of the medication employed. In general, when there is improvement, we see decreases in agitation, but no improvement in cognition. In some cases, the patient may become overly fatigued and show reduced behaviors in all areas.

Rapp, Flint, Herrmann, and Proulx (1992), in an excellent review, suggest that aggression, restlessness, delusions, hallucinations, and some inappropriate sexual behavior respond to medication, but that wandering or inappropriate noise does not. Since no drug seems to be more useful than any other (see Carlyle, Ancill, & Sheldon, 1993), the authors suggest the use of perphenazine or loxapine to minimize side effects. Drugs must be tried at their highest dose (equivalent to about 300 mg of chlorpromazine) for at least a month to test the effectiveness of a medication. Drug holidays are recommended as well. The authors found the antipsychotic medication to be greatly preferable to the benzodiazepines.

Clozapine is an atypical antipsychotic medication that has been suggested for those who cannot tolerate other antipsychotic medications. Oberholzer, Hendriksen, Monsch, Heierli, and Stahelin (1992) suggested its use as an alternative in the demented population, but data and controlled results again remain limited.

An alternative class of drugs that has been investigated restore serotogenic functions in the brain (Altman & Normile, 1988; Gottfries, Adolfsson, & Aquilonius, 1983; Strathmann, 1988). Early studies with traumatic dementias suggested that this class of drugs might be useful (Pinner & Rich, 1988; Simpson & Foster, 1986). Olafsson and colleagues (1992), however, failed to find significant improvement in patients with primary degenerative dementia.

Schneider and Sobin (1992) indicated that other classes of drugs have been used as well, including lithium and beta blockers. In general, findings with lithium have been disappointing; however, there have been no well-controlled studies at reasonable dosage levels. Similarly poor results have been found for beta-blockers even though they are often prescribed in nursing home and rehabilitation settings.

Rosen, Mulsant, and Wright (1992) emphasize the need for the physician (before using medications) to identify the roots of agitation and related behavior. These may include pain and discomfort, illness, delirium, depression, psychosis, distress, or caregiver burden or burnout. In the last case, treatment needs to be directed toward the caregiver rather than the patient. In the other cases, treatment should be geared toward the actual cause rather than providing general treatment with psychoactive medication.

Overall, the use of these medications has produced mediocre results that are only slightly better than use of placebos. Much of the use in clinical settings is ineffective in terms of monitoring and ability to improve patients' behavior without significant side effects. These drugs work in some patients, but placebos appear to work just as well in a significant minority of clients. Much more research is needed to identify when these medications can help and under what conditions. More careful methods of assessing the etiology of symptoms is also strongly recommended.

Behavioral and Environmental Intervention

Behavioral and environmental intervention attempt to evaluate what aspects of the environment precipitate behaviors in the client. Once these are identified, changes can be made in the environment so that cues that elicit the unwanted behavior are avoided or behavior modification techniques are employed to alter the response of the client to the environment. While behavior modification techniques can be used with dementia clients, more progress is made when environmental cues can be altered, as the rate of new learning in dementia is usually slow and uneven. Behavioral interventions may also be difficult when there is a lack of attention to "new cues" that might be used to signal appropriate behaviors. Such cues, although obvious to others, may not be noticed by an individual with perseverative tendencies or perceptual defects as is often seen in dementia.

Several aspects of the environment are easily identified as problems with dementia clients. One major area is changes in the environment. Individuals with dementia, by definition, have difficulties with memory and new learning. Such individuals must rely on old learning and habits to maintain appropriate behavior. When the environment changes, these behaviors may become inappropriate. For example, a dementia client may have lived in a given house for many years and knows the way to the bathroom from the bedroom. In an attempt to help the client, the house is altered or the client is moved to another residence to be nearer relatives or to an institution. The client's appropriate "spatial" behavior suddenly would become "inappropriate" because the path to the bathroom may now be the path to someone else's bedroom. The stroll to the store and back suddenly becomes roaming, as the individual is unable to reach the store or get back to home.

Thus, the basic rule is to change as little as possible. When confronted with tasks that depend only on overlearned skills, the mild to moderate dementia client can do well. However, this very reliance on overlearning impedes effectiveness in a new environment. Clients do better when left in their own environment than when given a new environment. (A new environment for client with motor deficits, but who is cognitively intact, is a very different situation which is often positive.) Clients moved into new environments may suddenly become identified as having dementia because of their inability to cope. This may be mistaken as a sudden onset dementia because of the environmental change, when in fact the disorder may have been slowly progressive.

This general rule applies to the full range of life activities. The early dementia client may be dissuaded from going to work or carrying on normal recreational activities, which simply adds to the client's dysfunction. In all of these cases, the client may need help: reduced hours at work, an aide at home to help in more complex areas, family support, help with recreational activities, and the like. Interventions that minimize the amount of change the person must endure are usually more effective.

The difficulty for caregivers is concern for safety of the client when remaining in the old environment versus increased safety and access to family or caregivers in a new environment. However, from both a cost perspective and a family health perspective, the hiring of aides or occasional family visits may work much more effectively. There are areas in which this becomes difficult, however: in clients with sufficient motor deficits to need 24-hour care and in driving. The combination of significant motor and cognitive deficit is an especially difficult one as the prior environment may be unsafe or unwieldy. However, because such clients are less likely to roam, some of these concerns become less of an issue. As much as possible, however, the client will do better in a familiar environment. The second major area of concern is driving. Because of overlearned skills, clients may drive without difficulty in areas they are familiar with, but easily get lost in other areas. Motor skills may appear adequate except in unusual driving situations. However, deficits will appear in emergency situations. Clients may even be able to pass routine driving tests, making driving decisions very difficult as well as debatable.

When changes are made, they need to be as small as possible. It is not surprising that moving a dementia client from a situation where he or she lives alone into a home with children and grandchildren may lead to irritability and aggressive behavior (on everybody's part). Moving into an institution where freedom is restricted can lead to aggression and roaming as can staff who treat clients as objects rather than people. It is important to recognize that individuals with dementia see and remember themselves as fully functional adults who are insulted and irritated when treated inappropriately. Combine this with emotional lability and judgment defects, and there is a high likelihood for inappropriate behavior. However, the change must be in the environment rather than the client.

When environments must change, the new environment should be as simple, concrete, and clear as possible so that the client gets adequate social and environmental support that emphasizes maximum independence and freedom. The more we ask the client to become institutionalized, the more we are likely to see outbreaks of inappropriate behaviors. Lines that allow the client to get from one place to another, access to simple kitchen activities, access to a wide range of recreational activities, access to reading material, papers, radio, television, music, and other normal aspects of life minimize negative reactions.

When negative reactions occur, a behavioral analysis is necessary to analyze the conditions and environmental cues involved. When environmental change is not possible, then the client's behavior must be changed. It is strongly recommended that the client be told of the problem and allowed to be involved as much as possible in a contract for the solution. This may involve allowing more access to tape players at certain types of the day, negative consequences for inappropriate sexual behavior, or any other intervention consistent with behavioral analysis. Active, simple, and very consistent behavioral programs have the highest likelihood of success. Any agreements or contracts must be written or recorded in a form that the client can review, because of the likely impact of memory problems on any agreement.

These suggestions sound basic, but they work well in a wide variety of conditions. However, one additional area is the question of the caregiver. Whether we deal with an aide, family members, or institutional staff there are many human interactions that can cause significant problems. Attention from one or more people in the environment may be dependent on acting out. Stimulation may also be received when acting out. The stress on a family unit that has a dementing relative move in may create severe psychological problems that are communicated to the patient. In many cases, patient behavior is manageable, but the effort is too much for the caregivers. Thus, close attention to the mental health of the caregiver (whether family or institutional or personal) is a clear and important aspect of any program.

This should include relief from the client, which might involve day programs or activities with friends or relatives. In an institution, staff rotation may be a useful technique. If the client is at home, no family member should be expected to give up his or her life to take care of a patient.

Sleep

Another important related area is the question of sleep. "Sundowning," or the loss of cognitive and emotional control as the day goes on, has been used as an explanation for many problems in the dementia client. Although sundowning is usually associated with sleep disturbance, Bliwise, Carroll, Lee, Nekich, and Dement (1993) have suggested that the behaviors included under "sundowning" exist throughout the day, but may have more impact on nursing staff as the day goes on. Sleep disturbance may produce sundowning in individuals who follow different circadian rhythms, so they are alert when we are asleep and vice versa. This alone will produce clients sleepy at different times, hungry at different times, irritable at different times, and ready for activities at different times, a combination that could lead to excessive problems in institutions that maintain schedules for the institution and its staff rather than for the individual client.

There are many reasons for sleep disturbance in the elderly in general and in the dementia patient (see Bliwise, 1993). These causes include problems in circadian rhythms and difficulty in adjusting biologically to new schedules. They also include sleep-related respiratory disturbance, REM sleep deprivation, naps and resting during the day, excessive time in bed during the day, lack of daily activity, depression, seizures, sleep apnea, neuroleptic induced akathisia, and deterioration of the suprachiasmatic nucleus. The presence of any number of these factors can seriously interfere with adequate sleep, leading to behavioral problems throughout the day. While some of these symptoms may appear to be helped by medication, medication may not allow for adequate REM sleep or actually change ill-fitting circadian patterns. Failure to adequately address these problems will result in continuing behavioral dysfunction, and indeed may increase the apparent level of dementia.

Practice

One of the great strengths of the brain is its ability to repair itself through reorganization of axonal connections and the development of new axonal connections among healthy neurons (Golden *et al.,* 1992). Swaab (1991) points out that in other organs of the body, the principle of "wear and tear" applies: the more you use it, the shorter time it will function properly. The brain, however, works on a "use it or lose it" principle. Skills we do not use simply disappear while those that we practice and reinforce remain with us longer.

This appears to arise out of the fact that abilities that are practiced will develop new underlying patterns of axonal representation that will allow them to continue. If a task is not practiced, there is no reason for the brain to maintain systems for that behavior. Hence, it is quickly lost as brain injury or deterioration occurs. As a consequence, individuals with dementia of any kind will do better the more active they are in the widest range of activities. As we give activities up, they are lost quickly in the degenerating brain, whereas those we practice can be better maintained or partially regained.

While practice does not maintain the brain itself or keep neurons from dying, practice maintains skills on a behavioral level and makes the best use of those areas of the brain that keep their function. The effects of practice cannot overcome the basics of neuronal loss that will limit the amount of behavior that can be retained, but it will allow for maximal performance. We see demented clients who have little left but can still play poker or sing or perform some other highly specific and overpracticed task.

Thus, the best programs at home or in institutions emphasize the patient's independence: doing as much as possible for themselves despite slowness or inaccuracy. This includes all basic skills: dressing and hygiene, food preparation, household care, recreation and the full range of ADLs discussed earlier. In some cases, the individual will need support and review. However, it is essential that caregivers not "take the easy way out" by doing something because it is easier than waiting for the client, or because the client becomes depressed and refuses.

An important aspect of any program that emphasizes supervision is safety. For example, in some clients, cooking needs to be restricted to microwaves and toasters because of dangers in using a stove (which can be easily inactivated by turning off gas supplies or removing fuses). Fireplace use and driving may require restrictions. Other problems may occur because of motor limitations, but there are literally thousands of "aids" that can help the patient with motor problems be more independent (although the presence of both motor and cognitive problems may limit their use). Independence involves some risk and creativity, but is well worth maximizing so as to maximize the quality of life of the client.

SUMMARY

As our society ages, dementia has become an increasingly common and serious problem both to the individual and to society as a whole. Dementias come in many different forms with many disparate etiologies. The diagnosis of dementia is dependent on identifying the central symptoms of a dementia (memory loss and cognitive loss) and on the more complex task of identifying the underlying etiology using history, a survey of ADL skills, medical and radiological examinations, screening tests, and neuropsychological examinations. Many forms of dementia are untreatable, but current research is attempting to identify medications that can improve motor, cognitive, and behavioral symptoms. Other treatment has focused on the need of the client for a familiar and stable environment, and using environmental manipulations along with behavior modification to control inappropriate behavior. The need for continued practice and independence is also emphasized.

REFERENCES

Alafuzoff I. (1992). The pathology of dementias: An overview. *Acta Neurologica Scandinavica, 139*, 8–15.

Alafuzoff, I., Ronnberg, A., & Asikainen-Gustafsson, S. (1991). Clinical to histopathological correlation of the diagnosis of dementia. *International Psychogeriatrics, 3*, 69–74.

Altman, H., & Normile, H. (1988). What is the nature of the role of the serotonergic nervous system in learning and memory: Prospects for the development of a treatment strategy for senile dementia. *Neurobiology of Aging, 9*, 627–639.

Alzheimer, A. (1898). Neuere Arbeiten uber die Dementia senilis und die auf atherimatoser Gefasserk rankung basierended Gehirnkrankheiten. *Monatsschrift fuer Psychiatrie und Neurologie, 3*, 101–115.

American Psychiatric Association. (1994). *Diagnostic and Statistical Manual of Mental Disorders* (4th ed.). Washington, DC: Author.

Anthony, J., LeResche, L., Niaz, U., von Korff, M., & Folstein, M. (1982). Limits of the mini-mental state as a screening test for dementia and delirium among hospital patients. *Psychological Medicine, 12*, 397–408.

Artola, A., & Singer, W. (1987). Long term potentiation and NMDS receptors in rat visual cortex. *Nature, 330*, 649–652.

Ashford, J. W., Kumar, V., Barringer, M., Becker, M., Bice, J., Ryan, N., & Vicari, S. (1992). Assessing Alzheimer severity with a global clinical scale. *International Psychogeriatrics, 1*, 55–74.

Ball, M. (1980). Features of Creutzfeldt–Jakob disease in brains of patients with familial dementia of the Alzheimer's type. *Canadian Journal of Neurological Sciences, 7*, 51–57.

Banfi, S., & Dorigotti, L. (1986). Experimental behavioral studies with oxiracetam on different types of chronic cerebral impairment. *Clinical Neuropharmacology, 9*, 519–526.

Beck, E., & Daniel, P. (1987). Neuropathology of transmissible spongiform encephalopathies. In S. Pruisner & M. McKinley (Eds.), *Prions: Novel infectious pathogens causing scrapie and Creutzfeldt–Jakob disease.* San Diego: Academic.

Berg, R., Franzen, M., & Wedding, D. (1994). *Screening for brain impairment.* New York: Springer.

Berman, M. (1990). Severe brain dysfunction: Alcoholic Korsakoff's syndrome. *Alcohol Health and Research, 14*, 120–129.

Biggins, C. A., Boyd, J., Harrop, F., Madeley, P., Mindham, R., Randall, J., & Spokes, E. (1992). A controlled longitudinal study of dementia in Parkinson's disease. *Journal of Neurology, Neurosurgery, and Psychiatry, 55*, 566–571.

Bliwise, D., Carroll, J., Lee, K., Nekich, J., & Dement, W. (1993). Sleep and "sundowning" in nursing home patients with dementia. *Psychiatry Research, 48*, 277–292.

Bliwise, D. L. (1993). Sleep in normal aging and dementia. *Sleep, 16*, 40–81.

Bonte, F. J., Ross, E. D., Chehabi, H. H., & Devous, M. D. (1986). SPECT study of regional cerebral blood flow in Alzheimer's disease. *Journal of Computed Assisted Tomography, 10*, 579–583.

Bottini, G., Vallar, G., Cappa, S., Monza, G. C., Scarpini, E., Baron, P., Cheldi, A., & Scarlato, G. (1992). Oxiracetam in dementia: A double blind, placebo-controlled study. *Acta Neurologica Scandinavica, 86*, 237–241.

Brandt, J., & Butters, N. (1986). The alcoholic Wernicke–Korsakoff syndrome and its relationship to long term alcohol abuse. In G. Grant & K. Adams (Eds), *Neuropsychological assessment of neuropsychiatric disorders.* New York: Oxford University Press.

Brenner, R., Ulrich, R., Spiker, D., Sclabassi, R., & Reynolds, C. (1986). Computerized EEG spectral analysis in elderly normal, demented, and depressed subjects. *Electroencephalography and Clinical Neurophysiology, 64*, 483–492.

Breslau, J., Starr, A., Sicotte, N., Higa, J., & Buchsbaum, M. (1989). Topographic EEG changes with normal aging and SDAT. *Electroencephalography and Clinical Neurophysiology, 40*, 281–289.

Brown, P. (1989). Central nervous system amyloidoses: A comparison of Alzheimer's disease and Creutzfeldt–Jakob disease. *Neurology, 39*, 1103–1105.

Burns, A., Philpot, M. P., Costa, D. C., Ell, P. J., & Levy, R. (1989). The investigation of Alzheimer's disease with single photon emission tomography. *Journal of Neurology, Neurosurgery and Psychiatry, 52*, 248–253.

Carlyle, W., Ancill, R., & Sheldon, L. (1993). Aggression in the demented patient: A double blind study of loxapine versus haloperidol. *International Clinical Psychopharmacology, 8*, 103–108.

Chanarin, I., Deacon, R., Lumb, M., & Perry, J. (1989). Cobalaminfolate interrelationships. *Blood Review, 3*, 211–215.

Copeland, J., Kelleher, N., Kellett, J., Gourlay, A., & Gurland, B. (1976). A semistructured clinical interview for the assessment of diagnosis and mental state in the elderly. *Psychological Medicine, 6*, 439–449.

Copeland, J. R., Dewey, N., Henderson, A., Kay, D., & Neal, C. (1988). The Geriatric Mental State (GMS) used in the community: Replication studies of the computerized diagnoses AGECAT. *Psychological Medicine, 18*, 219–223.

Corey-Bloom, J., Galasko, D., Hofstetter, R., Jackson, J., & Thal, L. (1993). Clinical features distinguishing large cohorts with possible AD, probable AD, and mixed dementia. *Journal of the American Geriatrics Society, 41*, 31–37.

Cummings, J., & Benson, D. (1992). *Dementia*. Toronto: Butterwirth-Heinemann.

Cutler, N. R., Fakouhi, D., Smith, W. T., Hendrie, H. C., Matsuo, F., Sramek, J. J., & Herting, R. L. (1993). Evaluation of multiple doses of milacemide in the treatment of senile dementia of the Alzheimer's type. *Journal of Geriatric Psychiatry and Neurology, 6*, 115–119.

DeCarli, C., Haxby, J., Gillette, J., Teichberg, D., Rapoport, S., & Schapiro, M. (1992). Longitudinal changes in lateral ventricular volume in patients with dementia of the Alzheimer type. *Neurology, 42*, 2029–2036.

Eberling, J. L., Jagust, W. J., Reed, B. R., & Baker, M. G. (1992). Reduced temporal lobe blood flow in Alzheimer's disease. *Neurobiology of Aging, 13*, 483–491.

Edwards, A. J. (1993). *Dementia*. New York: Plenum Press.

Evenhuis, H. M. (1992). Evaluation of a screening instrument for dementia in aging mentally retarded persons. *Journal of Intellectual Disability Research, 36*, 337–347.

Fields, S., Fulop, G., Sachs, C., Strain, J., & Fillit, H. (1992). Usefulness of the neurobehavioral cognitive status examination in the hospitalized elderly. *International Psychogeriatrics, 4*, 93–102.

Fischhof, P., Saletu, B., Ruther, E., Litschauer, G., Moslinger-Gehmayr, R., & Herrmann, W. (1992). Therapeutic efficacy of pyritinol in patients with senile dementia of the Alzheimer type (SDAT) and multi-infarct dementia (MID). *Neuropsychobiology, 26*, 65–70.

Folstein, M., Folstein, S., & McHugh, P. (1975). "Mini-mental state": A practical method for grading the cognitive states of patients for the clinician. *Journal of Psychiatric Research, 12*, 189–198.

Fratiglioni, L., Grut, M., Forsell, Y., Viitanen, M., & Winblad, B. (1992). Clinical diagnosis of Alzheimer's disease and other dementias in a population survey. *Archives of Neurology, 49*, 927–932.

Galasko, D., Klauber, M., Hofstetter, R., Salmon, D., Lasker, B., & Thal, L. (1990). The MMSE in the early diagnosis of Alzheimer's disease. *Archives of Neurology, 47*, 49–52.

Giurgea, C. (1972). Vers une pharmacologie de l'activite integrative du cerveau: Tentative du concept nootrope en psychopharmacologie. *Actual Pharmacology, 25*, 115–156.

Golden, C., Osmon, D., Moses, J., & Berg, R. (1981). *Interpretation of the Halstead–Reitan Neuropsychological Battery*. New York: Harcourt Brace Jovanovich.

Golden, C., Zillmer, E., & Spiers, M. (1992). *Neuropsychological assessment and intervention*. Springfield, IL: Thomas.

Goodwin, J. S., Goodwin, J. M., & Garry, P. J. (1983). Association between nutritional status and cognitive functioning in a healthy elderly population. *Journal of the American Medical Association, 249*, 2917–2921.

Gottfries, C. (1991). Classifying organic mental disorders and dementia—A review of historical perspectives. *International Psychogeriatrics, 3*, 9–17.

Gottfries, C., Adolfsson, R., & Aquilonius, S. (1983). Biochemical changes in dementia disorders of the Alzheimer type (AD/SDAT). *Neurobiology of Aging, 4*, 261–271.

Gunther, W., Giunta, R., Klages, U., Haag, C., Steinberg, R., Satzger, W., Jonitz, L., & Engel, R. (1993). Findings of electroencephalographic brain mapping in mild to moderate dementia of the

Alzheimer type during resting, motor, and music-perception conditions. *Psychiatry Research: Neuroimaging, 50,* 163–176.

Gurland, B., Kuriansky, J., Sharpe, L., Simon, R., & Stiller, P. (1977). The comprehensive assessment and referral evaluation (CARE). *International Journal of Aging and Human Development, 8,* 9–42.

Gustafson, L. (1992). Clinical classification of dementia conditions. *Acta Neurologica Scandinavica, 139,* 16–20.

Herrmann, W., & Stephan, K. (1992). Moving from the question of efficacy to the question of therapeutic relevance: An exploratory reanalysis of a controlled clinical study of 130 inpatients with dementia syndrome taking piracetam. *International Psychogeriatrics, 4,* 25–44.

Holttum, J., & Gershon, S. (1992). The cholinergic model of dementia, Alzheimer type: Progression from the unitary transmitter concept. *Dementia, 3,* 174–185.

Israel, J., Kozarevic, N., & Sarorius, N. (1984). *Source book of geriatric assessment.* Basel, Switzerland: Karger.

Jacobson, R., Acker, C., & Lishman, W. (1990). Patterns of neuropsychological deficit in alcoholic Korsakoff's syndrome. *Psychological Medicines, 20,* 321–334.

Jarvik, L. F. (1992). Possible biological basis for a major memory disorder. In J. Morley, R. Coe, R. Strong, & G. Grossbergs (Eds.), *Memory function and age related disorders.* New York: Springer.

Johnson, J. W., & Asher, P. (1987). Gylcine potentiates the NMDS response in cultured mouse brain neurons. *Nature, 325,* 31–35.

Jones, H., Hedley-White, T., & Friedberg, S. (1985). Ataxic Creutzfeldt–Jakob disease: Diagnostic techniques and neuropathological observations in early disease. *Neurology, 35,* 254–357.

Jung, R., & Solomon, K. (1993). Clinical practice and psychiatric manifestations of Pick's disease. *International Psychogeriatrics, 5,* 187–202.

Kay, D., Henderson, A., Scott, R., Wilson, J., Rickwood, D., & Grayson, D. (1985). Depression and dementia among the elderly living in the Hobart community. *Psychological Medicine, 15,* 771–788.

Kraepelin, E. (1896). *Psychiatrie: Ein Lehrbuch für Studierende und Aerzte.* Leipzig, Germany: Verlag von Johann Ambrosius Bath.

Kuhn, F. J., Schingnitz, G., Lehr, E., Montagna, E., Hansen, H. D., & Giachetti, A. (1988). Pharmacology of WEB-1881-F, a central cholinergic agent, which enhances cognition and cerebral metabolism. *Archives of Internal Pharmacodynamic Therapy, 292,* 13–34.

Kumar, A., Schapiro, M. B., Grady, C., Haxby, J. V., Wagner, E., Salerno, J. A., Friedland, R. P., & Rapoport, S. (1991). High-resolution PET studies in Alzheimer's disease. *Neuropsychopharmacology, 4,* 35–46.

Kurz, A., Haupt, M., Pollmann, S., & Romero, B. (1992). Alzheimer's disease: Is there evidence of phenomenological subtypes? Observations from a longitudinal study. *Dementia, 3,* 320–327.

Lamberty, G. J., & Bieliauskas, L. A. (1993). Distinguishing between depression and dementia in the elderly: A review of neuropsychological findings. *Archives of Clinical Neuropsychology, 8,* 149–170.

Levitt, A. J., & Karlinsky, H. (1992). Folate, vitamin B_{12}, and cognitive impairment in patients with Alzheimer's disease. *Acta Psychiatrica Scandinavica, 86,* 301–305.

Marsden, C., & Fahn, S. (1987). *Movement disorders II.* London: Butterworths.

Mendez, M., Selwood, A., Mastri, A., & Frey, W. (1993). Pick's disease versus Alzheimer's disease: A comparison of clinical characteristics. *Neurology, 43,* 289–292.

Mielke, R., Herholz, K., Grond, M., Kessler, J., & Heiss, W. (1992). Severity of vascular dementia is related to volume of metabolically impaired tissue. *Archives of Neurology, 49,* 909–913.

Miller, B., Cummings. J., Villanueva-Meyer, J., Boone, K., Mehringer, C., Lesser, I., & Mena, I. (1991). Frontal lobe degeneration: Clinical, neuropsychological, and SPECT characteristics. *Neurology, 41,* 1374–1382.

Miyauchi, T., Hagimoto, H., Ishii, M., Endo, S., Tanaka, K., Kajiwara, S., Endo, M., Kajiwara, A., & Kosaka, K. (1994). Quantitative EEG in patients with presenile dementia of the Alzheimer type. *Acta Neurologica Scandinavica, 89,* 56–64.

Mondadori, C., & Classen, W. (1984). Effect of oxiracetam on the performance of aged rates in a one way active avoidance situation. *Clinical Neuropharmacology, 1984,* 770–771.

Nissen, T., Mellgren, S., & Selseth, B. (1989). Demens evaluert med MMSE. *Tidsskrift for den Norske Laegeforening, 109,* 1158–1162.

Oberholzer, A., Hendriksen, C., Monsch, A., Hieierli, B., & Stahelin, H. (1992). Safety and effectiveness of low-dose clozapine in psychogeriatric patients: A preliminary study. *International Psychogeriatrics, 4,* 187–195.

Ohno, M., Yamamoto, T., Kitajima, I., & Ueki, S. (1990). WEB 1881 F ameliorates impairment of working memory induced by scopolamine and cerebral ischemia in the three panel runway task. *Japanese Journal of Pharmacology, 54,* 53–60.

Olafsson, K., Jorgensen, S., Jensen, H., Bille, A., Arup, P., & Andersen, J. (1992). Fluvoxamine in the treatment of demented patients: A double blind, placebo controlled study. *Acta Psychiatrica Scandinavica, 85,* 453–456.

Onofri, M., Gambi, D., Del Re, M., Fulgente, T., Bazzano, S., Colamartino, P., & Malatesta, G. (1991). Mapping of event related potentials to auditory and visual odd ball paradigms in patients affected by different forms of dementia. *European Neurology, 31,* 259–269.

Overall, J. E., & Schaltenbrand, R. (1992). The SKT neuropsychological test battery. *Journal of Geriatric Psychiatry and Neurology, 5,* 220–227.

Parsons, O., & Nixon, S. (1993). Neurobehavioral sequelae of alcoholism. *Neurologic Clinics, 11,* 205–218.

Pinner, E., & Rich, C. (1988). Effects of trazodone on aggressive behavior in seven patients with organic mental disorder. *American Journal of Psychiatry, 145,* 1295–1296.

Powell, A. L., Mezrich, R. S., Coyne, A. C., Loesberg, A., & Keller, I. (1993). Convex third ventricle: A possible sign for dementia using MRI. *Journal of Geriatric Psychiatry and Neurology,* 217–221.

Rapp, M. S., Flint, A., Herrmann, N., & Proulx, G. (1992). Behavioral disturbances in the demented elderly: Phenomenology, pharmacotherapy, and behavioural management. *Canadian Journal of Psychiatry, 37,* 651–657.

Roman, G., Tatemichi, T., Erkinguntti, T., Cummings, J., Masdeu, J., Garcia, J., Amaducci, L., Orgogozo, J., Brun, A., Hofman, A., Moody, D., O'Brien, M., Yamaguchi, T., Grafman, J., Drayer, B., Bennet, D., Fisher, M., Ogata, J., Kokmen, E., Bermejo, F., Wolf, P., Gorelick, P., Bick, K., Pageau, A., Bell, M., DeCarli, C., Culebras, A., Korczyn, Z., Bogousslavsky, J., Hartmann, A., & Scheinberg, P. (1993). Vascular dementia: Diagnostic criteria for research studies. *Neurology, 43,* 250–260.

Rosen, J., Mulsant, B., & Wright, B. (1992). Agitation in severely demented patients. *Annals of Clinical Psychiatry, 4,* 207–215.

Roth, M., Tym, E., Mountjoy, C., Huppert F., & Hendrie H. (1986). CAMDE: A standardized instrument for the diagnosis of mental disorder in the elderly with special reference to the early detection of dementia. *British Journal of Psychiatry, 149,* 698–709.

Sabe, L., Jason, L., Juejati, M., Leiguarda, R., & Starkstein, S. (1993). Sensitivity and specificity of the mini-mental state exam in the diagnosis of dementia. *Behavioural Neurology, 6,* 207–210.

Saletu, B., & Anderer, P. (1988). EEG Mapping in der psychiatrischen diagnose und therapieforschung. In B. Saletu (Ed.), *Biologische Psychiatrie.* New York: Springer-Verlag.

Saletu, B., Anderer, P., Fischhof, P., Lorenz, H., Barousch, R., & Bohmer, F. (1992). EEG mapping and psychopharmacological studies with deribufylline in SDAT and MID. *Biological Psychiatry, 32,* 668–681.

Sawada, H., Udaka, F., Kameyama, M., Seriu, N., Nishinaka, K., Shindou, K., Kodama, M., Nishitani, N., & Okumiya, K. (1992). SPECT findings in Parkinson's disease associated with dementia. *Journal of Neurology, Neurosurgery, and Psychiatry, 55,* 960–963.

Schneider, L., & Sobin, P. (1992). Non-neuroleptic treatment of behavioral symptoms and agitation in Alzheimer's disease and other dementias. *Psychopharmacology Bulletin, 28,* 71–79.

Schneider, L., Pollock, V., & Lyness, S. (1990). A metaanalysis of controlled trials of neuroleptic treatment in dementia. *Journal of the American Geriatric Association, 38,* 553–563.

Shorvon, S. D., Carney, M. W. P., Chanarin, I., & Reynolds, E. H. (1980). The neuropsychiatry of megaloblastic anaemia. *British Journal of Medicine, 281,* 1036–1038.

Shulman, R. (1967). Vitamin B_{12} deficiency and psychiatric illness. *British Journal of Psychiatry, 113,* 252–256.

Simpson, S., & Foster, D. (1986). Improvement in organically disturbed behavior with trazodone treatment. *Journal of Clinical Psychiatry, 47,* 191–193.

Skoog, I., Nilsson, L., Palmertz, B., Andreasson, L., & Svanborg, A. (1993). A population based study of dementia in 85 year olds. *New England Journal of Medicine, 328,* 153–158.

Sneath, P., Chanarin, I., Hodkinson, H. M., McPherson, C. K., & Reynolds, E. H. (1973). Folate status in a geriatric population and its relation to dementia. *Age and Aging, 2,* 177–182.

Spignoli, G., Pedata, F., Giovanelli, L., Banfi, S., Moroni, F., & Pepeu, G. (1986). Effect of oxiracetam and piracetam on central cholinergic mechanisms and active avoidance acquisition. *Clinical Neuropharmacology, 9,* S39–S47.

Strathmann, G. C. (1988). Possible neurotransmitter basis of behavioral changes in Alzheimer's disease. *Annals of Neurology, 23,* 616–620.

Swaab, D. F. (1991). Brain aging and Alzheimer's disease, "wear and tear" versus "use it or lose it." *Neurobiology of Aging, 12,* 317–324.

Urakami, K., Shimomura, T., Ohshima, T., Okada, A., Adachi, Y., Takahashi, K., Asakura, M., & Matsumura, R. (1993). Clinical effect of WEB 1881 (Nebracetam Fumurate) on patients with dementia of the Alzheimer type and study of its clinical pharmacology. *Clinical Neurophamacology, 16,* 347–358.

Van der Cammen, T., Van Harskamp, F., Stronks, D., Passchier, J., & Schudel, W. (1992). Value of the mini-mental status examination and informants' data for the detection of dementia in geriatric outpatients. *Psychological Reports, 71,* 1003–1009.

Zappoli, R., Ametoli, G., Paganini, M., Battaglia, A., Novellini, R., & Pamparana, F. (1991). Topographic bit-mapped event-related neurocognitive potentials and clinical status in patients with primary presenile mental decline chronically treated with nicergoline. *Current Therapeutic Research, 49,* 1078–1097.

Zaudig, M. (1992). A new systematic method of measurement and diagnosis of "mild cognitive impairment" and dementia according to *ICD-10* and *DSM-III-R* criteria. *International Psychogeriatrics, 4,* 203–239.

Zaudig, M., Mittelhammer, J., Hiller, W., Pauls, A., & Thora, C. (1991). SIDAM-A structured interview for the diagnosis of dementia of the Alzheimer type multi-infarct dementia, and dementias of other etiology according to *ICD-10* and *DSM-III-R. Psychological Medicine, 21,* 225–236.

CHAPTER 8

Substance Abuse Disorders

TED D. NIRENBERG, EDITH S. LISANSKY-GOMBERG, AND TONY CELLUCCI

INTRODUCTION

In 1996, the first "baby boomers" turned fifty years of age. During the next two decades as the baby boomers enter their 60s there will be an inexorable increase in the elderly population. The proportion of people 65 years of age and older in the general population is now approximately 13%. While the percentage of older persons will clearly increase, the effect of this historical phenomenon on alcohol and drug consumption among the older persons in future years remains to be seen. Up to now, the data show that alcohol drinking in general, and heavy alcohol use in particular, declines with aging (Adams, Garry, Rhyne, Hunt, & Goodwin, 1990; Fillmore, 1987; Fillmore *et al.*, 1991; Glynn, Bouchard, LoCastro, & Laird, 1985). There are differences within the older age group; for the "young elderly," those 60 to 74, there are modest changes, with some investigators reporting an increase in alcohol consumption during those years (Glynn et al., 1985; Gordon & Kannel, 1983). Beyond the age of 75, the drop in alcohol intake is considerable, and there are fewer drinkers and fewer heavy drinkers in the older years. It is believed that this decrease relates to increasing health problems and to the increased proportion of women in older population subgroups. As is true throughout the life span, older women drink less and abuse alcohol less than do older men (E. S. L. Gomberg, 1995b). There are also geographic differences: the prevalence of alcohol abuse ranges among older persons from 1.5 percent in North Carolina to 3.7 percent in Baltimore (Helzer, Burnham, & McEvoy, 1991).

TED D. NIRENBERG • Department of Psychiatry and Human Behavior, and Center for Alcohol and Addiction Studies, Brown University, and Department of Emergency Medicine, Rhode Island Hospital, Providence, Rhode Island 02908.   EDITH S. LISANSKY-GOMBERG • Alcohol Research Center, Department of Psychology, University of Michigan, Ann Arbor, Michigan 48104.   TONY CELLUCCI • Department of Psychology, Francis Marion University, Florence, South Carolina 29501-0547.

Handbook of Clinical Geropsychology, edited by Michel Hersen and Vincent B. Van Hasselt. Plenum Press, New York, 1998.

It is likely that with an increasing percentage of the population in the elderly group, there will be an increase in the number of elderly alcohol and drug abusers. Relatively unstudied are decisions about alcohol and drug use made by people as they age: some may choose to abstain, some to lower the quantity and frequency, some may continue exactly as they have been doing for decades, and others may increase the amount they use alcohol with the attendant risk of problems. Such decisions are part of the aging process; for example, older adults may need to decide whether to continue work or retire, work part-time or start new careers, where to live, whether to travel, and whether to become active in community institutions such as the church, elder hostels, or volunteer organizations. In a word, decisions have to be made about lifestyle, and decisions about alcohol and drug use are part of adaptation to aging. Health status, marital status, and income will play significant roles in these decisions.

Over the life span, there are biological changes in the body's response to different drugs. To learn about altered drug response in elderly persons, effects of age on pharmacokinetics and pharmacodynamics need to be studied. Gambert (1992) reviewed many of the physiological aspects of substance abuse in older persons. Such changes associated with aging may heighten the impact of alcohol and other drugs. For example, there is a decline in fluid relative to body mass, so drinking results in a higher blood alcohol concentration and greater CNS effects, including possible confusion and falls. Drug induced hypotension also may be greater and more prolonged at this time of life, thus increasing risk for cardiovascular problems. There is decreased respiratory functioning and exercise tolerance. In addition, neuroceptors may be more sensitive with advancing age, and the slow release of fat-soluble drugs into the bloodstream may cause protracted effects (Miller, Belkin, & Gold, 1991). As a result, tolerance is reduced in the elderly and withdrawal from dependence may be more severe. Therefore, older individuals may find that amount of alcohol or other drugs that they could easily tolerate when they were younger now results in adverse effects (Wartenberg & Nirenberg, 1994).

Elderly individuals also seem to be more susceptible to adverse drug reactions (ADRs). ADRs can result from multiple drug therapy, drug overuse or misuse, slowing of drug metabolism or elimination, or age-related chronic diseases. ADRs in older persons are more severe than among younger patients. Risk factors for ADRs include being female, living alone, multiple illnesses, multiple drug intake, and poor nutritional status.

Although use and abuse of alcoholic beverages gets the lion's share of research and media attention, use and abuse of substances other than alcohol are relevant. Although illicit drugs ("street drugs") are not often used by the elderly, the use and overuse of opiates in medical practice for pain control may be a concern. Tobacco is frequently used and has been implicated in many health problems found among older persons. Over-the-counter (OTC) drugs and prescribed medications have not been well researched, although there are significant problems associated with its use; for example, overprescribing of benzodiazepine, the frequent use of sedative drugs in nursing homes, and in general the issue of drug noncompliance among the elderly. Finally there is alcohol, a recreational substance easily available to adults, which may lead to significant problems for many older persons. Abuse of alcoholic beverages by elderly persons has been studied and described (Beresford & Gomberg, 1995; E. S. L. Gomberg, 1982; E. S. L. Gomberg, 1990; Wartenberg & Nirenberg, 1994). First, a review of the abuse of illicit drugs, tobacco, prescription and over-the-counter medications, and alcohol is presented. This is followed by a discussion of assessment and treatment implications.

Illicit Drugs

The use of drugs such as marijuana, heroin, and cocaine does occur among some older individuals, but it is a limited phenomenon. Of interest, though, are reports about a small group of opiate addicts who survive into old age (DesJarlais, Joseph, & Courtwright, 1985). Despite the widely held idea that addicts die or "mature out," there are addicts who survive into old age. DesJarlais and his colleagues (1985) described a group of heroin-dependent patients, 65 and older, attending methadone maintenance facilities. These long-term addicts survived by avoiding violence, using clean needles during IV use, and apparently being able to hold some drug supply in reserve. They also tend to avoid other drugs such as alcohol. Although we find such survivors among the heroin-dependent, it is less likely that we will find them among cocaine- or crack-dependent groups. In Michigan (Michigan Department of Public Health, 1994), treatment admissions for heroin-dependent people is 6% for those less than 60 years of age and 3% for those 60 years and older. Treatment admissions for those dependent on cocaine or crack is 18% for those under 60 and 2% of those 60 and older. In addition, opium smoking among older people is seen in some Oriental cultures. With increased immigration to the United States from Southeast Asia, this phenomenon may increase.

Tobacco

Men are more likely to be tobacco smokers than are women, although the gender gap has narrowed in the past three decades. The National Center for Health Statistics (1986) reported that in 1965, 28.5% of older men and 9.6% of older women were smokers. By 1985, percentages had become 19.6% for men and 13.5% for women. It is striking that the proportion of older men who smoke has decreased while the proportion of older women who smoke has increased. Among women aged 20 to 64, the percentage of current smokers has been dropping (not true among adolescent girls; Berman & Gritz, 1993). One may speculate that the female cohort that began smoking during and immediately after World War II is the current older population group. The price of such "liberated" behavior has been high: In the 1960s, female deaths from lung cancer began to rise. Since 1985, lung cancer has surpassed breast cancer as the chief cause of cancer death among women. However, it is difficult to establish the role of tobacco in the health status of older people. A study of drug metabolism (Sellers, Frecker, & Romach, 1982) concluded that the effects of aging, smoking, and drinking are confounded and difficult to disentangle.

Prescribed and Nonprescribed Psychoactive Drugs

In terms of prevalence, use of prescribed psychoactive drugs (e.g., sedatives, antidepressants, stimulants, anxiolytics) probably involves the greatest number of older persons. Although the elderly represent only approximately 13% of the general population, estimates are that they receive at least one third of all prescriptions. While such prescriptions include antibiotics, diuretics, cardiovascular medication, and analgesics, they also include significant amounts of psychoactive drugs (E. S. L. Gomberg, 1987).

Although treatment facilities report some elderly patients with drug-associated problems and dependence on prescribed psychoactive drugs, the issue has not evoked much interest among researchers, clinicians, or legislators. Older persons frequently associate their intake of psychoactive drugs with problems such as insomnia or depression and almost half of those taking such medication report that they could not perform their daily activities without the medication (Prentice, 1979). It is difficult to define what abuse of prescribed psychoactive drugs is. Kleber (1990) has differentiated primary low-dosage dependency, primary high-dosage dependency, and secondary dependency as patterns seen with benzodiazepine use. Individuals may use benzodiazepines in usually prescribed low therapeutic doses, in prescribed high doses, or in multiple drug use, frequently involving alcohol, to achieve a "high" or some form of self-prescribed release. Use in high doses or in multiple drug use usually involves withdrawal symptoms when drug use is terminated. Another classification of prescribed psychoactive drug use distinguishes appropriate use, unintentional misuse, and purposeful misuse.

There are a number of issues that may be raised about older individuals' use of prescribed psychoactive medication. First, questions have been raised about use of such medications in nursing homes. How certain can we be that medication given to ensure docility and compliance of the patient is given for that individual's own benefit? Second, as noted earlier, what is the risk of adverse drug reactions (ADRs)? It is estimated that the incidence of ADRs is two to three times more frequent among older patients. Studies suggest that several drugs (i.e., dioxin, diuretics, aspirin, cytoxins, nonsteroidal anti-inflammatory drugs, and psychotropics) in particular should be monitored for ADRs. ADRs may be a consequence of multiple drug therapies, drug interactions, changes in drug metabolism and elimination with age, noncompliance with prescribed use, incompatible food-drug combinations, or alcohol intake combined with medication use.

Noncompliance with prescribed drug regimens is an interesting and understudied phenomenon. In all age groups, noncompliance in use of prescribed medication is noted, but it commands more attention when manifested by older persons. Although noncompliance with medication by elderly persons is often attributed to cognitive impairment, it appears to be more complex than simple memory failure. Perhaps rebellion against authority or need for autonomy is involved. Noncompliance includes the following: (1) not obtaining the prescribed drug, possibly because of limited financial resources; (2) not completing the prescribed course of medication, often because of side effects or because the patient feels better; (3) incorrect dosage (more or less than prescribed); (4) improper timing or sequencing of medication; (5) combining the prescribed medication with OTC drugs; (6) sharing medications: using medications prescribed for another person; and (7) stockpiling or hoarding medications.

In a pilot study of patient medication compliance in a veterans hospital, male outpatients with a mean age of 58 reported stockpiling or hoarding medication as their major noncompliant behavior (E. S. L. Gomberg, Hsieh, & Adams, 1990). As pointed out by the investigators, such hoarding might well be construed as adaptive behavior for a low-income group threatened by budget cuts.

A comparison of different age groups in drug-associated emergencies is revealing. In the 43 major American cities for which emergency department data are included in the Drug Abuse Warning Network (Annual Medical Examiner Data, 1995), younger patients were more likely to die in emergencies relating to illicit drugs like cocaine than were older patients. Of those for whom the "drug mention" was cocaine, 74% were between the ages of 26 and 44. Among persons 55 and older, the most frequent "drug mentions" included nonbarbiturate and barbiturate sedatives, nonnarcotic analgesics, antidepressants, and tranquilizers. Also frequent were emergencies of older persons involving the use of such over-the-counter drugs as diphenhydramine.

Examination of the gender patterns in drug abuse deaths reported by the Drug Abuse Warning Network indicates that the proportion of drug abuse deaths reported for women in the 55 and older group is twice that for men in the same group: 6.5% for the men, 13.3% for women. This is striking, considering that men use emergency departments three times more frequently than do women. This gender difference is primarily a White phenomenon. Blacks show the same proportion of drug abuse deaths for men and women and Hispanics show twice as many for men as for women.

Nonprescription drugs (OTC) also are frequently used and abused by the older persons; in fact, two thirds of persons greater than 60 years of age take at least one OTC drug daily (Abrams & Alexopoulous, 1988). The most commonly purchased nonprescription drugs are analgesics, nutritional supplements (e.g., vitamins), antacids, and laxatives. The Food and Drug Administration has suggested special labeling for persons over 65 but the general response to age-related labeling on OTC drugs has been negative; the consensus is that labeling by specific medical conditions and symptoms is preferable. While generally viewed as less dangerous than prescribed medications, the OTC drugs are frequently misused—either underutilized, overutilized, or negatively interacting with another drug.

Alcohol

Although a large percentage of older people continue to drink moderately (and some, heavily), by and large the percentage of elderly who drink and the amount they drink diminish with age. There are, however, a number of recent reports that suggest that among some older groups, alcohol consumption remains steady or even increases (Eaton, Kramer, & Anthony, 1989; Gordon & Kannel, 1983; Huffine, Folkman, & Lazarus, 1989). Community survey findings vary with the age range studied, the gender ratio in the population, and the geographic site. There is some evidence that after declining, the rate of alcohol abuse among older males rises (Eaton et al., 1989); this confirms an early epidemiological study that reported a jump in the proportion of alcoholics among men in their seventies (Bailey, Haberman, & Alksne, 1965).

In all age groups, women tend to drink less than men, and it is apparently true with older cohorts. As noted earlier, there also are geographic differences among samples: whereas prevalence of alcohol abuse was reported as 1.5% in the Piedmont area of North Carolina, it was 3.7% in Baltimore (Helzer *et al.,* 1991). In California, 8.2% of respondents aged 65 to 74, and 6.4% aged 75 and over were "heavy drinkers" (Molgard, Nakamura, Stanford, Peddecord, & Morton, 1990). Retirement communities have reported a high prevalence (i.e., 20% or more) of heavy drinking (Alexander & Duff, 1988; Paganini-Hill, Ross, & Henderson, 1986). Explanations of lowered alcohol consumption among older persons in terms of historical experience with Prohibition and the Depression are increasingly inappropriate as this generation begins to die. Also, such explanations have always been limited by the fact that many western countries, which did not experiment with Prohibition, show similar rates and patterns of drinking by older age groups.

It is difficult to estimate the extent of alcohol abuse and dependence. Community surveys and hospital interviews produce some estimates ranging as high as 25% of the elderly. As always, it is a matter of definition, with some investigators addressing heavy drinking, others alcohol-associated problems, and still others clinically defined abuse and dependence. Helzer and his colleagues (1991) have pointed out that a much higher percentage of older people had less severe alcohol problems in the Epidemiologic Catchment Area data. When estimates of heavy or problem drinking are made, particularly in retirement communities, prevalence ranges from 20% (Alexander & Duff, 1988) to 31% of men and 22% of women 60 years of age and older (Paganini-Hill *et al.,* 1986). Clearly, alcohol use cannot be written off as irrelevant to the older age group simply because many of the heavy drinkers or problem drinkers have died or "matured out" of such behavior.

By and large, the patterns of drinking and alcohol-related problems do not seem very different for young and older problem drinkers (DeHart & Hoffman, 1995). Older problem drinkers are less likely to have work-associated problems, but they may have more alcohol-related health problems, more accidents, more concern about finances, and possibly more likelihood of binge drinking. Variations within the population of older problem drinkers, who range from unemployed, homeless Skid Row men (Rubington, 1982) to retired executives of corporations, suggest that the private versus public aspects of drinking, the beverages consumed, and the consequent difficulties vary widely.

Information specifically about elderly female problem drinkers is limited, but a recent report comparing problem drinking elderly men and women (E. S. L. Gomberg, 1995b) shows a remarkable consistency. The women, however, reported more marital disruption, although in this age group, it is more likely that widowhood is a major form of marital disruption. When queried about onset of their alcohol problem, more than a third of the women reported onset within the past ten years, compared with only 4% of the men studied. Women also are admitted to treatment programs with shorter duration of problem drinking than men in all age groups. Heavy or problem drinking by a spouse or significant other is, again, reported by more women than men—true of all age groups studied. Women report more drinking at home and men more drinking in public places. And, finally, as is true in all age comparisons, elderly women are more likely to report heavy use and dependency on prescribed psychoactive drugs than are men.

A comparison of black and white elderly alcoholic men in treatment shows some interesting differences (E. S. L. Gomberg & Nelson, 1995). Although drawn from the same clinical sources, the black patients had significantly less education and lower occupational status and income. In terms of drinking patterns, the black patients drank larger quantities, preferred distilled beverages, and were more likely to drink outdoors or in public places. Consequences of heavy drinking that were health-related were reported more often by black patients. Black men also reported more difficulty in the workplace and with the police. A regression model for social and community drinking consequences suggested that educational achievement, lifetime daily drinking average, drinking in public, and race had the greatest relevance. It is of interest to note that "objections from family members" was an area of similarity between elderly black and white men.

There is a fair amount of published literature on neuropsychological or cognitive loss as a consequence of heavy drinking. Deficits have been studied in terms of functions impaired, gender differences, the relationship to age, and heavy alcohol use. A "premature aging" hypothesis posited premature senescence brought on by heavy drinking; the hypothesis said little about elderly drinkers, but instead focused on middle-aged alcohol abusers. Cognitive impairment studies tend to focus on such specific functions as short-term memory and the ability to process new information. A significant clinical problem is the reversibility of cognitive loss; most clinicians agree that elderly alcohol abusers will, given sufficient time, regain most of their lost functioning. Older persons need more time than younger problem drinkers for such reversal to occur. However, some alcohol-dependent patients recovering from classic Wernicke's encephalopathy exhibit the selective memory disturbance of Korsakoff's amnestic syndrome, which involves long-term deficits in anterograde and retrograde memory and apathy (Kopelman, 1995; Victor, Adams & Collins, 1989).

Finally, there is a neglected, understudied group of elderly problem drinkers. Once called the chronic drunkenness offenders, this Skid Row group has become merged with the general homeless population. In past studies, a disproportionately high percentage of arrests for public intoxication was noted among men 60 years of age and older (Epstein, Mills & Simon, 1970). There have been significant changes since a Supreme Court decision of the 1960s in which arrests for public drunkenness were ruled a violation of rights under the 8th amendment of the Bill of Rights (i.e., cruel and unusual punishment for the disease of alcoholism). There has been a shift toward more available detoxification sites for this group (Rubington, 1982); unfortunately, without also providing rehabilitation, the detoxification sites have turned into the revolving door that jails once represented. This subgroup of elderly alcohol abusers still deserves study and rehabilitation effort.

Age of Onset

Clinical observations have led to classification of elderly problem drinkers and alcoholics on the basis of whether alcohol problems began earlier or later in their life: early versus late onset (Atkinson, Turner, Kofoed, & Tolson, 1985; Zimberg, 1974). The age cutoff used to delimit late-onset problem drinking typically ranges from 40 to 60 years (Atkinson, 1984). Late-onset problem drinking has been reported to account for between 28% and 40% of elderly problem drinkers found in clinical samples (Atkinson *et al.*, 1985; Rosin & Glatt, 1971; Zimberg, 1974). There is disagreement among researchers and clinicians about the specifics of this classification, in particular, the age that should be used to define late onset. If one uses 40 years of age as the cutoff of late onset, we would be including problem drinkers with a history of 25 or 30 years of alcohol abuse. Other efforts at classification attempt to capture more variation in drinking patterns by including categories for drinkers whose problems are transient or intermittent throughout the individual's lifetime, or that may vary over time with respect to the quantity and consequences of drinking (E. S. L. Gomberg, 1982; Dunham, 1981). An alternative definition of late onset views the problem drinking developed relatively recently as linked to adaptations and difficulties related to aging. Gomberg (1990) defined *recent* onset as the preferable term, the criterion being the beginning of alcohol-related problems within the past 10 years.

The epidemiological literature on risk factors predicting vulnerability to late-onset alcohol problems is limited (Douglas, 1984). Generally, late-onset patients are seen as having less family history of alcoholism and greater psychological resources (Atkinson, Tolson, & Turner, 1990). Some evidence suggests that late-onset alcohol problems are a maladaptive response to common personal, social, and environmental stressors that are correlates of the aging process (Atkinson, 1984; Finlayson, Hurt, Davis & Morse, 1988; Rosin & Glatt, 1971; Zimberg, 1974). Schonfeld and Dupree (1991) compared early- versus late-onset alcohol abusers, matched for age and gender. Although late-onset patients were more stable in terms of residence, both groups experienced the losses and stresses associated with aging, including diminished social support, loneliness, and feelings of depression. Zimberg (1995) has argued that although reactive drinking in response to the stressors of aging describes the late-onset alcoholic, such events also may prolong drinking problems in those patients with early-onset alcohol problems.

DIAGNOSIS

Substance-related disorders are classified by the *Diagnostic and Statistical Manual of Mental Disorders,* 4th edition (*DSM-IV;* American Psychiatric Association, 1994) into two groups: (1) Substance Use Disorders which include Substance Dependence and Substance Abuse and (2) Substance-Induced (S-I) disorders which include Substance Intoxication, Substance Withdrawal, S-I Delirium, S-I Persisting Amnestic Disorder, S-I Mood Disorder, S-I Anxiety Disorder, S-I Sexual Dysfunction, and S-I Sleep Disorder.

The general criteria for diagnosis of Substance Dependence include tolerance; withdrawal; substance use in larger amounts or over a longer period of time than was intended; persistent desire or unsuccessful efforts to cut down or control substance use; much time spent in activities necessary to obtain or use the substance or recover from its effects; social, occupational, or recreational activities given up or reduced because of substance use; and continued use despite knowledge of having a persistent or recurrent physical or psychological problem that is likely to have been caused or exacerbated by the substance. Criteria for Substance Abuse include recurrent substance use resulting in a failure to fulfill major role obligations at work, school, or home; recurrent substance use in situations in which it is physically hazardous; recurrent substance-related legal problems; and continued substance use despite having persistent or recurrent social or interpersonal problems caused or exacerbated by the effects of the substance. The S-I disorders, though frequently overlooked by clinicians, are highly relevant to the elderly patient. Although older persons may not exactly fit the criteria of dependence or abuse, their substance use may be the cause or one of the causes of another disorder.

Relevance of the *DSM-IV* diagnostic criteria to the older persons is questionable since the criteria were based primarily on younger age groups. Indeed, some of the criteria may not be relevant to many older individuals (King, Van Hasselt, Segal & Hersen, 1994). For some older people, absence of standard daily obligations (e.g., work, community service, school, and child rearing) and physical and medical problems may obscure signs of substance intoxication and withdrawal. Therefore, reliance on such criteria may lead to misdiagnosis and probably explains the apparent underdiagnosis and inconsistencies in reported prevalence rates. To address this problem, it has been suggested that the weight of these criteria for older people be changed (Atkinson, 1990) or that there be more focus on the elderly person's pattern of use.

Many of the assessment instruments that have been developed have been standardized on younger age groups. Only recently has the validity of these instruments for use with older persons been examined. For instance, Jones, Lindsey, Yount, Soltys, and Farani-Enayat (1993) examined the validity of the CAGE questionnaire (Ewing, 1984) and the Michigan Alcoholism Screening Test (MAST; Selzer, 1971) for patients 65 years of age or older. They found, by using the alcohol module of the Revised Diagnostic Interview Schedule (DIS-III-R) as the "gold standard," that the CAGE was more effective than the MAST in identifying elderly medical outpatients with alcohol abuse or dependence. However, the finding that both the CAGE and the MAST had low sensitivities at the conventional screening cutoffs suggests that cutoffs should be modified for older persons. Willenbring, Christensen, Spring, and Rasmussen (1987), however, in a comparison of four versions of the MAST used with an elderly sample found that the regular MAST had excellent sensitivity. F. C. Blow and colleagues (1992) introduced a geriatric version of the MAST. Although the scale needs further study, it is one of the first attempts to devise a screening tool that takes into account the unique characteristics of the elderly. Similarly, Finney, Moos, and Brennan (1991) developed the Drinking Problems Index, a 17-item test that assesses older persons' drinking problems over the past year. It includes such items as being intoxicated or drunk, feeling confused after drinking, feeling isolated from others due to drinking, and falling or having an accident because of drinking.

Further development and refinement of existing instruments that will be sensitive to older persons are warranted. Graham (1984) argues that older individuals may have memory impairments that affect the validity of self-reported alcohol use and abuse. Although memory impairment is clearly a correlate of severe dementia, very little is known about implications of moderate or mild dementia on self-reports (Fogel, Furino, & Gottlieb, 1990). Selecting appropriate measures and employing multiple measures is essential to ensure the validity of self-reports (Babor, Stevens, & Marlatt, 1987; Carp, 1989; Tucker, Gavornik, Vuchinich, Rudd, & Harris, 1989; Werch, 1989). Procedures should minimize response bias on alcohol and drug measures that are due to memory loss, for example, avoiding items that require mental averaging and increasing use of fixed-response choices (National Institute on Alcohol Abuse and Alcoholism, 1990; Babor et al., 1987).

In addition to self-report measures, investigators should (1) obtain collateral reports (i.e., from caregivers, spouse, children, and friends), (2) examine previous medical records, (3) use breath alcohol tests and drugs toxicology screens, (4) examine biochemical markers of alcohol abuse such as gama-glutamyl transpeptidase, and (5) assess medical conditions and psychosocial problems that might be correlated with substance abuse. Much of the literature on substance abuse and older persons discusses the need for treatment to take into account the unique biological and psychosocial factors associated with aging. Clearly, treatment recommendations and planning should be based on a comprehensive assessment, with a continuum of services available for both substance abuse and dependence.

TREATMENT

Despite prevalence data reviewed earlier, older persons are underrepresented in treatment settings (Lawson, 1989). The diagnosis of substance abuse problems reported by clinicians is less than prevalence rates as determined by the Epidemiologic Catchment area study (Miller *et al.,* 1991). Moos, Mertens, and Brennan (1993) found that older inpatients were less likely to be referred for rehabilitation, which is consistent with earlier studies suggesting underdiagnosis. For many reasons, older individuals also seek outpatient mental health services, including alcohol treatment, less readily than younger persons (Brennan & Moos, 1991; Carstensen, Rychtarik, & Prue, 1985). Generally, help seeking among older persons is more prevalent if they are female, have more negative life events and chronic stressors, report fewer friends who approve of drinking, use more avoidant coping, and have a history of prior use of treatment (Brennan, Moos, & Mertens, 1994; Finney & Moos, 1995).

There are a number of barriers that may prevent older adults from obtaining help (Lawson, 1989; Zimberg, 1995). First, there are differences in presentation and, as noted earlier, difficulties in diagnosis. Health care professionals often lack training and knowledge about substance abuse, especially patterns of substance abuse in this population (Lewis, 1995). There are also such patient characteristics as long-standing denial accompanied by severe medical complications. Medical and social problems of the elderly are often inappropriately seen as simply part of the aging process. Certainly, attitudes that substance abuse among older patients does not warrant or respond to treatment efforts reflect ageism. However, there also are practical problems involved including lack of financial resources and insurance, or limited transportation. Lawson (1989) has argued that older persons should be treated in the settings they frequent (e.g., senior centers, primary care facilities), and Zimberg (1995) perceives lack of treatment models alternative to traditional and 12-step programs as a limitation. There is a need for further research on possible impediments to engaging older problem drinkers in treatment.

There also has been little empirical study of the effectiveness of substance abuse treatment approaches with elderly patients, and much of the available information is retrospective (Institute of Medicine, 1990). Early studies (e.g., Janik & Dunham, 1983) found treatment effects for older patients to be comparable with those of younger patients in traditional programs. However, other clinical investigators have argued for programs specific to older people (Dupree, Broskowski, & Schonfeld, 1984; Zimberg, 1974, 1995). In a systematic examination of this issue, Kofoed, Tolson, Atkinson, Toth, and Turner (1987) compared use of elder-specific peer groups with a control group of patients seen in typical mixed-age outpatient groups. Those alcoholics (mean age 60.2 years) who received elder-specific treatment were more likely to remain in treatment despite lapses and were less likely to be drinking at discharge. A follow-up study of the same program revealed that 57% of patients completed one year of elder-specific outpatient treatment, in marked contrast to the 27% completion rate typical of many VA programs (Atkinson, Tolson, & Turner, 1993).

Krashner, Rodell, Ogden, Guggenheim, and Karson (1992) similarly compared an "older alcohol rehabilitation" (OAR) program to traditional treatment in a VA setting. The study population, described as mostly unmarried, white, with less than a high school education, and relatively poor, was randomly assigned to the two programs. OAR patients resided on a separate unit with specialized staff. Peer relationships and use of reminiscence therapy were emphasized, as opposed to traditional confrontation and problem solving. At a 1-year follow-up, OAR patients were significantly more likely to report abstinence and this difference increased with patient age.

Although these data suggest that there is therapeutic value in special programming for elders, findings from the National Drug and Alcoholism Treatment Unit survey indicated that such efforts are relatively rare. Only 9% of NIDA/NIAAA treatment units in 1982 reported offering specialized programs for elderly patients, with the proportion declining to 8% in 1987 (Institute of Medicine, 1990). Similarly, Nirenberg and Maisto (1990) in a survey of VA inpatient alcohol treatment programs found that only 3% of program directors reported providing special interventions in terms of minority issues or special populations.

Detoxification, Medical Complications, and Medication

In evaluating the need for detoxification, the patient's prior withdrawal experience, level of tolerance, and clinical status should be considered (Wartenberg & Nirenberg, 1995). The older patient may have fewer hyperautonomic signs, but may be at greater risk for associated complications. A recent study of withdrawal distress revealed that elderly patients experienced significantly more withdrawal symptoms for a longer time despite similar drinking histories prior to admission (Brower, Mudd, Blow, Young, & Hall, 1994). They also were more likely to experience cognitive impairment, daytime sleepiness, weakness, and high blood pressure. These latter symptoms may reflect underlying medical conditions. Wartenberg and Nirenberg (1995) generally recommend that the elderly patient in withdrawal be medically monitored. Treatment of acute withdrawal may involve administration of a short-acting benzodiazepine, usually lorazepam. The dose may need to be modified and the detoxification period extended for the elderly patient. Nutritional status should be assessed, with thiamine typically administered to prevent amnestic syndrome.

The elderly patient is more likely to have medical problems because of his or her association with chronic dependence and because of age-prevalent illnesses. Solomon, Manepalli, Ireland, and Mahon (1993) described the many medical consequences of alcoholism in the elderly, including peripheral neuropathy, acute and chronic pancreatitis, alcoholic liver disease, gastrointestinal bleeding, cardiomyopathy, cancer, and electrolyte and metabolic disturbances. An early review of the medical records of elderly patients with alcoholism found elevated rates of liver disease, peptic ulcers, psoriasis, and pulmonary disease (Hurt, Finlayson, & Morse, 1988). Gambert (1992) also listed age-prevalent diseases or conditions that may coexist with and are exacerbated by substance abuse. These include anemia, hypertension, gout, arrhythmias, diabetes, osteoporosis, dementia, and incontinence. Medical problems also may be caused by the interaction of alcohol and OTC medications (Lawson, 1989). A thorough evaluation of such medical problems is an important aspect of treatment, in that regaining and improving health status is often a goal the elderly substance abuser is motivated to work toward.

Certain medications (e.g., antabuse, naltrexone) are increasingly being recognized as having a legitimate role in substance abuse treatment, but little is known about their efficacy among elderly patients. In his review, Gorelick (1993) could not locate any medication trials that explicitly addressed pharmacological treatment of alcoholism in this population. While antabuse may be helpful in selected married, middle-aged men (Azrin, Sisson, Meyers, & Godley, 1982), it may be contraindicated in some medically compromised elderly patients. Zimberg (1995) also has discussed the importance of using antidepressants in treating depressed elderly patients who are also substance abusers.

Psychosocial Treatment

Evidence from general population surveys for the role of psychosocial stressors in development of excessive drinking among older persons has been conflicting (Jennison, 1992; Welte & Mirand, 1993). Jennison (1992) reported that subjects 60 years of age or above who experienced significant losses (e.g., divorce, lost employment, relative hospitalized or disabled) were more likely to drink excessively, although supportive resources (e.g., friends, family, church) had a stress buffering effect. However, Welte and Mirand (1993) did not find a relationship between acute stress and heavy drinking among older persons, although chronic stress did predict more drinking consequences and dependence. Krause (1995) found that drinking in later life tends to be a lifestyle factor rather than a coping response, with heavy drinking exacerbating the effect of salient role stressors on depressive symptoms. In a community hospital study of elderly inpatients on a general medical ward, neither alcohol consumption nor alcohol problems were found to be associated with the number of stressful life events reported (Laforge, Nirenberg, Lewis, & Murphy, 1993).

Yet, many elderly substance abuse patients present with recent psychosocial issues, and such events often are considered as contributing to late-onset substance abuse. For example, in an early study 81% of patients with late-onset alcoholism reported such life stressors as retirement, death of a spouse or relative, family conflict, and physical health problems (Finlayson *et al.,* 1988). Five of seven (71%) elderly late-onset alcohol patients in a VA sample were found to have recent difficulties adjusting to retirement (Carstensen *et al.,* 1985). Lawson (1989) has discussed the losses and other adjustments associated with aging as risk factors for substance abuse, although obviously not all stressed older persons become alcohol abusers. It may be that the clinically observed association between stressful life events and late-onset drinking problems is simply a reflection of the high rate of stressful events for the elderly population in general.

Considerable information has been generated about the personal characteristics, life circumstances, and coping responses of older individuals with drinking problems through the ongoing research program of Rudolf Moos and his colleagues (Brennan & Moos, 1995; Brennan *et al.,* 1994; Schutte, Brennan & Moos, 1994). A detailed assessment of selected elderly patients at several large medical facilities was used to obtain information about drinking status, health, and other life circumstances. The majority of the sample were white and well educated. Subjects were classified based on their Drinking Problem Index scores (Finney *et al.,* 1991) as either remitted problem drinkers, problem drinkers, or nonproblem drinkers. Problem drinkers reported more alcohol consumption and an average of five current drinking problems. In addition, they reported more negative life events and chronic stressors such as home difficulties, financial stress, and interpersonal conflict. Their life contexts involved fewer material resources and less social support from family and friends. Although problem drinkers and nonproblem drinkers reported similar types of stressors and coping strategies, the problem drinkers were more likely to react to stress with resignation and to use avoidance or emotion-focused coping. Not surprisingly, those elders in more stressful life contexts with fewer social resources had greater alcohol consumption, more drinking problems, and were more depressed. Moreover, greater use of avoidance coping was linked to chronic stress, fewer social resources, and eventually poorer functioning.

Importantly, personal and environmental risk factors also were found to interact. Heavier drinkers generally increased their consumption when they experienced more negative life events and, unlike lighter drinkers, did not reduce their consumption with new health events. Also, as with younger patients, association with peers who approve of drinking may sustain problem drinking status. This research suggests that intervention efforts should assess various domains of life functioning and aim for improved life circumstances, increased social resources, and adaptive coping skills.

Not all drinking problems among these older persons were stable; a sizable portion (approximately 20%–25%) of older individuals changed their drinking problem status over time. Most (70%) of those identified as remitted at 1 year maintained this status at a 4-year follow-up. A greater proportion of late-onset, as compared to early-onset, drinkers achieved stable remission. Patients who remitted generally included those with less consumption, fewer drinking problems, less spouse support, fewer friends who approved of drinking, more personal distress, and were more likely to have sought professional help. Correlates of remission also differed for early-onset versus late-onset problem drinkers with remission in the former group mostly associated with help-seeking efforts. Symptoms and life functioning of remitted drinkers relative to nonproblem drinkers continued to be poor early in their course of recovery, but were improved at the later follow-up, even though some deficits (e.g., marital strain and physical health) remained. This continuing research effort provides the clinician with a rich picture of the context, interactive nature, and course of late-life drinking problems.

Behavioral Treatment

To date, few treatment approaches have been evaluated for elderly substance abusers. Among these approaches is cognitive-behavioral skill training. A follow-up study of older patients treated in the alcohol treatment program in the Jackson Veterans Administration Hospital, which employed a social learning view of substance abuse, showed that many elderly responded positively to this approach (Carstensen *et al.,* 1985). In addition to medical attention, patients received alcohol education and counseling, which included training in self-management and problem-solving skills. Structured interviews with patients and collaterals revealed that 50% of these male veterans (aged 65–70) had successfully maintained abstinence for 2 to 3 years, with an additional 12% reporting significantly decreased intake.

The Gerontology Alcohol Project (GAP) in Florida is perhaps the most frequently cited reference (Dupree *et al.,* 1984) of behavioral treatment. This pilot day treatment program involved intensive assessment of 48 late-onset alcohol abusers (mean age 64) and a self-management treatment approach based on functional analysis of drinking, skill acquisition, and reestablishment of social support networks. Most of the subjects were either widowed, separated, or divorced, with generally poor social networks. In a community center for the aged, treatment using manuals was provided in a group format. Treatment consisted of various modules (e.g., analysis of the antecedents and consequences of drinking, self-management of high-risk situations, alcohol education, problem solving, building a social support network). In the original report, 17 patients chose abstinence and another 7 patients a treatment goal of limited, responsible drinking. Program success was conservatively defined as not violating these goals throughout the 12-month follow-up, with those lost in follow-up considered failures. Nevertheless, the program was 74% successful. There also was significant improvement in collateral ratings, community adjustment scores, and size of the patients' social networks. Of the few patients who slipped, none returned to their earlier abusive drinking pattern.

These reports support use of cognitive-behavioral treatment. However, the data are limited by the small sample sizes and by the problem of high treatment dropout rates. Moreover, in these studies there was little emphasis on cognitive intervention per se, although Glatz (1995) recently has suggested a method of applying the cognitive treatment model (see also Beck, Wright, Newman, & Liese, 1993) to the substance-abusing elderly.

Group Treatment

A second model that has been successfully employed with older substance abusers is supportive, social group treatment (Atkinson, 1995). There are many advantages of group treatment for this population, including counteracting feelings of loneliness and isolation, peer modeling and support, and opportunities to draw on the life experiences and leadership skills of the elderly. Lawson (1989) succinctly states that an important resource for older persons is older individuals themselves, and he discussed the need for therapists who genuinely like working with this population. Such groups have been described as positive and task oriented with the goal of making life more meaningful and enjoyable. Psychosocial themes explored in these groups include accepting the losses involved in aging, dealing with feelings of hopelessness and grief, confronting and solving life problems, and reviewing one's life or reminiscing. Physical fitness and social activities also may be included.

Zimberg (1995) suggested, for example, dividing weekly 2-hour group sessions into an informal socializing period with refreshments and a problem-solving time. While patients are told that they have a drinking problem that is probably related to the difficulties they are having in life adjustment, this is only one of the problem areas discussed. Zimberg has found that many elderly alcoholics are more comfortable in senior-oriented programs, although some may accept alcohol-specific treatment with the addition of such a psychosocial group focusing on the stresses of aging. A small survey of recovering elderly patients (Johnson, 1989) indicated that group treatment, especially elder-specific groups, was preferred by patients, who also made further recommendations to use large print materials and allow ample time for seniors to complete suggested projects. Such programs also may draw on community resources such as needed social services (e.g., home health and meals-on-wheels).

Much of the evaluation data supporting this approach have arisen from comparisons of elder-specific to mainstream treatment (Atkinson *et al.,* 1993; Kofoed *et al.,* 1987). Kofoed and colleagues (1987) reported on a sample of elderly (aged 55 to 76 years) in terms of program completion, known relapses, and successful treatment after relapses. The groups (containing 6 to 10 patients) met weekly in the afternoon, used a slower pace, and emphasized socialization and support versus confrontation. Sociotherapeutic processes included social bonding, shared reminiscences, alcoholism-related information, and efforts to resolve life problems. Abstinence was the stated goal for all patients. Seven of nine relapsing patients were successfully treated with only two patients drinking at discharge. In a 5-year study of the same program, 117 (57%) of 205 VA patients completed 1 year of outpatient treatment; this presumably translated into improved drinking status and psychological functioning (Atkinson *et al.,* 1993).

Although these reports have a different focus (e.g., predicting treatment compliance), the data have been used to support the use of such groups. More outcome information is needed on the impact of social treatment groups on other areas of life health besides drinking, and on comparisons with community samples. It is not advantageous to mix severely dependent and alcohol abusing patients who have different treatment perceptions and goals. Moreover, as yet no studies have compared supportive social groups to cognitive behavioral treatment (Atkinson, 1995).

Community Outreach

Community outreach programs are a third alternative for providing needed services to patients who may be unable or reluctant to leave their home. Graham and colleagues (1995) have recently published a report of their experience with the Community Older Persons Alcohol project in Toronto. This innovative, holistic program provided individualized assistance to seniors so as to maintain them in their homes and improve physical and emotional well-being (including a reduction or elimination of alcohol or other drug dependence or both). The intervention process included assessment, active treatment, and maintenance phases. A problem-centered, nonconfrontational approach was adopted using collaborative goal setting, counseling and other direct services, and case management. Monitoring data were reported on 56 treated clients (mean age 64). Most of the clients were drinking daily or nearly every day, although maximum average consumption was relatively low (i.e., 38% drinking five or more drinks per day). Use of psychoactive prescription drugs was high, with frequent problems related to poor medication compliance, side effects, and interactions with alcohol.

Overall, the investigators concluded that 40% of the clients showed improvement in both alcohol use and other life areas, with an additional 35% showing improvement in one area or the other. Life areas most consistently related to the status of alcohol problems were personal hygiene, activities of daily living, mental or cognitive health, and adequacy of diet. Also, physical health was the most likely to covary with other life areas, and it declined with the worsening of recent drinking status. Together the associations suggest a relationship between substance abuse and life areas related to maintaining clients in the community. An informal follow-up found that about half of the subjects maintained their gains after discharge. This thoughtfully conducted project exploring community outreach deserves careful reading and replication.

Family Treatment

Despite early discussion of the importance of family involvement (Dunlop, Skorney, & Hamilton, 1982), a literature search yielded few studies specifically evaluating family therapy for elderly substance abusers. Tabisz, Jacyk, Fuchs, and Grymonpre (1993) have described the Elders Health Program, an intervention program for chemically dependent seniors based in the emergency department of an acute-care hospital. About a third of the patients (65 years or older) were assessed as having active enablers in their family or social-professional networks, and this was particularly true of women in the sample. Although having an active enabler was not associated with outcome, patients with active enablers required greater intensity of effort. If spouses or families refused to cooperate, the coordinator stopped the intervention. Approximately half of the identified cases showed improvement after an individualized level of intervention. Although the enabling concept and Johnson Institute model have become widely accepted, there has been surprisingly little systematic research in this area (Liepman, Nirenberg, & Begin, 1989). There is a need for evaluating various models of working with family members whose older member continues to drink abusively, as well as the effectiveness of marital and family treatment for seniors (see O'Farrell, 1993).

Self-Help Groups

Elderly patients are frequently referred to Alcoholics Anonymous and other 12-step recovery groups, which have continued to grow in popularity (Weisner, Greenfield, & Room, 1995). In 1990, older men (age 50 or over) with dependency symptoms were more likely to go to Alcoholics Anonymous (AA) or a private physician than other types of treatment. Accompanying this growth in AA has been the development of specialized AA groups for elderly alcoholics in some communities (Zimberg, 1995). Although no research was found addressing the effectiveness of AA with elderly patients, current literature suggests the importance of preparing patients to affiliate with AA and matching selected patients to an appropriate group (McCrady & Miller, 1993).

Patient–Treatment Matching

The concept of patient–treatment matching has become more accepted selecting appropriate treatment. A study by Rice, Longabaugh, Beattie, and Noel (1993) is apparently the first one to report a significant age-by-treatment interaction. A mixed age group (18 to 76 years) of 229 patients was randomly assigned to cognitive-behavioral treatment, relationship enhancement, or an occupational focus condition. The percentage of abstinent and heavy drinking days was examined 3 to 6 months after treatment assignment. Although there were no overall differences between treatment conditions or defined age groups, the older patients (50 years or greater) did significantly better with cognitive-behavioral treatment as opposed to the occupational focus. The authors suggest that this may have been due to the reduced social influence and/or support associated with the workplace in later years. It seems reasonable to conclude that the effectiveness of treatment will vary with the perceived importance and influence of issues addressed at a particular stage in the life cycle. This speaks again to the importance of tailoring treatment programs to the psychosocial stressors involved in aging. Patient–treatment matching, however, also refers to the need to address important clinical and psychosocial issues found in selected subgroups of elderly patients (i.e., the medically ill, dually diagnosed, and women).

Medically ill alcoholics are generally older, unable to work, retired, frequently isolated or without family support, or combinations of these characteristics, and more often present with multiple health concerns to medical facilities. Frequently, they have refused referral to traditional treatment programs. Willenbring, Olson, Bielinski, and Lynch (1995) have described a demonstration project in an outpatient primary care center to reach these patients who have serious medical disorders, such as pancreatitis and liver disease. The goal was to reduce alcohol-related morbidity through interventions that reduce drinking and address psychosocial problems within the context of comprehensive medical treatment and follow-up. As with other chronic diseases, partial improvement and patient stabilization were seen as an acceptable goal in cases where permanent abstinence (although more desirable) had not been attained. Family and environmental interventions, asset management, and emergency hospitalization were used with the assumption that such patients would require long-term treatment planning and outpatient care.

In an initial evaluation, 30 male veterans admitted into the program were followed and their outcomes contrasted with a comparison group. Control patients met admission criteria but because of space limitations were treated elsewhere in the medical center; they were all offered but declined conventional alcoholism treatment. The mean age of the clinic patients was 61.5 years. For patients in the program, clinic visits significantly increased and hospitalization days declined. Moreover, there was less mortality (3%) relative to controls (31%) at a 13-month follow-up. In recognizing that patients continue to die from medical complications of alcohol dependence, these investigators challenged the field to consider what alternative but caring treatments might be provided to this difficult subgroup of elderly patients.

Those older persons who have comorbid psychiatric or organic disorders or both also pose a significant problem. The drinker whose cognitive or psychiatric problems appear to contribute to abusive drinking was one of three patient types discussed in Graham and colleagues' (1995) typology of clients in the Community Older Persons Alcohol project. Preexisting psychiatric disorder or intermittent cognitive problems interfered with their understanding of the need to control their drinking, often resulting in bizarre behavior and neglect of self-care. Stabilizing psychiatric treatment, increasing compliance with medicines, and dealing with the life sequelae of the person's drinking problem became the focus. Speer, O'Sullivan, and Schonfeld (1991) have discussed policy and planning issues that must be addressed as such patients increasingly enter the public mental health system.

Moos and colleagues (1993) found that such dually diagnosed older persons required more inpatient care as well as outpatient treatment after discharge and had higher 4-year readmission rates. Canter and Koretzky (1989) also reported that organically impaired older alcoholics were less likely to benefit from standard treatment and required a modified treatment approach. They suggested greater emphasis on stress reduction, with an individualized didactic approach to teaching about the physical and social impact of drinking. Also, there is a need to take into account the possible information-processing deficits of these patients, and evaluate the possible role of cognitive rehabilitation.

Finally, the distinct needs of older women with substance abuse problems deserve mention. Knowledge about women with substance abuse problems has proliferated with an increase in specialized treatment services (Galanter, 1995; E. S. Gomberg & Nirenberg, 1993; Szwabo, 1993). As discussed above, elderly women in treatment report more drinking problems among family members, have a later age of onset and shorter duration of alcohol abuse, report more depressive feelings, and are much more likely to be using prescribed tranquilizers in addition to alcohol (E. S. L. Gomberg, 1995b). Although it is not clear whether these patients are best provided services in treatment centers for women or specialized programs for the elderly, all treatment should be sensitive to gender issues.

Prevention

The need for research on health promotion and alcohol problem prevention among elderly persons is now just emerging as a national health care priority (Abdellah, 1988; Gilford, 1988; Noel & McCrady, 1984; Office of Technology Assessment, 1985). As a result, there have been few alcohol prevention studies targeted specifically toward older persons (Institute of Medicine, 1989; National Institute on Alcohol Abuse and Alcoholism, 1990). Existing studies focus on clinical samples of elderly alcoholics or problem drinkers to assess the need for or the differential impact of tertiary care, or both, or involve efforts to increase early detection (Beresford, Blow, Brower, Adams, & Hall, 1988; F. Blow, 1990; Curtis, Geller, Stokes, Levine, & Moore, 1989; Janik & Dunham, 1983; Kofoed *et al.*, 1987). Evaluative studies of health promotion and disease prevention programs with older persons drawn from other fields, however, generally provide evidence that health promotion education programs are usually well received by the elderly, and can lead to substantial improvements in health knowledge, skills performance, increased efforts to improve life-style, and improvements in the quality of life (Hersey, Glass, & Crocker, 1984; Nelson *et al.*, 1984).

As a group, older persons are very concerned with their health. Those aged 65 or over demonstrate greater compliance with many (but not all) recommended health behaviors (German, 1978; National Center for Health Statistics, 1986) and typically perceive those behaviors to be more efficacious than do persons under age 65 (Bausell, 1986; Nelson et al., 1984). Paradoxically, although older adults may be among the most health conscious, they also appear to be most in need of health information. Data from the 1985 Disease Prevention Health Promotion supplement to the National Health Interview survey indicate that persons aged 65 or over have the highest rates of "do not know/no opinion" responses to information items regarding the health effects of smoking, alcohol use, exercise, dietary, and dental behavior (National Center for Health Statistics, 1986). For example, at least 33% to 50% of all persons aged 65 or over responded "do not know" or "no opinion" to questions assessing knowledge of the association between alcohol consumption and the risk of throat, bladder or mouth cancer, arthritis, and blood clots. Such lack of information can be addressed through prevention initiatives focused on health promotion and health education.

Hospitals are an important community site for health promotion for older persons. Since 1979, the House of Delegates of the American Hospital Association has encouraged hospitals to identify target areas and population groups for hospital-based health promotion and disease prevention programs (American

Hospital Association, 1979), and older persons are among the most frequent target populations of these efforts. Studies suggest that more than 40% of hospitals have a health promotion program for older patients and their families (Longe, 1986). In addition to the enhanced availability of target populations, the hospital setting provides many unique opportunities for the identification, intervention, and prevention of alcohol problems (Babor, Ritson, & Hodgson, 1986; Institute of Medicine, 1990). Researchers consistently point to the general hospital as one of the best sites in which to identify and conduct alcohol problem prevention activities with at-risk elderly drinkers (Babor *et al.,* 1986; F. Blow, 1990; Brody, 1982). The hospital affords an opportunity to intervene with a captive population, who may be especially receptive to health promotion and problem prevention initiatives (Nutting, 1986). Techniques for screening and intervention have shown that the implementation of such programs is feasible and well accepted by general hospital patients (Lewis & Gordon, 1983). Further, the infrastructure of many hospitals already supports staff members who regularly conduct preventive interventions.

SUMMARY

The number of older persons in our communities will continue to grow over the next three decades. While available statistics as to prevalence of substance abuse among older individuals are only estimates, it is clear that older persons are not immune to this problem. In fact, due to biological and psychosocial characteristics, many older adults may be prone to developing substance abuse. Although it has been stated for years that elderly substance abusers (and for that matter many other special groups) require at least some degree of specialized care, to date the outcome data are lacking. However, interest in the elderly is evident and specialized programs may yet increase in number. There clearly is a need to develop a variety of intervention and treatment services for elderly patients with substance use or abuse problems, in keeping with their unique biopsychosocial factors and specific circumstances. Descriptive studies on this population should now give way to those testing specific treatments. The interventions and settings that work best for particular segments of the elderly population should be explored. The general finding that older patients in treatment do at least as well as younger patients (Atkinson, 1995), given the early stage of development of such programming, suggests that a great many more older persons with substance abuse difficulties can be effectively helped.

REFERENCES

Abdellah, F. G. (1988). *Surgeon General's workshop on health promotion and aging: Proceedings.* Department of Health and Human Services, U.S. Public Health Service, March 20–23.

Abrams, R. C., & Alexopoulous, G. S. (1988). Substance abuse in the elderly: Over-the-counter and illegal drugs. *Hospital and Community Psychiatry, 39,* 822–829.

Adams, W. L., Garry, P. J., Rhyne, R., Hunt, W. C., & Goodwin, J. S. (1990). Alcohol intake in the healthy elderly: Changes with age in a cross-sectional and longitudinal study. *Journal of the American Geriatric Society, 38,* 211–216.

Alexander, F., & Duff, R. W. (1988). Social interaction and alcohol use in retirement communities. *Gerontologist, 28,* 632–636.

American Hospital Association. (1979). *The hospital's responsibility for health promotion.* Policy statement from the American Hospital Association House of Delegates, Chicago.

American Medical Association. (1995). *Alcoholism in the elderly: Diagnosis, treatment, prevention: Guidelines for primary care physicians.* Chicago: Author.

American Psychiatric Association. (1994). *Diagnostic and statistical manual of mental disorders* (4th ed.). Washington, DC: Author.

Annual Medical Examiner Data 1993. (1995). Data from the Drug Abuse Warning Network (DAWN), Series 1, No. 13B (DHHS Publication No. (SMA) 95-3019). Rockville, MD: U.S. Department of Health and Human Services.

Atkinson, R. M. (1984). *Alcohol and drug abuse in old age.* Washington, DC: American Psychiatric Press.

Atkinson, R. M. (1990). Aging and alcohol use disorders: Diagnostic issues in the elderly. *International Psychogeriatrics, 2,* 55–72.

Atkinson, R. M. (1995). Treatment programs for aging alcoholics. In T. P. Beresford & E. Gomberg (Eds.), *Alcohol and aging* (pp. 186–210). New York: Oxford University Press.

Atkinson, R. M., Turner, J. A., Kofoed, L. L., & Tolson, R. L. (1985). Early versus late onset alcoholism in older persons: Preliminary findings. *Alcoholism: Clinical and Experimental Research, 9,* 513–515.

Atkinson, R. M., Tolson, R. L., & Turner, J. A. (1990). Late versus early onset problem drinking in older men. *Alcoholism: Clinical and Experimental Research, 14,* 574–579.

Atkinson, R. M., Tolson, R. L., & Turner, J. A. (1993). Factors affecting outpatient treatment compliance of older male problem drinkers. *Journal of Studies on Alcohol, 54,* 102–106.

Azrin, N. H., Sisson, R. W., Meyers, R., & Godley, M. (1982). Alcoholism treatment by disulfiram and community reinforcement therapy. *Journal of Behavior Therapy and Experimental Psychiatry, 13,* 105–112.

Babor, T. F., Ritson, E. B., & Hodgson, R. J. (1986). Alcohol-related problems in the primary health care setting: A review of early intervention strategies. *British Journal of Addiction, 81,* 23–46.

Babor, T. F., Stevens, R. S., & Marlatt, G. A. (1987). Verbal report methods in clinical research on alcoholism: Response bias and its minimization. *Journal of Studies on Alcohol, 48,* 410–424.

Bailey, M. P., Haberman, P. W., & Alksne, H. (1965). The epidemiology of alcoholism in an urban residential area. *Quarterly Journal of Studies on Alcohol, 26,* 19–40.

Bausell, R. B. (1986). Health-seeking behavior among the elderly. *Gerontologist, 26,* 556.

Beck, A. T., Wright, F. D., Newman, C. F., & Liese, B. S. (1993). *Cognitive therapy of substance abuse.* New York: Guilford.

Beresford, T. P., & Gomberg, E. S. L. (1995). *Alcohol and aging.* New York: Oxford University Press.

Beresford, T. P., Blow, F. C., Brower, K. J., Adams, K. M., & Hall, R. C. (1988). *Psychosomatics, 29,* 61–72.

Berman, B. A., & Gritz, E. R. (1993). Women and smoking: Toward the year 2000. In E. S. Lisansky-Gomberg & T. D. Nirenberg (Eds.), *Women and substance abuse* (p.p. 258–285), Norwood, NJ: Ablex.

Blow, F. (1990, April 6). *Screening for elderly alcohol problems.* Paper presented at Aging in the 1990s Alcohol and Other Drug Abuse Conference, Western Michigan University, Novi, MI.

Blow, F. C., Brower, K. J., Schulenberg, J. E., Demo-Dananberg, L. M., Young, K. J., & Beresford, T. P. (1992). The Michigan alcoholism screening test. Geriatric version (MAST-G): A new elderly-specific screening instrument [Abstract]. *Alcoholism Clinical & Experimental Research, 16* (2), 105, 372.

Brennan, P. L., & Moos, R. H. (1991). Functioning, life context, and help-seeking among late-onset problem drinkers: Comparisons with nonproblem and early-onset problem drinkers. *British Journal of Addiction, 86,* 1139–1150.

Brennan, P. L., & Moos, R. H. (1995). Life context, coping responses, and adaptive outcomes: A stress and coping perspective on late-life problem drinking. In T. P. Beresford & E. Gomberg (Eds.), *Alcohol and aging* (pp. 230–248). New York: Oxford University Press.

Brennan, P. L., Moos, R. H., & Mertens, J. R. (1994). Personal and environmental risk factors as predictors of alcohol use, depression, and treatment seeking: A longitudinal analysis of late-life problem drinkers. *Journal of Substance Abuse, 6,* 191–208.

Brody, J. A. (1982). Aging and alcohol abuse. *Journal of the American Geriatrics Society, 30,* 123–126.

Brower, K. J., Mudd, S., Blow, F. C., Young, J. P., & Hall, E. M. (1994). Severity and treatment of alcohol withdrawal in elderly versus younger patients. *Alcoholism: Clinical and Experimental Research, 18,* 196–201.

Canter, W. A., & Koretzky, M. B. (1989). Treatment of geriatric alcoholics. *Clinical Gerontologist, 9,* 67–70.

Carp, F. M. (1989). Maximizing data quality in community studies of older people. In M. P. Lawton & A. R. Regula (Eds.)., *Special research methods for gerontology.* Amityville, NY: Baywood.

Carstensen, L. L., Rychtarik, R. G., & Prue, D. M. (1985). Behavioral treatment of the geriatric alcohol abuser: A long term follow-up study. *Addictive Behaviors, 10,* 307–311.

Curtis, J. R., Geller, G., Stokes, E. J., Levine, D. M., & Moore, R. D. (1989). Characteristics, diagnosis, and treatment of alcoholism in elderly patients. *Journal of the American Geriatric Society, 37,* 310–316.

DeHart, S. S., & Hoffman, N. G. (1995). Screening and diagnosis of "alcohol abuse and dependence" in older adults. *The International Journal of the Addictions, 30,* 1717–1747.

DesJarlais, D. C., Joseph, H., & Courtwright, D. (1985). Old age and addiction: A study of elderly patients in methadone maintenance treatment. In E. Gottheil, K. A. Druley, T. E. Skoloda, & H. M. Waxman (Eds.)., *The combined problems of alcoholism, drug addiction, and aging* (pp. 201–209). Springfield, IL: Thomas.

Douglas, R. L. (1984). Aging and alcohol problems: Opportunities for socioepidemiological research. In M. Galanter (Ed.), *Recent developments in alcoholism* (Vol. 2, pp. 251–266). New York: Plenum.

Dunham, R. G. (1981). Aging and changing patterns of alcohol use. *Journal of Psychoactive Drugs, 13,* 143–151.

Dunlop, J., Skorney, B., & Hamilton, J. (1982). Group treatment for elderly alcoholics and their families. *Social Work in Groups, 5,* 87–92.

Dupree, L. W., Broskowski, H., & Schonfeld, L. (1984). The gerontology alcohol project: A behavioral treatment program for elderly alcohol abusers. *Gerontologist, 24,* 510–516.

Eaton, W. W., Kramer, M., & Anthony, J. C. (1989). The incidence of specific DIS/DSM-III mental disorders: Data from the N.I.M.H. Epidemiologic Catchment Area Program. *Acta Psychiatrica Scandinavia, 79,* 163–178.

Epstein, L. J., Mills, C., & Simon, A. (1970). Antisocial behavior of the elderly. *Comprehensive Psychiatry, 11,* 36–42.

Ewing, J. A. (1984). Detecting alcoholism: the CAGE questionnaire. *Journal of the American Medical Association, 252,* 1905–1907.

Fillmore, K. M. (1987). Prevalence, incidence, and chronicity of drinking patterns and problems among men as a function of age: A longitudinal and cohort analysis. *British Journal of Addiction, 82,* 77–83.

Fillmore, K. M., Hartka, E., Johnstone, B. M., Leino, E. V., Motoyoshi, M., & Temple, M. T. (1991). A meta-analysis of life course variation in drinking. *British Journal of Addiction, 86,* 1221–1268.

Finlayson, R. E., Hurt, R. D., Davis, N. J., & Morse, R. M. (1988). Alcoholism in elderly persons: A study of the psychiatric and psychosocial features of 216 inpatients. *Mayo Clinic Proceedings, 63,* 761–768.

Finney, J. W., & Moos, R. H. (1995). Entering treatment for alcohol abuse: A stress and coping perspective. *Addiction, 90,* 1223–1240.

Finney, J. W., Moos, R. H., & Brennan, P. L. (1991). The drinking problems index: A measure to assess alcohol-related problems among older adults. *Journal of Substance Abuse, 3,* 395–404.

Fogel, B. S., Furino, A., & Gottlieb, G. L. (1990). *Mental health policy for older Americans: Protecting minds at risk.* Washington, DC: American Psychiatric Press.

Galanter, M. (1995). *Recent developments in alcoholism: Alcoholism in women* (Vol. 12). New York: Plenum.

Gambert, S. R. (1992). Substance abuse in the elderly. In J. H. Lowinson, P. Ruiz, & R. B. Millman (Eds.), *Substance abuse: A comprehensive textbook* (2nd ed., pp. 843–851). Baltimore: Williams & Wilkins.

German, P. (1978). The elderly: A target group highly accessible to health education. *International Journal of Health Education, 21,* 267–272.

Gilford, D. M. (1988). *The aging population in the twenty-first century: Statistics for health policy.* Committee on National Statistics, Commission on Behavioral and Social Sciences and Education, National Research Council. Washington, DC: National Academy Press.

Glatz, M. D. (1995). Cognitive therapy with elderly alcoholics. In T. P. Beresford & E. Gomberg (Eds.), *Alcohol and aging* (pp. 211–229). New York: Oxford University Press.

Glynn, R. L., Bouchard, G. R., LoCastro, J. S., & Laird, N. M. (1985). Aging and generational effects on drinking behaviors in men: Results from the Normative Aging Study. *American Journal of Public Health, 75,* 1413–1419.

Gomberg, E. S., & Nirenberg, T. D. (Eds.). (1993). *Women and substance abuse.* Norwood, NJ: Ablex.

Gomberg, E. S. L. (1982). Alcohol use and alcohol problems among the elderly. Alcohol and Health Monograph 4 (NIAAA DHHS Publication No. (ADM) 82–1193). *Special population issues* (pp. 263–290). Rockville, MD: U.S. Department of Health and Human Services.

Gomberg, E. S. L. (1987). Drug and alcohol problems of elderly persons. In T. D. Nirenberg & S. A. Maisto (Eds.), *Developments in the assessment and treatment of addictive behaviors* (pp. 319–337). Norwood, NJ: Ablex.

Gomberg, E. S. L. (1990). Drugs, alcohol, and aging. In L. T. Kozlowski, H. M. Annis, H. D. Cappell, F. B. Glaser, E. M. Sellers, M. S. Goodstodt, Y. Israel, H. Kalatant, & E. R. Vingilis (Eds.), *Research advances in alcohol and drug problems* (Vol. 10, pp. 171–213). New York: Plenum.

Gomberg, E. S. L. (1992). Medication problems and drug abuse. In F. J. Turner (Ed.), *Mental health and the elderly* (pp. 355–374). New York: Free Press.

Gomberg, E. S. L. (1995a). Older alcoholics: Entry into treatment. In T. P. Beresford & E. Gomberg (Eds.), *Alcohol and aging* (pp. 169–185). New York: Oxford University Press.

Gomberg, E. S. L. (1995b). Older women and alcohol: Use and abuse. In M. Galanter (Ed.), *Recent developments in alcoholism* (Vol. 12, pp. 61–79). New York: Plenum.

Gomberg, E. S. L., & Nelson, B. W. (1995). Black and white older men: Alcohol use and abuse. In T. P. Beresford & E. S. L. Gomberg (Eds.), *Alcohol and aging* (pp. 307–323). New York: Oxford University Press.

Gomberg, E. S. L., Hsieh, G., & Adams, K. M. (1990). Patterns of drug use in a general medical care clinic for veterans. A pilot study. In B. B. Wilford (Ed.), *Balancing the response to prescription drug use* (pp. 119–132). Chicago: American Medical Association.

Gordon, T., & Kannel, W. B. (1983). Drinking and its relation to smoking, blood pressure, blood lipids, and uric acid. *Archives of Internal Medicine, 146,* 262–265.

Gorelick, D. A. (1993). Pharmacological treatment. In M. Galanter (Ed.), *Recent developments in alcoholism* (Vol. 11, pp. 413–427). New York: Plenum.

Graham, K. (1984). Identifying and measuring alcohol abuse among the elderly: Serious problems with existing instrumentation. *Journal of Studies on Alcohol, 47,* 253–262.

Graham, K., Saunders, S. J., Flower, M. C., Timney, C. B., White-Campbell, M., & Pietropaolo, A. Z. (1995). *Addictions treatment for older adults: Evaluation of an innovative client-centered approach.* New York: Haworth.

Helzer, J. E., Burnham, A., & McEvoy, L. T. (1991). Alcohol use and dependence. In L. N. Robins & D. A. Regier (Eds.), *Psychiatric disorders in America: The epidemiologic catchment area study* (pp. 81–115). New York: Macmillan.

Hersey, J. C., Glass, L. I., & Crocker, P. (1984). *Aging and health promotion behavior: Marketing research for public education.* Final report prepared under contract number DDS/OASH 282-83-105. Rockville, MD: U.S. Department of Health and Human Services.

Huffine, C., Folkman, S., & Lazarus, R. S. (1989). Psychoactive drugs, alcohol, and stress and coping processes in older adults. *American Journal of Drug and Alcohol Abuse, 15,* 101.

Hurt, R. D., Finlayson, R. E., & Morse, R. M. (1988). Alcoholism and elderly persons: Medical aspects and prognosis of 216 patients. *Mayo Clinic Proceedings, 63,* 753–760.

Institute of Medicine. (1989). *Prevention and treatment of alcohol problems: Research opportunities.* Report of a study by a Committee of the IOM, Division of Mental Health and Behavioral Medicine. Washington, DC: National Academy Press.

Institute of Medicine. (1990). *Broadening the base of treatment for alcohol problems.* Washington, DC: National Academy Press.

Janik, S. W., & Dunham, R. G. (1983). A nationwide examination of the need for specific alcoholism treatment programs for the elderly. *Journal of Studies on Alcohol, 44,* 307–317.

Jennison, K. M. (1992). The impact of stressful life events and social support on drinking among older adults: A general population survey. *International Journal of Aging and Human Development, 35,* 99–123.

Johnson, L. K. (1989). How to diagnose and treat chemical dependency in the elderly. *Journal of Gerontological Nursing, 15,* 22–26.

Jones, T. V., Lindsey, B. A., Yount, P., Soltys, R., & Farani-Enayat, B. (1993). Alcoholism screening questionnaires: Are they valid in elderly medical outpatients? *Journal of General Internal Medicine, 8,* 674–678.

King, C. J., Van Hasselt, V. B., Segal, D. L., & Hersen, M. (1994). Diagnosis and assessment of substance abuse in older adults: Current strategies and issues. *Addictive Behaviors, 19,* 41–55.

Kleber, H. D. (1990). The nosology of abuse and dependence. *Journal of Psychiatric Research, 24,* (Suppl. 2), 57–64.

Kofoed, L. L., Tolson, R. L., Atkinson, R. M., Toth, R. L., & Turner, J. A. (1987). Treatment compliance of older alcoholics: An elder-specific approach is superior to "mainstreaming." *Journal of Studies on Alcohol, 48,* 47–51.

Kopelman, M. D. (1995). The Korsakoff syndrome. *British Journal of Psychiatry, 166,* 154–173.

Krashner, T. M., Rodell, D. E., Ogden, S. R., Guggenheim, F. G., & Karson, C. N. (1992). Outcomes and costs of two VA inpatient treatment programs for older alcoholic patients. *Hospital and Community Psychiatry, 43,* 985–989.

Krause, N. (1995). Stress, alcohol use, and depressive symptoms in later life. *Gerontologist, 35,* 296–307.

Laforge, R. G., Nirenberg, T. D., Lewis, D.C., & Murphy, J. B. (1993). Problem drinking, gender, and stressful life events among hospitalized elderly drinkers. *Behavior, Health, and Aging, 3,* 129–138.

Lawson, A. W. (1989). Substance abuse problems of the elderly: Considerations for treatment and prevention. In G. W. Lawson & A. W. Lawson (Eds.), *Alcoholism and substance abuse in special populations* (pp. 95–113). Gaithersburg, MD: Aspen.

Lewis, D.C. (1995, October 2–5). *Training about alcohol and substance abuse for all primary care physicians.* Proceedings of conference, Phoenix, AZ. New York: Josiah Macy, Jr. Foundation.

Lewis, D.C., & Gordon, A. J. (1983). Alcoholism and the general hospital: The Roger Williams Intervention Program. *Bulletin—New York Academy of Medicine, 59,* 181–197.

Liepman, M. R., Nirenberg, T. D., & Begin, A.M. (1989). Evaluation of a program designed to help family and significant others to motivate resistant alcoholics into recovery. *American Journal of Drug and Alcohol Abuse, 15,* 209–221.

Longe, M. E. (1986). Elderly hospitalization programs. In K. Dychtwald (Ed.), *Wellness and health promotion for the elderly.* Rockville, MD: Aspen Systems.

McCrady, B. S., & Miller, W. R. (1993). *Research on alcoholics anonymous.* Piscataway, NJ: Rutgers Center of Alcohol Studies.

Michigan Department of Public Health. (1994). *Substance abuse services for older adults* (OA 089/10M9-84/NONOG). Lansing, MI: Author.

Miller, N. S., Belkin, B. M., & Gold, M. S. (1991). Alcohol and drug dependence among the elderly: Epidemiology, diagnosis, and treatment. *Comprehensive Psychiatry, 32,* 153–165.

Molgard, C.A., Nakamura, C. N., Stanford, E. P., Peddecord, K. M., & Morton, D. J. (1990). Prevalence of alcohol consumption among older persons. *Journal of Community Health, 15,* 239–251.

Moos, R. H., Mertens, J. R., & Brennan, P. L. (1993). Patterns of diagnosis and treatment among late-middle-aged and older substance abuse patients. *Journal of Studies on Alcohol, 54,* 479–487.

Moos, R. H., Mertens, J. R., & Brennan, P. L. (1994). Rates and predictors of four-year readmission among late-middle-aged and older substance abuse patients. *Journal of Studies on Alcohol, 55,* 561–570.

National Center for Health Statistics. (1986). Health promotion data for the 1990 objective: Estimates from the National Health Interview Survey of Health Promotion and Disease Prevention: United States, 1985, *Advance Data from Vital and Health Statistics,* No. 126 (DHHS Publication No. (PHS) 86-1250). Hyattsville, MD: U.S. Public Health Service.

National Institute on Alcohol Abuse and Alcoholism. (1990). *Alcohol and health: Seventh special report to the U.S. Congress.* Rockville, MD: Public Health Service, U.S. Department of Health and Human Services.

Nelson, E., McHugo, G., Schnurr, P., Devito, C., Roberts, E., Simmons, J., & Zubkoff, W. (1984). Medical self-care education for elders: A controlled trial to evaluate impact. *American Journal of Public Health, 74,* 1357–1363.

Nirenberg, T. D., & Maisto, S. A. (1990). The relationship between assessment and alcohol treatment. *The International Journal of the Addictions, 25,* 1275–1285.

Noel, N. E., & McCrady, B. S. (1984). Target populations for alcohol abuse prevention. In P. M. Miller & T. D. Nirenberg (Eds.), *Prevention of alcohol abuse* (pp. 55–96). New York: Plenum.

Nutting, P. A. (1986). Health promotion in primary care: Problems and potential. *Preventive Medicine, 15,* 537–548.

O'Farrell, T. J. (1993). *Treating alcohol problems: Marital and family interventions.* New York: Guilford.

Office of Technology Assessment. (1985). *Technology and aging in America* (OTA-B-A-264). Washington, DC: U.S. Government Printing Office.

Paganini-Hill, A., Ross, R. K., & Henderson, B. E. (1986). Prevalence of chronic disease and health practices in a retirement community. *Journal of Chronic Diseases, 39,* 699–707.

Prentice, R. (1979). Patterns of psychotherapeutic drugs use among the elderly. In *The aging process and psychoactive drug use* (pp. 17–41). National Institute of Drug Abuse. Washington, DC: U.S. Government Printing Office.

Rice, C., Longabaugh, R., Beattie, M., & Noel, N. (1993). Age group differences in response to treatment for problematic alcohol use. *Addiction, 88,* 1369–1375.

Rosin, A. J., & Glatt, M. M. (1971). Alcohol excess in the elderly. *Quarterly Journal of Studies on Alcohol, 32,* 53–59.

Rubington, E. (1982). The chronic drunkenness offender on Skid Row. In E. S. L. Gomberg, H. R. White, & J. A. Carpenter (Eds.), *Alcohol, science and society revisited* (pp. 322–336). Ann Arbor: University of Michigan Press.

Schonfeld, L., & Dupree, L. W. (1991). Antecedents of drinking for early- and late-onset elderly alcohol abusers. *Journal of Studies on Alcohol, 52,* 587– 592.

Schutte, K. K., Brennan, P. L., & Moos, R. H. (1994). Remission of late-life drinking problems: A four year follow-up. *Alcoholism: Clinical and Experimental Research, 18,* 835–844.

Sellers, E. M., Frecker, R. C., & Romach, M. L. (1982). *Drug metabolism in the elderly: Confounding of age, smoking and ethanol effects.* Substudy 1219. Toronto, Ontario, Canada: Addiction Research Foundation.

Selzer, M. L. (1971). The Michigan Alcoholism Test: The quest for a new diagnostic instrument. *American Journal of Psychiatry, 127,* 1653–1658.

Sobell, L. C., Sobell, M. B., & Nirenberg, T. D. (1988). Behavioral assessment and treatment planning with alcohol and drug abusers: A review with an emphasis on clinical application. *Clinical Psychology Review, 8,* 19–54.

Solomon, K., Manepalli, J., Ireland, G. A., & Mahon, G. M. (1993). Alcoholism and prescription drug abuse in the elderly: St. Louis University grand rounds. *Journal of the American Geriatric Society, 41,* 57–69.

Speer, D. C., O'Sullivan, M., & Schonfeld, L. (1991). Dual diagnosis among older adults: A new array of policy and planning problems. *Journal of Mental Health Administration, 18,* 43–50.

Szwabo, P. A. (1993). Substance abuse in older women. *Clinics in Geriatric Medicine, 9,* 197–208.

Tabisz, E. M., Jacyk, W. R., Fuchs, D., & Grymonpre, R. (1993). Chemical dependency in the elderly: The enabling factor. *Canadian Journal on Aging, 12,* 78–88.

Tucker, J. A., Gavornik, M. G., Vuchinich, R. E., Rudd, E. J., & Harris, C. V. (1989). Predicting the drinking behavior of older adults from questionnaire measures of alcohol consumption. *Addictive Behaviors, 14,* 655–658.

Victor, M., Adams, R. A., & Collins, G. H. (1989). *The Wernicke–Korsakoff syndrome and related disorders due to alcoholism and malnutrition,* Philadelphia: Davis.

Wartenberg, A. A., & Nirenberg, T. D. (1995). Alcohol and other drug abuse in older patients. In W. Reichel (Ed.), *Care of the elderly: Clinical aspects of aging* (4th ed., pp. 133–141). Baltimore: Williams & Wilkins.

Weisner, C., Greenfield, T., & Room, R. (1995). Trends in the treatment of alcohol problems in the U.S. general population, 1979–1990. *American Journal of Public Health, 85,* 55–60.

Welte, J. W., & Mirand, A. L. (1993). Drinking, problem drinking, and life stressors in the elderly general population. *Journal of Studies on Alcohol, 56,* 67–73.

Werch, C. (1989). Quantity-frequency and diary measures of alcohol consumption for elderly drinkers. *International Journal of the Addictions, 24,* 859–865.

Willenbring, M. L., Christensen, K. J., Spring, W. D., & Rasmussen, R. (1987). Alcoholism screening in the elderly. *Journal of the American Geriatric Society, 35,* 864–869.

Willenbring, M. L., Olson, D., Bielinski, J., & Lynch, J. (1995). Treatment of medically ill alcoholics in the primary-care setting. In T. P. Beresford & E. Gomberg (Eds.), *Alcohol and aging* (pp. 249–262). New York: Oxford University Press.

Zimberg, S. (1974). Two types of problem drinkers. *Geriatrics, 29,* 135–139.

Zimberg, S. (1995). The elderly. In A. M. Washton (Ed.), *Psychotherapy and substance abuse* (pp. 413–427). New York: Guilford.

CHAPTER 9

Schizophrenia

Stephen J. Bartels, Kim T. Mueser, and Keith M. Miles

INTRODUCTION

Overview

Schizophrenia is a severe and frequently debilitating illness that affects one percent of the population (Gurland & Cross, 1982). Not surprisingly, there is a substantial literature of the phenomenology, course, biology, and treatment of schizophrenia in young adults. However, there is a remarkable lack of data on this disorder in late life. In this chapter we provide an overview of the clinical features of schizophrenia and aging. First, we will discuss changing views on the onset and outcome of schizophrenia, including features of early- and late-onset schizophrenia in the elderly. Next, we will discuss factors that appear to be important in the long-term outcome of schizophrenia, including the role of age cohorts, family resources, antipsychotic medication, and medical comorbidity. Finally, we will outline the elements of a strategy for the treatment of schizophrenia in the elderly based on the application of a comprehensive biopsychosocial model.

A Changing View of Schizophrenia

Early views of schizophrenia maintained that the disorder always began in young adulthood and inevitably resulted in a progressive deterioration of function, thinking, and cognition. The term "dementia praecox" was introduced by Kraepelin (1919/1971) to describe this characteristic course and outcome of the

Stephen J. Bartels, Kim T. Mueser, and Keith M. Miles • Department of Psychiatry and Community and Family Medicine, New Hampshire–Dartmouth Psychiatric Research Center, Dartmouth Medical School, Concord, New Hampshire 03301.

Handbook of Clinical Geropsychology, edited by Michel Hersen and Vincent B. Van Hasselt. Plenum Press, New York, 1998.

disorder. However, his early view of schizophrenia has been replaced by a more optimistic and dynamic understanding of the disorder as the result of longitudinal research on schizophrenia and recent studies on schizophrenia in late life. Among the five studies of the long-term course of schizophrenia, the preponderance of the data suggests a remarkably favorable outcome over time, with 46% to 68% substantially improved, including 18% to 22% experiencing global recovery (Bleuler, 1974; Ciompi, 1980; Harding, Brooks, Ashigawa, Strauss, & Breier, 1987a,b; Huber, Cross, Schuttler, & Linz, 1989; M. Tsuang & Winokur, 1975). However, these studies fail to provide definitive data on the outcome of schizophrenia in old age, and they do not all agree that improvement occurs in all areas of functioning. For example, these studies have been widely interpreted to suggest a benign long-term outcome for most older individuals with schizophrenia, yet in four of the five studies the majority of patients were less than 65 years of age at follow-up. Furthermore, consensus is lacking on functional outcomes. For example, two of the five studies reported that social functioning was fair to poor for two thirds of the patients at follow-up (Ciompi 1980; M. Tsuang & Winokur, 1975). In general, however, these data indicate a historical shift to a more optimistic view of the long-term outcome of schizophrenia.

Views of treatment and systems for care for those with schizophrenia have also changed. Traditional institutional care models have been replaced by a different model of care emphasizing community treatment, with greater promise of normalized life functioning. Advances in mental health treatment and general medical care have resulted in more individuals with schizophrenia surviving into old age than before (Moak, 1996). However, this shift in the locus of treatment from institutional settings to the community has largely focused on younger adults and has included innovations in vocational rehabilitation, treatment of comorbid substance abuse, and the development of assertive case management teams. Despite advances in treatment of these disorders, service models specifically designed for the older adult with severe and persistent mental illness are still lacking (Light & Lebowitz, 1991). In this context, the current growth in the number of elderly persons with schizophrenia will present a major challenge to the health care system and society.

AGE AND THE ONSET OF SCHIZOPHRENIA

While onset of schizophrenia usually occurs in late adolescence or early adulthood, recent findings show that the disorder can begin in middle age and, less commonly, in old age. In a review of eight studies of late-onset schizophrenia, Harris and Jeste (1988) estimated that almost one quarter (23%) of patients with schizophrenia have onset of their disorder after age 40, including 13% between ages 40 and 50, 7% between the ages 50 and 60, and 3% after the age of 60. In a separate report of a 20-year study of first diagnosis of psychiatric disorders in the community in Camberwell catchment area of London, England, D. Castle, Wessely, Der, and Murray (1991) reported that 28% of patients with schizophrenia had an onset of the illness after age 44, and 12% after age 64. Overall, the annual incidence rate for late-onset schizophrenia was 12.6 per

100,000, approximately half of that for those aged 16 to 25. Differences in age of onset appear to relate to clinical features of schizophrenia, resulting in descriptive subtypes of schizophrenia in the elderly.

Based on age of onset, two broad groups of older adults with schizophrenia have been described with overlapping but different symptom profiles. One group of older individuals developed schizophrenia as young adults; they have early-onset schizophrenia (EOS). This group first became ill at an early age and continues to have symptoms of schizophrenia in old age. A second group, with late-onset schizophrenia (LOS), is composed of elderly adults who developed their illness in middle or old age. These individuals were largely free of symptoms of major mental illness during their early adult years, yet developed psychotic illness as they became older. In the following sections we first describe older individuals with lifelong schizophrenia (EOS), and then those with late-onset schizophrenia (LOS), illustrating the importance of the factors discussed above in assessment and treatment.

Early-Onset Schizophrenia

Individuals with early-onset schizophrenia (EOS) typically experience disordered thinking and unusual behavior that have a negative effect on their personal, social, and vocational lives. Although schizophrenia occurs with wide variation in the type and severity of symptoms in different individuals, common problems include difficulties in initiating and maintaining relationships, impaired role function (e.g., problems in education, employment), and deficits in basic self-care or community living skills (e.g., grooming, hygiene, managing finances). These problems generally develop following persistent symptoms of psychosis, although early signs of schizophrenia can also include progressive difficulties in social functioning. For example, the first onset of psychosis may be preceded by difficulties in social adjustment and interpersonal relationships with gradual signs of social withdrawal (Zigler & Glick, 1986). These early signs of schizophrenia generally develop over a period of months and can also include prodromal symptoms, such as depression, disordered thinking, and a decline in interest and spontaneity. Problems may appear in the workplace, school, or home setting, reflecting early difficulties in thinking and perceptions. Relationships with family members or friends may be affected by the patient's unusual behavior or by hostile or paranoid verbalizations.

The final onset of psychosis is often marked by dramatic and severe symptoms and functional difficulties. Three major symptom clusters are commonly described, including positive, negative, and affective symptoms.

Positive symptoms consist of the primary active symptoms of psychosis, most commonly delusions and hallucinations, but also including severely disordered thought processes such as illogical or unrelated thoughts or associations. Behavioral problems, such as bizarre behaviors, repetitive or ritualistic behaviors, and posturing, are also examples of positive symptoms. Positive symptoms are among the most common and noticeable signs of acute relapse and may indicate a need for more intensive treatment, including hospitalization. However, in the early stage of psychotic relapse, these symptoms can sometimes be identified and brought to the attention of care providers. Appropriate adjustments in medication dosage and crisis stabilization treatment may avert full symptomatic relapse and hospitalization. Increasingly, clinicians are using educational sessions with patients and their families to help them recognize early signs of relapse. Then changes can be implemented in treatment to avoid an acute psychotic episode (Herz, 1985) This clinical use of early symptoms to suggest treatment changes represents the more recent view of schizophrenia as subject to treatment and management by clinician, patient, and patient's family.

The term *negative symptoms* applies to symptoms characterized by a lack of active or spontaneous behaviors, emotions, or thoughts. This term was first used to describe the symptoms of neurologically impaired patients with frontal lobe brain damage who exhibited infrequent speech, passivity, and emotional unresponsiveness (Jackson, 1984). The concept of negative symptoms was subsequently applied to a subgroup of patients with schizophrenia who had severe deficits in social, emotional, and cognitive functioning, but often lacked prominent active positive symptoms of psychosis. A useful construct is to consider this cluster of symptoms as consisting of the five A's of negative symptoms in schizophrenia:

- Blunted or flat *affect* (lack of emotional expression)
- *Alogia* (reduced amount of speech or poverty of content)
- *Asociality* (social withdrawal)
- *Apathy* (lack of interest or spontaneity or psychomotor retardation).
- *Attentional* impairment (difficulty concentrating or performing sequential tasks)

Severe negative symptoms have been shown to be relatively stable over time (R. R. J. Lewine, 1990; Mueser, Douglas, Bellack, & Morrison, 1991; Mueser, Sayers, Schooler, Mance, & Haas, 1994) and strongly associated with poor social functioning (Bellack, Morrison, Wixted, & Mueser, 1990). Negative symptoms are also typically the most resistant to treatment, although the newer atypical antipsychotic medications (e.g., clozapine) have a greater effect on negative symptoms compared to traditional agents (Salzman, Vaccaro, & Lief, 1995).

In addition to positive and negative symptoms, schizophrenia can also include *affective symptoms*. One important affective symptom in schizophrenia is depression. Postpsychotic or secondary depression occurs after 25% of acute schizophrenic episodes, and approximately 60% of individuals with schizophrenia suffer a major depression at some time during the course of their illness. Depression is associated with poor outcomes, including increased rate of relapse, longer duration of hospitalization, poorer response to pharmacological treatments, and chronicity (Bartels & Drake, 1988). In addition, suicide is a catastrophic outcome associated with depression in schizophrenia. Approximately 50% of persons with schizophrenia attempt suicide at some time during their lives, with a 10% rate of mortality (Roy, 1986).

Identification of specific subtypes and causes of depression in schizophrenia is a critical step in evaluating appropriate treatment alternatives. Elsewhere, we have postulated three broad subtypes to describe depression in schizophrenia: depressive symptoms secondary to organic factors (e.g., medication side effects, alcohol and substance abuse, medical disorders); depressive symptoms associated with acute psychosis; and depressive symptoms in chronic states, including secondary major depression, negative symptoms, chronic demoralization, and prodromal precursors to acute psychotic episodes (Bartels & Drake, 1988). Identifying the specific subtype of depression is critical in determining and implementing effective treatment approaches (Bartels & Drake, 1989).

Late-Onset Schizophrenia

The diagnosis of late-onset schizophrenia evolved from early descriptions of a disorder called paraphrenia. Kraepelin (1919/1971) used the term paraphrenia to describe a group of older patients with symptoms similar to dementia praecox, but with fewer negative and cognitive symptoms. Kay and Roth (1961) later described "late paraphrenia" as a paranoid syndrome occurring in late life that was not accompanied by co-occurring dementia. Late paraphrenia was characterized by an onset after age 45 of a well-organized paranoid delusional system, with or without auditory hallucinations, and it often occurred with preserved personality (Herbert & Jacobson, 1967). More recently, psychiatric diagnostic criteria have been revised to reclassify most individuals formally diagnosed with late paraphrenia as having late-life schizophrenia. For example, recent revisions of the *Diagnostic and Statistical Manual of Mental Disorders* allow for a diagnosis of schizophrenia with the first onset of symptoms after age 45 (e.g., American Psychiatric Association, 1994).

Symptoms of LOS typically include relatively well-circumscribed, nonbizarre delusions without a formal disorder in thought processes. In most instances, the individual with LOS exhibits speech and thought processes that are indistinguishable from other older adults who do not have a major mental illness. In contrast, many individuals with EOS display disorganized speech symptomatic of a prominent underlying thought disorder. Delusions and hallucinations are also common symptoms in late-onset schizophrenia, and occur at a rate comparable to those found in adults with early-onset schizophrenia. Delusions tend to be paranoid and are often systematized (Almeida, Howard, Levy, & David, 1995a, 1995b; Howard, Castle, Wessely, & Murray, 1993; Kay & Roth, 1961). Auditory hallucinations are substantially more common than visual or somatic hallucinations, similar to young adults with EOS (Almeida *et al.*, 1995a, 1995b). In contrast to EOS, LOS is significantly less likely to manifest formal thought disorder, negative symptoms, or inappropriate affect (Almeida *et al.*, 1995a, 1995b; Howard *et al.*, 1993; Kay & Roth, 1961; Pearlson & Rabins, 1988; Pearlson *et al.*, 1989).

In the diagnosis of late-onset schizophrenia, one should consider a variety of alternatives. Other disorders should be ruled out before assigning a diagnosis of LOS. For example, special consideration should be given to ruling out psychiatric disorders secondary to medical causes (formerly organic mental disorders), major affective disorders, and delusional (paranoid) disorders (Harris & Jeste, 1988). As previously discussed, medical disorders can present with symptoms of psychosis that are entirely caused by the underlying medical illness. Major affective disorders, including bipolar disorder and delusional depression, can also mimic signs and symptoms of late-onset schizophrenia.

Delusional disorder shares some characteristics with LOS but can be differentiated by the presence of prominent nonbizarre delusions and nonprominent (or absent) hallucinations. Nonbizarre delusions, for example, involve situations that may occur in real life, such as being poisoned, followed, having a disease, or being deceived by a spouse or lover. In contrast, bizarre delusions involve phenomena that are considered totally implausible within one's culture, such as being possessed by aliens or having one's thoughts or actions controlled by implanted electronic devices (American Psychiatric Association, 1994; Yassa & Suranyl-Cadotte, 1993). Individuals with LOS are more likely to show better premorbid occupational adjustment and higher marriage rates compared to those with EOS (Post, 1966). However, individuals with LOS may have schizoid or paranoid premorbid personalities and are frequently socially isolated compared to normal comparison groups (Kay & Roth, 1961; Harris & Jeste, 1988).

A final symptom associated with LOS is the presence of sensory impairment that appears to predate onset of the disorder. In a review of 27 articles evaluating visual and hearing abilities in elderly with late-onset disorders, Prager and Jeste (1993) found that sensory deficits are overrepresented in the elderly LOS population. A specific relationship between visual impairment and late-onset paranoid psychosis remains controversial, although an association between visual impairment and visual hallucinations is suggested by the literature. On the other hand, the literature does support an association between hearing deficits and late-onset paranoid psychosis. Approximately 40% of those with late onset paranoid psychoses have been found to have moderate to severe hearing deficits (Kay & Roth, 1961; Herbert & Jacobson, 1967). It is possible that deafness may precipitate or exacerbate symptoms, since significant reductions in psychotic symptoms have been reported for some individuals with late-onset paranoid disorders after being fitted with a hearing aid (Almeida, Förstl, Howard, & David, 1993).

Gender and Age of Onset

Differences have been found between men and women in a number of areas related to onset and course of schizophrenia. R. J. Lewine (1988) found that mean age of onset of schizophrenia in women is approximately 5 years later than in men, a finding consistent with many other studies documenting a later age of onset of schizophrenia for women (Häfner *et al.*, 1993). In a comprehensive review of the literature, Harris and Jeste (1988) found that virtually all studies report a greater proportion of women than men with late-onset schizophrenia, with the ratio of women to men ranging from 1.9:1 to 22.5:1. In contrast, most studies of EOS report similar proportions of women to men. Several explanations for this difference have been proposed. One view suggests that EOS and LOS are different forms of schizophrenia with different characteristics, including different rates among men and women. An alternative view suggests that biological factors are responsible for a later onset of schizophrenia in women, resulting in an overrepresentation of women compared to men for LOS. In a community study which included EOS and LOS, D. J. Castle and Murray (1993) found that 16% of males had the onset of schizophrenia after age 45, compared with 38% of females. Speculation about the difference in age of on-set between men and women includes a possible protective effect of estrogens or a precipitating effect of androgens (D. J. Castle & Murray, 1993).

J. M. Goldstein (1988) and Seeman (1986) suggest that male gender, by it-self, may represent a risk factor to poorer outcome in schizophrenia. Possible explanations for increased risk include biological causes such as differences in male and female brain structure (R. R. J. Lewine, Gulley, Risch, Jewart, & Houpt, 1990), or differences in protective hormonal levels such as estrogen (Seeman & Lang, 1990). An alternative explanation suggests that comorbid disorders, such as substance abuse, that are more prevalent in men result in poorer functioning and outcomes for men compared with women. Substance abuse has been asso-ciated with a variety of poor outcomes, including increased use of hospitalization and emergency services (Bartels *et al.,* 1993), aggressive and hostile behaviors (Bartels, Drake, Wallach, & Freeman, 1991), and housing instability and home-lessness (Drake, Osher, & Wallach, 1989). Prevalence of comorbid substance use disorders diminishes over time, yet these disorders continue to be important risk factors in older mentally ill patients (Bartels & Liberto, 1995). Finally, dif-ferences in social support and social skill between men and women with schiz-ophrenia may be associated with better outcomes. Women with schizophrenia are more likely to marry (Test & Berlin, 1981), are more likely to maintain con-tact with their children (Test, Burke, & Wallisch, 1990), and hence may tend to have stronger family social networks compared with men with schizophrenia. Mueser and associates (1990) found that women with schizophrenia are more socially skilled than men, perhaps leading to less social isolation and better functioning in the community.

KEY FACTORS AFFECTING TREATMENT OUTCOMES IN OLDER ADULTS WITH SCHIZOPHRENIA

The Role of Cohort

An important factor in considering different functional outcomes for elderly persons with schizophrenia is the "cohort effect." The concept of cohort reflects the fact that individuals born at a particular time share a unique set of historical experiences. Most importantly, these individuals experienced these events at a similar point in their life cycle. In this respect, cohort effect is the product of an interaction between the age and the historical period resulting in common ex-periences of key life events (Fischer, 1996). For the older person with schizo-phrenia, there are dramatic differences in life and treatment experience among those who entered the treatment system before the mid-1950s and those first treated after 1960. Before 1955, antipsychotic medications were not available and the standard treatment for severe and persistent psychotic illness was long-term hospitalization in mental asylums. Many individuals entering the state hospital system before this time were hospitalized for decades. In the 1960s use of antipsychotic medications became widespread, and a wave of mental health care reform resulted in deinstitutionalization of many individuals in the state hospital system, and the development of community mental health services. For the older patient with schizophrenia, these two experiences of the treatment system had dramatic long-term effects on functional and symptom outcomes.

The Institutional Treatment Cohort

Among the elderly who currently have schizophrenia are a group of individuals who are severely functionally impaired and who remain in long-term care units in state mental hospitals or nursing homes. Three factors are likely to be associated with their poor long-term outcomes. First, this group of individuals became ill before development of antipsychotic medication. Extensive reviews of outcome studies suggest that treatment with antipsychotic medication results in acute symptom improvement and long-term benefits in better outcomes (Hogarty *et al.*, 1986; Wyatt, 1991). Recent studies on first-onset psychosis also suggest that treatment occurring in the early stages of severe psychotic disorders may result in better long-term outcomes (Szymanski, Canoon, Gallacher, Erwin, & Gur, 1996). Second, it is likely that long-term institutionalization results in poor social skills, severe limits in functional abilities, and loss of social supports outside of the institutional setting. Independent living skills may become atrophied, with substantial dependence on care providers for basic needs.

Third, although many of the chronic deficits common in these individuals have been attributed to long-term institutionalization, it is likely that some individuals who remain in institutions are among the most severely mentally ill and have the most intractable and disabling form of the illness. These individuals may have been considered too ill to be discharged to community settings. For example, Ciompi (1980) found that long-term outcome of schizophrenia was characterized by severe functional deficits and symptoms for one third of the individuals. Some of these individuals remain in state hospitals (Davidson *et al.*, 1995), while others have been "transinstitutionalized" to nursing homes. Elderly schizophrenic patients who continue to require treatment in late life in nursing homes, compared to those in the community, were more severely impaired, both functionally and physically, and had more severe negative symptoms, cognitive impairment, and behavioral problems (Bartels, Miles, Dain, & Smyer, 1998). Regardless of the cause of these more severe symptoms and functional problems, little is known about the potential for rehabilitation for persistently institutionalized individuals.

The Community Treatment Cohort

In contrast to older individuals with schizophrenia who have been chronically institutionalized, a more recent and younger group of aging patients with severe mental illness entered the treatment system in an era of antipsychotic medication treatment and a declining use of institution-based care. These individuals are the "young-old" (in their 60s) and were among the first wave of severely mentally ill patients who became ill when states were closing their long-term wards and shifting treatment into the community. Some of these individuals were beneficiaries of early forms of community support and psychosocial rehabilitation services (Harding *et al.,* 1987a, 1987b). Others undoubtedly gained experience in developing adaptive coping and living skills through the assistance of family members or other social supports. Many of these individuals reside in the community with little or no need of mental health services. However, a substantial minority of older individuals with schizophrenia in the community remains highly symptomatic and still has substantial difficulties in many areas of functioning (Bartels, Mueser, Miles, 1997). Compared to older adults with other mental disorders, these patients use considerably greater and different types of mental health services (Bartels *et al.,* 1998). Comprehensive community support services and social supports appear to be essential to assisting many of these more severely impaired individuals in living in the community.

The Importance of Family and Social Supports

One of the major differences between older individuals with severe mental illness residing in the community, compared with those in nursing homes and other institutions, is the presence of family and social supports (Meeks *et al.,* 1990). Persons with schizophrenia are less likely to marry, are less likely to have children, and are less likely to work compared with persons without a severe psychiatric disorder. Social networks of persons with schizophrenia tend to be smaller than those of normal subjects and tend to diminish with age (Cohen, 1995). Thus, many older adults with schizophrenia do not have the supports that are often available to older persons without severe mental illness who reside in the community with the assistance of family members. The literature on family supports is also replete with reports of aging parents (usually mothers) caring for their middle-aged children with schizophrenia (e.g., Bulger, Wandersman, & Goldman, 1993; MacGregor, 1994; Platt, 1985) or supplementing financial resources (Salokangas, Palo-Oja, & Ojanen, 1991). The aging and eventual death of parents who are key supports places these individuals at risk for decompensation and loss of ability to continue to reside in individual placement in the community. When the parent becomes ill or dies, the offspring, frequently in his or her forties, must become accustomed to a dramatic reduction in financial and social support, which may also coincide with, or directly result in, a loss of residence. The need to bolster family capacity and social supports is an important component to consider in service planning.

The Older Adult With Schizophrenia and Antipsychotic Medications

Older persons are especially sensitive to the adverse side effects of medications; therefore, careful attention is required in choosing the appropriate type and dosage of medication. For example, age and duration of exposure to antipsychotic medications are extensively documented as primary risk factors for the development of tardive dyskinesia (J. Kane *et al.,* 1992). Tardive dyskinesia is a neurological syndrome characterized by persistent abnormal involuntary movements. Annual incidence rate of tardive dyskinesia in elderly with schizophrenia is 26% to 45%, depending on the criteria for tardive dyskinesia that are applied (Jeste, Lacro, Gilbert, Kline, & Kline, 1993). The more conservative estimate of 26% is nearly six times the rate reported for younger patients (J. Kane, Woerner, & Lieberman, 1988). Other common side effects of antipsychotic medications include extrapyramidal side effect, such as medication-induced Parkinson's syndrome (akinesia) and akathisia. Akinesia is characterized by muscle rigidity, shuffling gait, lack of spontaneous facial expressions, and severe resting tremor of the arms, hands, head, and legs. Akathisia is characterized by severe restlessness or pacing behavior. Older adults may be more vulnerable to all of these side effects due to greater sensitivity to lower doses of medication and co-occurring neurological disorders. Aging is associated with increased prevalence of extrapyramidal nervous system side effects (EPS) due to biological changes in neuroreceptor sensitivity and declining amounts of dopamine occurring with age. Hence, ongoing, close monitoring of side effects and neurological status is imperative.

More recently, alternatives to standard antipsychotic medications have become available that have reduced (or negligible) risk of extrapyramidal side effects. These atypical antipsychotic agents include medications such as clozapine, risperidone, and olanzapine. Initial trials of the class of agents in elderly patients with psychotic symptoms are promising, with evidence supporting their effects on both positive and negative symptoms (Salzman *et al.,* 1995). Clozapine was the first of these agents and has been limited by a variety of side effects such as excess sedation, positional hypotension (low blood pressure), and the need to closely monitor potentially life-threatening side effects such as agranulocytosis (dramatic decreases in white blood cell count) and spontaneous seizures. But it is also the only atypical antipsychotic medication that does not appear to cause tardive dyskinesia. Fortunately, the newer atypical agents risperidone and olanzapine appear to be safer and easier to monitor, while maintaining many of the benefits of clozapine (Pickar, 1995).

The Interaction of Psychiatric and Medical Illness—Comorbidity

Comorbidity is one of the major characteristics distinguishing the older person with schizophrenia from younger individuals with the disorder. Whereas younger patients have symptoms that often can be understood on the basis of a single disorder, the older patient with schizophrenia typically presents with multiple problems resulting from their symptoms and functional disabilities (Moak, 1996). These comorbid disorders include co-occurring medical illness and dementia.

Serious health problems are common in schizophrenia and are often undiagnosed and undertreated (Cohen, 1993). Often, people with schizophrenia are more likely to have difficulty obtaining medical services and are more likely to receive poor care (Koran *et al.,* 1989; Koranyi, 1979). Emerging medical problems may be misinterpreted as a worsening of psychiatric symptoms. For example, symptoms of agitated or bizarre behavior may be due to worsening physical pain or delirium. Symptoms of depression may be caused by thyroid hormone deficiency or an occult carcinoma. Common medical conditions affecting older patients include hypertension, heart disease, arthritis, diabetes, chronic lung disease, anemia, gastrointestinal disease, and neurological disorders including stroke, movement disorders, and seizure disorders. Worsening of psychiatric symptoms may be the first signs of underlying medical illness.

Just as medical disorders can cause or exacerbate psychiatric conditions, the converse may also be true. A worsening of psychotic symptoms may precipitate a deterioration in medical function. For example, an acute psychotic episode in a patient with brittle diabetes may result in failure to adhere to scheduled insulin injections, dietary restrictions, and adequate hydration, causing a severe and potentially life-threatening decompensation. In addition, the older patient with severe psychiatric symptoms may have difficulty communicating their medical concerns and may refuse needed medical evaluations and procedures. Behavioral problems, including severe social withdrawal, negativism, and aggression, can make it extremely difficult for medical providers to conduct appropriate physical examinations, medical tests, and treatments (Moak, 1990).

Other factors that contribute to poor physical health include health-damaging behaviors such as smoking (Hughes, Hatsukami, Mitchell, & Dahlgren, 1986), substance abuse (Bartels & Liberto, 1995), limited access to good health care because of financial constraints, and a delay in seeking medical treatment as a result of possible differences in pain threshold found in some persons with schizophrenia (Dworkin, 1994). Mortality rates in persons with schizophrenia are higher than nonpsychiatric comparison groups (M. T. Tsuang, Woolson, & Fleming, 1980). In addition to relatively high rates of suicide (Drake, Gates, Whitaker, & Cotten, 1985), the physical health of many persons with schizophrenia is similar to those much older (Mulsant *et al.*, 1993). Thus, assessment of physical health and the adequacy of their health care services are critical elements in the assessment of older persons with schizophrenia.

Another important factor that can complicate diagnosis and treatment in older adults is the development of co-occurring cognitive impairment disorders in late life. Several studies suggest that a subset of individuals with schizophrenia is prone to develop dementia in late life (Davidson *et al*, 1995; Lesser *et al.*, 1993), although the cause and prevalence of dementia in schizophrenia is controversial (Goldberg, Hyde, Kleinman, & Weinberger, 1993; Heaton *et al.*, 1994). For individuals in the community, comorbid cognitive impairment is associated with substantially higher use of psychiatric services and community supports (Bartels et al., 1998). When cognitive impairment becomes severe, symptoms of dementia can overshadow the psychosis and become the primary source of functional impairment in late life. For these individuals a supported, supervised setting becomes a necessity, and without the availability of 24-hour care, nursing home care may be unavoidable (Moak, 1996).

A TREATMENT APPROACH TO SCHIZOPHRENIA IN OLDER ADULTS: THE BIOPSYCHOSOCIAL MODEL

Remarkably little is known about effective treatments for the older person with schizophrenia, although potential directions are suggested by longitudinal outcome studies and by studies of younger patients with the disorder. Longitudinal studies have shown that the course of schizophrenia is usually episodic, with some residual impairment between exacerbations. However, there is a trend for gradual improvement and, in some cases, total remission later in life (Ciompi, 1980; Harding *et al.*, 1987a, 1987b). Long-term studies of the natural history of schizophrenia suggest that the first ten years of the illness are marked by exacerbations and remissions, but symptoms substantially remit in more than half of the individuals with schizophrenia in later life.

This improvement likely is a result of many factors. For example, biological changes, such as age-related decreases in the neurotransmitter dopamine, may result in symptom reductions. In addition, individuals may acquire illness management skills, such as strategies for reducing stress and improving symptom recognition and medication compliance (Herz, 1985). Other factors include reduction in substance use with age that can improve patients' symptoms and level of functioning (Zisook *et al.*, 1992). Overall, there is greater optimism for favorable long-term outcomes for many individuals afflicted with schizophrenia, although a subgroup remains that continues to require intensive treatment and supervision in late life.

Treatment of schizophrenia in late life is best considered within the framework of a biopsychosocial perspective. This perspective posits that biological, psychological, and social aspects of the person must be considered for an optimal assessment and treatment. This three-pronged approach is essential for the older person with schizophrenia. First, the older person commonly has multiple medical problems and is likely to be on a number of different medications that can substantially complicate assessment and treatment. Biological changes associated with aging directly affect medication metabolism and result in a higher prevalence of medication side effects and interactions with other drugs. Second, the psychological impact of mental illness and the effects of aging must be carefully weighed in designing a treatment program. The individual's cognitive abilities must be comprehensively assessed in order to inform the choice of intervention. Prior history of mental illness, psychological strengths, and emotional vulnerabilities need to be systematically evaluated. Finally, social supports and stressors are a major consideration in assessing needed services. One of the most important factors determining whether an older person with schizophrenia remains in the community or permanently resides in a nursing home is the presence of social and instrumental supports (Meeks *et al.*, 1990). In summary, the biopsychosocial perspective should be the foundation to ensure a comprehensive clinical assessment and effective plan of treatment. In the following section, we summarize biological and psychosocial approaches to treatment developed and studied largely in younger populations but adapted for older persons with schizophrenia.

Biological Treatment

Virtually any psychiatric symptom can be caused or exacerbated by an underlying medical illness (Bartels, 1989), underscoring the importance of an initial thorough medical evaluation in the biological treatment of the older adult with schizophrenia. The underdiagnosis of medical disorders among individuals with severe mental illness necessitates a careful review of current physical complaints and health status. Adequate assessment and treatment can be especially challenging when complex physical problems occur in individuals who are delusional, cognitively impaired, lacking in social or communication skills, or physically threatening (Moak, 1996). Nonetheless, comorbid medical illness must be thoroughly assessed in order to address symptoms that may be caused or exacerbated by medical conditions or medication toxicity.

There are few data on the pharmacological treatment of elderly with schizophrenia (Jeste et al., 1993; Jeste et al., 1996). A review of the few available studies states that most report that antipsychotic medications result in a reduction of symptoms and earlier discharge from the hospital (Jeste et al., 1993). Efficacy of antipsychotic medications for patients with schizophrenia has been demonstrated in numerous controlled studies. Older adults with LOS have been shown to be as responsive to antipsychotic medications as young patients with schizophrenia when treated with appropriate agents and dosages. For example, response rates of late-onset schizophrenia to antipsychotic medications range from 62% (Post, 1966) to 86% (Rabins, Pauker, & Thomas, 1984).

Antipsychotics serve two primary purposes in the treatment of schizophrenia. First, they reduce acute symptoms that appear during an exacerbation, including both positive and negative symptoms (J. M. Kane & Marder, 1993). Second, administration of antipsychotics lowers the probability of subsequent relapses by 30% to 60% (J. M. Kane, 1989). Low doses of antipsychotic medication have been shown to be effective at lowering risk of relapse (Van Putten & Marder, 1986), suggesting that it is possible to reduce patients' vulnerability to long-term side effects of these medications (e.g., tardive dyskinesia). Also, recent improvements in the development of atypical antipsychotic medications (e.g., clozapine, risperidone, olanzapine), have shown that the functioning of patients who are treatment refractory to the standard antipsychotics can be improved (Meltzer, 1990, 1994; Pickar, 1995; Jeste et al., 1996).

Physiological changes of aging contribute to increased risk of acute adverse side effects to antipsychotic medications in the elderly. Age-related alterations in drug distribution and metabolism may result in higher plasma levels of antipsychotic medications in elderly compared to younger schizophrenic patients. In addition, age-related changes in receptors and neurotransmitters may cause elderly patients to be more sensitive to the effects of medications. Hence, effective serum levels of medication in elderly patients are achieved with substantially lower doses of antipsychotic medication.

Because age is associated with remission of symptoms in more than half of individuals with schizophrenia (Harding et al., 1987a, 1987b), some elderly individuals may be spared the risks of continued exposure to antipsychotic medications. Jeste and colleagues (1993) reviewed six double-blind studies of antipsychotic drug withdrawal followed for a mean of 6 months in older adults with schizophrenia and found an average relapse rate of 40%, compared to a relapse rate of 11% for those who continued on medication. The authors concluded that stable, chronic outpatients without a history of antipsychotic discontinuation should be considered for a carefully monitored trial of antipsychotic withdrawal. In summary, although the need remains for effective psychosocial interventions for schizophrenia, antipsychotic medications continue to be the mainstay in all treatment programs for schizophrenia.

Psychosocial Interventions

The stress-vulnerability model for schizophrenia offers one approach to understanding the role of psychosocial treatment (Liberman, Mueser, Wallace, Jacobs, *et al.*, 1986; Nuechterlein & Dawson, 1984). In this model, biological vulnerability, psychological coping, and environmental stress contribute in combination to the presence and severity of schizophrenic symptoms. Genetic and other biological factors are thought to determine biological vulnerability early in life, whereas environmental stressors may include exposure to high levels of negative emotion, life events such as the death of a significant other, and an absence of structure or support. Stressful life events can directly contribute to psychotic relapse in schizophrenia (Ventura, Nuechterlein, Lukoff, & Hardesty, 1989). Coping and living skills can help to offset an underlying psychological vulnerability to stress.

The stress-vulnerability model calls for an approach to treatment consisting of (1) reducing vulnerability, (2) reducing environmental stress, and (3) enhancing coping skills. For example, biological vulnerability can be lessened by providing antipsychotic medications and decreasing substance abuse. Individual treatment approaches, such as social skills training (Liberman, DeRisi, & Mueser, 1989) tend to focus mainly on improving patients' coping skills, whereas psychosocial interventions, such as family interventions, are directed toward a reduction of environmental stress (Mueser & Glynn, 1995; Tarrier *et al.*, 1988). Most treatments for schizophrenia share one or more of these goals.

Social skills training has not been evaluated in older patients with schizophrenia, but effectiveness of this approach for younger individuals suggests that it may have a role in psychosocial treatment of elderly with severe mental illness. The fundamental premise of social skills training is that the social impairments of schizophrenia can be decreased through systematically teaching the behavioral components of social skills (Bellack & Mueser, 1993; Bellack, Turner, Hersen, & Luber, 1984; Dobson, McDougall, Busheikin, 1995; Liberman, Mueser, & Wallace, 1986; Marder *et al.*, in press). Many individuals with schizophrenia require outpatient interventions, such as social skills training, that can be provided on a group or individual basis (Taylor & McDowell, 1986). These skills can be learned through a combination of therapist modeling (i.e., demonstration of the skill), patient behavioral rehearsal (i.e., role playing), positive and corrective feedback, and homework assignments. Subsequently, clinicians and family members can assist the individual in generalizing these skills to the natural environment. Targeted social skills span a wide range of adaptive interpersonal and self-care behaviors, including the expression of feelings, conflict resolution skills, and medication management.

Overall, controlled studies on social skills training for schizophrenia provide some support for its efficacy, especially when treatment is provided over the long term (Mueser, Wallace, & Liberman, 1995). It is clear that skills training can improve social skills, and there is some evidence supporting its effect on social functioning. The impact of social skills training on the symptoms of schizophrenia is less clear, but it remains an important avenue for improving social functioning.

Family interventions directed toward reduction of environmental stress and enhancement of adaptive behaviors can also be important in reducing the risk of relapse in individuals with schizophrenia (Tarrier *et al.*, 1988). As institutional long-term care becomes rare, family interventions have taken on increasing importance. Several studies have demonstrated that a stressful family environment is associated with increased rates of relapse (Brown, Birley, & Wing, 1972; Vaughn & Leff, 1976; Vaughn, Snyder, Jones, Freeman, & Falloon, 1984; see Kavanagh, 1992). In particular, relapse has been associated with living environments where there are higher levels of critical comments, hostility, overinvolvement or "expressed emotion" (EE). Although high EE may play a role in precipitating relapse, it is also likely that living with a relative with frequent psychotic relapses may result in family caregivers' experiencing increased levels of stress, resulting in high EE (Glynn *et al.*, 1990). In either case, the treatment literature establishes that family-based interventions can have a significant, positive impact on many patients with schizophrenia and, frequently, on their relatives as well (I. Falloon *et al.*, 1982; Hogarty *et al.*, 1986; Leff, Kuipers, Berkowitz, Eberlein-Weis, & Sturgeon, 1982; Randolph *et al.*, 1994; Xiong *et al.*, 1994). Unfortunately, these studies have largely focused on younger patients with severe mental illness (generally with older parent care providers), and implications of this technology for the older patient with schizophrenia are unknown, particularly as the dynamic between family and patient is complicated by the medical deficits of the older adult.

Another focus of family-based treatment are interventions that enhance the coping skills of caregivers (e.g., Abramowitz & Coursey, 1989; Solomon, Draine, Mannion, & Meisel, 1996a, 1996b). Within the general population, one in six adults provide care to aging parents. In general, adult daughters are most likely to become care providers, with the average American woman spending 18 years helping aging parents (Stone & Kemper, 1989). The burden of caring for an aging parent or spouse has been associated with clinical depression and anxiety disorders, increased use of psychotropic medications, and increased stress-related disorders including immunological dysfunction, in addition to the cost of lost income and other opportunities (Cohen, 1993; Eisdorfer, 1991; Wright, Clipp, & George, 1993). The inability of family care providers to cope with the care needs of aging parents is a major risk factor for eventual placement of the older individual in a long-term care institutional setting.

One means of delaying nursing home placement may be through direct interventions that enhance the coping skills and support of spouse-caregivers. For example, Mittelman and colleagues (Mittelman, Ferris, Shulman, & Steinberg, 1996) conducted a randomized trial consisting of 206 spouse caregivers of Alzheimer's disease to assess the effectiveness of six sessions of individual and family counseling followed by support groups over 31/2 years. Alzheimer patients in the intervention group had a community tenure 329 days longer than the control group, with control group spouses being two thirds as likely to place their spouses in a nursing home at any time. This type of community-based intervention developed for family care providers of patients with Alzheimer's dementia may hold promise in the treatment of the older patient with severe mental illness, who may present significant challenges in late life to the family care provider.

Finally, there is also an important role for direct interventions to enhance coping skills in the person who has schizophrenia. A growing body of evidence has emerged that patients with schizophrenia employ a wide range of different strategies for coping with positive and negative symptoms. Coping efficacy appears to be strongly related to the number of coping strategies employed by the patient (Carr, 1988; Falloon & Talbot, 1981; Mueser, Valentiner, & Agresta, in press). Over the process of growing older, many individuals learn ways to cope with symptoms and psychosocial stressors though trial and error (Wing, 1987). Observed strategies include use of positive self-talk (to overcome unwanted thoughts), meditation, relaxation techniques, and engaging in distracting activities (Brier & Strauss, 1983; Cohen & Berk, 1985). Individuals with schizophrenia may benefit from systematic instruction in coping strategies. For example, Tarrier and colleagues (1993) found that patients with residual psychotic symptoms who were taught coping strategies experienced significant reductions in positive symptoms compared with patients who received training in problem-solving skills.

Overall, data on psychosocial interventions come largely from studies on younger patients. However, it is evident from the literature on older adults with schizophrenia that there is a substantial need for treatment approaches that address the considerable psychosocial needs of older patients and their families. Many of these approaches appear well suited to the older person and should be adapted and tested in clinical settings.

SUMMARY

Although schizophrenia among younger adults is a seriously debilitating disorder that has received considerable study, remarkably little is known about factors affecting the course or outcome of schizophrenia in older adults (Belitsky & McGlashan, 1993). Recent studies have begun to advance the base of knowledge on the phenomenology and treatment of schizophrenia in late life. Schizophrenia in late life can be part of a life-long illness (early-onset schizophrenia), or may first appear in older age (late-onset schizophrenia). Individuals with late-onset schizophrenia experience symptoms similar to those of early-onset schizophrenia, yet are more likely to report better premorbid functioning and exhibit fewer negative symptoms or symptoms of formal thought disorder. Treatment studies suggest that response to antipsychotic medication for LOS is comparable to that in early-onset schizophrenia. For either disorder, use of low dosages and trials of the newer atypical antipsychotic medications are likely to be preferred, as the risk of adverse side effects such as tardive dyskinesia and acute extrapyramidal side effects increases substantially with age.

The long-term outcome of schizophrenia is favorable for most individuals, yet outcomes are heterogeneous across individuals. Several factors appear to be especially important in the outcome of schizophrenia in late life. For older adults with early-onset schizophrenia, the effect of treatment cohort may have long-term consequences. The oldest of the old are likely to have spent many years in institutional care, whereas younger treatment cohorts are likely to have been exposed to antipsychotic medications early in the course of their illness and have acquired independent living skills through the assistance of community support and rehabilitation models of services. Comorbid medical illness and comorbid cognitive impairment are common in older adults with schizophrenia and require comprehensive medical assessment and specific attention to develop the necessary services to address acute and long-term care needs associated with these disorders. Finally, treatment approaches to schizophrenia in late life should follow from a biopsychosocial perspective. Appropriate use of antipsychotic medications should consider the increased vulnerability to adverse side effects and the potential advantages of the newer atypical antipsychotic agents. Psychological approaches to treatment should be tailored to the needs of the older adult and assist in developing coping and living skills that support optimal functioning and quality of life. Social interventions are needed that enhance the availability of social and family supports and the development of adaptive social skills.

In spite of growing attention to the issues of aging, there is a paucity of research on treatments and services for older persons with severe and persistent mental illness. In particular, little attention has focused on the individual with lifelong early-onset schizophrenia who is now in late middle age or old age. Further research is needed to determine the most effective and appropriate pharmacological and psychosocial interventions for the older person with schizophrenia.

REFERENCES

Abramowitz, I. A., & Coursey, R. D. (1989). Impact of an educational support group on family participants who take care of their schizophrenic relatives. *Journal of Consulting and Clinical Psychology, 57,* 232–236.

Almeida, O. P., Förstl, H., Howard, R., & David, A. S. (1993). Unilateral auditory hallucinations. *British Journal of Psychiatry, 162,* 262–264.

Almeida, O. P., Howard, R. J., Levy, R., & David, A. (1995a). Psychotic states arising in late life (late paraphrenia): The role of risk factors. *British Journal of Psychiatry, 166,* 215–228.

Almeida, O. P., Howard, R. J., Levy, R., & David, A. (1995b). Psychotic states arising in late life (late paraphrenia): Psychopathology and nosology. *British Journal of Psychiatry, 166,* 205–214.

American Psychiatric Association. (1994). *Diagnostic and statistical manual of mental disorders* (4th ed.) Washington, DC: Author.

Bartels, S. J. (1989). Organic mental disorder: When to suspect medical illness as a cause of psychiatric symptoms. In J. M. Ellison (Ed.), *Psychopharmacology: A primer for the psychotherapist* (pp. 205–239). Chicago: Year Book Medical Publishers.

Bartels, S. J., & Drake, R. E. (1988). Depressive symptoms in schizophrenia: Comprehensive differential diagnosis. *Comprehensive Psychiatry, 29,* 467–483.

Bartels, S. J., & Drake, R. E. (1989). Depression in schizophrenia: Current guidelines to treatment. *Psychiatric Quarterly, 60,* 333–345.

Bartels, S. J., & Liberto, J. (1995). Dual diagnosis in the elderly. In A. F. Lehman & L. B. Dixon (Eds.), *Double jeopardy: Chronic mental illness and substance use disorders* (pp. 139–158). Chur, Switzerland: Harwood Academic.

Bartels, S. J., Drake, R. E., Wallach, M. A., & Freeman, D. H. (1991). Characteristic hostility in schizophrenic outpatients. *Schizophrenia Bulletin, 17,* 163–171.

Bartels, S. J., Teague, G. B., Drake, R. E., Clark, R. E., Bush, P., & Noordsy, D. L. (1993). Service utilization and costs associated with substance abuse among rural schizophrenic patients. *Journal of Nervous and Mental Disease, 181,* 227–232.

Bartels, S. J., Miles, K. M., Dain, B., & Smyer, M. A. (1998). *Community mental health service use by elderly with severe mental illness.* Manuscript under review.

Bartels, S. J., Mueser, K. T., & Miles, K. M. (1997). A comparative study of elderly patients with schizophrenia and bipolar disorder in nursing homes and the community. *Schizophrenia Research, 27*(2–3), 181–190.

Bartels, S. J., Mueser, K. T., & Miles, K. M. (1997). Functional impairments in elderly patients with schizophrenia and major affective disorder living in the community: Social skills, living skills, and behavior problems. *Behavior Therapy, 28,* 43–63.

Belitsky, R., & McGlashan, T. H. (1993). The manifestations of schizophrenia in late life: A dearth of data. *Schizophrenia Bulletin, 19,* 683–689.

Bellack, A. S., & Mueser, K. T. (1993). Psychosocial treatment of schizophrenia. *Schizophrenia Bulletin, 19,* 317–336.

Bellack, A. S, Turner, S. M., Hersen, M., & Luber, R. F. (1984). An examination of the efficacy of social skills training for chronic schizophrenic patients. *Hospital and Community Psychiatry, 35,* 1023–1028.

Bellack, A. S., Morrison, R. L., Wixted, J. T., & Mueser, K. T. (1990). An analysis of social competence in schizophrenia. *British Journal of Psychiatry, 156,* 809–818.

Bleuler, M. (1974). The long-term course of the schizophrenic psychoses. *Psychological Medicine, 4,* 244–254.

Brier, A.M., & Strauss, J. S. (1983). Self-control of psychotic behavior. *Archives of General Psychiatry, 40,* 1141–1145.

Brown, G. W., Birley, J. L. T., & Wing, J. K. (1972). Influence of family life on the course of schizophrenic disorders: A replication. *British Journal of Psychiatry, 121,* 241–258.

Bulger, M. W., Wandersman, A., & Goldman, C. R. (1993). Burdens and gratifications of caregiving: Appraisal of parental care of adults with schizophrenia. *American Journal of Orthopsychiatry, 63,* 255–265.

Carr, V. (1988). Patients' techniques for coping with schizophrenia: An exploratory study. *British Journal of Medical Psychology, 61,* 339–352.

Castle, D., Wessely, S., Der, G., & Murray, R. (1991). The incidence of operationally defined schizophrenia in Camberwell, 1965 to 1984. *British Journal of Psychiatry, 159,* 790–794.

Castle, D. J., & Murray, R. M. (1993). The epidemiology of late-onset schizophrenia. *Schizophrenia Bulletin, 19,* 691–700.

Ciompi, L. (1980). The natural history of schizophrenia in the long term. *British Journal of Psychiatry, 136,* 413–420.

Cohen, C. I. (1993). Poverty and the course of schizophrenia: Implications for research and policy. *Hospital and Community Psychiatry, 44,* 951–958.

Cohen, C. I. (1995). Studies on the course and outcome of schizophrenia in later life. *Psychiatric Services, 46,* 877–889.

Cohen, C. I., & Berk, I. L. (1985). Personal coping styles of schizophrenic outpatients. *Hospital and Community Psychiatry, 36,* 407–410.

Davidson, M., Harvey, P. D., Powchick, P., Parrella, M., White, L., Knobler, H. Y., Losonczy, M. F., Keefe, R. S., Katz, S., & Frecska, E. (1995). Severity of symptoms in chronically institutionalized geriatric schizophrenic patients. *American Journal of Psychiatry, 152,* 197–207.

Dobson, D. J. G., McDougall, G., Busheikin, J., & Aldous, J. (1995). Social skills training and symptomatology in schizophrenia. *Psychiatric Services, 46,* 376–380.

Drake, R. E., Gates, C., Whitaker, A., & Cotten, P. G. (1985). Suicide among schizophrenics: A review. *Comprehensive Psychiatry, 26,* 90–100.

Drake, R. E., Osher, F. C., & Wallach, M. A. (1989). Alcohol use and abuse in schizophrenia: A prospective community study. *Journal of Nervous and Mental Disease, 177,* 408–414.

Dworkin, R. H. (1994). Pain insensitivity in schizophrenia: A neglected phenomenon and some implications. *Schizophrenia Bulletin, 20,* 235–248.

Eisdorfer, C. (1991). Care giving: An emerging risk factor for emotional and physical pathology. *Bulletin of the Meninger Clinic, 55,* 238–247.

Falloon, I., Boyd, J., McGill, C., Razani, J., Moss, H., & Gilderman, A. (1982). Family management in the prevention of exacerbations of schizophrenia. *New England Journal of Medicine, 306,* 1437–1440.

Falloon, I. R. H., & Talbot, R. E. (1981). Persistent auditory hallucinations: Coping mechanisms and implications for management. *Psychological Medicine, 11,* 329–339.

Fischer, W. H. (1996). Mental health services for an aging population: What history cannot teach us in planning for the twenty-first century. In S. M. Sorreff (Ed.), *Handbook for the treatment of the seriously mentally Ill* (pp. 503–515). Seattle, WA: Hogrefe & Huber.

Glynn, S., Randolph, E., Eth, S., Paz, G., Shaner, A., Strachan, A. (1990). Patient psychopathology and expressed emotion in schizophrenia. *British Journal of Psychiatry, 157,* 877–880.

Goldberg, T. E., Hyde, T. M., Kleinman, J. E., & Weinberger, D. R. (1993). Course of schizophrenia: Neuropsychological evidence for a static encephalopathy. *Schizophrenia Bulletin, 19,* 797–804.

Goldstein, J. M. (1988). Gender differences in the course of schizophrenia. *American Journal of Psychiatry, 145,* 684–689.

Gurland, B. J., & Cross, P. S. (1982). Epidemiology of psychopathology in old age. *Psychiatric Clinics of North America, 5,* 11–26.

Häfner, H., Riecher-Rössler, A., An der Heiden, W., Maurer, K., Fätkenheuer, B., & Löffler, W. (1993). Generating and testing a causal explanation of the gender difference in age at first onset of schizophrenia. *Psychological Medicine, 23,* 925–940.

Harding, C. M., Brooks, G. W., Ashikaga, T., Strauss, J. S., & Breier, A. (1987a). The Vermont longitudinal study of persons with severe mental illness, I: Methodology, study sample, and overall status 32 years later. *American Journal of Psychiatry, 144,* 718–726.

Harding, C. M., Brooks, G. W., Ashikaga, T., Strauss, J. S., & Breier, A. (1987b). The Vermont longitudinal study of persons with severe mental illness. II: Long-term outcome of subjects who retrospectively met DSM-III criteria for schizophrenia. *American Journal of Psychiatry, 144,* 727–735.

Harris, M., & Jeste, D. (1988). Late-onset schizophrenia: An overview. *Schizophrenia Bulletin, 14,* 39–55.

Heaton, R., Paulsen, J. S., McAdams, L. A., Kuck, J., Zisook, S., Braff, D., Harris, M. J., & Jeste, D. V. (1994). Neuropsychological deficits in schizophrenics: Relationship to age, chronicity, and dementia. *Archives of General Psychiatry, 51,* 469–476.

Hegarty J. D., Baldessarini, R. J., Tohen, M., Waternaux, C., & Oepem, G. (1994). One hundred years of schizophrenia: A meta-analysis of the outcome literature. *American Journal of Psychiatry, 151,* 1409–1416.

Herbert, M., & Jacobson, S. (1967). Late paraphrenia. *British Journal of Psychiatry, 113,* 461–469.

Herz, M. I. (1985). Prodromal symptoms and prevention of relapse in schizophrenia. *Journal of Clinical Psychiatry, 46,* 22–25.

Hogarty, G. E., Anderson, C. M., Reiss, D. J., Kornblith, S. J., Greenwald, D. P., Javna, C.D., & Madonia, M. J. (1986). Family psychoeducation, social skills training, and maintenance chemotherapy in the aftercare treatment of schizophrenia. I: One-year effects of a controlled study on relapse and expressed emotion. *Archives of General Psychiatry, 43,* 633–642.

Howard, R., Castle D., Wessely, S., & Murray, R. (1993). A comparative study of 470 cases of early- and late-onset schizophrenia. *British Journal of Psychiatry, 163,* 352–357.

Huber, G., Cross, G., Schuttler, R., & Linz, M. (1989). Longitudinal studies of schizophrenic patients. *Schizophrenia Bulletin, 6,* 592–605.

Hughes, J. R., Hatsukami, D. K., Mitchell, J. E., & Dahlgren, L. A. (1986). Prevalence of smoking among psychiatric outpatients. *American Journal of Psychiatry, 143,* 993–997.

Jackson, J. H. (1984). Remarks on the evolution and dissolution of the nervous system. *Journal of Mental Science, 33,* 25–48.

Jeste, D. V., Lacro, J. P., Gilbert, P. L., Kline, J., & Kline, N. (1993). Treatment of late-life schizophrenia with neuroleptics. *Schizophrenia Bulletin, 19,* 817–830.

Jeste, D. V., Eastham, J. H., Lacro, J. P., Gierz, M., Field, M. G., & Harris, M. J. (1996). Management of late-life psychosis. *Journal of Clinical Psychiatry, 57*(Supp. 3), 39–45.

Kane, J., Woerner, M., & Lieberman, J. (1988). Tardive dyskinesia: Prevalence, incidence, and risk factors. *Journal of Clinical Psychopharmacology, 8,* 52–56.

Kane, J., Jeste, D., Barnes, T., Casey, D., Cole, J., Davis, J., Gualtieri, C., Schooler, N., Sprague, R., & Wettstein, R. (1992). *Tardive dyskinesia: A task force report of the American Psychiatric Association.* Washington, DC: American Psychiatric Association.

Kane, J. M. (1989). Innovations in the psychopharmacologic treatment of schizophrenia. In A. S. Bellack (Ed.), *A clinical guide for the treatment of schizophrenia* (pp. 43–75). New York: Plenum.

Kane, J. M., & Marder, S. R. (1993). Psychopharmacologic treatment of schizophrenia. *Schizophrenia Bulletin, 19,* 287–302.

Kavanagh, D. J. (1992). Recent developments in expressed emotion and schizophrenia. *British Journal of Psychiatry, 160,* 601–620.

Kay, D., & Roth, M. (1961). Environmental and hereditary factors in the schizophrenias of old age ('late paraphrenia') and their bearing on the general problem of causation in schizophrenia. *Journal of Mental Science, 107,* 649–686.

Koran, L. M., Sox, H. C., Marton, K. I., Molzen, S., Sox, C. H., Kraemer, H. C., Imai, K., Kelsy, T. G., Rose, T. G., & Levin, L. C. (1989). Medical evaluation of psychiatric patients. *Archives of General Psychiatry, 46,* 733–740.

Koranyi, E. K. (1979). Morbidity and rate of undiagnosed physical illnesses in a psychiatric clinic population. *Archives of General Psychiatry, 36,* 414–419.

Kraepelin, E. (1971). *Dementia praecox and paraphrenia* (R. M. Barclay, Trans.). Huntington, NY: Kreiger. (Original work published in 1919)

Leff, J., Kuipers, L., Berkowitz, R., Eberlein-Vries, R., & Sturgeon, D. (1982). A controlled trial of social intervention in the families of schizophrenic patients. *British Journal of Psychiatry, 141,* 121–134.

Lesser, I., Miller, B., Swartz, R., Boone, K., Mehringer, C., & Mena, I. (1993). Brain imaging in late-life schizophrenia and related psychoses. *Schizophrenia Bulletin, 19,* 773–782.

Lewine, R. J. (1988). Gender in schizophrenia. In H. A. Nasrallah (Ed.), *Handbook of Schizophrenia* (Vol. 3, pp. 379–397). Amsterdam: Elsevier.

Lewine, R. R. J. (1990). A discriminant validity study of negative symptoms with a special focus on depression and antipsychotic medication. *American Journal of Psychiatry, 147,* 1463–1466.

Lewine, R. R. J., Gulley, L. R., Risch, S. C., Jewart, R., & Houpt, J. L. (1990). Sexual dimorphism, brain morphology, and schizophrenia. *Schizophrenia Bulletin, 16,* 195–203.

Liberman, R. P., Mueser, K. T., & Wallace, C. J. (1986). Social skills training for schizophrenic individuals at risk for relapse. *American Journal of Psychiatry, 143,* 523–526.

Liberman, R. P., Mueser, K. T., Wallace, C. J., Jacobs, H. E., Eckman, T., & Massel, H. K. (1986). Training skills in the psychiatrically disabled: Learning coping and competence. *Schizophrenia Bulletin, 12,* 631–647.

Liberman, R. P., DeRisi, W. J., & Mueser, K. T. (1989). *Social skills training for psychiatric patients.* Needham Heights, MA: Allyn & Bacon.

Light, E., & Lebowitz, B. D. (1991). *The elderly with chronic mental illness.* New York: Springer.

MacGregor, P. (1994). Grief: The unrecognized parental response to mental illness in a child. *Social Work, 39,* 160–166.

Marder, S. R., Liberman, R. P., Wirshing, W. C., Mintz, J., Eckman, T. A., & Johnston-Cronk, H. (in press). Management of risk relapse in schizophrenia. *American Journal of Psychiatry.*

Meeks, S., Carstensen, L. L., Stafford, P. B., Brenner, L. L., Weathers, F., Welch, R., & Oltmanns, T. F. (1990). Mental health needs of the chronically mentally ill elderly. *Psychology and Aging, 5,* 163–171.

Meltzer, H. Y. (1990). Clozapine: Mechanism of action in relation to its clinical advantages. In A. Hales, C. N. Stefanis, & J. Talbott (Eds.), *Recent advances in schizophrenia* (pp. 237–256). New York: Springer-Verlag.

Meltzer, H. Y. (1994). An overview of the mechanism of clozapine. *Journal of Clinical Psychiatry, 55* (Suppl. B), 47–52.

Mittelman, M., Ferris, S., Shulman, E., Stenberg, G., Mackell, J., & Ambinder, A. (1994). Efficacy of a multicompont individualized treatment to improve the well-being of AD caregivers. In E. Light, G. Niederehe, & Lebowitz (Eds.), *Stress effects on family caregivers of Alzheimer's patients* (pp. 185–204). New York: Springer.

Mittelman, M. S., Ferris, S. H., Shulman, E., Steinberg, G. & Levin, B. (1996). A family intervention to delay nursing home placement of patients with Alzheimer disease: A randomized controlled trial. *Journal of American Medical Association, 276* (21), 1725–1731.

Moak, G. S. (1990). Discharge and retention of psychogeriatric long-stay patients in a state mental hospital. *Hospital and Community Psychiatry, 41,* 445–448.

Moak, G. S. (1996). When the seriously mentally ill patient grows old. In S. M. Sorreff (Ed.), *Handbook for the treatment of the seriously mentally Ill* (pp. 279–294). Seattle: Hogrefe & Huber.

Mueser, K. T., & Glynn, S. M. (1995). *Behavioral family therapy for psychiatric disorders.* Needham Heights, MA: Allyn & Bacon.

Mueser, K. T., Yarnold, P. R., Levinson, D. F., Singh, H., Bellack, A. S., Kee, H., Morrison, R. L., & Yadalam, K. G. (1990). Prevalence of substance abuse in schizophrenia: Demographic and clinical correlates. *Schizophrenia Bulletin, 16,* 31–56.

Mueser, K. T., Douglas, M. S., Bellack, A. S., & Morrison, R. L. (1991). Assessment of enduring deficit and negative symptom subtypes in schizophrenia. *Schizophrenia Bulletin, 17,* 565–582.

Mueser, K. T., Sayers, S. L., Schooler, N. R., Mance, R. M., & Haas, G. L. (1994). A multi-site investigation of the reliability of the Scale for the Assessment of Negative Symptoms. *American Journal of Psychiatry, 151,* 1453–1462.

Mueser, K. T., Wallace, C. J., & Liberman, R. P. (1995). New developments in social skills training. *Behavior Change, 12,* 31–40.

Mueser, K. T., Valentiner, D. P., & Agresta, J. (in press). Coping with negative symptoms of schizophrenia: Patient and family perspectives. *Schizophrenia Bulletin.*

Mulsant, B. H., Stergiou, A., Keshavan, M. S., Sweet, R. A., Rifai, A. H., Pasternak, R., & Zubenko, G. S. (1993). Schizophrenia in late life: Elderly patients admitted to an acute care psychiatric hospital. *Schizophrenia Bulletin, 19,* 709–721.

Nuechterlein, K. H., & Dawson, M. E. (1984). A heuristic vulnerability/stress model of schizophrenic episodes. *Schizophrenia Bulletin, 10,* 300–312.

Pearlson, G. D., & Rabins, P. V. (1988). The late-onset psychoses—Possible risk factors. *Psychiatric Clinics of North America, Psychosis and Depression in the Elderly, 11,* 15–33.

Pearlson, G. D., Kreger, L., Rabins, P. V., Chase, G. A., Cohen, B., Wirth, J. B., Schlaepfer, T. B., & Tune, L. E. (1989). A chart review study of late-onset and early-onset schizophrenia. *American Journal of Psychiatry, 146,* 1568–1574.

Pickar, D. (1995). Prospects for the pharmacotherapy of schizophrenia. *Lancet, 4,* 345 (8949), 557–562.

Platt, S. (1985). Measuring the burden of psychiatric illness on the family: An evaluation of some rating scales. *Psychological Medicine, 15,* 383–393.

Post, F. (1966). *Persistent persecutory states of the elderly.* London: Pergamon.

Prager, S., & Jeste, D. V. (1993). Sensory impairment in late-life schizophrenia. *Schizophrenia Bulletin, 19,* 755–772.

Rabins, P. V., Pauker, S., & Thomas, J. (1984). Can schizophrenia begin after age 44? *Comprehensive Psychiatry, 25,* 290–293.

Randolph, E. T., Eth, S., Glynn, S. M., Paz, G. G., Leong, G. B., Shaner, A. L., Strachan, A., Van Vort, W., Escobar, J. I., & Liberman, R. P. (1994). Behavioral family management in schizophrenia: Outcome of a clinic-based intervention. *British Journal of Psychiatry, 164,* 501–506.

Roy, A. (1986). Suicide in schizophrenia. In A. Roy (Ed.), *Suicide* (pp. 97–112). Baltimore: Williams & Wilkins.

Salokangas, R. K. R., Palo-Oja, T., & Ojanen, M. (1991). The need for social support among outpatients suffering from functional psychosis. *Psychological Medicine, 21,* 209–217.

Salzman, C., Vaccaro, B., & Lief, J. (1995). Clozapine in older patients with psychosis and behavioral disruption. *American Journal of Geriatric Psychiatry, 3,* 26–33.

Seeman, M. V. (1986). Current outcome in schizophrenia: Women vs. men. *Acta Psychiatrica Scandinavica, 73,* 609–617.

Seeman, M. V., & Lang, M. (1990). The role of estrogens in schizophrenia gender differences. *Schizophrenia Bulletin, 16,* 185–194.

Solomon, P., Draine, J., Mannion, E., & Meisel, M. (1996a). Impact of brief family psychoeducation on self-efficacy. *Schizophrenia Bulletin, 22,* 41–50.

Solomon, P., Draine, J., Mannion, E., & Meisel, M. (1996b). The impact of individualized consultation and group workshop family psychoeducation interventions on ill relative outcomes. *Journal of Nervous and Mental Disease, 184,* 252–255.

Stone, R., & Kemper, P. (1989). Spouses and children of disabled elders: How large a constituency for long-term care reform? *Milbank Quarterly, 67,* 485–506.

Szymanski, S. R., Canoon, T. H., Gallacher, F., Erwin, R. J., & Gur, R. E. (1996). Course of treatment response in first-episode and chronic schizophrenia. *American Journal of Psychiatry, 153,* 519–525.

Tarrier, N., Barrowclough, C., Vaughn, C., Bamrah, J., Porceddu, K., Watts, S., & Freeman, H. (1988). The community management of schizophrenia: A controlled trial of a behavioral intervention with families to reduce relapse. *British Journal of Psychiatry, 153,* 532–542.

Tarrier, N., Beckett, R., Harwood, S., Baker, A., Yusupoff, L., & Ugarteburu, I. (1993). A trial of two cognitive behavioral methods of treating drug-resistant residual psychotic symptoms in schizophrenic patients. I. Outcome. *British Journal of Psychiatry, 162,* 524–532.

Taylor, A., & Dowell, D. A. (1986). Social skills training in board and care homes. *Psychosocial Rehabilitation Bulletin, 10,* 55–69.

Test, M. A., & Berlin, S. B. (1981). Issues of special concern to chronically mentally ill women. *Professional Psychology, 12,* 136–145.

Test, M. A., Burke, S. S., & Wallisch, L. S. (1990). Gender differences of young adults with schizophrenic disorders in community care. *Schizophrenia Bulletin, 16,* 331–344.

Tsuang, M., & Winokur, G. (1975). The Iowa 500: Field work in a 35-year follow-up of depression, mania and schizophrenia. *Canadian Psychiatric Association Journal, 20,* 359–365.

Tsuang, M. T., Woolson, R. F., & Fleming, J. A. (1980). Premature deaths in schizophrenia and affective disorders. *Archives of General Psychiatry, 37,* 979–983.

Van Putten, T., & Marder, S. R. (1986). Low-dose treatment strategies. *Journal of Clinical Psychiatry, 47* Suppl. 5), 12–16.

Vaughn, C., & Leff, J. (1976). The influence of family and social factors on the course of psychiatric illness. *British Journal of Psychiatry, 129,* 125–137.

Vaughn, C., Snyder, K., Jones, S., Freeman, W., & Falloon, I. (1984). Family factors in schizophrenia relapse. *Archives of General Psychiatry, 41,* 1169–1177.

Ventura, J., Nuechterlein, K. H., Lukoff, D., & Hardesty, J. P. (1989). A prospective study of stressful life events and schizophrenic relapse. *Journal of Abnormal Psychology, 98,* 407–411.

Wing, J. H. (1987). Long term social adaptation in schizophrenia. In N. E. Miller & G. D. Cohen (Eds.), *Schizophrenia and aging* (pp. 183–199). New York: Guilford.

Wright, L., Clipp, E., & George, L. (1993). Health consequences of caregiver stress. *Medicine. Exercise, Nutrition, and Health, 2,* 181–195.

Wyatt, R. J. (1991). Neuroleptics and the natural course of schizophrenia. *Schizophrenia Bulletin, 17,* 325–351.

Xiong, W., Phillips, M. R., Hu, X., Ruiwen, W., Dai, Q., Kleinman, J., & Kleinman, A. (1994). Family-based intervention for schizophrenic patients in China: A randomised controlled trial. *British Journal of Psychiatry, 165,* 239–247.

Yassa, R., & Suranyl-Cadotte, B. (1993). Clinical characteristics of late-onset schizophrenia and delusional disorder. *Schizophrenia Bulletin, 19,* 701–707.

Zigler, E., & Glick, M. (1986). *A developmental approach to adult psychopathology.* New York: Wiley.

Zisook, S., Heaton, R., Moranville, J., Kuck, J., Jernigan, T., & Braff, D. (1992). Past substance abuse and clinical course of schizophrenia. *American Journal of Psychiatry, 149,* 552–553.

CHAPTER 10

Depression

PATRICIA A. AREÁN, HEATHER UNCAPHER,
AND DEREK SATRE

INTRODUCTION

For many decades our society believed that to be old was to be depressed. To some extent the myth is still pervasive that with old age comes problems with health, finances, and loss of friends, family, and purpose. If one thinks this way, one would certainly believe that the later years of life constitute a bleak time that is hopeless and bereft of any joy. However, recent research has indicated that this belief is not an accurate picture of later life. According to the McArthur Foundation Successful Aging studies, the process of aging is variable; not everyone who ages becomes disabled, dissatisfied with life, or depressed (Curb et al., 1990). These findings are further corroborated by the results of the Epidemiological Catchment Area Study, which demonstrated that Major Depression (one of the most serious and widely studied of the mood disorders) is less prevalent in people over the age of 65 than it is in younger age groups: 1% of older adults had a lifetime prevalence of Major Depression whereas 6% of younger adults had a Major Depressive Episode in their lives (Robins et al., 1984).

If depressive disorders are so uncommon in late life, then why bother studying them? Even though only a small percentage of older adults will ever become depressed, those few people who do become depressed are very disabled by the symptoms of these disorders. For instance, research indicates that older adults who have Major Depressive Disorder will die sooner from an illness than nondepressed older adults with the same physical illness. Older adults with minor depression (one of the Depressive Disorders Not Otherwise Specified (NOS) are more disabled, report more physical pain, and use more health services than older adults without any depressive symptoms (Callahan,

PATRICIA A. AREÁN AND DEREK SATRE • Department of Psychiatry, University of California–San Francisco, San Francisco, California 94143-0984   HEATHER UNCAPHER, Department of Psychology, University of California–Berkeley, Berkeley, California, 94720.

Handbook of Clinical Geropsychology, edited by Michel Hersen and Vincent B. Van Hasselt. Plenum Press, New York, 1998.

Hui, Nienaber, Musick, & Tierney, 1994; Ganzini, Lee, Heintz, Bloom, & Fenn, 1994). Moreover, senior citizens who attempt to take their lives are more successful at completing a suicide than any other age group: nearly half of all suicide attempts are completed. Depressive disorders in late life constitute a major public health concern.

Depressive disorders (Major Depression, Dysthymia, and Depression NOS) are among the most widely studied psychiatric phenomena in geriatrics, second only to Alzheimer disease and other dementias. In the past ten years, substantial research has been carried out to understand the etiology, prevalence, presentation, and treatment of depression in community-dwelling older adults. However, considerable controversy remains as to the etiology of late-life depression, how to assess and recognize depressive disorders in older adults, and what interventions are most useful for treating depression in late life. Further, the research into the course, cause, and prevalence of these disorders in minorities, frail elderly, and other special populations is still preliminary. The purpose of this chapter, then, is to review the current research on late-life depression, discuss the controversies, and discuss treatment outcome studies.

DEPRESSIVE DISORDERS DEFINED

Classification

The *Diagnostic and Statistical Manual of Mental Disorders*, 4th ed. (*DSM-IV*; American Psychiatric Association, 1994) classifies depressive disorders into three groups: Major Depressive Disorder (MDD), Dysthymia, and Depressive Disorder NOS (DDN: includes Minor Depression, Depression due to Medical Conditions or Substance Use). These disorders have overlapping symptoms and presentations, but differ in their prevalence, course, and symptom severity. MDD is the most serious of the three. *DSM-IV* describes an episode of MDD as consisting of feelings of depression and/or lack of interest in pleasant activities for two weeks, every day, nearly all day, and five or more of the following symptoms: appetite or weight disturbance, sleep disturbance, psychomotor retardation or agitation, fatigue, difficulty concentrating, feelings of guilt or worthlessness, thoughts of death or suicide. As stated earlier, only 1% of older adults in community samples experienced an episode of MDD during their lifetimes (Regier *et al.*, 1988). However, MDD appears to be quite prevalent in ambulatory medical settings: 10% according to Koenig and Blazer (1992) and Areán and Miranda (1995). As many as 12.3% of seniors in nursing homes suffer from MDD (P. A. Parmalee, Katz, & Lawton, 1991).

Minor Depression (one of the DDN subgroups) is the most common disorder in late life, with as many as 30% of older adults having experienced an episode during their lifetimes, regardless of setting (Areán & Miranda, 1995; Parmalee, Katz, & Lawton, 1989). This disorder is similar to but less severe than MDD, with only three of the depressive symptoms mentioned above present nearly every day for at least two weeks.

Dysthymia is a mild, yet more chronic depressive disorder, in which the above-mentioned symptoms of depression exist for two years or more but are experienced on occasion throughout a week. Dysthymia is also more prevalent than MDD, but less so than Minor Depression, with only 10% of the elderly population having experienced an episode during their lifetimes (Regier *et al.,* 1988). Rates of this disorder in medical and skilled nursing settings is unknown.

Late Versus Early Onset

Although *DSM-IV* does not include a special classification for geriatric depression, there is speculation that depressive disorders that first occur after the age of 65 are different from disorders with an earlier onset in terms of their etiology and presentation. Gerontologists refer to this phenomenon as *late-life,* or *geriatric, depression* (Blazer, 1990; Devanand *et al.,* 1994). Research differentiating late- and early-onset depressions is preliminary. However, we do know that people with geriatric depression present with more extreme weight loss, hypochondriacal preoccupation, trouble falling asleep, agitation, and preoccupation with guilt (Brown *et al.,* 1984). Moreover, differences between geriatric depression and early-onset depressions indicate that older adults who have had a previous episode of depression were more likely to have a personality disorder than were older adults with geriatric depression (Devanand *et al.,* 1994). People with geriatric depression are less likely to suffer another depressive episode, but geriatric depressives who do relapse show symptoms within 2 months of treatment. Older adults with early-onset depression tend to relapse within 6 months (Baldwin & Jolley, 1986).

ETIOLOGY

Many geriatricians believe that late-life depressive disorders result from chronic life stressors, genetic, biological, and endocrinological factors, and physical illnesses. In older adults, the main risk factors for depression are a previous history of depression, current physical illness, recent stressful life events, social and economic deprivation, and living alone (Henderson, 1989). The course and prognosis of depressive disorders vary. Some studies show that older adults have poorer treatment outcomes and higher rates of relapse than younger people (Alexopoulos, Young, Meyers, Abrams, & Shamolan, 1988), whereas more recent research suggests that course and prognosis of MDD in older adults is similar to that of younger adults. According to Brodarty and colleagues (1993), people with geriatric depression tend to show greater improvements over time, respond better to treatments for depression than younger patients, and are less likely to relapse than younger adults or older adults with an early-onset depression. These findings are preliminary, and more prospective and longitudinal research is needed to understand the course of geriatric depression and depressive disorders in older adults.

Psychosocial Factors in Depression in Older Adults

Older adults often identify a stressful life event as the precursor to their depressive episode. The most common stressful life events are physical disability, financial stress, caring for a chronically ill family member, and grief over the loss of a social role or important family member (Markides & Cooper, 1989). However, many older adults faced with these problems do not become depressed. Theorists suggest that amount of preparation and social support one has in dealing with a stressful life event may determine whether a senior citizen will become depressed. For instance, loss of a loved one or retirement do not affect the well-being of older adults as much as they do younger adults, who may be less prepared for such types of stressors (George, 1989). Senior citizens who plan ahead for retirement or illness are less likely to suffer psychologically than those who do not prepare.

Some studies indicate that depressed seniors are more likely to be socially isolated and have fewer social outlets than older adults who are not depressed. In addition, perceived social support (whether older adults feel they have people they can turn to) mediates the impact of a stressful life event on depressive symptoms (Husiani *et al.*, 1991). Krause (1987) found that depressed seniors had less emotional support for their problems and fewer social contacts than seniors who were not depressed. Although the causal direction of the relationship between social support and late-life depression is not known, it is likely that those older adults who are at greatest risk for becoming depressed are those who feel they have no one to turn to in times of stress.

In addition to stressful life events and few social supports, many depressed older adults tend to have limited problem-solving skills. Only a few studies have investigated the role coping skills play in depression in older adults, but preliminary evidence suggests that senior citizens who are active problem solvers (assertively pursuing information about a problem and then developing a plan to solve it) are less likely to be depressed than seniors with more passive and unassertive coping styles (Fry, 1989; Thompson & Gallagher-Thompson, 1993). Moreover, seniors who are religious or cope better with uncontrollable events, such as a chronic medical illness, are also less likely to be depressed than those older adults who are not religious (Koenig *et al.*, 1989).

Late-life depression has also been found to be associated with both social and biological changes. From a psychosocial perspective, geriatric depression is due to the inability to cope with life problems specific to aging. Older adults have never had to face many of the medical and financial problems that can occur in late life, and therefore are unprepared for and ill equipped to deal with these events (Areán & Miranda, 1997). Repeated exposure to the inability to solve problems then results in learned helplessness reactions, which subsequently lead to depression (Yost *et al.*, 1986).

In summary, older adults are more likely to become depressed if they are faced with stressors for which they are unprepared, have few social supports, and are relatively passive problem solvers. Therefore, older adults most vulnerable to depressive disorder are those who are more isolated socially and encounter stressful situations with which they are unable to deal. Therapies aimed at increasing social supports and coping abilities would be beneficial in treating depression in the elderly.

Biology and Neuroendocrinology

There has been much research investigating the biology of late-life depression, particularly geriatric onset depressions. Such research suggests that biological variables responsible for onset of a depressive episode in late life include severe lesions in the frontal deep white matter and basal ganglia of the brain (Krishnan, 1991), dysregulation of endocrine function (specifically, increased cortisol levels; D. Blazer, 1990), and a dearth of cerebral neurotransmitters such as serotonin. The most compelling of these arguments is the role of cortisol in the development of depression. High levels of cortisol have been consistently related to physical illness, stress, and depression (Blazer, 1990). Cortisol levels increase with age, as does dysregulation of the endocrine system. This may make older adults vulnerable to depression (Blazer, 1990). However, because depression is a relatively rare disorder in older adults, the cortisol hypothesis does not explain all depression, but this hypothesis may explain why physically ill elderly (who have even more increased cortisol) are more likely to be depressed.

The neurotransmitter hypothesis indicates that depression in older adults may be due to, or correlated with, a depletion of essential neurotransmitters in the brain. For years a lack of neurotransmitters norepinephrine and serotonin has been associated with depression. It is not clear whether lack of these chemicals is the cause or consequence of developing a depressive disorder, but they do seem to play an important role.

From a biological perspective, there is evidence to suggest that people with late-onset depression are more likely to have cerebral changes and injuries than older adults who are not depressed. For instance, researchers have found that those with geriatric depression have a higher incidence of cerebral vascular disease, significant delays in the auditory evoked response, and anatomic changes such as ventricular dilation and cortical atrophy (Alexopoulos et al., 1988). There is also evidence to demonstrate that people with geriatric depression are more likely to develop subsequent dementing illness. Most researchers are still uncertain as to the significance of these correlations, but most believe that there is a biological component to late-onset depression.

Physical Illness

Depression is highly prevalent in patients of all ages with acute and chronic medical illness. Older adults are particularly susceptible because they are more likely to be sick than younger adults. In older adults with cardiac, pulmonary, endocrine, and neurological disorders, functional disability, and cancer, high prevalence rates of depression are reported (Dreyfus, 1988).

Many possible causes of depression in ill people have been identified. Substances (e.g., drug, alcohol, lead) and medications (e.g., antihypertensives, digitalis, benzodiazepines, analgesics, l-dopa, antimicrobial agents, cardiovascular agents, hypoglycemic agents, and steroids) can produce depressive symptoms because of the physiological changes these disorders create. Medical conditions, diseases, and physiologic disturbances can also cause depressive symptoms through brain tissue damage. For instance, cerebrovascular accidents (stroke), seizure disorders, dementia (e.g., Alzheimer's disease), postconcussive syndrome, normal pressure hydrocephalus, and cerebral hypoxia have all been identified as contributing to depression in some older patients. Poststroke depressions are particularly prevalent up to two years after a cerebral incident (Robinson & Price, 1982). In addition, coronary artery disease and chronic obstructive pulmonary disorder are two medical conditions in which depression may significantly predict disability (Weaver & Narsavage, 1992).

Cancer and diabetes are also associated with depression. The prevalence of depression in cancer patients has been estimated to be from 4.5% to 58% (Massie, Gagnon, & Holland, 1994). Other diseases, such as Alzheimer's and Parkinson's disease, infectious diseases (e.g., AIDS, encephalitis, meningitis, syphilis, hepatitis), and autoimmune diseases or inflammatory conditions (e.g., arthritis, pancreatitis, multiple sclerosis, and systemic lupus erythematosus) are accompanied by high rates of depression and are thought to play a role in the onset of depression in older adults (Evans, Copeland, & Dewey, 1991). Many of these diseases create physiological changes resulting in depressive disorder, but they also create psychosocial difficulties, such as financial drain, disability, and pain. Gerontologists believe that physical illness impacts depressive symptoms directly through physiological change and indirectly through psychological stress.

Comments

Depression in older adults appears to be a function of several factors. Research suggests that older adults who are sick, are stressed financially and socially, who have few social supports, poor coping skills, and are biologically vulnerable are more likely to become depressed. Age of onset also appears to be important, and early evidence suggests that late-onset depression may have a strong biological component. The field of geriatrics would benefit from studies examining the relative impact that all these factors play in depressive disorders in senior citizens so that treatment decisions and preventive measures can be implemented.

ASSESSMENT OF DEPRESSION IN THE ELDERLY

Overview

Depression in late life is not easy to diagnose, largely because 75% of older adults have at least one chronic medical illness that may mimic or share symptoms of depressive disorders (G. Klerman, 1989). For many years, geropsychologists have struggled over the best way to recognize these disorders in older populations. In order to appreciate the difficulty in recognizing late-life depression, one should be familiar with the criteria for making a diagnosis of MDD.

Many reports describe difficulties in establishing a concise symptom profile of depression in the elderly. Certain vegetative symptoms that contribute to a diagnosis of depression, (e.g., insomnia, early morning awakening, and decreased appetite), are likely to be present in nondepressed as well as depressed older adults. In addition, although depressed older adults may present with apathy, fatigue, weight loss, sleep disturbance, and lack of initiative (Achte, 1988), older adults with poor physical health might present with the same symptoms, and not be depressed (Neese, 1991). Older adults vary widely in their functional capacity, social support, cognitive functioning, activity, sleep, and appetite. Thus an important aspect of diagnosis is to determine whether the constellation of symptoms is impairing the older adult's normal baseline functioning. Patients are asked whether any of these potential symptoms are recent changes and whether these changes have resulted in an impairment of usual functioning.

Researchers and clinicians disagree on how to consider physical symptoms in the diagnosis of depression. Some clinicians and researchers emphasize that physical symptoms or illness and depression occur together so often that they should be evaluated together (Caine, Lyness, King, & Conners, 1991). Some suggest that physical symptoms might be indicative of depression in older adults. For example, sleep disturbance (Gallo, Anthony, & Muthen, 1994), appetite disturbance, and weight loss appear to be more prevalent in older versus younger patients with Major Depressive Disorder (Blazer, Bachar, & Hughes, 1987) and may be important signs of depression in late life.

Variations in definition of depression are reflected in various standardized interviews and diagnostic categories. The *DSM-IV*, ICD-10 and the Diagnostic Interview Schedule (DIS) (Robins, Helzer, Croughan, & Ratcliff, 1981) all exclude symptoms of depression from a diagnosis of Major Depressive Disorder if they are considered to be due to a physical illness or condition. Exclusion of these symptoms may have clinical and research implications. For example, excluding physical symptoms from a diagnosis of depression may result in underestimation of depression in physically ill older adults (Newmann, 1989). These considerations all need to be taken into account when conducting an unstructured interview to diagnose depression in older adults.

Debate continues as to the constellation of symptoms that characterize geriatric depression in an unstructured interview. Depression might be qualitatively different in the elderly and involve symptoms not considered standard diagnostic criteria, such as helplessness (Depue & Monroe, 1978), hopelessness (Abramson, Metalsky, & Alloy, 1989), real or perceived cognitive deficit (Weiss, Nagel, & Aronson, 1986), or anxiety. Some investigators suggest that dysphoric mood may be a less salient feature in some older adults (Areán & Miranda, 1992; Gallo *et al.*, 1994). Others have reported that older patients with depression endorsed dysphoric mood (Koenig *et al.*, 1992), so the issue remains controversial and in need of clarification.

Methods of Assessment

Because of difficulties surrounding diagnosis of depression in older adults with an unstructured interview, gerontologists often rely on standardized instruments to help clarify a diagnosis of depressive disorder. There is a variety of methods for assessing depression in late life, including self-report scales and structured interviews.

Self-report scales are questionnaires that can either be read to or by the patient to determine the severity of depressive symptoms. Answers to specific questions are added to determine an overall depression score. These instruments are meant to be sensitive enough to identify everyone who is depressed. The Geriatric Depression Scale (GDS; Brink *et al.*, 1982), and the Zung Self-Rating Depression Scale (SRS; Zung, 1965) have been created specifically for adults. The GDS is a 30-item scale that asks about symptoms of depression in a True/False format. The Zung is a 20-item scale in which each item has a four-choice format ranging from "none of the time" to "all of the time." Both of these scales have excellent reliability and validity and they are equally useful in detecting depression in older adults (Hickie & Snowdon, 1987). However, one study compared the GDS to the SRS and found that although they were equally effective in identifying depression in older adults, the GDS was the easiest scale for the older subjects to complete (Dunn & Sacco, 1989). The GDS, therefore, may be preferable because of its simple response format.

Other self-report measures, such as the Beck Depression Inventory (BDI; Beck *et al.*, 1961), and the Center for Epidemiological Studies—Depression Scale (CES-D; Radloff, 1977) also appear to have sound psychometric properties for detecting depression in the elderly. However, given that such studies are sparse, it may be prudent to rely on scales developed exclusively for the geriatric population.

The main drawback of self-report measures for detecting depression is their tendency to overestimate presence of MDD in older adults. For research purposes, several structured clinical interviews exist that provide a strict guideline and list of questions for clinicians to adhere to when conducting a diagnostic interview. Included in these interviews are The Structured Clinical Interview for *DSM-IV* (SCID; First *et al.*, 1994), the Schedule for Affective Disorders and Schizophrenia (SADS; Spitzer *et al.*, 1988), and the Diagnostic Interview Schedule (DIS; Robins, 1981). All of these interviews follow a similar format. The questions are structured around the *Diagnostic and Statistical Manual of Mental Disorders*, 3rd ed., rev. (*DSM-III-R;* American Psychiatric Association, 1987) or *DSM-IV* criteria for diagnosing depressive disorders, are meant to be administered by trained clinicians, and provide an objective means of determining a diagnosis. Dolores Gallagher-Thompson reviewed six of these structured interviews: the SADS, the DIS, the Comprehensive Assessment and Referral Evaluation (CARE) (Gurland *et al.*, 1983), the Older Americans Resources and Services (OARS) Multidimensional Functional Assessment Questionnaire (MFAQ) (Duke University Center for the Study of Aging, 1978), the Longitudinal Interval Follow-up Evaluation (LIFE) (Shapiro & Keller, 1979), and the Hamilton Rating Scale for Depression (HRS-D) (Hamilton, 1960). The SADS was the most reliable and valid diagnosis of depression in community older adults (Gallagher, 1986).

Comment

Assessing depression in older adults is complex. We know that older adults may present or emphasize different depressive symptoms from younger patients. For instance, older depressed adults seem to be more hopeless, anxious, dysphoric, and have more somatic changes, such as sleep and appetite disturbance. Somatic symptoms need to be evaluated carefully so that the normal process of aging is not confused with depression. Additionally, a physical examination should always be conducted to determine whether there is a physiological cause. As a final note, the importance of assessing for suicidal ideation in this population is underscored by the relatively high successful suicide rate in older adults. It is imperative that clinicians ask their older patients directly about potential suicidal feelings and plans. Asking about suicide will not put the idea in an older person's mind.

TREATMENT OF GERIATRIC DEPRESSION

Despite difficulties in diagnosing depression in late life, MDD is easily treated in older adults. Pharmacotherapy, electroconvulsive therapy, and psychotherapeutic approaches have all been successful in treating depression in senior citizens.

The Use of Psychotherapy for Geriatric Depression

Psychosocial treatments used with older adults include cognitive, behavioral, psychodynamic, reminiscence, and interpersonal therapy. Many clinical reports have been published over the past 40 years demonstrating efficacy of psychological interventions for older adults (Smyer, Zarit, & Qualls, 1990; Weiss & Lazarus, 1993). Based on a review of the treatment literature, the November 1991 National Institutes of Health (NIH, 1992) Consensus Development Conference on Diagnosis and Treatment of Depression in Late Life (Washington, DC) recommended that psychotherapy be used after a trial of pharmacotherapy and electroconvulsive therapy. The panel indicated that this recommendation was based on the lack of studies investigating the efficacy of psychotherapy in older adults. There are now several studies of note that indicate the efficacy of psychotherapy in late-life depression. One metanalysis identified 17 articles examining the efficacy of psychosocial interventions for treating depression in older adults (Scogin & McElreath, 1994). The results suggest that psychosocial interventions are highly effective for treating both geriatric major depression and minor levels of depression.

Conducting Therapy With an Older Person

In all types of therapy with the older adult, the therapist should educate the person about therapy, keep the pace slower, and attempt to prevent relapse and recurrence through booster sessions (Gallagher-Thompson & Thompson, 1992).

Some geriatricians will often help patients remember the elements of their therapy by providing the older client with a journal and written materials, and sometimes reminder calls are given during the week to provide the older adult with additional support around completing out-of-session assignments. A therapist should also keep in mind that not all older people have the same developmental experiences. An octogenarian is 20 years older than a person who is 60, and clearly grew up with different experiences and values. Therapists must remain flexible and educate themselves about their older patients' developmental experiences.

Cognitive-Behavioral Psychotherapy:

Theory and Process. One of the more empirically validated forms of therapy with older adults is cognitive-behavioral psychotherapy (see Teri, Curtis, Gallagher-Thompson, & Thompson, 1994, for review), a combination of cognitive models (Beck, Rush, Shaw, & Emery, 1979), and behavioral models of psychopathology (Lewinsohn, Biglan, & Zeiss, 1976). The cognitive-behavioral model takes into account how a person's cognitive, affective, and behavioral responses to life events contribute to the development of depression. Specifically, depression is due to the interaction of stress, coping abilities, problem-solving skills, people's belief about whether they can cope with their problems, and how supportive the world is around them. Issues from childhood or the past are discussed only as to how they apply to problems occurring now. The goal of therapy is to teach new coping strategies and to identify and challenge cognitions that interfere with effective coping. This is achieved through collaborative discussion of life problems, generating strategies to solve or cope with the problems, and implementing new strategies during the time between therapy sessions, so that new skills can be practiced and reinforced.

Outcome Studies. Several studies have demonstrated the utility of CBT in treating late-life depression (Areán *et al.,* 1993; Beutler *et al.,* 1987). CBT has been compared to interpersonal therapy, finding positive change in depression in all conditions, with the patients in the cognitive or behavioral conditions scoring better on outcome depression scales 1 year later (Gallagher & Thompson, 1982; Thompson, Gallagher, & Breckenridge, 1987). CBT has also been compared with pharmacotherapy (Desipramine) alone and combined with CBT, indicating that medication combined with therapy was more effective than cognitive therapy alone, and that cognitive therapy alone was more effective than medication alone (Thompson & Gallagher-Thompson, 1993).

Interpersonal Psychotherapy

Theory and Process. Interpersonal psychotherapy (ITP) (G. L. Klerman, Weissman, Rounsaville *et al.,* 1984) combines aspects of psychodynamic and cognitive psychotherapy to focus on the patient's social roles and relationships in the production, exacerbation, and maintenance of depression. ITP was designed to address four specific areas: guilt, interpersonal disputes, role transitions, and interpersonal deficits. The depressed older adult may experience abnormal grief reactions, role transitions, and social problems that are addressed by this form of treatment. Variations of IPT treatment were developed for older adults: interpersonal psychotherapy for late-life depression (IPT-LL) and interpersonal psychotherapy for the maintenance treatment of recurrent depression in late life (IPT-LLM) (Frank *et al.*, 1993). Included in these variations are age-specific adaptations: a more flexible session, a more active role for the therapist including problem solving and coping with disagreements. In the interpersonal form of therapy, treatment begins with identifying important relationships in the patient's life. Problem areas and the nature of the identified relationships and their contributions to depression are explored. Eight general techniques assist this process, including the use of therapeutic relationship, exploratory and directive techniques, encouragement of affect, analyzing communication patterns, clarification, and behavior change techniques.

Outcome Studies.   Preliminary positive findings of IPT use with clients in midlife and those aged 50 to 65 were reported (Schneider *et al.,* 1986). In evaluations on midlife adults, IPT-M was not found to enhance imipramine treatment, but it was significant alone or with placebo compared to a placebo and medical clinic visits (Frank *et al.,* 1993). More studies are needed to evaluate the effectiveness of IPT for older adults. Treatment studies comparing IPT with other forms of psychotherapy will enhance future evaluations.

Psychodynamic Psychotherapy.

Theory and Process.   Psychodynamic psychotherapy originated with the work of Freud and his emphasis on intrapsychic processes. At first not recommended for older adults because of a number of assumptions, including rigidity of character and defenses (Freud, 1959), psychodynamic psychotherapy is now considered a viable form of treatment with older adults (Myers, 1991). Given that the older patient has a willingness and ability to work with unconscious issues, an ability to connect with the therapist, and a motivation to change, psychodynamic therapies explore themes of object relatedness, unconscious drives, self-esteem, self-worth, and resulting behaviors and relationships (Myers, 1991). There are no variations of this form of therapy specifically for older adults.

Outcome Studies.   Individual psychodynamic psychotherapy is effective in older adults (Altshuler, 1989). L. W. Lazarus and colleagues (1984, 1987) studied the effectiveness of individual psychodynamic psychotherapy for depressed older adults, and found lower distress, lower depression and defenses, and increased self-esteem following treatment. However, very few empirical studies exist.

Reminiscence Psychotherapy

Theory and Process.   According to Eric Erikson (1959), throughout life people are continually faced with syntonic and dystonic conflicts that create a process of psychopathology until balance is reached between these conflicts

(Disch, 1988). In older adults, this struggle is between integrity (coming to terms with coming to the end of life) and despair over past and present successes and failures. This despair can often result in depression, and only through life review and acceptance can depression be treated. To support this theory, several studies have demonstrated that older adults who are depressed tend to engage in less active reminiscing (or life review) than do those who are not depressed (Blum & Tross, 1988). According to Lewis and Butler (1974), the most effective type of reminiscing takes place when memories are used to (1) reframe past experience, (2) achieve resolution, (3) resolve regrets about unattained goals, (4) accept death and refocus on living, and (5) instruct the next generation. Rattenberg and Stones (1989) have found that the best way to treat depression through this process is in a group setting, so that reminiscences of one person can stimulate those of another.

Reminiscence therapy can take many forms, but the usual structure of this therapy is to stimulate life review by discussing milestones in one's life and the meaning those events have for the person. Discussion can be stimulated by providing prepared topics and bringing photographs and music from the older person's generation. Discussion and reminiscence are guided to reflect upon these events and then to work toward reframing the events, accepting them, and finding ways for such experiences to be instructional.

Outcome Studies. In one of the few empirical studies, Haight (1992) compared individual life review with supportive and no treatment conditions in a sample of 52 older adults, and reported increased life satisfaction and decreased depressive symptoms. Reviewed often and very popular in geriatric settings, RT appears to be most suitable for healthy adults. Although efficacy of reminiscence therapy is supported by a few studies (e.g. Areán *et al.*, 1993), more empirical research is needed.

Comment

Overall, clinical and empirical evidence suggests that depressed elderly have positive responses to the four main types of psychotherapy discussed here. Similar to studies of young adults, studies of older adults to date have not demonstrated empirical evidence for differences in treatment effects among the four main approaches. All four are effective in reducing symptoms of depression in older adults.

Biological Interventions

The defining feature of biological interventions is to alter brain functioning in depressed older adults. This is achieved by changing the neurochemistry of the brain through inducing a shock (electroconvulsive therapy; ECT) or through inducing higher levels of neurotransmitters in the brain (antidepressant medication). Because these interventions produce a direct biological change, they pose risks that should always be considered before using them. Below we review the action, utility, and risks of these interventions.

Electroconvulsive Therapy (ECT)

Action and Indications. ECT remains a controversial treatment for depression, although it is often described in the research literature as safe and effective for older adults (Burke, Zubin, Zorumski, & Wetzel, 1987; Kramer, 1987; Rubin, Kinscherf, Figiel, & Zorumski, 1993). ECT involves the passing of an electrical current through the brain, either bilaterally or unilaterally, inducing a generalized seizure and unconsciousness in the patient. Although not well understood, induction of the seizure, rather than the electricity itself, may result in therapeutic benefits, relieving symptoms of depression.

ECT may be employed as a last resort with severely depressed patients who have not responded to antidepressant medications or for whom such medications are contraindicated. Other possible indications for ECT include refusal to eat or drink and high suicide risk (Karlinsky & Schulman, 1984). For elderly patients who fall into these categories, ECT may be the only feasible treatment.

Outcome Studies. Whereas some investigators have concluded that ECT is even more effective in the elderly than in younger patients (Weiner, 1992), others have found no correlation between age and response rates (Karlinsky & Schulman, 1984). Most studies of ECT with the elderly show significant decreases in depressive symptoms. In one study, 63.3% of depressed elderly patients who had not previously responded to antidepressant medications showed significant improvement on symptoms of depression. Yet, this same study also found very high rates of relapse, with 28% of patients treated with ECT rehospitalized for depression within one year (Stoudemire *et al.,* 1991).

Risks and Contraindications. The risk of cardiovascular complications needs to be carefully investigated in elderly patients being considered for treatment with ECT, since heart failure is the principal ECT-related medical complication and the most frequent cause of death during treatment. Patients taking cardiovascular medications appear to be at higher risk for complications during ECT (Burke *et al.,* 1987). Two recent studies suggest that careful monitoring of patients during and after treatment can minimize this risk even in patients with severe cardiovascular disease (Rice, Sombrotto, Markowitz, & Leon, 1994). But such additional monitoring may add to the already considerable expense and hospitalization requirements of ECT. Rice and her associates concede that "lowering the risk for patients with cardiac impairment who receive ECT may be possible only in settings with highly specialized medical services" (1994). ECT has also been associated with increased risk of falling in the elderly (Burke *et al.,* 1987).

Perhaps the most serious drawback to the use of ECT is the risk of permanent memory loss. Few studies have adequately addressed the extent of this and other cognitive side effects in the elderly, although the risk of cognitive dysfunction may be greater than in younger patients (American Psychiatric Association, 1990). The higher doses of electricity necessary to induce seizures in the elderly may be a factor in this increased danger. Some researchers have suggested that the risk of memory loss and confusion in elderly patients receiving ECT may be reduced by using brief pulse wave forms rather than sine wave forms (Kramer, 1987). However, further study of the extent and nature of these serious side effects in the elderly is necessary.

Comment. ECT remains a treatment of last resort, due to the risk factors just described, its expense and hospitalization requirements, and the invasive nature of the procedure. Although many studies demonstrate effectiveness of ECT in the short term, the high rate of relapse is disturbing. Investigation of long-term effectiveness and possible types of maintenance treatments following ECT in elderly people remains to be done. Studies of the efficacy and side effects of ECT in those of very advanced age (over 80) have also yet to be conducted.

Pharmacotherapy

Of all the options for the treatment of depressed elders, use of antidepressant medications has been the most thoroughly researched. Because many of these studies have demonstrated usefulness of these medications, they should be considered when evaluating treatment options for depressed elderly individuals. There are currently three major categories of these drugs: tricyclics (TCAs), monoamine oxidase inhibitors (MAOIs), and serotonin enhancers (SSRIs). All of these drugs have shown some usefulness in clinical trials, and there are also concerns common to all of them. In particular, side effects of these medications are frequent and sometimes severe (Dunner, 1994). Preexisting medical conditions may also interfere with successful treatment with antidepressants, causing intolerable side effects particularly in severely ill medical patients (Koenig *et al.,* 1989).

When prescribing medications to older patients, clinicians must be careful to avoid adverse interactions with other drugs that patients are already taking. Because the elderly are more likely than younger people to be taking multiple medications, risk of adverse interactions is increased. Another general concern in prescribing antidepressant medications is greater compliance problems in the elderly. Presence of cognitive impairment may increase the risk of adverse effects, particularly if patients are not able to remember specific prescription requirements.

Another consideration in prescription decisions is patient age. Descriptions of successful research findings for use of antidepressants in the elderly are not necessarily generalizable to patients of very advanced age. A recent review of 400 reported controlled trials or case studies of antidepressant treatment in the elderly found that while pharmacotherapy has been examined in more than 5000 individuals over 55 years old, only 45 subjects aged 80 and older have been included in these trials (Salzman, 1994). Clinicians clearly should monitor dosages and side effects in these oldest individuals with additional care if treatment with antidepressants is decided.

In all elderly patients, initial dosage and increases in psychoactive medication should be small. Patients should be carefully monitored for worsening of symptoms and for potential side effects. Phamacokinetic effects of antidepressants may differ in elderly persons as compared with younger people: reduced rates of absorption, metabolism, and excretion lead to longer drug half-lives (the time it takes for the amount of medication in the blood plasma to be reduced by half). Because the drug stays in the older patient's body longer, there is a prolonged risk of side effects. As a result, doses should begin at approximately one half to one third of that normally prescribed for younger patients (Volz & Moller, 1994).

Tricyclics

Action and Indications. Tricyclic antidepressants (TCAs) block the presynaptic terminals' reuptake of the neurotransmitters norepinephrine and serotonin. The most frequently prescribed tricyclics include nortriptyline, amitriptyline, desipramine, imipramine, doxepin, and maprotiline. Desipramine may be the most appropriate of this group for depressed elders not experiencing anergia and anhedonia. Nortriptyline may be preferred for patients requiring more sedation or who are especially sensitive to a decline in blood pressure (Salzman, 1994).

Outcome Studies. Studies investigating effectiveness of treating elderly patients with TCAs frequently report good immediate response rates, coupled with high levels of side effects. Cohn and colleagues (1990) found that amitriptyline alleviated depressive symptoms in 62.5% of subjects as measured by the Hamilton Rating Scale for Depression (HRSD), but 35% of the subjects withdrew from the study because of side effects.

Common side effects in Cohn's study for subjects receiving amitriptyline included dry mouth (71.3%), dizziness (37.5%), constipation (27.5%), and fatigue (22.5%). Similar levels of these side effects in the elderly have also been reported for doxepin, such that only 39% of subjects receiving it completed the trial (Feighner & Cohn, 1985). There is some evidence that nortriptyline may cause fewer side effects in elderly patients than other TCAs (McCue, 1992). One study showed a 62% response rate, with only 4% of subjects dropping out due to side effects (Georgotas *et al.*, 1987).

Risks and Contraindications. Cardiac complications are a potentially serious risk in treating elderly patients with TCAs. Possible problems include increased heart rate, orthostatic hypotension, and arrhythmia (Glassman & Roose, 1994). These reactions have been correlated with high plasma levels of tricyclics (Preskorn, 1993). As a result, use of tricyclics in the elderly may involve serious risk (Goldman, Alexander, & Luchins, 1986). High plasma levels may also lead to central nervous system toxicity, including delirium and seizures. Elderly patients can develop these side effects at lower plasma levels than would be required in younger patients (Preskorn, 1993).

Tricyclics may also lead to adverse reactions caused by pharmacodynamic interaction with sedatives, including alcohol and antihistaminic agents often found in nonprescription medication (Preskorn, 1993). They may also lead to increased risk of falling, particularly among elderly women (Ruthazer & Lipsitz, 1993). Finally, tricyclics are highly toxic in overdose (Rickels & Schweizer, 1993), and should not be prescribed in situations of high suicide risk or if there is a possibility of accidental overdose.

Monoamine Oxidase Inhibitors (MAOIs)

Action and Indications. The oldest of the antidepressants, MAOIs increase synaptic concentrations of norepinephrine, serotonin, and dopamine by blocking oxidative enzymes in synaptic terminals. Commonly used MAOIs include phenylzine, tranylcypromine, and isocarboxazid. MAOIs are often used for elderly patients who are mildly to moderately depressed and whose symptoms include extreme anergia, fatigue, and anxiety (Salzman, 1992). They also may be useful for patients who are not eating enough or who are having trouble sleeping.

MAOIs may be the best pharmacological treatment for atypical depression, which is associated with increased appetite, weight gain, hypersomnia, anxiety, neurotic symptoms, and hysteroid dysphoria. Symptoms of atypical depression may worsen in the evening for patients who have trouble sleeping (Mendels, 1993).

Outcome Studies. There have been few controlled studies of MAOIs in elderly populations. In one study by R. Lazarus (1986), which tested only 15 subjects, 47% of patients receiving phenylzine had an improvement of 25% or better on the HRSD. Orthostatic hypotension was a common side effect. Another study by Georgotas, McCue, Friedman, & Cooper (1987) found that 61.1% of subjects receiving phenylzine had scores reduced from 16 or higher to 10 or lower on the HRSD.

Risks and Contraindications. Orthostatic hypotension and low blood pressure are common side effects of MAOIs (Goldman, 1986; Preskorn, 1993). Another concern is the pharmacodynamic interaction with serotonin-active agents and foods containing high levels of tyramine, such as cheese (Preskorn, 1993).

Selective Serotonin Reuptake Inhibitors (SSRIs)

Action and Indications. SSRIs are the newest of the three major categories of antidepressants. They act by slowing the reuptake of serotonin by presynaptic terminals, and include fluoxetine, sertraline, and paroxetine. Because SSRIs lack cardiovascular complications, do not cause anticholinergic side effects such as dry mouth and constipation, are less dangerous with respect to overdosing, and do not interfere with cognitive functioning, they may have significant advantages over tricyclics and MAOIs in the treatment of elderly patients (Dunner, 1994; Preskorn, 1993). They may be particularly useful for individuals exhibiting symptoms of inertia, extreme fatigue, and lack of motivation (Salzman, 1994).

Outcome Studies. Comparison of fluoxetine and doxepin in elderly patients found the two drugs to be equally efficacious. Common side effects of fluoxetine included nervousness or anxiety, or both, and nausea, although fluoxetine appeared to be better tolerated than doxepin (Feighner & Cohn, 1985). Dunner and colleagues (1992) compared paroxetine and doxepin in two double-blind studies, and found both to be effective in reducing symptoms of depression, with fewer and less severe side effects in paroxetine. One recent study comparing fluoxetine to paroxetine in elderly patients found paroxetine to be significantly more effective, with the two drugs equally well tolerated (Geretsegger, Bohmer, & Ludwig, 1994).

Risks and Contraindications. Use of SSRIs should not overlap with MAOIs, because the interaction between the two drugs can be fatal. Because of the particularly long half life of SSRIs, a washout period of at least 5 weeks is necessary before treatment with MAOIs is begun (Preskorn, 1993).

Comment

Antidepressant medications should be considered in the treatment of depressed elders. As the research discussed above indicates, medication should be selected carefully to minimize medical risk and distressing side effects, and should be regularly monitored. Further research on the use of antidepressants remains to be done, particularly in the treatment of medically ill patients and those of very advanced age. Also, most outcome studies report effectiveness of antidepressant treatment in isolation, rather than in conjunction with other forms of intervention such as psychotherapy. Further research into such combinations may reveal that medication alone is not the best course of treatment for depression in the elderly.

SUMMARY

The discussion of depression in older adults in this chapter is based on the literature that exists at the time of writing. From this literature, we know that depressive disorders in older adults vary in their prevalence. Older adults seen in medical clinics and nursing homes have higher rates of depression than do older adults sampled from the community. In addition, we know that older adults exhibit agitation, relatively higher rates of appetite and sleep disturbance, hopelessness, and guilt when they are depressed. We also know that there may be a unique type of depression in late life with its own etiology and prognosis. Many methods for treating these disorders exist and are generally successful in alleviating symptoms of depression. We still need to study issues such as the roles that gender and ethnicity have on the development, presentation, and treatment of depressive disorders, whether some methods of treating depression in older adults are more useful than others, and how effective these interventions are in treating depressive disorders in special populations (e.g., medically ill or frail elderly people). Research on these questions should help to further shape our understanding of depressive disorders in late life.

REFERENCES

Abramson, L. H., Metalsky, G. I., & Alloy, L. B. (1989). Hopelessness depression: A theory based subtype of depression. *Psychological Review, 96,* 358–372.

Achte, K. (1988). Suicidal tendencies in the elderly. *Suicide and Life-Threatening Behavior, 18,* 55–65.

Alexopoulos, G. S., Young, R., Meyers, B., Abrams, R., & Shamoian, C. (1988). Late onset depression. *Psychiatric Clinics of North America, 11* (1), 101–115.

Altshuler, K. Z. (1989). Will the psychotherapies yield differential results? *American Journal of Psychiatry, 43*, 310–320.

American Psychiatric Association (APA Task Force on ECT). (1990). The practice of electroconvulsive therapy: Recommendations for treatment, training, and privileging. Washington, DC: American Psychiatric Press.

American Psychiatric Association (1994). *Diagnostic and statistical manual of mental disorders* (4th ed.). Washington, DC: Author.

Areán, P. A., & Miranda, J. (1997). The utility of the Center for Epidemiological Studies–Depression Scale in older primary care patients. *Aging & Mental Health, 1*(1), 47–56.

Areán, P. A., & Miranda, J. (1995, September). *Prevalence and comorbidity of psychiatric disorders in low-income elderly.* Paper presented at the Ninth International Conference of Mental Health Service Research, Bethesda, MD.

Areán, P. A., Perri, M. G., Nezu, A. M., Schein, R. L., Christopher, F., & Joseph, T. X. (1993). Comparative effectiveness of social problem-solving therapy and reminiscence therapy as treatments for depression in older adults. *Journal of Consulting and Clinical Psychology, 61*(6), 1003–1010.

Baldwin, R. & Jolley, D. (1986). The prognosis of depression in old age. *British Journal of Psychiatry, 149*, 574–583.

Beck, A. T., Ward, C. H., Mendelson, M., Mock, J., & Erbaugh, J. (1961). An inventory for measuring depression. *Archives of General Psychiatry, 4*, 561–571.

Beck, A. T., Rush, A. J., Shaw, B., & Emery, G. (1979). *Cognitive therapy of depression.* New York: Guilford.

Beutler, L. E., Scogin, F., Kirkish, P., Schretlen, D., Corbishley, A., Hamblin, D., Meredith, K., Potter, R., Bamford, C. R., & Levenson, A. I. (1987). Group cognitive therapy and Alprazolam in the treatment of depression in older adults. *Journal of Consulting and Clinical Psychology, 55*, 550–556.

Birren, J. E., & Deutchman, D. E. (1991). *Guiding autobiography groups for older adults: Exploring the fabric of life.* Baltimore: Johns Hopkins University Press.

Blazer, D. (1990). *Emotional problems in later life: Intervention strategies for professional caregivers.* New York: Springer.

Blazer, D. G., Bachar, J. R., & Hughes, D. C. (1987). Major depression with melancholia: A comparison of middle-aged and elderly adults. *Journal of the American Geriatrics Society, 35*, 927–932.

Blum, J. E., & Tross, S. (1988). Psychodynamic treatment of the elderly: A review of issues in theory and practice. In C. Eisdorfer (Ed.), *Annual Review of Gerontology and Geriatrics* (vol. 1). New York: Springer.

Brink, T. L., Yesavage, J. A., Lum, O., Heersema, P. H., Adey, M., & Rose, T. L. (1982). Screening tests for geriatric depression. *Clinical Gerontologist, 1*, 37–43.

Brodaty, H., Harris, L., Peters, K., Wilhelm, K., Hickie, I., Boyce, P., Mitchell, P., Parker, G., & Eyers, K. (1993). Prognosis of depression in the elderly: A comparison to younger patients. *British Journal of Psychiatry, 163*, 589–596.

Brown, R. P., Sweeney, J., Loutsch, E., Kocsis, J., & Frances, A. (1984). Involutional melancholia revisited. *American Journal of Psychiatry, 141*, 24–28.

Burke, W. J., Rubin, E. H., Zorumski, C. F., & Wetzel, R. D. (1987). The safety of ECT in geriatric psychiatry. *Journal of the American Geriatrics Society, 35*, 516–21.

Caine, E. D., Lyness, J. M., King, D. A., & Conners, L. (1991). Clinical and etiological heterogeneity of mood disorders in elderly patients. In L. S. Schneider, C. F. Reynolds, B. Lebowitz, & A. FriedHoff, (Eds.), *Diagnosis and treatment of depression in late-life: Results of the NIH consensus development conference.* Washington, DC: American Psychiatric Press.

Callahan, C. M., Hui, S. L., Nienaber, N. A., Musick, B. S., & Tierney, W. M. (1994). Longitudinal study of depression and health services use among elderly primary care patients. *Journal of the American Geriatrics Society, 42*, 833–838.

Cohn, C. K., Shrivastava, R., Mendels, J., Cohn, J. B., Fabre, L., Claghorn, J. L., Dessain, E. C., Itil, T. M., & Lautin, A. (1990). Double-blind, multicenter comparison of sertraline and amitriptyline in elderly depressed patients. *Journal of Clinical Psychiatry, 51*, (Supp. B), 28–33.

Curb, J. D., Guralnik, J. M., LaCroix, A. Z., Korper, S. P., Deeg, D., Miles, T., & White, L. (1990). Effective aging: Meeting the challenge of growing older. *Journal of the American Geriatric Society, 38*, 827–828.

Depue, R. A., & Monroe, S. M. (1978). Learned helplessness in the perspective of the depressive disorders: Conceptual and definitional issues. *Abnormal Psychology, 87,* 3–20.

Devanand, D. P., Nobler, M. S., Singer, T., Kiersky, J. E., Turret, N., Roose, S. P., & Sackeim, H. A. (1994). Is dysthymia a different disorder in the elderly? *American Journal of Psychiatry, 151* (11), 1592–1599.

Disch, R. (Ed.). (1988). Twenty-five years of life review: Theoretical and practical considerations. *Journal of Gerontological Social Work, 12* [Special issue] 1–148.

Dreyfus, J. K. (1988). Depression assessment and interventions in medically ill frail elderly. *Journal of Gerontological Nursing, 14,* 27–36.

Dunn, V. K., & Sacco, W. P. (1989). Psychometric properties of the Geriatric Depression Scale and the Zung Self-Rating Depression Scale using an elderly community sample. *Psychology and Aging, 4* (1), 125–126.

Dunner, D. L. (1994). Therapeutic considerations in treating depression in the elderly. *Journal of Clinical Psychiatry, 55* (Supp.), 48–58.

Dunner, D. L., Cohn, J. B., Walsh, T., Cohn, C. K., Feighner, J. P., Fieve, R. R., Halikas, J. P., Hartford, J. T., Hearst, E. D., Settle, E. C., Menolascino, F. J., & Muller, D. J. (1992). Two combined, multicenter double-blind studies of paroxetine and doxepin in geriatric patients with major depression. *Journal of Clinical Psychiatry, 53* (Supp.), 57–60.

Erikson, E. H. (1959). *Identity and the life cycle.* New York: Norton.

Evans, M. E., Copeland, J. R. M., & Dewey, M. E., (1991). Depression in the elderly in the community: Effect of physical illness and selected social factors. *International Journal of Geriatric Psychiatry, 6,* 787–795.

Feighner, J. P., & Cohn, J. B. (1985). Double-blind comparative trials of fluoxetine and doxepin in geriatric patients with major depressive disorder. *Journal of Clinical Psychiatry, 46,* 20–25.

First, M. (1994). Structured Clinical Interview for DSM-IV.

Frank, E., Frank, N., Cornes, C., Imber, S. D., Miller, M. D., Morris, S. M., & Reynolds, C. F. (1993). Interpersonal psychotherapy in the treatment of late-life depression. In G. L. Klerman & M. M. Weissman (Eds.), *New applications of interpersonal psychotherapy* (pp. 167–198). Washington, DC: American Psychiatric Press.

Freud, S. (1959). On psychotherapy. In S. J. London (Ed.), *The standard edition of the complete psychological works of Sigmund Freud* (Vol. 7, pp. 257–268). London: Hogarth. (Original work published 1905)

Fry, P. (1989). Mediators of perceptions of stress among community elders. *Psychological Reports, 65,* 307–314.

Gallagher, D. (1986). Assessment of depression by interview methods and psychiatric rating scales. In L. W. Poon (Ed.), *Handbook for clinical memory assessment of older adults* (pp. 202–212). Washington, DC: American Psychological Association.

Gallagher, D., & Thompson, L. (1982). Treatment of major depressive disorder in older adult outpatients with brief psychotherapies. *Psychotherapy: Theory, Research, and Practice, 19,* 482–490.

Gallagher-Thompson, D., & Thompson, L. W. (1992). The older adult. In A. Freeman & F. Dattilio (Eds.), *Comprehensive casebook of cognitive therapy* (pp. 193–200). New York: Plenum.

Gallo, J. J., Anthony, J. C., & Muthen, B. O. (1994). Age differences in the symptoms of depression: A latent trait analysis. *Journal of Gerontology: Psychological Issues, 49* (6), P251–P264.

Ganzini, L., Lee, M. A., Heintz, R. T., Bloom, J. D., & Fenn, D. S. (1994). The effects of depression treatment on elderly patients' preferences for life-sustaining medical therapy. *American Journal of Psychiatry, 151* (11), 1631–1636.

George, L. K. (1989). Stress, social support, and depression over the life course. In K. S. Markides & C. L. Cooper (Eds.), *Aging, stress, and health.* New York: Wiley.

Georgotas, A., McCue, R. E., Friedman, E., & Cooper, T. (1987). Response of depressive symptoms to nortriptyline, phenelzine, and placebo. *British Journal of Psychiatry, 151,* 102–107.

Geretsegger, C., Bohmer, F., & Ludwig, M. (1994). Partoxetine in the elderly depressed patient: Randomized comparison with fluoxetine of efficacy, cognitive and behavioural effects. *International Clinical Psychopharmacology, 9,* 25–29.

Glassman, A. H., & Roose, S. P. (1994). Risks of antidepressants in the elderly: Tricyclic antidepressants and arrhythmia-revising risks. *Gerontology, 40* (Supp. 1), 15–20.

Goldman, L. S. (1986). Monoamine oxidase inhibitors and tricyclic antidepressants: Comparison of their cardiovascular effects. *Journal of Clinical Psychiatry, 47,* 225–229.

Goldman, L. S., Alexander, R. C., & Luchins, D. J. (1986). MAOIs and tricylic antidepressants: Comparison of their cardiovascular effects. *Journal of Clinical Psychiatry, 47*(5), 225–229.

Gurland, B. (1997). The Comprehensive Assessment and Referral Evaluation (CARE): Rationale, development and reliability. *International Journal of Aging and Human Development, 8* (1), 9–42.

Gurland, B. J., Copeland, J. R., Kurlansky, J., Kelleher, M. J., & Sharpe, L. (1983). *The mind and mood of aging.* New York: Hawthorne Press.

Haight, B. K. (1992). Long-term effects of a structured life review process. *Journal of Gerontology: Psychological Sciences Section, 47*, 312–315.

Hamilton, M. (1960). A rating scale for depression. *Journal of Neurology, Neurosurgery and Psychiatry, 23*, 56–62.

Hamilton, M. (1986). The Hamilton Rating Scale for Depression. In N. Sartorius & T. A. Ban (Eds.), *Assessment of depression.* New York: Springer-Verlag.

Henderson, A. S. (1989). Psychiatric epidemiology and the elderly. *International Journal of Geriatric Psychiatry, 4*, 249–253.

Hickie, C., & Snowdon, J. (1987). Depression scales in the elderly: Geriatric Depression Scale Gilleard, Zung. *Clinical Gerontologist, 6* (3), 51–53.

Husaini, B. A., Moore, S. T., Castor, R. S., Neser, W., Whitten-Stovall, R., Linn, G., & Griffin, D. (1991). Social density, stressors, and depression: Gender differences among Black elderly. *Journals of Gerontology: Psychological Sciences, 46* (5), P236–P242.

Karlinsky, H., & Schulman, K. I. (1984). The clinical use of electroconvulsive therapy in old age. *Journal of the American Geriatrics Society, 32*, 183–186.

Klerman, G. L. (1989). Efficacy of a brief psychosocial interventions for symptoms of stress and distress in primary care. *Medical Care, 25* (11), 1078–1088.

Klerman, G. L., Weissman, M. M., & Rounsaville, B. J., (1984). *Interpersonal psychotherapy of depression.* New York: Basic Books.

Koenig, H. G., & Blazer, D. G (1992). Epidemiology of geriatric affective disorders. *Clinics in Geriatric Medicine, 8* (2), 235–251.

Koenig, H. G., Blazer, D. G., Cohen, H. J., Meador, K. G., & Westlund, R. (1992). A Briez depression scale for use in the medically ill. *International Journal of Psychiatry in Medicine, 22*(2), 183–195.

Koenig, H. G., Veeraindar, G., Shelp, F., Kundler, H. S., Cohen, H. J., Meador, K. G. & Blazer, D. G. (1989). Antidepressant use in elderly medical inpatients: Lessons from an attempted clinical trial. *Journal of General Internal Medicine, 4*, 499–508.

Kramer, B. A. (1987). Electroconvulsive therapy use in geriatric depression. *Journal of Nervous and Mental Disease, 175*, 233–235.

Krause, N. (1987). Life stress, social support, and self-esteem in an elderly population. *Psychology and Aging, 2*, 185–192.

Krishnan, K. R. R. (1991). Organic bases of depression in the elderly. *Annual Review of Medicine, 42*, 261–266.

Krishnan, K., Doraiswamy, P., Fifiel, G., Husain, M. (1991). Hippocampal abnormalities in depression. *Journal of Neuropsychiatry and Clinical Neuroscience, 3* (4), 387–391.

Lazarus, L. W., Groves, L., Newton, N., Gutmann, D., Ripeckyj, A., Frankel, R., Grunes, J., & Havasy-Galloway, S. (1984). Brief psychotherapy with the elderly: A review and preliminary study of process and outcome. In L. W Lazarus (Ed.), *Clinical approaches to psychotherapy with the elderly* (pp. 15–35), Washington, DC: American Psychiatric Press.

Lazarus, L. W., Groves, L., Gutmann, D., Ripeckyj, A., Frankel, R., Newton, N., Grunes, J., & Havasy-Galloway, S. (1987). Brief psychotherapy with the elderly: A study of process and outcome. In J. Sadavoy & M. Leszcz (Eds.), *Treating the elderly with psychotherapy* (pp. 265–293). Madison, CT: International Universities Press.

Lazarus, R. (1986). Coping Strategies. In S. McHugh & T. M. Vallis (Eds.). *Illness behavior: A multidisciplinary approach.* New York: Plenum.

Lazarus, R. S., & Folkman, S. (1984). *Stress, appraisal, and coping.* New York: Springer.

Lewinsohn, P. M., Biglan, T., & Zeiss, A. (1976). Behavioral treatment of depression. In P. Davidson (Ed.), *Behavioral management of anxiety, depression, and pain* (pp. 91–146). New York: Bruner/Mazel.

Lewis, C. N., & Butler, R. N. (1974). Life review therapy: Putting memories to work in individual and group therapy. *Geriatrics, 29*, 165–173.

Markides, K., & Cooper, C. (1989). *Aging, stress, and health.* New York: Wiley.

Massie, M. J., Gagnon, P., & Holland, J. C. (1994). Depression and suicide in patients with cancer. *Journal of Pain and Symptom Management, 9* (5), 325–340.

McCue, R. E. (1992). Using tricyclic antidepressants in the elderly. *Clinics in Geriatric Medicine, 8,* 323–334.

Mendels, J. (1993). Clinical management of the depressed geriatric patient: Current therapeutic options. *American Journal of Medicine, 94* (Supp. 5A), 13S–18S.

Myers, W. A. (1991). Psychoanalytic psychotherapy and psychoanalysis with older patients. In W. A. Myers (Ed.), *New techniques in the therapy of older patients.* Washington, DC: American Psychiatric Press.

National Institutes of Health (NIH) Consensus Development Panel on Depression in Late Life. (1992). Diagnosis and treatment of depression in late life. *Journal of the American Medical Association, 268,* 1018–1024.

Neese, J. B. (1991). Depression in the general hospital. *Nursing Clinics of North America, 26,* 613–622.

Newmann, J. P. (1989). Aging and depression. *Psychology and Aging, 4,* 150–166.

Parmalee, P., Katz, I., & Lawton, P. (1989). Depression among institutionalized aged: Assessment and prevalence estimation. *Journals of Gerontology, 44,* M22–M29.

Parmalee, P. A., Katz, I. R., & Lawton, M. P. (1991). The relation of pain to depression among institutionalized aged. *Journals of Gerontology, 46,* 15–21.

Preskorn, S. H. (1993). Recent pharmacologic advances in antidepressant therapy for the elderly. *American Journal of Medicine, 94,* S(Supp. 5A), 2S–12S.

Radloff, L. S. (1977). The CES-D scale: a self-report depression scale for research in the general population. *Applied Psychological Measurement, 1,* 385–401.

Rattenberg, C., & Stones, M. J. (1989). A controlled evaluation of reminiscence and current topics discussion groups in a nursing home context. *The Gerontologist, 29*(6), 768–777.

Regier, D. A., Hirschfeld, R. M. A., Goodwin, F. K., Burke, J. D., Lazar, J. B., & Judd, L. L. (1988). The NIMH Depression Awareness, recognition and treatment program: Structure, aims and scientific basis. *American Journal of Psychiatry, 145*(11), 1351–1357.

Rice, E. H., Sombrotto, L. B., Markowitz, J. C., & Leon, A. C. (1994). Cardiovascular morbidity in high-risk patients during ECT. *American Journal of Psychiatry, 151,* 1637–1641.

Rickels, K., & Schweizer, E. (1993). Anxiolytics: Indications, benefits and risks of short and long term benzdiazepine therapy: Current research data. *NIDA Research Monographs, 131,* 51–67.

Robins, L. N., Helzer, J. E., Croughan, J., & Ratcliff, K. S. (1981). National Institute of Mental Health Diagnostic Interview Schedule: Its history, characteristics, and validity. *Archives of General Psychiatry, 38,* 381–389.

Robins, L. N., Helzer, J. E., Weissman, M. M., Orvaschel, H., Gruenberg, E., Burke, J. D., & Regier, D. A. (1984). Lifetime prevalence of specific psychiatric disorders in three sites. *Archives of General Psychiatry, 41,* 949–958.

Robinson, R. G., & Price, T. R. (1982). Post-stroke depressive disorders: A follow-up of 103 patients. *Stroke, 13,* 335–341.

Rubin, E. H., Kinscherf, D. A., Figiel, G. S., & Zorumski, C. F. (1993). The nature and time course of cognitive side effects during ECT in the elderly. *Journal of Geriatric Psychiatry and Neurology, 6*(2), 78–83.

Ruthazer, R., & Lipsitz, L. (1993). Antidepressants and falls among elderly people in long-term care. *American Journal of Public Health, 83,* 746–49.

Salzman, C. (1992). Monoamine oxidase inhibitors and atypical antidepressants. *Clinics in Geriatric Medicine, 8*(2), 335–348.

Salzman, C. (1994). Pharmacological treatment of depression in elderly patients. In L. Schneider, C. Reynolds, B. Lebowitz, & A. J. Friedhoff (Eds.), *Diagnosis and treatment of depression in late life: Results of the NIH Consensus Development Conference,* (pp. 181–244). Washington, DC: American Psychiatric Press.

Schneider, L. S., Sloane, R. B., Staples, F. R., & Bender, M. (1986). Pre-treatment orthostatic hypotension as a predictor of response to nortriptyline in geriatric depression. *Journal of Clinical Psychopharmacology, 6,* 172–176.

Scogin, F., & McElreath, L. (1994). Efficacy of psychosocial treatments for geriatric depression: A quantitative review. *JCCP, Journal of Consulting and Clinical Psychology, 62* (1), 69–74.

Shapiro, R. N., & Keller, M. B. (1981). Initial 6-month follow-up of patients with major depressive disorders. *Journal of Affective Disorders, 3*(3), 205–220.

Smyer, M., Zarit, S., & Qualls, S. H. (1990). Psychological intervention with the aging individual. In J. Birren & K. W. Schaie (Eds.), *Handbook of the psychology of aging* (3rd ed., pp. 375–403). New York: Academic.

Spitzer, R. L. , Williams, J. B. W., Gibbon, M., & First, M. B. (1988). *Structured clinical interview for DSM-III-R Patient Version (SCID-P 6/1/88)*. New York: Biometrics Research Department, New York State Psychiatric Institute.

Stoudemire, A., Moran, M. G., & Fogel, B. S. (1991). Psychotropic drug use in the medically ill. Part II. *Psychosomatics, 32*(1), 34–46.

Teri, L., Curtis, J., Gallagher-Thompson, D., & Thompson, L. W. (1994). Cognitive/behavioral therapy with depressed older adults. In L. S. Schneider, C. F. Reynolds, B. Lebowitz, & A. Friedhoff (Eds.), *Diagnosis and treatment of depression in late life*. Washington DC: American Psychiatric Press.

Thompson, L. W., & Gallagher-Thompson, D. (1993, November). *Comparison of Desipramine and cognitive-behavioral therapy in the treatment of late- life depression: A progress report*. Paper presented at the 27th annual American Association of Behavior Therapy Convention, Atlanta, GA.

Thompson, L. W., Gallagher, D., & Breckenridge, J. S. (1987). Comparative effectiveness of psychotherapy for depressed elders. *Journal of Consulting and Clinical Psychology, 55* (3), 385–390.

Volz, H.-P., & Moller, H.-J. (1994). Antidepressant drug therapy in the Elderly—A critical review of the controlled clinical trials since 1980. *Pharmacopsychiatry, 27*, 93–100.

Weaver, T. E., & Narsavage, G. L. (1992). Physiological and psychological variables related to functional status in chronic obstructive pulmonary disease. *Nursing Research, 41*, 286–191.

Weiner, R. D. (1992). The role of electroconvulsive therapy in the treatment of depression in the elderly. *Journal of the American Geriatrics Society, 30*, 710–712.

Weiss, I. K., Nagel, C. L., & Aronson, M. K. (1986). Applicability of depression scales to the old old person. *Journal of the American Geriatric Association, 34*(3), 215–218.

Weiss, L. J., & Lazarus, L. W. (1993). Psychosocial treatment of the geropsychiatric patient. *International Journal of Geriatric Psychiatry, 8*, 95–100.

Yost, E. B., Beutler, L. E., Corbishely, M. A., & Allender, J. L. (1986). *Group cognitive therapy: A treatment manual for depressed older adults*. New York: Pergamon.

Zung, W. W. K. (1965). A self-rating depression scale. *Archives of General Psychiatry, 12*, 63–70.

CHAPTER 11

Anxiety Disorders

Melinda A. Stanley and J. Gayle Beck

INTRODUCTION

In the past two decades, major advances have been made regarding the psychopathology and treatment of anxiety disorders (Barlow, 1988; Beidel & Turner, 1991). The negative impact of these disorders on life function has been well documented, and epidemiological data have suggested that anxiety disorders comprise the second most common form of psychiatric disturbance over the lifetime in the United States, following only substance abuse disorders (Robins *et al.,* 1984). Despite the voluminous amount of data available regarding anxiety disorders in the general population, however, the nature and treatment of these in older adults has received relatively little empirical attention. The need for additional work in this area has been emphasized on many occasions (e.g., Carstensen, 1988; Hersen & Van Hasselt, 1992; Salzman & Lebowitz, 1991), and a small body of relevant literature has begun to accumulate. The purpose of this chapter is to review the available scientific literature that addresses the epidemiology, psychopathology, assessment, and treatment of anxiety in the elderly. Given that this literature is in an early developmental stage, directions for future research also are suggested.

EPIDEMIOLOGY

Prevalence

As noted, the National Institute of Mental Health (NIMH) Epidemiological Catchment Area (ECA) survey conducted during the 1980s found that across all age groups surveyed, lifetime prevalence rates for anxiety disorders in the United States were second only to those for substance abuse disorders (Robins

MELINDA A. STANLEY • Department of Psychiatry and Behavioral Sciences, University of Texas Mental Sciences Institute, Health Science Center at Houston, Houston, Texas 77030.   J. GAYLE BECK • Department of Psychology, State University of New York, Buffalo, New York 14260.

Handbook of Clinical Geropsychology, edited by Michel Hersen and Vincent B. Van Hasselt. Plenum Press, New York, 1998.

et al., 1984). When 1-month prevalence rates were examined, anxiety disorders actually were the most prevalent of all groups of psychiatric conditions (Regier *et al.,* 1988; Regier, Narrow, & Rae, 1990). A similar pattern emerged when data were examined for the 30.7% of participants who were 65 years of age or older (*n* = 5702). In this group, anxiety disorders also were most common, with a 1-month prevalence rate of 5.5% across five sites (Regier *et al.,* 1988, 1990). The majority of anxiety disorders assigned were classified as phobias (4.8%), including agoraphobia, social phobia, and simple phobia. Much lower prevalence rates were recorded for obsessive-compulsive disorder (0.8%) and panic disorder (0.1%). Six-month prevalence rates from the Yale University site, which oversampled older adults (*n* = 2588), were similar (Weissman *et al.,* 1985). At this site, an overall rate of 4.6% was found for anxiety disorders in older adults, with 3.9% of diagnoses classified as phobias, 0.7% as obsessive-compulsive disorder, and 0.1% as panic disorder.

It is notable that Wave I of the ECA survey, conducted in 1982 and 1983, omitted consideration of prevalence rates for posttraumatic stress disorder (PTSD) and generalized anxiety disorder (GAD). (GAD was omitted because it had not been recognized as a distinct psychiatric entity at the time [American Psychiatric Association, 1980]). In Wave II of the survey, conducted 1 year later, a subset of participants were reinterviewed, with questions included to address the prevalence of PTSD and GAD. Data from the Duke University site, wherein older adults were oversampled, indicated 6-month and lifetime prevalence rates of 1.9% and 4.6% for GAD in adults aged 65 years or older (Blazer, George, & Hughes, 1991). These figures omitted consideration of individuals with a concurrent diagnosis of major depression or panic disorder, however, and thus may have underestimated the true prevalence of GAD. (Only overall population prevalence estimates were provided for PTSD [Helzer, Robins, & McEvoy, 1987].)

In a review of ECA data and seven other community surveys that provided figures for older adults (aged 60 years and older), overall prevalence rates for anxiety disorders ranged from 0.7% to 18.6% (Flint, 1994). Prevalence rates for phobic disorders ranged from 0.0% to 10.0%, GAD from 0.7% to 7.1%, obsessive-compulsive disorder from 0.0% to 1.5%, and panic disorder from 0.1% to 1.0%. The wide variations in rates for some disorders likely results from the range of survey methods, case definitions, and diagnostic procedures used to establish anxiety disorder diagnoses (Flint, 1994). For example, some surveys utilized self-report measures to establish diagnoses, whereas others relied on semistructured clinical interviews. In addition, some diagnostic criteria were based on widely accepted standards (e.g., American Psychiatric Association, 1980), while others used more idiosyncratic procedures. As a result, although criticisms have been registered regarding the methodology used in the ECA survey (Beidel & Turner, 1991; McNally, 1994), these data represent the best figures currently available to estimate the prevalence of anxiety disorders in the elderly.

ECA data consistently have indicated that prevalence rates for anxiety disorders in older adults are lower than those from younger adult samples (Blazer *et al.,* 1991; Regier *et al.,* 1988). Nonetheless, the figures just noted indicate that anxiety disorders pose a significant mental health problem for the elderly. In addition, ECA data may have underestimated the percentage of older adults with significant anxiety problems given the tendency of these individuals to underreport psychological symptoms (Oxman, Barrett, Barrett, & Gerber, 1987). For some time, depression in older persons has been emphasized as a serious public health issue (Reynolds, Lebowitz, & Schneider, 1993). However, ECA Wave I data attested that anxiety disorders in this population (excluding GAD) are more than twice as prevalent as affective disorders, in general, and 4 to 8 times more frequent than major depression (Regier *et al.*, 1988; Weissman *et al.*, 1985). When estimated prevalence rates for GAD are added, anxiety disorders emerge as an even more serious concern for the growing population of elders in the United States.

In addition to epidemiological investigations focusing on the prevalence of diagnosable anxiety disorders, another set of studies has addressed the frequency of distressing anxiety symptoms in older adults. These surveys have utilized standardized self-report inventories, such as the Hopkins Symptoms Checklist (HSCL; Derogatis, Lipman, Rickels, Uhlenhuth, & Covi, 1973) and the Spielberger Trait Anxiety Inventory (STAI; C. Spielberger, Gorsuch, & Lushene, 1970), to identify individuals with significant anxiety symptoms, using cutoff scores based on standard deviations from mean scores in normal and psychiatric samples. This type of methodology has yielded prevalence rates of 16.3% to 20.0% in community samples (Feinson & Thoits, 1986; Himmelfarb & Murrell, 1984) and 8.0% to 10.0% in a primary care setting (Oxman *et al.*, 1987). When relevant comparisons have been made, these figures again suggest that the prevalence of anxiety in older adults generally is lower than in younger adult samples (Feinson & Thoits, 1986; Oxman *et al.*, 1987), although a substantial number of older persons report distressing symptoms in this domain.

Age of Onset

At least two reports have suggested that many phobias in older adults are of recent onset (Eaton *et al.*, 1989; Lindesay, 1991). In the ECA study, for example, estimated incidence figures for phobias were unrelated to age, with similar frequencies of onset across age groups over a 1-year period (Eaton *et al.*, 1989). In another community survey of older adults, simple phobias generally were reported to have their onset in childhood (Lindesay, 1991), as has been reported in the younger adult literature (Thyer, Parrish, Curtis, Nesse, & Cameron, 1985). However, the majority of older adults with agoraphobic fears (e.g., of enclosed places, crowds, public transportation, going away from home) indicated recent onset, most often following an episode of physical illness (e.g., myocardial infarction, fractures, cerebrovascular accident) or traumatic experience (e.g., muggings, a fall at home). Given the types of onset frequently reported in this sample, diagnoses of agoraphobia in some cases may be questioned. Specifically, realistic fears or physical limitations rather than anticipation of panic may have motivated the symptoms reported (see McNally, 1994, for a similar discussion of diagnostic issues in younger adults). Further, a high incidence of depression in Lindesay's (1991) sample suggests that agoraphobic fears reported by participants in this study may have represented social withdrawal associated with depressive symptomatology (Flint, 1994). Therefore, conclusions regarding onset of phobias in the elderly from this report should be interpreted cautiously.

ECA data implied that panic disorder and obsessive-compulsive disorder, which occurred infrequently in community samples of older adults, typically did not begin in older age (Eaton *et al.,* 1989). In a chart review of 51 elderly clinic patients with panic disorder, however, Raj, Corvea, and Dagon (1993) found that more than half of the sample reported onset at age 60 years or later. No notable differences between older adults with late-onset or early-onset (i.e., at age 59 or younger) panic disorder were reported.

According to ECA Wave II data, age of onset for GAD in older persons appears to have a bimodal distribution, with 39% of patients reporting a duration of 21 years or more and 50% reporting onset within the prior 5 years (Blazer *et al.,* 1991). A similar biomodal distribution of onset was obtained in a clinical sample of older adults with GAD (Beck, Stanley, & Zebb, 1996). In this report, few differences in psychopathological features (e.g., anxiety, depression, fears) were noted in a comparison of early- and late-onset subsamples.

Demographic Correlates

As has been demonstrated in younger adults (Regier *et al.,* 1990), anxiety disorders in older individuals generally occur more often in women than men, with a particularly large male/female ratio for phobic disorders (e.g., Blazer *et al.,* 1991; Regier *et al.,* 1988; Weissman *et al.,* 1985). A similar pattern has been found in surveys targeting prevalence of anxiety symptoms rather than disorders. For example, in two community surveys, more women than men met preestablished cutoffs for notable anxiety symptoms (e.g., Himmelfarb & Murrell, 1984), and women reported greater overall fearfulness than men (Liddell, Locker, & Burman, 1991).

With regard to ethnic distribution, problems with sampling strategies for some minority groups in the ECA studies have been noted (Beidel & Turner, 1991), making it difficult to draw conclusions about the relationship between ethnicity and the prevalence of anxiety disorders in any age group. Among older adults, Weissman and colleagues (1985) reported lower rates of psychiatric disorders in general among blacks than among whites, although similar data were not made available for anxiety disorders separately. ECA Wave II data, however, indicated equivalent prevalence rates of GAD in older black and white adults (Blazer *et al.,* 1991). Two survey studies assessing the prevalence of anxiety symptoms in older adults reported no significant relationship between anxiety and ethnicity (Feinson & Thoits, 1986; Himmelfarb & Murrell, 1984), although in one of these studies, minority groups were underrepresented relative to the general population (Feinson & Thoits, 1986), and in the other, no data regarding ethnic distribution of the sample were provided (Himmelfarb & Murrell, 1984). Further research in this domain is clearly warranted.

Prevalence and/or severity of anxiety symptoms in older adults also has been related to marital status, with fewer symptoms reported by married persons than unmarried persons (Feinson & Thoits, 1986). A more complicated relationship between marital status, gender, and anxiety symptoms among the elderly was demonstrated by Himmelfarb and Murrell (1984), with highest levels of anxiety among never-married men and lowest anxiety scores among never-married women. Finally, significant inverse relationships have been noted between income and anxiety among the elderly (Feinson & Thoits, 1986; Himmelfarb & Murrell, 1984; Liddell *et al.*, 1991), and in some cases between educational attainment and anxiety (Himmelfarb & Murrell, 1984; Liddell *et al.*, 1991). These patterns are similar to relationships demonstrated among younger adults with anxiety disorders (Regier *et al.*, 1990).

PSYCHOPATHOLOGY

Much is known about the psychopathology of anxiety disorders in younger adults, although a full review of this literature is beyond the scope of this chapter (see reviews by Barlow, 1988; Beidel & Turner, 1991; Rapee & Barlow, 1991). However, an overview of issues relevant to unique aspects of anxiety in older adults is provided here.

Nature of Anxiety

A number of issues deserve special attention in the diagnosis of anxiety disorders in the elderly. First, differentiating physiological symptoms of anxiety from the medical problems that often are associated with advancing age needs to be considered carefully. This issue is particularly important given that older adults often attribute anxiety-related difficulties to physical illnesses and consequently deny symptoms or seek treatment in a primary care facility rather than a psychiatric clinic (Gurian & Miner, 1991). Consequently, primary care physicians need to be aware of the signs and symptoms of anxiety in their patients, providing appropriate treatment or referrals when warranted. Similarly, clinicians in psychiatric settings need to be careful not to attribute somatic complaints to anxiety difficulties when diagnosis and treatment of a medical condition might alleviate reported symptoms. Second, careful attention needs to be paid to differentiating anxiety disorders from realistic fears that may accompany the aging process. In this case, qualifiers used regularly to describe fears that meet criteria for anxiety disorders (e.g., "excessive," "unrealistic") need to be considered carefully in light of real-life circumstances that may exist for older individuals, such as decreasing independence and increasing health problems. It can be tempting for practitioners, however, to overattribute anxiety and fears in older adults to the normal aging process, thereby overlooking or ignoring treatable psychiatric symptomatology (Weiss, 1994). In this regard, examination of normal versus abnormal fears in elderly samples becomes paramount. A small body of literature has begun to address this issue.

The majority of work examining the nature of fears in older persons has focused on worry, most likely because generalized anxiety is one of the most prevalent forms of anxiety observed in older adults (Blazer *et al.*, 1991). Available studies have assessed characteristics of worry in both normal, community samples and diagnosed clinical groups. In one community survey of worry topics among adults, Person and Borkovec (1995) categorized participants' "most important problems, worries or concerns" into five categories: (1) family-home-interpersonal, (2) illness-health-injury, (3) work-school, (4) finances, and (5) miscellaneous. Results demonstrated that older adults (aged 65 years or older) worried most about health and least about work, whereas younger adults (aged 25 to 64) worried most about family and finances. The authors reported a linear relationship between worries and age, noting that worries about family, work, and finances decreased with age while concerns about health and miscellaneous issues increased with age (Person & Borkovec, 1995). Thus, common worries across various age groups appeared to represent changing life circumstances.

In another community survey of worries among younger and older adults, older persons reported few worries overall, with significantly fewer worries about social events and finances than in a college-age comparison group (Powers, Wisocki, & Whitbourne, 1992). Elderly participants in this survey worried most about health, although scores in this domain were similar for older and younger cohorts. Again, reported fears for both groups appeared to represent developmentally appropriate real-life concerns. However, it is notable that in this community sample of older adults, worries occurred infrequently, suggesting that older age is not necessarily associated with significantly increasing anxiety, despite the relatively high prevalence rates reviewed above (Powers *et al.*, 1992). Similarly, in a broader examination of anxiety characteristics in 94 older adult volunteers without diagnosable psychiatric symptomatology, scores on a series of self-report anxiety measures were significantly lower than those reported in younger community samples (Stanley, Beck, & Zebb, 1996). In particular, older adults demonstrated lower levels of worry, state and trait anxiety, specific fears, and obsessive-compulsive symptomatology, suggesting that many older adults are functioning well with regard to various anxiety symptoms. In addition, these data accentuate the need for age-appropriate norms to interpret self-report measures of anxiety symptoms in older adults (see the following section, "Assessment").

In addition to documenting normal patterns of worry in the elderly, it also is of interest to examine the psychopathological features associated with various anxiety disorders in well-diagnosed clinical samples (Hersen & Van Hasselt, 1992). One of the first studies in this domain examined the clinical characteristics of GAD in 44 older adults diagnosed according to a semistructured interview (Beck *et al.*, 1996). Comparisons with a matched sample free of psychiatric disorders were made to assess severity of worry and associated symptoms. Results revealed that GAD in older persons was associated with elevated anxiety, worry, social fears, and depression. Of particular interest is the fact that elderly GAD patients were comparable with younger samples with GAD on various demographic variables (e.g., gender, ethnicity, education) and clinical features (e.g., severity of worry, anxiety, and depression). Similar findings were reported in a retrospective chart review of elderly patients with panic disorder (Raj *et al.*, 1993). Although the focus of this report was on the overlap between patients with early- or late-onset disorders, the authors noted that older adults with panic disorder were similar to younger patients with the same diagnosis on various demographic and clinical features. Thus, although the body of literature at present is quite small, anxiety disorders appear to be associated with similar psychopathological features across the lifespan.

Overlap With Depression and Medical Problems

Overlap between the anxiety disorders and depression has long been an important issue in psychiatric diagnosis, with high frequencies of coexisting pathology and symptom overlap demonstrated repeatedly in younger adult samples (e.g., Cloninger, 1990; Copp, Schwiderski, & Robinson, 1990; Feldman, 1993). Specifically, 6-month prevalence data from the ECA study indicated that 21% of participants with an anxiety disorder also met criteria for an affective disorder, and one third of individuals with affective disorders also were diagnosed with an anxiety disorder (Regier *et al.,* 1990). In recent reviews, significant overlap between anxiety and depression in the elderly also has been highlighted (Alexopoulos, 1991; Flint, 1994). In particular, a community survey by Lindesay, Briggs, and Murphy (1989) reported that 90.9% of older adults diagnosed with GAD and 39.3% of those assigned a diagnosis of phobia also met criteria for depression. (In this report, *ICD-8* diagnoses were assigned based on a semistructured clinical interview). Not surprisingly, significant correlations also were noted between measures of anxiety and depression. Finally, in a retrospective chart review of elderly clinic patients with *Diagnostic and Statistical Manual of Mental Disorders,* 3rd ed., rev. (*DSM-III-R;* American Psychiatric Association, 1987), panic disorder, Raj and colleagues (1993) found that 45% met criteria for comorbid major depression. When older adults with depressive disorders have been assessed, more than one third have been assigned a coexistent anxiety disorder diagnosis (Alexopoulos, 1991). Even greater percentages of depressed patients have been reported to experience both psychic and somatic symptoms of anxiety (Alexopoulos, 1991; Ben-Aire, Swartz, & Dickman, 1987; Parmelee, Katz, & Lawton, 1992). Thus, although frequency estimates vary considerably across studies (probably because of differing methodological procedures), data consistently show a significant amount of overlap between anxiety and depressive disorders and symptoms in older persons.

As noted earlier, another issue that is highly salient for the evaluation of anxiety disorders in older adults is the overlap between anxiety symptoms and the manifestations of various medical diseases. In particular, anxiety-like symptoms can be produced by a range of physical conditions including cardiovascular disease, chronic obstructive pulmonary disease, hyperthyroidism, and sensory impairments involving both the visual and auditory systems (Cohen, 1991). In addition, high rates of anxiety disorders have been reported among elderly patients with these types of physical conditions (Cohen, 1991). In fact, ECA data indicated that anxiety disorders were significantly more prevalent among older adults who reported being confined to their homes than others who were more mobile, with statistical effects explained by variations in physical functioning and not socioeconomic status (Bruce & McNamara, 1992). As noted, the frequency of significant anxiety symptoms in older adults seen in a primary care setting has been estimated at 8% to 10% (Oxman *et al.,* 1987). Older adults with anxiety disorders or symptoms also report high levels of physical complaints. For example, Lindesay (1991) found that older adults with phobic disorders endorsed significantly more physical symptoms than control participants. Similarly, significant positive correlations have been noted between severity of anxiety and extent of physical health problems in both community (Himmelfarb & Murrell, 1984) and nursing home samples (Parmelee *et al.*, 1992). Thus, although the amount of available literature is limited, the overlap between anxiety problems and medical illness is clearly an important issue that warrants attention in all psychiatric evaluations among older adults.

ASSESSMENT

Of central importance to any future work addressing the nature and treatment of anxiety disorders in the elderly is the development of psychometrically sound assessment strategies for this population. In younger adults, a broad range of assessment instruments has been established to measure anxiety symptoms (Nietzel, Bernstein, & Russell, 1988). One popular strategy for assessment research with older adults has involved examination of psychometric properties for measures that already have been demonstrated reliable and valid in younger adults. This strategy has both advantages and disadvantages. First, further examination of preexisting measures is economical in terms of time and expense. In addition, this approach allows for potential comparisons of symptoms in older and younger samples. However, it also has been noted that the phenomenological experience of anxiety among the elderly may not be well represented by measures for younger adults (Sheikh, 1991). In particular, assessment instruments for use with the elderly may need to be particularly sensitive to certain symptom patterns that are more prevalent in this population (e.g., worries about health, Person & Borkovec, 1995), as well as potential overlap between the symptoms of anxiety and medical illness and the comorbidity between anxiety and depression (Hersen, Van Hasselt, & Goreczny, 1993; Sheikh, 1991). Given the potentially unique experience of some facets of anxiety in the elderly, another assessment strategy has involved creation of new measures specifically targeting anxiety symptoms in older adults. These two strategies have produced a small body of literature addressing the utility of various anxiety measures for older adults.

Clinician-Rated Instruments

Clinician-rated instruments are used regularly to assist in the diagnosis of anxiety disorders among younger adults. The most popular diagnostic interview in this regard is the Anxiety Disorders Interview Schedule (ADIS), the most recent version of which (ADIS-IV; Brown, DiNardo, & Barlow, 1994) was created to establish anxiety disorder diagnoses according to *DSM-IV* (American Psychiatric Association, 1994). Interrater agreement for an earlier version of this instrument has been well documented in younger adult samples (e.g., DiNardo, Moras, Barlow, Rapee, & Brown, 1993). Nonetheless, the instrument has been used only recently to identify anxiety disorders in the elderly. Specifically, in a set of studies designed by the authors and their colleagues to investigate the nature and treatment of GAD in older adults (Beck, Stanley, & Zebb, 1995; Beck *et al.*, 1996; Stanley, Beck, & Glassco, 1996; Stanley, Beck, & Zebb, 1996), the ADIS-R (DiNardo & Barlow, 1988) was used to establish principal *DSM-III-R* diagnoses of GAD and to identify coexistent anxiety and unipolar affective disorders. All ADIS-R interviews in a total sample of 50 GAD patients (aged 55 years and older) were videotaped, with 28% selected randomly for evaluation by a second clinician to estimate interrater agreement. Diagnostic agreement of 100% was noted for GAD, most likely due to extensive prescreening of potential participants and the use of videotaped interviews rather than administration of two separate interviews (Borkovec & Costello, 1993). Kappa coefficients for coexistent diagnoses indicated excellent reliability (1.00) for social phobia, simple phobia, and panic disorder, and moderate reliability (.58) for major depression. Thus, although the sample upon which these data were based was small and somewhat homogeneous with regard to diagnostic picture, the resultant coefficients provide some support for the utility of the ADIS-R as a tool for diagnosing anxiety disorders in the elderly.

Segal, Hersen, Van Hasselt, Kabacoff and Roth (1993) provided support for the utility of the Structured Clinical Interview for *DSM-III-R* (SCID; Spitzer, Williams, Gibbon, & First, 1988), a more broad-based semistructured interview for diagnosing Axis I disorders, in older adults. This interview was administered to 33 adults, aged 55 years and older, seen through university-affiliated psychiatric outpatient and residential facilities. All interviews were taped and reviewed by a second clinician to estimate interrater agreement for diagnostic categories with base rates above 10%. Kappa coefficients revealed excellent interrater agreement for major depression (.70) and the broad categories of anxiety disorders (.77) and somatoform disorders (1.00). In a follow-up study (Segal, Kabacoff, Hersen, Van Hasselt, & Ryan, 1995), SCID interviews were administered to another sample of 40 older adults recruited from the same settings. Results replicated prior findings of strong interrater agreement (kappa) for major depression (.79) and the broad categories of anxiety and somatoform disorders (.73, .84), and also provided support for the interrater agreement on panic disorder diagnoses (.80). Thus, the SCID also appears to be a useful instrument for the establishment of anxiety disorders in older adults, although future studies will need to examine its utility in larger samples with higher base rates of various anxiety disorders.

Clinician-rated instruments also are used regularly to evaluate the severity of anxiety, irrespective of diagnosis, in the younger adult literature. The most routinely used measure in this domain is the Hamilton Anxiety Rating Scale (HARS; Hamilton, 1959), a 14-item instrument which measures largely somatic symptoms of anxiety. Interrater agreement for this instrument in younger adults is well established, although revisions have been suggested to improve its internal consistency and discriminant validity (Riskind, Beck, Brown, & Steer, 1987). It has been suggested that overendorsement of somatic symptoms may pose a problem for use of the HARS with elderly samples (Sheikh, 1991). However, a recent report (Beck *et al.*, 1996, August) demonstrated adequate interrater agreement for the HARS in a sample of 44 older adults with GAD ($r = .82$). This investigation also presented the first set of normative scores for the HARS in two older adult samples, one with GAD and one without diagnosable psychiatric complaints, both of which were categorized according to the ADIS-R. It also is notable that the HARS significantly differentiated these two samples of older adults, with nearly perfect classification of participants into groups as a result of a discriminant function analysis. Thus, the HARS appears to be a viable measure for use with older anxious adults, although correlations with the Hamilton Rating Scale for Depression (Hamilton, 1960) were high (Beck *et al.*, 1996, August), and its utility for differentiating anxiety and depression in the elderly has yet to be investigated.

Self-Report Measures

Self-report measures for the assessment of anxiety in younger adults have been established to target a wide range of symptom types, including (but not limited to) generalized anxiety, worry, obsessive-compulsive symptoms, and specific fears. A small collection of literature has emerged that examines the utility of some of these instruments in older adults.

To evaluate measures of generalized anxiety in the elderly, data have addressed the psychometric properties of the Spielberger State-Trait Anxiety Inventory (STAI; Spielberger *et al.*, 1970), the Hopkins Symptom Checklist (SCL-90; Derogatis *et al.*, 1973), and the Self-Rating Anxiety Scale (SAS; Zung, 1971). In an initial study, the STAI and the STAI for Children (STAIC; Spielberger, Edwards, Lushene, Montouri, & Platzek, 1973) were administered to 51 older adults, ages 55 to 87 years, who were participating in a mental health gerontology program (Patterson, O'Sullivan, & Spielberger, 1980). The STAIC was selected given that its simpler format and vocabulary were thought to be more appropriate for some elders who had difficulty completing the STAI. Approximately half of the sample were in day treatment and half were residential clients. Results revealed significant positive correlations among all STAI and STAIC subscales, with coefficients ranging from .65 to .82. All STAI and STAIC scores also correlated positively and significantly with a clinician-rated measure of anxiety from the Missouri Inpatient Behavioral Scale (MIBS; Sletten & Ulett, 1972), although the magnitude of these correlations was low (.34 to .44). Thus, the data provided some evidence for convergent validity of the STAI and STAIC in older adults. In addition, nonsignificant correlations were noted between the anxiety measures and other MIBS ratings, indicating support for the divergent validity of the STAI and STAIC. The authors concluded that these two instruments could be considered parallel forms in the evaluation of older adults (Patterson *et al.*, 1980). As noted by Hersen and Van Hasselt (1992), however, results of this report are limited by the small and diagnostically heterogeneous sample, many of whom were heavily medicated and none of whom were categorized based on semistructured interviews.

In a second study with the STAI, Himmelfarb and Murrell (1983) administered the trait subscale to 109 geriatric inpatients and 279 community residents aged over 55 years. Results provided normative data for both groups and revealed adequate internal consistency in both subsamples (coefficient alpha = .87, .93, respectively). Significant, positive correlations also were noted between the STAI-Trait and measures of depression, life satisfaction, well-being, and affect balance. As expected, the inpatient group had a significantly higher mean score on the STAI-Trait than the community sample, even when significant differences between the groups on age, gender, health status, and marital status were controlled. However, discriminant analyses indicated that measures of well-being and depression were the best predictors of group membership, with no significant additional contribution of trait anxiety. The data thus provided mixed support for the reliability and validity of the STAI for older adults, although the inpatient group was diagnostically heterogeneous and no semi-structured interviews were used to categorize participants.

In a more recent study (Stanley, Beck, & Zebb, 1996), the STAI was administered to two groups of older adults (aged 55 to 82 years), both of which were selected based on the ADIS-R. One group ($n = 50$) met *DSM-III-R* criteria for GAD, while the other group ($n = 94$) had no diagnosable psychiatric complaints. Results revealed adequate internal consistency for the STAI Trait and State subscales in both groups (alpha = .79 to .84). Test–retest reliability, assessed over a 2- to 4-week interval in a subgroup of 46 control participants, was strong for the STAI-Trait subscale ($r = .84$), but weaker for the State subscale ($r = .62$), as would be expected. Evidence for convergent validity in the normal control group was strong, as demonstrated by significant correlations with measures of worry, obsessive-compulsive symptoms, and specific fears. However, convergent validity in the patient group was mixed, possibly demonstrating some degree of independence among these symptom types in patients with GAD. In a separate analysis of data from the same study, Beck *et al.* (1996) demonstrated significant differences between STAI scores for older adults with GAD and a matched group of normal controls. Discriminant analyses revealed, however, that the STAI did not contribute significantly to the prediction of group membership.

Other measures of general anxiety that are used regularly with younger adults have been examined in a preliminary fashion with elderly samples. For example, Magni and DeLeo (1984) administered the SCL-90 anxiety and depression scales to 178 elderly hospital patients. The data provided normative scores for the sample and indicated that older adults reported fewer anxiety symptoms than a comparison group of younger adult hospital patients. Results failed to demonstrate a significant relationship between anxiety and type of medical illness in either sample. Although these data provided some information regarding the evaluation and nature of anxiety in older adults, as Hersen and Van Hasselt (1992) noted, the study failed to address the utility of the SCL-90 in older psychiatric patients. In another report, Zung (1980) administered the SAS to a normal sample of 91 adults aged 65 and over. Descriptive data revealed a mean score similar to that for younger adults (aged 20 to 64). However, no other psychometric or demographic data were provided in this report.

In addition to data regarding measures of general anxiety, other studies have begun to examine the psychometric properties of self-report instruments that assess more specific types of anxiety symptoms in older samples. Again, available data have addressed the utility of measures developed for younger samples. In particular, the psychometric properties of the Penn State Worry Questionnaire (PSWQ; Meyer, Miller, Metzger, & Borkovec, 1990), the Padua Inventory (PI; Sanavio, 1988), and the Fear Questionnaire (FQ; Marks & Mathews, 1979) have been examined in samples of older adults (aged 55 to 82) with GAD or no diagnosable psychiatric symptomatology based on the ADIS-R (Beck *et al.*, 1995; Stanley, Beck, & Zebb, 1996). The PSWQ is a 16-item scale designed to assess a person's tendency to worry, without focus on specific content of the worry. The PI is a 60-item questionnaire that evaluates obsessive-compulsive symptoms, with subscales assessing the severity of contamination and checking rituals, as well as fears of losing control over mental activities and motor behaviors. The FQ is a well-known 15-item inventory assessing severity of avoidance related to agoraphobic, social, and blood-injury fears.

In both the GAD and normal control samples, the PSWQ demonstrated strong internal consistency (coefficient alpha > .80; Beck *et al.,* 1995). Adequate convergent validity for this instrument also was demonstrated by significant correlations with other measures of anxiety and depression (Beck *et al.,* 1995). In addition, factor analyses suggested a two-factor structure for the PSWQ in both groups, with items loading on the first factor appearing to assess a tendency to worry and items on the second factor assessing an absence of worry. However, it should be noted that internal consistency for the second factor in the GAD group was marginal (alpha = .60). In a separate analysis, scores on the PSWQ were significantly different in the GAD sample and a matched normal control group, and this measure had a very high positive loading in a discriminant function analysis that successfully separated these two subsamples (Beck *et al.,* 1996).

Internal consistency of the PI generally was adequate in both samples (alpha = .74 to .95), with the exception of the Behavior Control subscale in the normal control group (alpha = .19), wherein a restricted range of scores may have created subscale instability (Stanley, Beck, & Zebb, 1996). Internal consistency for the FQ Total and Bodily Injury subscales were adequate in both groups (alpha = .73 to .85), although alpha coefficients for the FQ Social Phobia subscale in both samples and the Agoraphobia subscale in the GAD group were marginal (.60 to .67). Coefficients of test–retest reliability, assessed in a subsample of normal control participants over a 2- to 4-week interval, suggested that the Total and some subscale scores of the PI assessed stable, traitlike features while other subscales estimated more statelike clinical symptoms (r = .61 to .80). Stability over time for the FQ in general was poor (r = .41 to .64), with post hoc comparisons revealing a pattern of decreasing fear over the test–retest interval, indicating the possibility of regression to the mean on this measure for older adults without anxiety complaints. Adequate convergent validity was demonstrated for the PI, with significant correlations between this instrument and other measures of worry and anxiety in both the GAD and normal control groups. The FQ, however, failed to correlate significantly with other measures of anxiety symptoms in the GAD group, possibly due to potential reliability problems with this instrument in older adults.

In general, available data suggest that the STAI, PSWQ, and PI, which have been used routinely in samples of younger adults, also should be useful for further investigations of psychopathology and treatment in samples of older anxious adults. Additional data are needed, however, to address the utility of these measures for discriminating older adults with GAD from those with other anxiety disorders (e.g., panic disorder, specific phobias), alternative psychiatric syndromes (e.g., depression), or serious medical conditions. In addition, given mixed reliability data for the FQ, further consideration should be given to the measurement of specific fears in older adults (Stanley, Beck, & Zebb, 1996).

As an alternative to addressing the utility of instruments previously used in younger adults, another psychometric strategy involves the development of new measures specifically targeting anxiety symptoms in the elderly. Wisocki and her colleagues have developed the Worry Scale (WS; Wisocki, Handen, & Morse, 1986), a 35-item self-report measure that targets financial, health, and social worries commonly associated with aging. Preliminary reports provided some support for the concurrent validity of the WS in community-dwelling and homebound older adults (Powers *et al.*, 1992; Wisocki *et al.*, 1986; Wisocki, 1988). In a study previously described (Stanley, Beck, & Zebb, 1996), additional psychometric data were collected for the WS in two samples of older adults with GAD or no diagnosable psychiatric symptomatology. Coefficients of internal consistency were adequate in both groups (alpha = .76 to 94). Two- to 4-week test–retest reliability, assessed in a subsample of normal control participants, also was adequate (r = .69 to .80), with the exception of the Health subscale (r = .58). It was suggested that this subscale may have assessed sensitivity to real physical complaints which varied over time for nonanxious older adults, whereas financial and social issues remained more stable for individuals in this group. Adequate convergent validity for the WS also was demonstrated in both groups, with significant correlations between this measure and instruments assessing obsessive-compulsive symptoms and general anxiety (Stanley, Beck, & Zebb, 1996). In a separate analysis of an overlapping dataset (Beck *et al.*, 1996), WS scores were significantly different in the GAD sample and a matched normal control group, and the Social Phobia subscale was one of four variables that successfully differentiated these groups in a discriminant function analysis. Thus, the WS also appears useful for future investigations of the nature and treatment of anxiety in older adult samples, although again, further work is needed to examine the utility of this instrument for discriminating older anxious adults from those with other psychiatric disorders or significant medical problems.

TREATMENT

Utilization of Services

Despite relatively high prevalence rates of anxiety disorders among older persons and the severity of interference in life function that may result, very few older adults with anxiety problems seek assistance from mental health professionals. In particular, ECA data indicated that only 0.6% of adults over age 65 with agoraphobia and 2.2% with other phobias had sought services from a mental health provider in the 6 months prior to interview (Thompson *et al.*, 1988). A greater percentage of older adults in these groups had sought assistance for mental health problems from alternative sources (e.g., general physicians, clergy), but even across these settings, older adults with agoraphobia were significantly less likely to have sought treatment of any type for emotional problems than were adults aged 25 to 64 (Thompson *et al.*, 1988). Similarly, Lindesay (1991) reported that only 3% of older adults classified with phobias had ever received any form of treatment specifically for their phobic symptoms. Finally,

Blazer *et al.* (1991) noted that only 38% of older adults with GAD (identified during Wave II of the ECA survey) reported utilization of outpatient mental health services during the year prior to interview. Thus, it is clear that only a minority of older adults with anxiety disorders seek and utilize available mental health services. This pattern is consistent with reports that mental health resources in general are severely underutilized by the elderly (Lasoski, 1986).

Explanations for these patterns of underutilization have included the reluctance of older adults to define their difficulties in psychological terms or to seek social services of any kind, the relative lack of treatment providers available to offer services to this population, and practical barriers including transportation problems, financial difficulties, and limited outreach or publicity for services (Lasoski, 1986; McCarthy, Katz, & Foa, 1991). Also, as mentioned previously, it often is tempting for older adults and mental health providers to attribute the signs and symptoms of anxiety to a normal aging process, thereby overlooking treatable psychiatric disorders (Weiss, 1994). As a result of these factors, the empirical literature addressing the efficacy of treatments for anxiety in older people is quite limited. Nonetheless, there appears to be some support for the utility of both pharmacological and cognitive-behavioral interventions.

Pharmacological Treatment

Treatment of anxiety in older adults typically begins in a primary medical care setting (Blazer *et al.,* 1991; McCarthy *et al.,* 1991) and most often involves the use of antianxiety medication, typically the benzodiazepines. In fact, older adults report more frequent use of these medications than younger samples (Blazer *et al.,* 1991), with figures from 17% to 50% reported (Salzman, 1991). Despite such widespread use, literature addressing the efficacy of benzodiazepines in older adults is limited in terms of both number of studies available and methodological rigor. In a review of 14 studies of benzodiazepine treatment for anxiety in older adults, Salzman (1991) noted some evidence for the efficacy of chlordiazepoxide, diazepam, lorazepam, and oxazepam. Other data have attested to the effects of alprazolam relative to placebo (Cohn, 1984). However, conclusions from these studies are seriously limited by methodological problems including the use of diagnostically heterogeneous samples selected via unstructured clinical interviews, failure to differentiate participants with primary anxiety symptoms from those with anxiety secondary to depression or medical disease, failure to distinguish anxiety disorders from behavioral agitation resulting from dementia or psychosis, omission of appropriate controls for medical illnesses or concomitant drug treatment, and variations in outcome criteria and treatment duration (Salzman, 1991).

Despite these serious limitations, recommendations regarding the use of benzodiazepines in the elderly have been made routinely (Fernandez, Levy, Lachar, & Small, 1995; Markovitz, 1993; Weiss, 1994), generally on the basis of studies addressing the use of anxiolytics in younger adults, pharmacokinetic properties of the medications in nonsymptomatic elderly, and anxiolytic toxicity in older adults (Salzman, 1991). Recommendations have been consistent, suggesting that short half-life benzodiazepines be used for as brief a duration as possible, with some authors noting the need to consider psychosocial interventions whenever appropriate (Lader, 1986; Wengel, Burke, Ranno, & Roccaforte, 1993). Recommended benzodiazepine doses for the elderly are lower than those prescribed for younger adults given age-related alterations in the absorption, distribution, metabolism, and elimination of these medications that lead to increased sensitivity to therapeutic effects and adverse events (Lader, 1986). Because of these pharmacokinetic changes, significant attention has been given to concerns regarding cognitive impairment, respiratory depression, and psychomotor slowing that may be associated with benzodiazepine use in the elderly (Weiss, 1994; Wengel *et al.,* 1993). In particular, it has been noted that use of benzodiazepines may create amnesia, delayed recall, confusion, disorientation, and agitation among older adults, and that psychomotor slowing or oversedation may lead to increased rates of falls and hip fractures (Wengel *et al.,* 1993). These symptoms in turn also may exacerbate anxiety symptoms (in particular, worry). Other pharmacotherapy-related concerns include potential drug interactions, given increased rates of medical illness among older adults, and medication compliance. Survey data have pointed to an increased risk of alterations in medication doses or schedules when more than three drugs are prescribed per day (Salzman, 1995). Given that 25% of elders are prescribed multiple (3 or more) medications, compliance problems are of central importance in the pharmacological treatment of anxiety among older adults.

Although benzodiazepines remain the most frequently prescribed drugs for anxiety among older adults, pharmacological recommendations also include consideration of other types of medications. The greatest amount of attention has been given to the effects of buspirone. At least four open trials have documented the utility of this medication for the treatment of anxiety among older persons (Salzman, 1991). Clinical recommendations generally have noted that the therapeutic effects of buspirone are comparable to those of the benzodiazepines, although side effects are preferable for buspirone given its negligible potential for tolerance, withdrawal, or serious overdose toxicity (Weiss, 1994). However, due to the lack of well-controlled treatment trials comparing the effects of buspirone to placebo or benziodiazepines among the elderly, these recommendations are without strong empirical support.

Clinical recommendations based on empirical studies with younger adults also have noted the potential efficacy of beta blockers and antidepressants for the treatment of anxiety in older adults, and the possible utility of antihistamines has been mentioned (Fernandez *et al.,* 1995; Markovitz, 1993). Given that no empirical support for these medications in older adults has been reported, these recommendations must be considered very carefully. In general, the dearth of data addressing the pharmacological treatment of anxiety disorders among the elderly suggests that significant work is yet to be done in this domain to establish standards of treatment for the different anxiety disorders in this population.

Cognitive Behavioral Treatments

Although treatment with medication may be effective for reducing anxiety, chronic and widespread use of benzodiazepines in this population may not be optimal treatment given the potential problems noted earlier. Furthermore, a pharmacological approach to treatment typically neglects potentially important psychosocial factors such as social support, coping skills, and interpersonal relationships. Thus, the development of psychosocial adjuncts or alternatives for the treatment of anxiety in older persons is highly desirable. Although a significant number of studies have addressed the utility of psychosocial interventions for the treatment of depression in older adults (e.g., Areán *et al.,* 1993; Thompson, Gallagher, & Breckenridge, 1987), relatively little attention has been paid to the development of psychosocial treatments for anxiety disorders in this population. Given the well-developed literature supporting the utility of cognitive behavior therapy (CBT) for anxiety among younger adults (e.g., Barlow, 1988; Beidel & Turner, 1991), it is not surprising that initial efforts to identify effective psychosocial treatments in older samples have concentrated on these approaches. However, the majority of literature currently available is limited to clinical case studies or group comparisons with nonclinical volunteers who report general anxiety complaints.

Case studies have addressed the utility of cognitive-behavioral interventions with elderly adults who meet diagnostic criteria for generalized anxiety disorder (King & Barrowclough, 1991), panic disorder (Rathus & Sanderson, 1994), specific phobias (Thyer, 1981), and obsessive-compulsive disorder (Calamari, Faber, Hitsman, & Poppe, 1994; Carmin, Ownby, & Pollard, 1995; Junjinger & Ditto, 1984). Treatment approaches have followed closely those validated empirically in younger samples, with results documenting the utility of various forms of exposure, response prevention, breathing retraining, and cognitive restructuring. Conclusions from these case reports are limited, of course, by the lack of appropriate methodological controls. Nonetheless, these types of reports provide some support for the benefits of further empirical investigation into the usefulness of cognitive behavioral treatments for anxiety in older persons.

A number of controlled group comparisons with nonclinical volunteers reporting anxiety complaints have provided additional support for the potential use of CBT with older adults. In one of the earliest of these studies, 36 female volunteers (aged 63 to 79) with complaints of anxiousness, tension, fatigue, insomnia, sadness, and somatic symptoms were assigned randomly to receive one of two versions of relaxation training or an attention control condition (DeBerry, 1982). Participants were selected from a prescreening procedure that followed a discussion about stress at a senior citizen center. Results demonstrated that relaxation training led to significant decreases in state and trait anxiety on the STAI, although no changes were noted in the control condition. On the other hand, depressive symptoms (measured by the Zung depression scale) were not diminished in any group.

In a similar comparison, 24 community volunteers (aged 60 years and older) with both anxiety and depressive symptoms were selected from attendants at a series of self-improvement workshops (Sallis, Lichstein, Clarkson, Stalgaitis, & Campbell, 1983). Participants were assigned randomly to receive behavioral treatment for anxiety (relaxation training), cognitive behavioral treatment for depression (pleasant events scheduling and rational emotive procedures), or a nonspecific control condition that involved self-disclosure and reflection of feelings. Results revealed significant improvement in both anxiety and depression, as measured by the STAI and the Beck Depression Inventory (BDI), for participants in all groups.

Subsequently, DeBerry and colleagues (DeBerry, Davis, & Reinhard, 1989) compared the effects of relaxation training, cognitive restructuring, and an attention control condition in 32 nonclinical volunteers (aged 65 to 70 years) with various anxiety-related complaints. Results indicated that only relaxation training was effective in decreasing STAI state anxiety scores, although STAI trait anxiety and BDI scores were improved across all conditions. More recently, progressive and imaginal relaxation training were compared with a wait-list control group in 71 older adults (aged 60 years and older) with subjective tension or anxiety or both (Scogin, Rickard, Keith, Wilson, & McElreath, 1992). Results revealed significantly greater decreases in anxiety, as measured by the STAI state anxiety scale and the SCL-90-R, following both types of relaxation training relative to the control condition. Treatment gains also were maintained at 1-year follow-up (Rickard, Scogin, & Keith, 1994).

Taken together, these studies suggest some efficacy of cognitive behavioral interventions, in particular relaxation training, for the treatment of anxiety in older adults. However, results are limited by small sample sizes and the focus on nondiagnosed community volunteers. Only recently has a group comparison study addressed the utility of cognitive behavioral interventions for a sample of older adults diagnosed via semistructured clinical interview.

Following findings from the younger adult literature, Stanley, Beck, and Glassco (1996) conducted a comparison of CBT and nondirective supportive psychotherapy (SP) in a sample of 48 older adults with generalized anxiety disorder (GAD). Participants were recruited through the community and diagnosed according to the ADIS-R. CBT and SP were conducted in a small group format, with weekly meetings over a 14-week period. CBT included three major components: progressive deep muscle relaxation (sessions 1 through 5), cognitive therapy (session 6 through 10), and exposure treatment (sessions 11 through 14). SP focused on nondirective group discussion of anxiety symptoms and experiences, with the therapist assuming a supportive, facilitative role. Results indicated significant pre-to-post decreases in measures of worry (e.g., PSWQ, global severity of GAD, time spent worrying), anxiety (STAI, HARS), and depression (BDI, HRSD) for participants in both treatment groups. Some evidence for a preferential effect of CBT on measures of specific fears (FQ) was noted, although potential problems with the psychometric properties of the FQ limit this conclusion. Six-month follow-up analyses revealed maintenance of treatment gains on measures of anxiety and depression, with some continued improvement in severity of worry for both groups. Correlational analyses further suggested that pretreatment severity of anxiety and ratings of treatment credibility (provided after treatment procedures had been explained) correlated significantly with outcome. In particular, higher levels of pretreatment anxiety and lower estimates of treatment credibility were associated with poorer response at posttreatment. Conclusions from this study are limited by the omission of a no-treatment or wait-list control condition. However, this study is the first to document the potential viability of psychosocial treatment procedures for older adults with well-diagnosed anxiety disorders. Future studies will need to include appropriate control conditions and assess the effects of cognitive behavioral and other psychosocial interventions for older adults with GAD and other *DSM-IV* anxiety disorders.

SUMMARY

Anxiety disorders are the most prevalent of all psychiatric conditions among the elderly, with phobias and generalized anxiety disorder the most commonly assigned diagnoses. Current prevalence estimates, along with the degree of interference in life function that can result from significant anxiety problems, suggest that these disorders pose a serious public health problem for older adults. Additional epidemiological data are needed, however, regarding the ethnic distribution of anxiety disorders among the elderly. More information also is needed to address issues of differential diagnosis in this population, with specific attention to the overlap between anxiety, depression, and medical illness, as well as the distinction between anxiety disorders and symptoms of anxiety that may be associated with the normal aging process. In this regard, the need for age-appropriate norms for standardized assessment tools is paramount.

With regard to psychopathology, recent studies have begun to identify features of anxiety disorders in the elderly that suggest overlap with younger adult samples as well as those characteristics of anxiety that may be unique to older individuals. To date, the majority of this work has focused on worry and associated symptoms. However, more attention will need to be given to these issues in elderly patients with a range of anxiety disorders. To do so, further research will need to address the development of appropriate and psychometrically sound assessment tools. One strategy has involved examination of the psychometric characteristics of instruments commonly used with younger adults. Some support has been obtained for the reliability and validity of both self-report and clinician-rated measures of worry, anxiety, and obsessive-compulsive symptoms. Given the potentially unique experience of some facets of anxiety in the elderly, another assessment strategy has involved creation of new measures specifically targeting anxiety symptoms in older adults. This approach has yielded one measure of worry that appears useful for future investigations. More data are needed, however, to establish a broad range of measures that can be used routinely for evaluation of elderly samples in both research and clinical settings. Normative data with both community and clinical samples will be needed, with study participants classified carefully according to structured interview procedures (Hersen & Van Hasselt, 1992).

With the establishment of psychometrically sound assessment procedures, it should be possible to extend the treatment literature dramatically. At present, studies regarding the effects of pharmacological and psychosocial (primarily cognitive behavioral) interventions are severely limited by the omission of appropriate control groups and the use of diagnostically heterogenous clinical groups or samples of nonclinical community volunteers with vague anxiety complaints. Future studies will need to be conducted with samples of carefully diagnosed participants who are assigned randomly to the treatments of interest and appropriate control conditions. Emphasis will need to be placed on the effects of treatment not only on symptom reduction, but also on the transfer effects of interventions on associated depression, social functioning, and quality of life. Durability of treatment response over long-term follow-up intervals also will need to be targeted, as will generalizability of findings to patients recruited from a wide array of settings (e.g., psychiatric clinics, primary care facilities) and from diverse sociocultural backgrounds.

REFERENCES

Alexopoulos, G. S. (1991). Anxiety and depression in the elderly. In C. Salzman & B. D. Lebowitz (Eds.), *Anxiety in the elderly: Treatment and research* (pp. 63–77). New York: Springer.

American Psychiatric Association. (1980). *Diagnostic and statistical manual of mental disorders* (3rd ed.). Washington, DC: Author.

American Psychiatric Association. (1987). *Diagnostic and statistical manual of mental disorders* (3rd ed.–revised). Washington, DC: Author.

American Psychiatric Association. (1994). *Diagnostic and statistical manual of mental disorders* (4th ed.). Washington, DC: Author.

Areán, P. A., Perri, M G., Nezu, A. M., Schein, R. L., Christopher, F., & Joseph, T. X. (1993). Comparative effectiveness of social problem-solving therapy and resminiscence therapy as treatments for depression in older adults. *Journal of Consulting and Clinical Psychology, 61,* 1003–1010.

Barlow, D. H. (1988) *Anxiety and its disorders.* New York: Guilford.

Beck, J. G., Stanley, M. A., & Zebb, B. J. (1995). Psychometric properties of the Penn State Worry Questionnaire in older adults. *Journal of Clinical Geropsychology, 1,* 33–42.

Beck, J. G., Stanley, M. A., & Zebb, B. J. (1996). Characteristics of generalized anxiety disorder in older adults: A descriptive study. *Behavior Research and Therapy, 34,* 225–234.

Beck, J. G., Stanley, M. A., & Zebb, B. J. (1996, August). *How do the Hamiltion scales perform with geriatric GAD patients?* Paper presented at the Annual Convention of the American Psychological Association, Toronto, Ontario.

Beidel, D. C., & Turner, S. M. (1991). Anxiety disorders. In M. Hersen & S. M. Turner (Eds.), *Adult psychopathology and diagnosis* (pp. 226–278). New York: Wiley.

Ben-Arie, O., Swartz, L., & Dickman, B. J. (1987). Depression in the elderly living in the community: Its presentation and features. *British Journal of Psychiatry, 150,* 169–174.

Blazer, D., George, L. K., & Hughes, D. (1991). The epidemiology of anxiety disorders: An age comparison In C. Salzman & B. D. Lebowitz (Eds.), *Anxiety in the elderly: Treatment and research* (pp. 17–30). New York: Springer.

Borkovec, T. D., & Costello, E. (1993). Efficacy of applied relaxation and cognitive-behavioral therapy in the treatment of generalized anxiety disorder. *Journal of Consulting and Clinical Psychology, 61,* 611–619.

Brown, T. A., DiNardo, P. A., & Barlow, D. H. (1994). *Anxiety Disorders Interview Schedule for DSM-IV.* Albany, NY: Phobia and Anxiety Disorders Clinic, Center for Stress and Anxiety, State University of New York.

Bruce, M. L., & McNamara, R. (1992). Psychiatric status among the homebound elderly: An epidemiologic perspective. *Journal of the American Geriatrics Society, 40,* 561–566.

Calamari, J. E., Faber, S. D., Hitsman, B. L., & Poppe, C. J. (1994). Treatment of obsessive compulsive disorder in the elderly: A review and case example. *Journal of Behavior Therapy and Experimental Psychiatry, 25,* 95–104.

Carmin, C. N., Ownby, R. L., & Pollard, C. A. (1995, November). *Effects of cognitive behavioral treatment of obsessive compulsive disorder in geriatric versus younger adult patients.* Paper presented at the annual convention of the Association for Advancement of Behavior Therapy, Washington, DC.

Carstensen, L. L. (1988). The emerging field of behavioral gerontology. *Behavior Therapy, 19,* 259–281.

Cloninger, C. R. (1990). Comorbidity of anxiety disorders. *Journal of Psychopharmacology, 10,* 43–46.

Cohen, G. D (1991). Anxiety and general medical disorders In C. Salzman & B. D. Lebowitz (Eds.), *Anxiety in the elderly: Treatment and research* (pp. 47–62). New York: Springer.

Cohn, J. B. (1984). Double-blind safety and efficacy comparison of alprazolam and placebo in the treatment of anxiety in geriatric patients. *Current Therapeutic Research, 35,* 100–112.

Copp, J. E., Schwiderski, U. E., & Robinson, D. S. (1990). Symptom comorbidity in anxiety and depressive disorders. *Journal of Clinical Psychopharmacology, 10,* 52–60.

DeBerry, S. (1982). The effects of meditation-relaxation on anxiety and depression in a geriatric population. *Psychotherapy: Theory, research, and practice, 19,* 512–521.

DeBerry, S., Davis, S., & Reinhard, K. E. (1989). A comparison of meditation-relaxation and cognitive behavioral techniques for reducing anxiety and depression in a geriatric population. *Journal of Geriatric Psychiatry, 22,* 231–247.

Derogatis, L. R., Lipman, R. S., Rickels, K., Uhlenhuth, E. H., & Covi, L. (1973). The Hopkins Symptom Checklist (HSCL): A self-report inventory. *Behavioral Science 19,* 1–15.

DiNardo, P. A., & Barlow, D. H. (1988). *Anxiety Disorders Interview Schedule–Revised (ADIS-R).* Albany, NY: Phobia and Anxiety Disorders Clinic, State University of New York.

DiNardo, P. A., Moras, K., Barlow, D. H., Rapee, R. M., & Brown, T. A. (1993). Reliability of DSM-III-R anxiety disorder categories: Using the Anxiety Disorders Interview Schedule–Revised (ADIS-R). *Archives of General Psychiatry, 50,* 251–256.

Eaton, W. W., Kramer, M., Anthony, J. C., Dryman, A., Shapiro, S., & Locke, B. Z. (1989). The incidence of specific DIS/DSM-III mental disorders: Data from the NIMH Epidemiologic Catchment Area Program. *Acta Psychiatrica Scandinavia, 79,* 163–178.

Feinson, M. C., & Thoits, P. A. (1986). The distribution of distress among elders. *Journal of Gerontology, 41,* 225–233.

Feldman, L. A. (1993). Distinguishing depression and anxiety in self-report: Evidence from confirmatory factor analysis on nonclinical and clinical samples. *Journal of Consulting and Clinical Psychology, 61,* 631–638.

Fernandez, F., Levy, J. K., Lachar, B. L., & Small, G. W. (1995). The management of depression and anxiety in the elderly. *Journal of Clinical Psychiatry, 56,* 20–29.

Flint, A. J. (1994). Epidemiology and comorbidity of anxiety disorders in the elderly. *American Journal of Psychiatry, 151,* 640–649.

Gurian, B. S., & Miner, J. H. (1991). Clinical presentation of anxiety in the elderly. In C. Salzman & B. D. Lebowitz (Eds.), *Anxiety in the elderly: Treatment and research* (pp. 31–44). New York: Springer.

Hamilton, M. (1959). The assessment of anxiety states by rating. *British Journal of Medical Psychology, 32,* 50–55.

Hamilton, M. (1960). A rating scale for depression. *Journal of Neurology, Neurosurgery, and Psychiatry, 23,* 56–62.

Helzer, J. E., Robins, L. N., & McEvoy, L. (1987). Post-traumatic stress disorder in the general population. *New England Journal of Medicine, 317,* 1630–1634.

Hersen, M., & Van Hasselt, V. B. (1992). Behavioral assessment and treatment of anxiety in the elderly. *Clinical Psychology Review, 12,* 619–640.

Hersen, M., Van Hasselt, V. B., & Goreczny, A. J. (1993). Behavioral assessment of anxiety in older adults. *Behavior Modification, 17,* 99–112.

Himmelfarb, S., & Murrell, S. A. (1983). Reliability and validity of five mental health scales in older persons. *Journal of Gerontology, 38,* 333–339.

Himmelfarb, S., & Murrell, S. A. (1984). The prevalence and correlates of anxiety symptoms in older adults. *Journal of Psychology, 116,* 159–167.

Junjinger, J., & Ditto, B. (1984). Multitreatment of obsessive-compulsive checking in a geriatric patient. *Behavior Modification, 8,* 379–390.

King, P., & Barrowclough, C. (1991). A clinical pilot study of cognitive-behavioral therapy for anxiety disorders in the elderly. *Behavioural Psychotherapy, 19,* 337–345.

Lader, M. (1986). The use of hypnotics and anxiolytics in the elderly. *International Clinical Psychopharmacology, 1,* 273–283.

Lasoski, M. C. (1986). Reasons for low utilization of mental health services by the elderly. In T. L. Brink (Ed.), *Clinical gerontology: A guide to assessment and intervention* (pp. 1–18). New York: Haworth.

Liddell, A., Locker, D., & Burman, D. (1991). Self-reported fears (FSS-II) of subjects aged 50 years and over. *Behavior Research and Therapy, 29,* 105–112.

Lindesay, J. (1991). Phobic disorders in the elderly. *British Journal of Psychiatry, 159,* 531–541.

Lindesay, J., Briggs, K., & Murphy, E. (1989). The Guy's/Age Concern Survey: Prevalence rates of cognitive impairment, depression and anxiety in an urban elderly community. *British Journal of Psychiatry, 155,* 317–329.

Magni, G, & De Leo, D. (1984). Anxiety and depression in geriatric and adult medical inpatients: A comparison. *Psychological Reports, 55,* 607–612.

Markovitz, P. J. (1993). Treatment of anxiety in the elderly. *Journal of Clinical Psychiatry, 54,* 64–68.

Marks, I. M., & Mathews, A. M. (1979). Brief standardized self-rating for phobic patients. *Behavior Research and Therapy, 17,* 263–267.

McCarthy, P. R., Katz, I. R., & Foa, E. B. (1991). Cognitive-behavioral treatment of anxiety in the elderly: A proposed model. In C. Salzman & B. D. Lebowitz (Eds.), *Anxiety in the elderly: Treatment and research* (pp. 197–214). New York: Springer.

McNally, R. J. (1994). *Panic disorder: A critical analysis.* New York: Guilford.

Meyer, T. J., Miller, M. L., Metzger, R. L., & Borkovec, T. D. (1990). Development and validation of the Penn State Worry Questionnaire. *Behavior Research and Therapy, 28,* 487–495.

Nietzel, M. T., Bernstein, D. A., & Russell, R. L. (1988). Assessment of anxiety and fear. In A. S. Bellack & M. Hersen (Eds.), *Behavioral assessment: A practical handbook* (3rd ed., pp. 280–312). New York: Pergamon.

Oxman, T. E., Barrett, J. E., Barrett, J., & Gerber, P. (1987). Psychiatric symptoms in the elderly in a primary care practice. *General Hospital Psychiatry, 9,* 167–173.

Parmelee, P. A., Katz, I. R., & Lawton, M. P. (1992). Anxiety and its association with depression among institutionalized elderly. *American Journal of Geriatric Psychiatry, 1,* 46–58.

Patterson, R. L., O'Sullivan, M. J., & Spielberger, C. D. (1980). Measurement of state and trait anxiety in elderly mental health clients. *Journal of Behavioral Assessment, 2,* 89–97.

Person, D. C., & Borkovec, T. D. (1995, August). *Anxiety disorders among the elderly: Patterns and issues.* Paper presented at the 103rd annual meeting of the American Psychological Association. New York.

Powers, C. B., Wisocki, P. A., & Whitbourne, S. K. (1992). Age differences and correlates of worrying in young and elderly adults. *Gerontologist, 32,* 82–88.

Raj, B. A., Corvea, M. H., & Dagon, E. M. (1993). The clinical characteristics of panic disorder in the elderly: A retrospective study. *Journal of Clinical Psychiatry, 54,* 150–155.

Rapee, R. M., & Barlow, D. H. (1991). *Chronic anxiety: Generalized anxiety disorder and mixed anxiety-depression.* New York: Guilford.

Rathus, J. H., & Sanderson, W. C. (1994, November). *Cognitive behavioral treatment for panic disorder in geriatric patients.* Paper presented at the annual convention for the Association for Advancement of Behavior Therapy, San Diego.

Regier, D. A., Boyd, J. H., Burke, I. D., Rae, D. S., Myers, J. K., Kramer, M., Robins, L. N., George, L. K., Karno, M., & Locke, B. Z. (1988). One-month prevalence of mental disorders in the United States: Based on five epidemiologic catchment area sites. *Archives of General Psychiatry, 45,* 977–986.

Regier, D. A., Narrow, W. E., & Rae, D. S. (1990). The epidemiology of anxiety disorders: The Epidemiologic Catchment Area (ECA) experience. *Journal of Psychiatric Research, 24,* 3–14.

Reynolds, C. F., Lebowitz, B. D., & Schneider, L S (1993). Diagnosis and treatment of depression in late life. *Psychopharmacology Bulletin, 29,* 83–85.

Rickard, H. C., Scogin, F., & Keith, S. (1994). A one-year follow-up of relaxation training for elders with subjective anxiety. *Gerontologist, 34,* 121–122.

Riskind, J. H., Beck, A. T., Brown, G., & Steer, R. (1987). Taking the measure of anxiety and depression: Validity of the reconstructed Hamilton Scales. *Journal of Nervous and Mental Disease, 175,* 474–479.

Robins, L. N., Helzer, J. E., Weissman, M. M., Orvaschel, H., Gruenberg, E., Burke, J. D., & Regier, D. A. (1984). Lifetime prevalence of specific psychiatric disorders in three sites. *Archives of General Psychiatry, 41,* 949–958.

Sailis, J. F., Lichstein, K. L., Clarkson, A. D., Stalgaitis, S., & Campbell, M. (1983). Anxiety and depression management for the elderly. *International Journal of Behavioral Geriatrics, 1,* 3–12.

Sanavio, E. (1988). Obsessions and compulsions: The Padua Inventory. *Behavior Research and Therapy, 26,* 169–177.

Salzman, C. (1991). Pharmacologic treatment of the anxious elderly patient. In C. Salzman & B. D. Lebowitz (Eds.), *Anxiety in the elderly: Treatment and research*. New York: Springer.

Salzman, C. (1995). Medication compliance in the elderly. *Journal of Clinical Psychiatry, 56,* 18–22.

Salzman, C., & Lebowitz, B. D. (1991). *Anxiety in the elderly: Treatment and research*. New York: Springer.

Scogin, F., Rickard, H. C., Keith, S., Wilson, J., & McElreath, L. (1992). Progressive and imaginal relaxation training for elderly persons with subjective anxiety. *Psychology and Aging, 7,* 419–424.

Segal, D. L., Hersen, M., Van Hasselt, V. B., Kabacoff R. I., & Roth, L. (1993). Reliability of diagnosis in older psychiatric patients using the Structured Clinical Interview for DSM-III-R. *Journal of Psychopathology and Behavioral Assessment, 15,* 347–356.

Segal, D. L., Kabacoff, R. I., Hersen, M., Van Hasselt, V. B., & Ryan, C. F. (1995). Update on the reliability of diagnosis in older psychiatric outpatients using the Structured Clinical Interview for DSM-III-R. *Journal of Clinical Geropsychology, 1,* 313–321.

Sheikh, J. I. (1991). Anxiety rating scales for the elderly. In C. Salzman & B. D. Lebowitz (Eds.), *Anxiety in the elderly: Treatment and research* (pp. 251–265). New York: Springer.

Sletten, I. W., & Ullett, G. A. (1972). The present status of automation in a state psychiatric system. *Psychiatric Annals, 2,* 77–80.

Spielberger, C. D., Gorsuch, R., & Lushene, R. (1970). *STAI Manual for the State-Trait Anxiety Inventory*. Palo Alto, CA: Consulting Psychologists Press.

Spielberger, C. D., Edwards, C. D., Lushene, R. E., Montouri, J., & Platzek, D. (1973). *STAIC: Preliminary manual for the State-Trait Anxiety for children*. Palo Alto, CA: Consulting Psychologists Press.

Spitzer, R. L., Williams, J. B. W., Gibbon, M., & First, M. B. (1988). *Structured Clinical Interview for DSM-III-R—Patient Version (SCID-P 6/1/88)*. New York: Biometrics Research Department, New York State Psychiatric Institute.

Stanley, M. A., Beck, J. G., & Glassco, J. D. (1996). Treatment of generalized anxiety in older adults: A preliminary comparison of cognitive-behavioral and supportive approaches. *Behavior Therapy, 27,* 565–581.

Stanley, M. A., Beck, J. G., & Zebb, B. J. (1996). Psychometric properties of four anxiety measures in older adults. *Behaviour Research and Therapy, 34,* 827–838.

Thompson, L. W., Gallagher, D., & Breckenridge, J. S. (1987). Comparative effectiveness of psychotherapies for depressed elders. *Journal of Consulting and Clinical Psychology, 55,* 385–390.

Thompson, J. W., Burns, B. J., Bartko, J., Boyd, J. H., Taube, C. A., & Bourdon, K. H. (1988). The use of ambulatory services by persons with and without phobia. *Medical Care, 26,* 183–198.

Thyer, B. A. (1981). Prolonged in vivo exposure therapy with a 70-year-old woman. *Journal of Behavior Therapy and Experimental Psychiatry, 12,* 69–71.

Thyer, B. A., Parrish, R. T., Curtis, G. C., Nesse, R. M., & Cameron, O. G. (1985). Ages of onset of DSM-III anxiety disorders. *Comprehensive Psychiatry, 26,* 113–121.

Weiss, K. J. (1994). Management of anxiety and depression syndromes in the elderly. *Journal of Clinical Psychiatry, 55,* 5–12.

Weissman, M. M., Myers, J. K., Tischler, G. L., Holzer, C. E., Leaf, P. J., Orvaschel, H., & Brody, J. A. (1985). Psychiatric disorders (DSM-III) and cognitive impairment among the elderly in a U.S. urban community. *Acta Psychiatric a Scandinavia, 71,* 366–379.

Wengel, S. P., Burke, W. J., Ranno, A. E., & Roccaforte, W. H. (1993). Use of benzodiazepines in the elderly. *Psychiatric Annals, 23,* 325–331.

Wisocki, P. A. (1988). Worry as a phenomenon relevant to the elderly. *Behavior Therapy, 19,* 369–379.

Wisocki, P. A., Handen, B., & Morse, C. K. (1986). The Worry Scale as a measure of anxiety among homebound and community active elderly. *Behavior Therapist, 9,* 91–95.

Zung, W. W. K. (1971). A rating instrument for anxiety disorders. *Psychosomatic, 12,* 371–370.

Zung, W. W. K. (1980). How normal is anxiety? In *Current concepts*. Kalamazoo, MI: Scope.

CHAPTER 12

Sexual Dysfunction

Nathaniel McConaghy

AGE AND SEXUAL FUNCTIONING

Age and Decline of Sexuality

The general decline of frequency of sexual activity with age has been consistently documented since it was reported by Kinsey and his colleagues (Kinsey, Pomeroy, & Martin, 1948; Kinsey, Pomeroy, Martin, & Gebhard, 1953). The Kinsey and Hunt (1974) surveys of nonrepresentative samples reported median weekly frequencies of intercourse declining from 2.5 to 3.3 for people aged 16 to 25 to 0.5 to 1 for those aged 46 to 60 (Seidman & Rieder, 1994). Pfeiffer, Verwoerdt, and Davis (1972) investigated 261 White men and 241 White women aged 46 to 71 chosen randomly from membership lists of the local medical group, so that they were broadly representative of the middle and upper socioeconomic levels of the community. Ninety-eight percent of the men and 71% of the women were married. Cessation of sexual intercourse was reported by 14%, 61%, and 73% of women and 0%, 20%, and 24% of men in the age ranges 46 to 50, 61 to 65, and 66 to 71; and frequencies of 2 to 3 or more times a week by 21%, 5%, and 0% of women and 33%, 7%, and 2% of men in these age ranges. Of 91 German women of slightly above average education, cessation of intercourse was reported by 26%, 77%, 79%, and 100% of those in the four age ranges from 50 to 59 to 80 to 91. The percentages in these age ranges without sexual partners were 15, 44, 75, and 92 (von Sydow, 1995).

Laumann, Gagnon, Michael, and Michaels (1994) surveyed 3,432 subjects, of whom 3,159 were a 78% representative sample of English-speaking 18–59-year-olds living in households in the United States. They found number of subjects reporting frequencies of partnered sexual activity in the past year of two or more times a week declined in men from a maximum of 48% of those aged 25 to 29 to 18% of those aged 55 to 59, and in women from 48% of those aged 25

Nathaniel McConaghy • Psychiatric Unit, Prince of Wales Hospital, Randwick 2031, New South Wales, Australia.

Handbook of Clinical Geropsychology, edited by Michel Hersen and Vincent B. Van Hasselt. Plenum Press, New York, 1998.

to 29 to 7% of those aged 55 to 59. The percentage reporting no partnered activity in the past year increased from 7% of men and 4% of women aged 25 to 29 to 16% of men and 41% of women aged 55 to 59. Laumann and colleagues reported data for older subjects from the general Social Surveys for 1988 to 1991 and for 1993. These surveys were conducted on about 1,500 respondents yearly, approximately 75% of probability samples of individuals aged 18 or over, living in households. The percentage with no partnered sexual activity in the past year increased steadily with age, being reported by 45%, 75%, and 95% of women aged 60 to 64, 70 to 74, and 80 to 84, respectively, and by 16%, 40%, and 55% of men in these age ranges. Lewontin (1995a), in his trenchant criticism of the validity of self-report of sexual behavior, was scornful of the authors' acceptance "without the academic equivalent of a snicker" of this finding that 45% of men aged 80 to 84 still have sex with a partner; Sennett (1995) was interested and cheered by the finding, "even if the aged have confused fantasy with fact" (p 43). Lewontin (1995b) suggested that "facing the abyss, old people need to affirm themselves even more than the young. In a culture that is obsessed with youth, physical vigor, and sexuality, one form of affirmation is surely sexual boasting" (p. 56). These statements indicated a confident belief that few if any older people continue sexual activity; this belief was considered widespread by the men and women aged 50 to over 70 investigated by Brecher (1984). More than 3,000 agreed and less than 500 disagreed with the statement that "Society thinks of older people as nonsexual." Findings demonstrating that the survey evidence to the contrary has some validity were reported by Persson and Svanborg (1992). Forty-five (56%) of a representative sample of 81 married men reported having sexual intercourse at the age of 70. Five years later 25 had ceased, 21 due to factors in themselves. Vasculogenic and stress factors had been present 5 years earlier in 10 of the 21, compared to one of the 20 who were continuing intercourse. Hence, these factors were predictive of the subjects' reports at 75, supporting their validity.

Duration of the last partnered sexual event, and occurrence in that event of active and receptive oral sex were also found to decline with age in Laumann and colleagues' (1994) study. However, anal sex was reported in that event by 42% of men and 1.4% of women aged 55 to 59, both figures higher than the means for the entire sample. Aging may be associated with an increased acceptance of anal stimulation; 16% of the heterosexual subjects in Brecher's (1984) study of 4,246 socially advantaged men and women reported having had their anus stimulated during sex since age 50, 86% of the men and 67% of the women reporting this stating that they liked it.

Investigation of 436 male-partnered women, aged 35 to 59 years, 87% of a random sample of 600 women registered with two general practices in England, found age associated not only with reduced frequency of sexual intercourse and of experiencing orgasm in partnered sexual activity in the preceding 3 months, but found it was also associated with reduced enjoyment of such activity (Hawton, Gath, & Day, 1994). No enjoyment was reported by 2% of women aged 35 to 39, but 28% of women aged 55 to 59; the activity was considered unpleasant on all occasions by 1.1% and 11.3% of women in these age ranges. Brecher (1984) reported the prevalence of high enjoyment of sex to reduce with age in his older but health advantaged subjects, from 71% of women and 90% of men in their

50s to 61% of women and 75% of men aged 70 and older. Brecher pointed out that this decline was less than the decline in the frequency of sexual activity; prevalence of its weekly incidence reduced from 73% to 50% in women and 90% to 58% in men in the two age ranges. Hawton and colleagues (1994) found that age of the partner was at least as important as that of the women in determining frequency of sexual intercourse.

Cohort Effects

These studies reporting decline in sexual activity with age were cross-sectional rather than longitudinal in nature; that is to say, they examined the relationship in subjects of different ages at one point in time. In cross-sectional studies, the effects of aging are confounded with the effects of belonging to a particular age group or cohort. Findings of the studies reported cannot exclude the possibility that sexual activity of the older subjects had always been less than that of the younger subjects due, for example, to such factors as different socialization experiences and religious and moral values. However, although the subjects investigated by Kinsey and colleagues (1948, 1953), Hunt (1974), and Pfeiffer and colleagues. (1972) were less representative than those of Laumann and colleagues (1994), the fact that 40 and 20 years previous to recent studies they reported comparable declines in sexual activity with age suggests it is unlikely that such declines could be accounted for solely by a cohort effect. Pfeiffer and colleagues (1972) attempted to examine the effect of age in isolation by asking subjects if they were aware of a change in their sexual interest and activity. The number who reported awareness of a decline in sexual interest and activity increased with age, the largest increase being found between subjects in the age groups 46 to 50 and 51 to 55. Decline was reported by 58% of women aged 46 to 50, 78% of women aged 51 to 55, and 96% of women aged 66 to 71; and by 49% of men aged 46 to 50, 71% of men aged 51 to 55, and 88% of men aged 66 to 71. In what could seem a conflicting report, Adams and Turner (1985) stated that they found that women more than men reported increases from young adulthood to old age on one or more sexual measures. They should have said the minority of their subjects who reported increases consisted more of women than of men. They asked 62 women and 40 men aged 60 to 85 years to rate the sexual measures currently and when they were age 20 to 30. The highest percentage reporting an increase were 17% of women in regard to frequency of orgasm; 5% of men reported an increase. However, frequency was reported to stay low or decrease by 70% of women and 62% of men. Frequency of orgasm in women tends to increase from early adulthood until middle age (McConaghy, 1993), so a more meaningful comparison for the current rating would have been with their rating when they were aged 35 to 45. Brecher (1984) found more women than men aged 50 and over reported increase in interest in sex compared to when they were aged approximately 40. However, the majority of both sexes reported interest in sex was about the same or had decreased.

Longitudinal studies, that is, studies following up the same subjects over time, are methodologically the most appropriate to investigate the influence of age independent of cohort effects. Hallstrom and Samuelsson (1990) investigated initially and 6 years later 497 Swedish women living with their spouse or other partner who were part of an 89% representative sample of a town population. At follow-up in only a minority of each age group, 7%, 26%, 31%, and 37% of those finally aged 44, 52, 56, and 60 respectively, had the strength of sexual desire declined over the 6 years. George and Weiler (1981) investigated frequency of sexual intercourse in 108 married women and 170 married men, studied earlier by Pfeiffer and colleagues (1972). No decline over 6 years was present in 62%, 56%, and 33% of the women finally aged 52 to 61, 62 to 71, and 72 to 77, respectively. No sexual activity over the previous 6 years was reported by 5% of women finally aged 52 to 61 and 62 to 71, and by 33% of those finally aged 72 to 77; a further 5%, 22%, and 33% respectively, of those in these three age ranges ceased intercourse during the same period. In the men followed up, as in the women, frequency of sexual intercourse remained stable over the 6 years in the majority of those finally aged 52 to 71; it was also stable in 42% of men finally aged 72 to 77. No activity was reported from the commencement of the period of the study by 0%, 9%, and 12% of men finally aged 52 to 61, 62 to 71, and 72 to 77 respectively, and a further 5%, 7%, and 18% of men in these age groups ceased activity. Cessation of sexual activity in the 66% of women and 30% of men finally aged 72 to 77 in this study of economically advantaged married subjects could be in part a cohort effect, as the follow-up was only over 6 years. As Marsiglio and Donnelly (1991) pointed out in their report of what they believed was the first nationally representative data on the sexual frequency patterns of elderly persons, this effect can only be assessed when future representative data become available.

Importance of an Established Partner for Sexual Activity in Older Women

Pfeiffer and colleagues (1972) reported 97 women and 35 men who gave reasons for why they ceased sexual relations: 90% of the women attributed responsibility for stopping intercourse to absence of a spouse due to death, separation, or divorce, or to his illness or inability to perform sexually. Seventy-one percent of the 35 men who reported cessation of intercourse accepted that they were responsible due to illness, loss of interest, or inability to perform sexually. Regression analysis showed a number of factors to be associated with reduced current sexual activity in men (Pfeiffer & Davis, 1972). These included less past sexual activity, age, poor health status, lower social class, taking of antihypertensive medication, and reduced life satisfaction. Markedly fewer factors were associated with reduced sexual activity in women, but accounted for a greater percentage of the total variance than did the larger number of factors in men. Those for women were principally no intact marriage and age. Less education, being unemployed, and postmenopausal status made small contributions. As could be expected, in their 6-year follow-up of the subjects studied by Pfeiffer and colleagues (1972), George and Weiler (1981) reported that both the (married) men and women overwhelmingly attributed cessation of sexual relations to attitudes or physical condition of the male partner. They considered this testified to the importance of the man's role as initiator of sexual behavior among current cohorts of middle-aged and older adults. Findings supporting this conclusion were reported by Persson and Svanborg (1992). Of 25 men who ceased having sexual intercourse with their wives between the ages of 70 and 75, 21 attributed cessation to factors in themselves: lack of ability in 8, own illness in 4, and loss of interest in 9. Bretschneider and McCoy (1988) investigated by anonymous questionnaire 202 upper-middle-class White men and women, aged 80 to 102, living in retirement facilities for the healthy elderly, none of whom were taking regular medication. One of the six most frequently experienced sexual problems reported by 30% of women was their partner's inability to achieve or maintain erection. Lack of sexual interest was reported by 25% of the women but was not one of the six most common problems of men. Despite the women, in Pfeiffer and colleagues' (1972) study considering absence of an effective partner responsible for cessation of intercourse, they reported a much greater reduction of sexual interest in relation to their age than did the men. A quarter of women in their 50s and 50% in their 60s reported no sexual interest; corresponding figures for men in these two age ranges were less than 5% and 10%. It would seem that in the absence of an effective partner many women lose sexual interest and cease all sexual activity. The importance of an intact marriage in maintaining women's sexual activity, that is, partnered sex or masturbation, was demonstrated in Brecher's (1984) questionnaire investigation of 4,246 men and women 50 to over 70 years of age who were above average in education, health and income. The percentages of married women who were sexually active were 95, 89 and 81 for the age ranges 50 to 59, 60 to 69 and 70 and over; percentages of sexually active unmarried women of the same ages were 88, 63, and 50. Equivalent percentages for married and unmarried men were 98, 93, and 81, and 95, 85, and 75.

Although the relationship of marriage and sexual activity does not appear to have been investigated in representative population samples of older people, fewer unmarried as compared with married women must have reported having sexual activity to account for disparities in the percentages of subjects reporting no partnered sexual activity in the representative studies of married subjects reported by Marsiglio and Donnelly (1991) and of the total population reported by Laumann and colleagues (1994). In the former study, of the 66% who answered the question, 35%, 45%, 55%, and 76% respectively of those aged 61 to 65, 66 to 70, 71 to 75, and 76 or older reported they had not had sex with their spouse in the past month. The percentage of women stating they had not had sex was only slightly less than that of the men, consistent with the authors' statement that any time a husband has sex a wife also will be having sex. Laumann and colleagues reported for comparable age ranges that 45%, 60%, 75%, and 80% of women and 16%, 25%, 40%, and 45% of men reported no partnered sexual activity in the past year. Laumann and colleagues also reported that by the age of 60, more than 20% of men and women report frequencies of a few times a year. Hence, a significant number of these subjects would be included in Marsiglio and Donnelly's (1991) but not in Laumann and colleagues' (1994) study as not having sex. Despite Laumann and colleagues' study including this 20% of women in the percentage having partnered sex, it still found a much higher percentage of married and unmarried women combined not having partnered sex than did Marsiglio and Donnelly's (1991) study of married women only.

Inclusion in Marsiglio and Donnelly's (1991) study of many of the men having partnered sex a few times a year in the percentage of men not having it would account for their finding a higher percentage of married men not having partnered sex than the married and single men in Laumann and colleagues' (1994) study. Not allowing for their different treatment of men having partnered sex a few times a year, the findings of the two studies would indicate that a higher percentage of unmarried than married older men had partnered sex. Allowing for the different treatment, the findings still indicate that marriage is not a major factor determining maintenance of partnered sex in older men. Evidence that marriage is a major determinant of partnered sex in older women but not men was also found in a Swedish study of 70-year-old subjects cited by Bretschneider and McCoy (1988); 46% of the men and 14% of the women were sexually active; only 2% of the unmarried women but 36% of married women and 52% of married men reported having sexual intercourse. Commenting on the dearth of older unmarried men compared to women, Brecher (1984) pointed out that official figures in the United States at the time were that for people over 50 years of age there were 2.7 unmarried women for every unmarried man, and for those 65 or older, the figures were 3.3 for one. He added that these figures seriously underestimated the problem. More unmarried men than women were already involved (in his study 57% of men compared to 33% of women had a regular sexual partner); and more considered themselves homosexual (10% compared to 1% of unmarried women in his study). Applying these percentages to the official figures, Brecher concluded that there were five unattached heterosexual women for every unattached heterosexual man in his subjects over 50 years of age. The unmarried women's regular male partners were mainly married or much older or both; those of unmarried men were mainly much younger women. Von Sydow (1995) investigated use of what she termed unconventional relationships by 91 German women aged 50 to 91 to compensate for the shortage of single male partners. Nine were in such relationships, one with a woman, four with younger men, and four with men living with their wives. She found the women in the relationships had been in similar relationships when younger so there was little evidence that they had adopted these patterns as solutions to the dilemma of being elderly and without an appropriate male partner.

Additional differences between the sexes reflecting men's greater sexual opportunities were Brecher's (1984) finding that of unmarried subjects 34% of men and 13% of women had had sex with one or more casual partners in the previous year, and older men were presumed more likely than women to have sex with prostitutes. Of the 2,402 men he investigated 34% reported experiences with female prostitutes prior to age 50, and 7% since, 2.5% in the last year. Brecher suggested that low use of female prostitutes by men in part resulted from their ability to find voluntary women partners. Older homosexual men may be less able to find suitable voluntary partners; 20% of the 86 men in his study who reported homosexual activity since the age of 50 had used male prostitutes. Women respondents were not asked about activities with prostitutes. Johnson, Wadsworth, Wellings, Field, and Bradshaw (1994) in their 60% representative sample of British men and women aged 16 to 59 found that the odds ratio for payment of women by men for sex increased rapidly with age and was significantly more likely for men who were cohabitees, widowed, separated, or divorced than for married men. Pfeiffer and Davis (1972) considered the remedy for the lack of sexual partners for older women to lie in efforts to prolong the vigor and life span of men.

Sexual Activities Apart from Intercourse

Although frequency of sexual activities apart from intercourse have been investigated in older persons it is not clear to what extent they are employed as substitutes when intercourse ceases due to inability or absence of a partner. Studies frequently do not adequately define terms leaving it uncertain, for example, whether masturbation is carried out alone, with a partner watching, or as mutual masturbation, whether sexual activity includes unpartnered masturbation, and whether partnered sexual activity requires penetrative intercourse. Reiss (1995) pointed out, in regard to the survey by Laumann and colleagues (1994), that the definition of sexual activity used specified that it did not require that intercourse or orgasm occur. However, subjects were given the definition after completing a questionnaire containing questions about sexual activity, but before a face-to-face interview. Yet very few differences were found in the number of partners reported in the two procedures, causing Reiss to conclude that the subjects were not following the definition in the interview and were ignoring partners with whom they had only genital petting. The issue is of importance in regard to the sexuality of the elderly, as many therapists encourage them to adopt other sexual practices when they cannot maintain penetrative intercourse.

Of the 202 advantaged subjects investigated by Bretschneider and McCoy (1988), 53% percent of the men and 25% of the women said they had at least one regular sex partner, including the 29% of men and 14% of women who were married. Of those with partners, 82% of the men and 64% of the women were at least mildly happy with them as lovers. Seventy percent of all the men and 50% of all the women fantasized or daydreamed often or very often about being close, affectionate, and intimate with the opposite sex. Forty-seven percent of the women and 22% of the men considered sex of no importance. Touching and caressing without sexual intercourse was the most common activity for men (83%) and women (64%), then masturbation for men (72%) and women (40%), followed by sexual intercourse for men (62%) and women (30%). Masturbation, as investigated in this study, was presumably not a partnered activity. Genital petting was assessed separately, and many of the subjects did not answer concerning masturbation, the percentage reported being based on the answers of those who did. Frequency of the activities investigated correlated positively, suggesting that none was a substitute for others. Current frequency and enjoyment of the activities was less than in the past, reduction being most marked in relation to intercourse and least marked in relation to masturbation.

Brecher (1984) reported anecdotal evidence of men and women aged 50 and over using masturbation, at times with vibrators, when penetrative intercourse became impossible, but did no report of the percentage who did so as part of sexual activity with a partner. More single than married subjects in his study masturbated presumably alone: 63% versus 52% of men and 54% versus 36% of women. The most frequent reason given was absence of an acceptable partner. Incidence declined with age from 66% of men and 47% of women in their 50s to 43% of men and 33% of women 70 and older, indicating that most women and men do not use masturbation to compensate for cessation of coitus. The percentage of women and men having sex with their spouses declined from 88% to 65% and 87% to 59%, respectively, for those in the same age ranges. The mean frequency in subjects who continued masturbation declined from 1.2 to 0.7 per week in men but remained the same in women in these age ranges; Brecher commented that it was the only one of the measures of sexual activity reported that did not show a decade-by-decade decline. He did not report the relationship of the use of masturbation to cessation of coitus. However, of his 38 women subjects aged 80 and over, sexual intercourse was reported by 3, other partnered sexual activity by a further 2, and unpartnered sexual activity, pre-sumably masturbation, by 10. Of his 76 male subjects, sexual intercourse was reported by 25, other partnered sexual activity by a further 4, and nonpartnered sexual activity by 17; 29 said they masturbated, presumably including 12 of those having partnered sex Brecher reported that an unstated percentage of men with erectile difficulty used "stuffing," inserting the inadequately erect penis into the vagina. He considered his subjects' use of sexual fantasy and sexually explicit material as countermeasures to the decline in sexuality with aging. Use of sexual fantasy was reported by 89% and 61% of his male and 74% and 52% of his female subjects during masturbation and partnered sex, respectively. The content was stated to include homosexual and "ego-alien" material. Use of sex-ually explicit reading material and hard-core pornographic films or photos was reported respectively by 37% and 18% of the women and 56% and 42% of the men. These prevalence figures are in the same range as those found in younger subjects (McConaghy, 1993), so that use of these stimuli as a continuation of earlier practices would need to be excluded before it can be accepted that they are adopted as compensatory by older people.

A Danish questionnaire study, mainly of men aged 51 to 95, found that only 3% of those in their 90s reported having coitus, although 28% had part-ners and 35% reported that they were still interested in sex (Hegeler & Mortensen, 1978). Prevalence of cessation of coitus with age increased more rapidly after the age of 70. Prevalence of cessation of masturbation increased more slowly; it was reported by 60% of men aged 51 to 55 years and 23% of those aged 90 to 95 "confessed" to its use. A further 31% in that age group did not answer concerning masturbation; the authors interpreted comments made as indicating that considerable guilt still existed about masturbation, suggesting the masturbation assessed was not a partnered activity. In their investigation of healthy married men, Weizman and Hart (1987) found that 51% of those aged 66 to 71, but only 27% of those aged 60 to 65 reported masturbation; 26% of the older and 9% of the younger men masturbated more than four times a month. Intercourse was reported by 64% of both groups, 64% of the younger and 47% of the older men reporting frequencies of more than four times a month. The re-lationship of presence and frequency of masturbation and intercourse was not reported, but the authors assumed that they were negatively related. As stated previously, Bretschneider and McCoy (1988) found them positively related in their study of older persons, as did Martin (1981) in 188 mostly White well-educated married men aged 60 to 79 years who had volunteered for a Baltimore study of aging.

Masturbation was reported by 37%, 33%, 29%, and 8%, respectively, of 91 German women of slightly above average education in the four age ranges from 50 to 59 through 80 to 91; the reduction in prevalence somewhat paralleled that of intercourse, which was 74%, 23%, 21% and 0% of subjects in the same age ranges (von Sydow, 1995). The author did not comment as to what extent masturbation was a continuation of its earlier use rather than compensatory for the decline in intercourse. Leiblum, Bachmann, Kemmann, Colburn, and Swartzman (1983) reported of the 52 postmenopausal women aged 50 to 65, that those having intercourse three or more times monthly masturbated more frequently than those having intercourse less than ten times yearly. They also had higher frequencies of giving and receiving manual and oral genital stimulation.

In Martin's (1981) study, coitus and masturbation in the past year was reported by 93% and 32%, respectively, of the sexually most active men, and by 40% and 17%, respectively, of the sexually least active. However, on the basis of their assumption of a negative relationship between frequency of coitus and masturbation, Weizman and Hart (1987) concluded that with advanced age interest in sexuality continues but the form of sexual expression changes from active sexual intercourse to masturbation even with the availability of the same partner. They attributed at least part of the change to decline in social status and self-confidence in masculinity due to retirement. All the younger men were working full-time and all the older men were retired. A possible influence of increased leisure time associated with retirement on the use of masturbation was not considered and indeed does not seem to have been explored in relation to the sexual activity of the elderly. Of the 60–85-year-old subjects investigated by Adams and Turner (1985), masturbation was reported by 46% and 56%, respectively, of the unmarried women and men and 13% and 16% of the married women and men. Adams and Turner found that in men, but not women, masturbation represented a continuation from their earlier life; the authors concluded that the older women's sexuality was more plastic. Their figure of 16% of elderly married men reporting masturbation was considerably below that of the studies reviewed previously, which were all of subjects of above-average health and socioeconomic level. Their subjects may have been more representative of the total population in these respects. Laumann and colleagues (1994) found that percentages of subjects in their representative sample who reported privately masturbating at least once a week in the previous year declined from about 30 in the younger men to about 12 in those aged 50 to 59; and from about 10 in the younger women to 2.4 in those aged 50 to 59. The percentage reporting not masturbating at all over the past year fell from 41% and 64% of the youngest men and women to 28% of men aged 30 to 34 and 50% of women aged 40 to 44, to rise again to 50% of men and more than 70% of women aged 50 to 59. Although the relationship with socioeconomic status as a whole was not reported there was a strong positive relationship of level of education and use and frequency of masturbation. Like Bretschneider and McCoy's (1988) study of upper- middle-class subjects aged 80 to 102, that of Laumann and colleagues (1994) found little evidence that masturbation was used as a substitute for intercourse. This was also the case in the 60–85-year-old subjects who reported change in their preferred sexual activity from the age of 20–30 (B. F. Turner & Adams, 1988). Of the 26 who ceased to prefer heterosexual intercourse, only 4 preferred masturbation; 15 selected petting, 3, dreaming, 2, daydreaming, 1, homosexual activity, and 1, other activity. An interesting finding in Brecher's (1984) study of advantaged subjects 50 years and older was that 61% of women but only 18% of men reported higher frequencies of experiencing orgasm with masturbation than with partnered sex, 16% of women and 26% of men reported the reverse, and the remaining 24% of women and 56% of men reported the same frequencies for the two activities. If replicated, the finding indicates that at least older women experience orgasm more readily with masturbation than with partnered sex. It might seem that this would encourage older women to use masturbation if partnered sex is unavailable, but this is contrary to the evidence discussed. Their failure to do so is consistent with the conclusion that women's sexuality is much more dependent than is men's on the existence of an emotional relationship with a partner (McConaghy, 1993).

Health and Socioeconomic Status and Partnered Sex

Bretschneider and McCoy (1988) concluded that people experienced a small steady increase in loss of interest in sex and cessation of intercourse from their late 40s, an increase which continued in men into their 90s, but ceased in women after they reached the age of 80. They reached this conclusion from comparison of their subjects aged 80 to 102 with the 66–71-year-old subjects of Pfeiffer and colleagues (1972). Percentages of older women without interest in sex or who were not having intercourse (about 45% and 70%, respectively) were the same or less than those of the younger women, whereas equivalent percentages of older men (about 20% and 37% respectively) were higher than those of the younger men. Bretschneider and McCoy (1988) further concluded that the major decline in sexual activity occurred in women in their late 50s and early 60s and could be related to the menopause and the associated fall in hormone levels. Their conclusions, based on a possibly invalid comparison of these two groups of nonrepresentative subjects who were above average in health and socioeconomic advantage, were not supported by Brecher (1984). He found prevalence of any sexual activity in 38 women and 76 men aged 80 and over was 39% and 61%, respectively lower than the equivalent prevalences of 65% and 79% in his subjects aged 70 and over, which in turn were lower than the prevalences of 81% and 91% in those in their 60s, and 93% and 98% of those in their 50s. The sexual activity of the 80–102-year-old subjects investigated by Bretschneider and McCoy (1988) was higher than that of comparably aged subjects studied by Brecher (1984). In the former study 62% of the men and 30% of the women reported having sexual intercourse, compared with 33% of men and 8% of women aged 80 or more investigated by Brecher, and 72% of men and 40% of the women reported masturbation, compared with 43% of men and 33% of women aged 70 and older in Brecher's study. Although the subjects in both groups were advantaged in health and socioeconomic status compared with the normal population, the degree of advantage may have been greater in those studied by Bretschneider and McCoy (1988). Certainly Bretschneider and McCoy's findings in regard to sexual activity of older persons cannot be generalized. Percentages of their healthy subjects who maintained partnered sexual activity after the age of 80 was markedly higher than those of the representative sample reported by Laumann and colleagues (1994), which were 45% of men and 5% of women. Of 250 residents of nursing homes in Texas whose mean age was greater than 80, 91% were sexually inactive; that is, they had not masturbated or had intercourse in the previous month (White, 1982). All were able to be interviewed in that they could give valid responses to a mental status questionnaire and to the interview questions; about two thirds were women. Of the sexually inactive, 17% said they would be interested in being sexually active but lacked opportunity, having no partner or lacking privacy.

In contrast to the findings of higher frequencies of sexual activity in groups of healthy as compared to less healthy older persons, Brecher (1984) reported that when the effect of age was statistically controlled for, the decade-by-decade increase in impaired health of his subjects had only a weak relationship with the parallel decline observed in most measures of sexual activity. His finding could have resulted from the limited range of degree of health of the subjects, which was better than average. This explanation would not account for Marsiglio and Donnelly's (1991) finding, in their study of a representative population sample of subjects more than 60 years of age, that regression analysis demonstrated a relationship with the spouse's but not the subject's health and the likelihood of their engaging in sex; the health of neither was related to frequency. Subjects assessed their health in relation to that of others of their age. This may be a poor measure of subjects' actual level of health. Johnson and colleagues (1994), using a similar question, found only a moderate relationship between health and age in their subjects aged 16 to 59; of those with health problems more than one in five considered their health good. They found a weak relationship between reduced frequency of heterosexual intercourse and poor health. Laumann and colleagues (1994) asked their subjects whether they would say their health was excellent, good, fair, or poor. They found a strong relationship between their subjects' health on this measure and their interest in having sex. Also 43% of 60–80-year-old men and women who reported very good health stated that sexuality was important to them, significantly more than the 15% stating this who reported bad physical health (Bergstrom-Walan & Nielsen, 1990).

It would seem that although older middle-aged women report less sexual interest and activity than younger ones, the difference in the majority of the healthy and socially advantaged is not great. They can expect their sexual interest and frequency of coitus to remain relatively unchanged into their 60s provided they have an active sexual partner, although some will experience a reduced ability to enjoy sexual activity or reach orgasm The decline in frequency of coitus in these women during and following their 60s appears to be largely determined by reduced ability or interest or loss of their male partners.

Biological Factors and Sexual Activity

Biological factors may play a larger role in the decline in sexuality with age in men as compared with women. Martin (1981) investigated possible reasons for the different levels of sexual interest and activity in 188 well-educated married men aged 60 to 79. Twenty-six percent had not experienced marital coitus for at least a year. Combining frequency of coitus, masturbation, nocturnal emissions, and homosexual activity, Martin found this measure of sexual expression was independent of marital adjustment, sexual attractiveness of wives, and sexual attitudes, but strongly related to the subjects' reported frequency of sexual behaviors from the age of 20. The relationship of current and earlier levels of sexual activity was also found in men in their 40s or older in studies Martin reviewed, including that of Pfeiffer and Davis (1972). When the men in Martin's (1981) study were asked if they would seek treatment to obtain greater sexual vigor if such treatment were possible, 29% of the least and 31% of the most sexually active men said they would do so. Martin concluded that the finding that the large majority of his subjects were well satisfied with the current sexual situation was compatible with the observation that their decline in sexual functioning with age resulted from a corresponding decline in motivation, and the finding that most respondents had maintained comparatively high or low rates of activity over a large part of their lives suggested they did so because of characteristic differences in level of motivation. These differences could result in part from biological determinants. White (1982) reported a relationship in 250 nursing home residents, of whom about two thirds were female, between their reported frequency of feeling sexually aroused and of sexual intercourse, but not of masturbation, with their self-assessment of level of sexual activity throughout life. However, Pfeiffer and Davis (1972) did not find a relationship between frequency of sexual activity in early and later life in women. Also, Martin pointed out that Christenson and Gagnon (1965) found that women in their 50s and 60s who were married to older men were much less active sexually than women married to younger men.

Tsitouras, Martin, and Harman (1982) investigated 183 men aged 60 to 79 years who were part of the Baltimore longitudinal study on aging and were of above-average health. They found the usual reduction in sexual activity with increased age but no reduction in total testosterone levels. Tsitouras and colleagues cited other studies that also found no reduction in testosterone levels of healthy older men and suggested that when it was found it was due to such accompanying factors as obesity, alcoholism, chronic disease, and stress (all of which were known to affect the level of the hormone). Although Tsitouras and colleagues found a relationship between their subjects' testosterone levels and amount of coital and masturbatory activity, it was much less than the relationship of the level of these activities with age. Testosterone levels did not show a significant relationship with their subjects' erectile ability, consistent with the evidence that reduction of levels of total testosterone to 30% of subjects' previous levels reduces sexual interest but not erectile ability (McConaghy, 1993). In a contrasting finding to that of Tsitouras and colleagues (1982), Korenman and colleagues (1990) found that healthy and sexually potent men (mean age 65) showed significantly lower levels of total and bioavailable testosterone compared to 57 healthy potent men aged 20 to 44. Using limits of 10.5 and 2.3 nmol/L for the total and bioavailable testosterone assessments, respectively (2.5 *SD* below the means of the younger men), 24% and 48% of the older men were hormonally hypogonadal. Korenman and colleagues did not report their subjects' sexual interest and activity levels. Chambers and Phoenix (1982) pointed out that the decline in the sexual performance of aging males is a general phenomenon found in several different mammalian species, including rodents, farm animals, and nonhuman primates, as well as in human beings. They noted that decline in aged rhesus monkeys could not be attributed to reduction in testosterone levels, as there is no change in these levels with age.

SPECIFIC SEXUAL DYSFUNCTIONS

DSM-IV Classification

As classified in the *Diagnostic and Statistical Manual of Mental Disorders* (*DSM-IV*; American Psychiatric Association, 1994) the sexual dysfunctions include the Sexual Desire Disorders of Hypoactive Sexual Desire and Sexual Aversion; the Sexual Arousal Disorders of Female Sexual Arousal Disorder, inability to attain or maintain an adequate genital lubrication-swelling response of sexual excitement until completion of sexual activity, and Male Erectile Disorder; the Orgasm Disorders of Female and Male Orgasmic Disorders and Premature Ejaculation; and the Sexual Pain Disorders of Dyspareunia, genital pain in either males or females before, during, or after sexual intercourse, and Vaginismus (involuntary spasm of the musculature of the outer third of the vagina that interferes with sexual intercourse). To receive the diagnosis of sexual disorder in these four categories, *DSM-IV* criterion A requires that the condition be recurrent or persistent, and criterion B that the disturbance causes marked distress or interpersonal difficulty. Criterion B presumably allows absence of orgasmic capacity to not be considered a dysfunction in at least some of the women in many surveys who reported that they enjoyed intercourse very much although they did not reach orgasm (McConaghy, 1993). The various criteria comprising A instruct the clinician to take into account such factors as the person's age, adequacy in focus, intensity, and duration of the sexual experience, and the novelty of the sexual partner or situation. However, the criterion gives no operationally defined guidelines as to how to take these factors into account, making it unlikely that the reliability of the diagnoses made by different clinicians using these criteria will be high.

Prevalence

Information concerning prevalence of sexual dysfunctions in representative groups of older subjects is limited; few studies of the prevalence of sexual disorders in the adult population have been undertaken; and those that have been tended to use different diagnostic criteria and exclude older subjects. Laumann and colleagues (1994) asked their 18–59-year-old subjects whether in the previous

12 months there had ever been a period of several months or more when they experienced particular sexual dysfunctions. There was a marked difference between prevalences of lack of interest in sex and inability to achieve orgasm in (1) representative American women subjects surveyed, (2) the representative sample of Swedish women living with their husbands or other partners in whom Hallstrom (1979) investigated prevalence of total inability to achieve orgasm, and (3) in Hallstrom and Samuelsson's (1990) investigation of prevalence of absence of sexual desire. Prevalence of both dysfunctions in the Swedish women showed a marked increase with age in those older than 46. In the American women prevalence of orgasmic dysfunction showed no clear relationship with age, and that of having trouble lubricating reduced until age 45, after which it showed a moderate increase, which remained at relatively the same level over the age range 45 to 59. Also, prevalences in the Swedish women aged 38 and those aged 46 of absence of desire (3%–4%) and anorgasmia (10%–12%) were much lower than those in women aged 35 to 44 in Laumann and colleagues' (1994) study (36% and 23% respectively). These findings seem related to prevalences in older women showing a marked increase in the Swedish study but remaining relatively unchanged in the American study. The disparities seem too great to have resulted from the fact that all the Swedish women were partnered; 29% of the married women in Laumann and colleagues' study reported lack of interest and 22% reported inability to achieve orgasm. The disparities also seem unexplained by differences in the eliciting questions. Laumann and colleagues (1994) asked about a period of several months or more in the past 12 months, and Hallstrom and Samuelsson (1990) about present experience. The Swedish women were representative of the population of an industrial town, again a difference that seems unlikely to explain the disparities. They could reflect cultural differences in the assessment of sexual activities. Osborn, Hawton, and Gath (1988) investigated percentage of women aged 35 to 59 years registered with two general practices in England, who reported impaired sexual interest and anorgasmia in partnered sexual activity in the past 3 months. They reported a prevalence more similar to that found by Hallstrom and Samuelsson (1990), though onset of its increase was more gradual and commenced earlier from the age of 40. The dearth of studies of the prevalence of dysfunctions in representative samples of older people clearly requires correction to clarify the causes of disparities in those studies available.

Laumann and colleagues (1994) found that lack of interest in having sex, not finding sex pleasurable, being unable to come to a climax, and experiencing physical pain during intercourse were reported by a much higher percentage of women than men in all age ranges. Coming to a climax too quickly and feeling anxious about their ability to perform sexually was reported by more men than women. Having trouble achieving or maintaining an erection was reported by fewer younger, but the same percentage of older men as the percentage of women reporting having trouble lubricating. Erectile difficulty was the dysfunction in men that showed the clearest relationships to age. It was reported by as many as 10% of men aged 18 to 49 but 21% of men aged 50 to 59. Its prevalence in most studies of men selected for health or who were socioeconomically advantaged was little different. Rates in the largely healthy men investigated by Kinsey, Pomeroy, and Martin (1948) were 1% at 30, 2% at 40, 7% at 50, 18% at 60, 27% at 70, 55% at 75, and 76% at 80 years of age. Of men above average in health and in a stable relationship, 23% of those aged 55 to 64 and 32% of those aged 65 to 74 reported difficulty in achieving vaginal insertion in 50% or more of coital attempts in the preceding 6 months (Schiavi, Schreiner-Engel, Mandeli, Schanzer, & Cohen, 1990); 36% of healthy happily married men aged 60 to 71 reported absence of erection during sexual activity (Weizman & Hart, 1987). Inability to attain an erection was present in 28% and inability to maintain an erection in 33% of upper-middle-class men aged 80 to 102 (Bretschneider & McCoy, 1988). The percentage with one or the other was not given. Lack of spontaneous erections during day or night was reported by 65% of men in Weizman and Hart's (1987) study. It was not stated whether such lack included difficulty in achieving erection without manual stimulation of the penis during sexual activity with a partner, a difficulty increasingly experienced by men after the age of about 50 (Brecher, 1984). Its prevalence does not appear to have been specifically documented. Other erectile changes in men aged 50 and over were longer refractory period, taking longer to get erections, erections less rigid, and more frequent loss of erection during sex, reported respectively by 65%, 50%, 44%, and 32% of Brecher's subjects. Brecher also pointed out that ejaculation may be less forceful with fewer contractions and reduction in amount of ejaculate. Men concerned about such changes need to be informed that they are normal aspects of aging.

Despite impairment of the genital lubrication-swelling response of women being regarded as the sexual arousal disorder equivalent to erectile dysfunction in men, its prevalence has been less frequently investigated so that there is little evidence to determine whether it is lower in subjects who are more healthy than those representative of the total population. However, it is established that its prevalence increases with age. Having trouble lubricating was reported by 21% to 24% of the representative sample of women in the age ranges 45 to 59, higher than the percentage of younger women reporting the problem (Laumann et al., 1994). Osborn and colleagues (1988) reported that the prevalence of vaginal dryness in English women attending two general practices increased steadily from 8% in women aged 35 to 39 to 26% in women aged 50 to 54, and then reduced to 22% in women aged 55 to 59. It was one of the most common six problems in advantaged women aged 80 to 102, being reported by 30% (Bretschneider & McCoy, 1988). The percentage of advantaged women studied by Brecher (1984) who reported "about the right amount" of vaginal lubrication during sexual arousal decreased from 48% of those in their 50s to 23% of those aged 70 and over.

Prevalence of inability to orgasm showed no relation with age in men and a small decline in women in a representative sample of subjects in the United States aged 18 to 59 (Laumann et al., 1994). It was present in just over 10%, just under 10%, 15%, and 25% of women aged 38, 46, 50, and 54, of the representative sample of partnered Swedish women (Hallstrom, 1979). As discussed earlier, the much higher prevalence of inability to achieve orgasm in younger women in the former compared to those in the latter study could account for opposite trends that the two studies reported in the relationship of the prevalence of anorgasmia to age in women. The decline in orgasmic ability with age found in the Swedish study was also found in studies of nonrepresentative samples whether or not selected for health and socioeconomic advantage. In English women attending general practitioners anorgasmia in partnered sexual activity in the past 3 months was present in 5%, 8%, 14%, 21%, and 35%, respectively, in the five age ranges from 35 to 39 through 53 to 59 (Hawton *et al.*, 1994). The percentage always reaching orgasm declined steadily from 24% to 12% over the same age range. Degree of ability to regularly reach orgasm reported by male veterans was over 80%, 72%, 61%, 48%, 40%, and 21%, in those aged 30 to 49, 50 to 59, 60 to 69, 70 to 79, 80 to 89, and 90 to 99, respectively (Mulligan & Moss, 1991). This dysfunction was one of the six most frequent problems of the advantaged subjects aged 80 to 102 with regular partners studied by Bretschneider and McCoy (1988), being experienced by 30% of women and 28% of men. These percentages were higher compared with the 22% of women and 9% of men aged 55 to 59 years who had the dysfunction in Laumann colleagues (1994) study, but comparable for women with the 35% of partnered women aged 55 to 59 years reporting anorgasmia who saw two general practitioners (Hawton *et al.*, 1994). The advantaged subjects investigated by Brecher (1984) reported a lower prevalence of anorgasmia than the subjects of the same age more representative of the total population investigated in the studies mentioned. In Brecher's study only 1% of men and 19% of women aged 50 to 59 reported seldom or never reaching orgasm in partnered sex; the percentages rose to 10 and 28, respectively, in those aged 70 and over. Seldom or never experiencing orgasm with masturbation was reported by fewer women but more men: 7% and 14% women and 4% and 13%, respectively, of men in these two age ranges. It appears that orgasmic ability is maintained at a higher level in the more healthy elderly compared to subjects of the same age more representative of the general population.

Prevalence of lack of interest in sex showed a slightly stronger increase with age in the male compared to the female subjects studied by Laumann and colleagues (1994). It was reported by about 35% of women aged 35 to 59 compared with about 31% of women aged 18 to 34 and about 22% of men aged 50 to 59 compared with about 16% of men aged 18 to 49. A marked increase in prevalence with age in women was found by Hallstrom and Samuelsson (1990). Absence of desire was reported by 4%, 3%, 9%, and 21%, and at 6-year follow-up by 0%, 7%, 16%, and 29% of their representative sample of partnered Swedish women finally aged 44, 52, 56, and 60. Prevalence of impaired sexual interest increased with age in the partnered English women who attended two general practices who were studied by Hawton and colleagues (1994), from 4% in those aged 35 to 39 to 28% of those aged 50 to 59. Of the American advantaged subjects studied by Pfeiffer and colleagues (1972) and Brecher (1984), no sexual interest was reported by 0%, 3%, and 11% of men and 7%, 25%, and 50% of women aged 46 to 50, 51 to 60, and 61 to 71, respectively, in the former study, and by 1%, 2%, and 8% of the men and 4%, 10%, and 18% of the women in their 50s, 60s, and 70s, respectively, in the latter study. Lack of interest was reported by 25% of women but not mentioned as one of their six most common problems by men in an American advantaged group aged 80 to 102 investigated by Bretschneider and McCoy (1988). Sexual interest was consistently higher in the advantaged men than those of the same age more representative of the normal population. A similar trend for women was present in the studies of Bretschneider and McCoy and Brecher (1984) but not that of Pfeiffer and colleagues (1972).

Laumann and colleagues (1994) found that the percentage of women reporting climaxing too early declined with age from 14% of those 18 to 24 to 8% of those 55 to 59, whereas percentage of men reporting this increased with age from 27% to 35% for the same age groups. Brecher (1984) reported statements of a number of men 50 to 70 years and greater that they had ceased to suffer from premature ejaculation, but commented that aging was not always a cure for the condition and that "a few of our old men continue to be afflicted with it" (p. 324). Only 3 of the 188 advantaged men aged 60 to 79 in Martin's study (1981) reported that premature ejaculation was recently a problem.

Percentages of women and men surveyed by Laumann and colleagues (1994) reporting anxiety about performance reduced markedly with age, from 18 to 4 of women and 21 to 11 of men in the age ranges 18 to 24 to 55 to 59 respectively. In advantaged subjects aged 80 to 102 fear of poor performance was not one of the six most common sexual problems reported by women, but it was the most common in men, being reported by 37% (Bretschneider & McCoy, 1988). The much higher prevalence in the advantaged men was presumably related in part to the prevalence of erectile dysfunction, reported by 33%, compared with 21% of the 55–59-year-old men in Laumann and colleagues' (1994) study. However, the marked difference in prevalence of performance anxiety suggests that many more advantaged men are concerned about their reduced function than are those representative of the normal population. This behavior is consistent with that of Martin's (1981) subjects, which led him to the conclusion referred to earlier, that many older men were comfortable with their reduced level of sexual activity.

Laumann and colleagues (1994) found prevalences of pain during sex and not finding sex pleasurable showed consistent and marked decreases with age in women, from 21% to 8% and 27% to 16% respectively, of those aged 18 to 24 and 50 to 59. Hawton and colleagues (1994) reported a contrary trend in English women seeing general practitioners as to prevalence of not finding sex pleasurable. The percentage who considered making love with a partner unpleasant on all occasions in the preceding 3 months increased with age from 1.1% of those aged 35 to 39 to 11.3% of those aged 55 to 59. Over the ages of 18 to 59 the men in the study by Laumann and colleagues (1994) reported prevalences of pain during sex ranging from 1.9% to 5.7% and of not finding sex pleasurable ranging from 5.6% to 9.7%. Neither prevalence showed a clear relationship with age, although that of pain during sex was highest in the youngest and oldest groups: 5.7% of those aged 18 to 24 and 4.6% in those aged 55 to 59. These two sexual dysfunctions do not appear to have been investigated in studies of subjects above average in health.

It would appear that in subjects of the same age superior health may result in lower incidence of orgasmic difficulties and, particularly in men, of loss of sexual interest, but not of erectile dysfunction or lack of vaginal lubrication. It does not prevent the incidence of all these dysfunctions increasing with age. A direct relationship between poor health and the prevalence of sexual dysfunctions was reported by Laumann and colleagues (1994). Seven percent of their subjects aged 18 to 24 but 25% of those aged 55 to 59 reported their health to be fair or poor. Those who reported this were much more likely also to report having at least one of the seven sexual problems investigated. The relationship was much stronger in men. Although women in fair or poor health reported higher prevalence of all the problems than did women in excellent health, the difference was never more than twice as great. Few men reported poor health, but prevalence of all the problems in those with fair health was up to four times greater than those in excellent health. Hence, although prevalence of erectile dysfunction or lack of vaginal lubrication was not found to be reduced in subjects selected for greater health compared with people of the same age more representative of the normal population, within the latter group a clear relationship was found between the subjects' self-assessed health status and the prevalence of both dysfunctions.

Sexual Dysfunctions and Sexual Satisfaction

The lack of relationship between sexual dysfunctions and sexual satisfaction found in younger adults (McConaghy, 1993) also has been found in older subjects. Schiavi and colleagues (1990) commented that advantaged 45–74-year-old men in stable relationships, although they reported decrease in several functional dimensions of male sexuality with age, also reported that their enjoyment of marital sex and their satisfaction with their own sexuality did not change. Male-partnered women aged 35 to 59 seeing two general practitioners in England reported reduced frequency of orgasm but no decrease in their sexual satisfaction with increasing age; strangely, this occurred despite the fact that increasing age was associated with a higher percentage of women reporting more occasions on which sexual activity was unpleasant and fewer occasions on which it was enjoyed (Hawton *et al.*, 1994). As many women at times prefer tender caressing to intercourse (McConaghy, 1993), the satisfaction of the older women may have been maintained by the caressing accompanying their sexual activity. Multivariate analysis revealed that their marital adjustment made the major contribution to their reports of sexual activity being pleasant and of sexual satisfaction. Brecher (1984) found that 90% of husbands and wives 50 years of age and over who were having intercourse, and 67% of wives and 71% of husbands who were not, reported being happily married; this was also reported by 92% of subjects who experienced orgasm in all or almost all sexual relationships compared with 83% of those who did so on half or fewer occasions. The increased prevalences of having intercourse and of reaching orgasm could have been a result of, rather than a contribution to, the happy marriage. A somewhat stronger correlation with marital happiness was found with being comfortable discussing sexual matters with spouses. Of men and women who reported this, 92% were happily married compared with 64% of wives and 70% of husbands who did not.

Laumann and colleagues (1994) did not report the relationship of the presence of sexual problems with sexual satisfaction, but in what could appear a contrasting finding, they found strong relationships between the presence of the sexual dysfunctions they investigated and feelings of being mainly unhappy. However, there also was a strong relationship between subjects' levels of health and happiness, so in view of the correlations between sexual dysfunctions and poor health, health rather than the dysfunctions could have been responsible for the unhappiness of subjects with sex problems.

Reluctance to seek help for sexual dysfunctions found in younger adults (McConaghy, 1993) is also evident in studies of older people. Of men attending a medical outpatient clinic, 401 of 1,080 admitted on questioning to having erectile dysfunction (Slag *et al.,* 1983). Prior to the inquiry only 6 had been identified as having the dysfunction. The authors commented that subjects were reluctant to call attention to the dysfunction but were eager to discuss and seek evaluation for it when the physicians broached the topic. In fact, only 188, slightly less than half, accepted the offer of evaluation. Their mean age was 59 years, comparable with the mean of 56.5 years of the functional men; the mean age of those who refused evaluation was 67 years. Of the 60–79-year-old male volunteers of a Baltimore study of aging who had potency problems, only 10% sought medical advice for the condition (Martin, 1981). Martin considered that the majority were uninterested, due to low sexual motivation. They were virtually free from performance anxiety, feelings of sexual deprivation, and loss of self-esteem. Solstad and Hertoft (1993) administered a questionnaire to 439 Danish men aged 51, whom they considered representative of the population; 20% reported occasional to total erectile dysfunction with intercourse. When 100 were subsequently interviewed a further 7 reported the dysfunction more than occasionally; 32 reported other sexual problems. However, of the total of 39 of the 100 interviewed who reported problems, only 7% considered them abnormal for their age and only 5% planned to consult a therapist. Of 142 English women, 87 of whom were 50 years old and older, who reported impaired sexual interest, vaginal dryness, infrequency of orgasm, or dyspareunia or a combination, only 32 considered they had a sexual problem, as did a further 10 of 294 with no dysfunctions (Osborn *et al.,* 1988). Of the 42 who considered they had a problem, 16 said they wished treatment if it was available. One was receiving it.

A factor increasing older people's sexual satisfaction could be what Brecher (1984) termed the "empty nest honeymoon": the experiences of older couples who became more free in their sexual activity when their children left home. He found that 87% of couples without, as compared with 80% of those with dependent children living at home, reported being happily married. Anecdotal evidence indicated that both men and women continued to go to considerable lengths to conceal their sexual activity from children into their adulthood. He found little evidence of the "empty nest syndrome" invoked by health professionals to explain a variety of problems experienced by women whose children have left home. However, before the syndrome is dismissed as another example of faulty post hoc, ergo proper hoc reasoning, the possibility needs to be considered that Brecher's conclusion may be relevant only to the subjects he studied who were above average in education, health, and income. Less educated women might obtain more of their satisfaction in life from their children and hence experience more dissatisfaction when they leave home.

Etiology

Most elderly men seeking help for sexual difficulties do so for erectile difficulties. Elderly women rarely seem to seek help directly for sexual problems, except as part of menopausal symptoms.

The 401 (34%) of 1,080 men who reported erectile dysfunction (Slag *et al.,* 1983) would appear to be one of the most representative samples studied, having been selected from those attending a medical clinic, and so not limited to those presenting with the dysfunction. The mean ages of both the functional and dysfunctional men were 61 years, so that percentage impotent was less than double the approximately 20%, which would be expected in a representative sample of the normal population of this age (McConaghy, 1993). In the 188 who agreed to evaluation, hormonal abnormalities were the most common organic cause, primary or secondary hypogonadism in 19%, diabetes in 9%, and hyperprolactinaemia, or hyper- or hypothyroidism, in 10%. Medications were considered responsible in 25%, those most often implicated being diuretics, antihypertensives, and vasodilators. Neurological causes were diagnosed in 7%, urological causes in 6%, and other medical conditions in 4%. Fourteen percent were considered to have a psychological cause, and no cause was found in 7%. The majority of the men with erectile dysfunction reported a gradual onset of the condition, with continuance of their normal libido, consistent with the evidence discussed earlier of the persistence of sexual interest in most older men. Nearly half of the dysfunctional men without diabetes or hyperprolactinaemia were having erections either in relation to sexual stimulation or spontaneously, but they were of inadequate turgidity for coitus. Slag and colleagues found that a number of patients who experienced erectile dysfunction with medications had stopped them, but were hesitant to tell their physician why they had, and hence were often considered noncompliant.

Absence of any cases of erectile dysfunction specifically attributed to vascular pathology in the study of Slag and colleagues (1983) appears inconsistent with the significance attributed to this condition by other workers. They did report that 81% of the dysfunctional men as compared to 54% of the functional men had diagnosed hypertension prior to the study. Apparently these investigators did not evaluate their subjects' penile blood pressure index (PBI) and the ratio of their penile to brachial systolic blood pressure. Gewertz and Zarins (1985) considered that vascular occlusive disease was too frequently overlooked as a cause of erectile dysfunction in middle-aged and older patients, and recommended PBI screening to avoid this omission. In men having intercourse with their wives at the age of 70, hypertension was present in 10 and hypertriglyceridemia in 2 of the 21 who ceased intercourse, and in 1 and 0, respectively, of the 25 who continued the activity, over the following 5 years (Persson & Svanborg, 1992). The authors pointed out that both conditions were risk factors for arterial disease.

In an investigation of 121 male veterans aged 60 to 85 years (mean age 68) who sought treatment, Mulligan and Katz (1989) found that 87% had a discernible organic cause and 9% a psychogenic cause. Coexistence of neurological and vascular disorders, present in 30%, was the most frequent organic cause. Vascular disease alone was responsible for 21%, diabetic neuropathy for 17%, and nondiabetic neuropathy for 10%. Hypogonadism was present in 2.6%. The much lower incidence of hormonal causes apart from diabetes in these subjects, compared with those evaluated by Slag and colleagues (1983), could be related in part to the latter subjects' being more representative of the total population of men with erectile dysfunction. Differences in diagnostic criteria could also be involved. Mulligan and Katz (1989) stated that they diagnosed hypogonadism only when a therapeutic response to testosterone was present. Salmimies, Kockott, Pirke, Vogt, and Schill (1982) found that the threshold of total testosterone in hypogonadal men below which sexual function is impaired varied between 2 and 4.5 ng/ml; some with levels of above 3 ng/ml showed reduced frequency of erections and ejaculations, which then increased in response to administration of testosterone. Korenman and colleagues (1990) reported that 267 men with erectile dysfunction (mean age 64) who attended a sex dysfunction clinic, 39% were hypogonadal based on bioavailable testosterone levels below 2.3 nmol/L, and 12% were hypogonadal based on total testosterone levels lower than 10.5 nmol/L (3 ng/ml). A higher percentage of a healthy potent control group of men aged 65 were hypogonadal on both criteria. The authors concluded that both hormonal hypogonadism and impotence were common but independent in older men, consistent with the evidence that the level of testosterone to maintain erectile function is markedly below that necessary to maintain sexual interest (McConaghy, 1993). They did not, however, assess their subjects' level of sexual interest. Studies of representative population samples are necessary to determine the relationship of testosterone levels with age and erectile dysfunction.

In addition to diseases specifically impairing sexual functioning, those associated with pain, or that produce debility, anxiety, or depression, are likely to reduce sexual interest significantly. Wabrek and Burchell (1980) found that, of men hospitalized for myocardial infarction, most of whom were aged 50 to 69, two thirds reported a sexual problem, predominantly erectile dysfunction, prior to the infarction. Possibly due to the belief then current that almost all sexual problems were psychologically caused, the authors considered that the infarction was secondary to the stress of the erectile dysfunction, rather than that the dysfunction was due to associated vascular disease and medication. Dhabuwala, Kumar, and Pierce (1986) found that 42% of 50 mostly elderly men who had suffered infarction 2 years to 6 months previously reported erectile dysfunction, defined as failure to have intercourse within the last 2 years despite attempts; 48% of a control group matched for age, hypertension, diabetes, and smoking reported the same complaint, indicating that infarction of itself was not a significant cause of the dysfunction.

Though pointing out the high incidence of hysterectomy in older women, at that time 43% in women aged 70, Brecher (1984) found only a small reduction of sexual activity and enjoyment in his subjects who had undergone it, in comparison with those selected to be of good health. This was also true of those who had both ovaries removed, many of whom were not taking replacement estrogen, and of those who had undergone mastectomy. Thirteen percent of his male subjects, including 42% of those aged 80 or over, had undergone prostate surgery, either transurethral resection or prostatectomy. Following surgery 83% reported being sexually active and 81% reported high enjoyment of sex compared to 94% and 87% of the healthy comparison group. Brecher did not report whether the nature of the sexual activity had changed following surgery, but did record sequelae of erectile dysfunction and lack of ejaculation.

Segraves and Segraves (1992) reviewed the literature reporting associations of erectile dysfunction with a wide variety of pharmacological agents and drugs of abuse. They pointed out the paucity of adequately designed studies to establish these associations but considered independent studies of large numbers of men experiencing the problem made the association highly probable. Brecher (1984) found in his subjects that, compared with those selected to be in good health, both men and women on antihypertensive medication reported lower levels of sexual activity and of enjoyment of sex. Riley, Steiner, Cooper, and McPherson (1987), in a study of subjects attending a hypertension clinic, concluded that treated hypertensive men had a higher incidence of both erectile and ejaculatory dysfunction than untreated men, but that treatment did not have a significant effect in women on the prevalence of arousal or orgasmic dysfunction. They commented that high prevalence of dysfunctions in women may have obscured such an effect. Segraves and Segraves (1992) considered that, of the commonly prescribed hypotensive agents, propranolol, methyldopa, clonidine, and guanethidine were highly likely, and prazosin, hydralazine, atenolol, labetalol, and especially captopril unlikely to produce erectile dysfunction. Of the psychiatric drugs, sexual problems were more common with most antipsychotics, particularly thioridazine, and tricyclic antidepressants, particularly amitriptyline and clomipramine, but less so with haloperidol, desipramine, carbamazepine, monoamine oxidase inhibitors, and minor tranquilizers. However, in their controlled study Harrison, Rabkin, and Ehrhardt (1986) found that monoamine oxidase inhibitors produced a high incidence of sexual problems compared to placebo in depressed patients. These conclusions are clearly relevant to the treatment of the large number of elderly subjects with hypertension or depression.

There appears to be little evidence from surveys of impotent men to support the commonly reported clinical observation that alcohol is an important contributing factor (McConaghy, 1993). Slag and colleagues (1983) found prevalence of alcoholism in older men evaluated for erectile dysfunction was far lower than in functional men, but similar to that in the general population. Of the representative married men who were having intercourse with their wives at the age of 70, the 25 who were continuing to have intercourse 5 years later indicated more heavy alcohol use than the 21 who ceased intercourse over this period due to factors in themselves (Persson & Svanborg, 1992).

A possible role for constitutional factors influencing prevalence of sexual dysfunctions independent of aging was suggested by Martin's (1981) finding in socioeconomically advantaged married men aged 60 to 79 years. In relation to level of sexual activity throughout their lives, 75% percent of the least active, 46% of the moderately active, and 19% of the most active were partially or totally impotent; 21% of the least active as compared with 8% of the most active had experienced long-term problems with premature ejaculation.

Investigation of the etiology of older women's reduced sexual interest and frequency of orgasm has largely focused on the relationship of these symptoms to menopause. Plotting levels of sexual interest of 562 partnered Swedish women aged 38, 46, 50, and 54 in relation to whether they were in the premenopausal, perimenopausal, or early or late postmenopausal phases, Hallstrom (1979) found a strong and significant association between these phases and decline in sexual interest; there were only small differences in decline with age when menopausal phases were held constant. Comparison of women seeing two general practitioners in Oxford, England, revealed that 57% of 34 postmenopausal and 33% of 34 age-matched premenopausal women reported low sexual interest in the past year (Hawton *et al.*, 1994). However, the difference failed to reach statistical significance, and the authors decided that their finding was somewhat at variance with that of Hallstrom (1979)—a likely Type 2 error resulting from the inappropriate significance attached to statistical significance when subject numbers are small. Twenty-nine percent of the postmenopausal but none of the premenopausal women reported never enjoying sexual activity (a significant difference). N. L. McCoy and Davidson (1985) in a longitudinal study investigated 16 perimenopausal women aged 45 to 54 from 22 months before to 23 months after their final cycles. Following menopause the women had fewer sexual fantasies and less vaginal lubrication during sex, and were less satisfied with their partners as lovers. N. McCoy, Cutler, and Davidson (1985) reported a close association in 43 perimenopausal women, probably including many of those in the study discussed, between increasing irregularity of menstrual cycles, hot flushes, declining estradiol levels, and declining frequency of intercourse. They suggested that discomfort from hot flushes and other symptoms may reduce interest in sexual activity, that reduction of estrogens associated with the menopause may result in hot flushes and reduced sexual interest, or that sexual activity may protect against hot flushes by releasing hormones. Myers and Morokoff (1986) found that vaginal lubrication and sexual arousal to an erotic film to be significantly greater in premenopausal women and postmenopausal women receiving replacement estrogen compared with postmenopausal women who were not. Degree of both responses to the film were significantly related to their estradiol levels. The sexual functioning of hysterectomized women receiving estrogen replacement was higher than those not receiving it, 94% reporting being sexually active compared with 72% not taking estrogen (Brecher, 1984). The sexual functioning of those taking estrogen was equivalent to that of women with superior levels of health. Brecher reported anecdotal evidence from six women of an association between cessation of estrogen replacement and occurrence of atrophic vaginitis with dyspareunia and remission of these conditions with resumption of estrogen. Of all the postmenopausal women in his study, 408 were taking estrogen and 1,356 were not. Sexual activity was reported by 93% of the former and 80% of the latter; other measures of sexual functioning were also greater in the women taking estrogen. Brecher pointed out that women taking estrogen were slightly younger but he did not attempt statistical control of this major variable.

There is no general agreement as to whether vasomotor symptoms (hot flushes and sweating) and atrophic vaginitis and associated reduction in vaginal lubrication are the only true symptoms of menopause and that they result from fall in estradiol levels. Workers holding this view consider that depression and reduced sexual interest, when present in women of menopausal age, are secondary to these symptoms or to stereotyped beliefs concerning the effects of menopause; an alternative view is that atrophic vaginitis results from reduced sexual activity which is associated with fall in androgen levels (McConaghy, 1993). Menopausal symptoms are related to the length of time since menopause, with vasomotor symptoms declining in severity, while genital symptoms such as atrophic vaginitis worsen (Walling, Andersen, & Johnson, 1990). These authors reviewed the literature on hormonal replacement therapy for postmenopausal women but did not find convincing evidence of a direct hormonal effect on the women's sexual interest, consistent with the lack of evidence of a clear effect on premenopausal women's sexuality of the fluctuations in hormonal levels accompanying the menstrual cycle (McConaghy, 1993).

There was no obvious change in the representative women studied by Laumann and colleagues (1994) in prevalence of sexual dysfunctions around the time of menopause apart from having trouble lubricating, which increased in those 45 and older. However, as discussed earlier, prevalence of sexual dysfunctions in younger women in this study was very high compared to that in other surveys. Prevalence of pain during intercourse in Laumann and colleagues' 18–59-year-old female subjects declined consistently with age from 21.5% to 8.7%. It was low in the representative partnered Swedish women aged 38, 46, 50, and 54; 5% occasionally, 1% usually, and 2% always experienced external dyspareunia with sexual intercourse (Hallstrom, 1979). Hawton and colleagues (1994) cited studies indicating that gynecological symptoms other than those of major surgery and serious disease had surprisingly little effect on women's sexual function, except for an association of sexual dysfunctions with the psychological symptoms of premenstrual syndrome and with stress incontinence. In their study of partnered women, after controlling for age effects, they found positive relationships between reduced frequency of orgasm and number of physical premenstrual symptoms in all the women, and between rarely or never enjoying intercourse and experienced hot flushes in the preceding month, in women aged 55 to 59.

MANAGEMENT

Assessment

As discussed earlier, only 6 of 401 medical outpatients with erectile dysfunction had informed their physicians concerning it, and when it was identified on direct questioning only 188 (mean age 59) accepted the offer of evaluation. The mean age of those who refused evaluation was 67 years (Slag *et al.,* 1983). Few men, aged 51 and 60 to 79 years respectively, identified in surveys by Solstad and Hertoft (1993) and Martin (1981) as having the dysfunction, intended to seek treatment. On examination, 142 of 436 English women mainly 50 had a sexual dysfunction; only 42 considered they had a sexual problem and only 16 wanted treatment if it was available (Osborn *et al.,* 1988). If older people's sexual dysfunctions are to be identified health professionals need to inquire directly about them. The findings of Slag and colleagues suggest that this is uncommon. Patterson and Dupree (1994), in discussing the diagnostic interviewing of older adults, stressed the importance of avoiding ageism, with its tendency to overlook the mental health of these adults. They made no reference to a need to investigate the sexual activity of older people. Rather than pointing out the requirement for direct inquiry, they advised "do not hesitate to discuss intimate data if presented" (p. 391). The finding of Solstad and Hertoft (1993) that many more men reported sexual problems at interview than in a previously administered questionnaire indicates some validity for direct inquiry in assessing sexual problems in the elderly.

Physical examination and laboratory assessments are virtually routinely carried out in elderly men with erectile dysfunction, as it is rarely situational and hence purely psychogenically determined. Situational erectile disorder is that occurring with some but not other partners, or with all partners but not in private masturbation where no pressure to produce an erection is experienced. Physical examination is indicated to exclude such conditions as Peyronie's disease and hypogonadism, and blood and urine screening to exclude diabetes, hyperprolactinaemia, and thyroid dysfunction. Karacan (1978) recommended nocturnal penile tumescence (NPT) assessment of subjects with erectile dysfunction as he considered that if they showed erections during dream or rapid eye movement sleep similar to those of normal men, their dysfunction was due to a psychological, not an organic cause. The procedure was conducted in a sleep laboratory over three consecutive nights. Men who showed erections were awakened on the third night for them to assess the fullness and to have the rigidity determined by the pressure necessary to produce buckling. Apart from evidence questioning the validity of the procedure in men of all ages (McConaghy, in press), Schiavi (1992) considered assessment of penile buckling to be impractical in older subjects because of rapid penile detumescence on testing. Adequacy of penile blood flow is commonly assessed by determination of subjects' penile-brachial index (PBI), the ratio of the blood pressure in the penile arteries, commonly measured by Doppler ultrasound probe, and conventionally measured blood pressure in the brachial artery in the arm. The reliance of clinicians on NPT and PBI assessment of erectile dysfunction was questioned by Saypol, Peterson, Howards, and Yazel (1983). They reported close agreement between diagnoses of the psychiatrist and urologist based on clinical examination alone, and diagnoses based on the results of the patients' fasting blood sugar and testosterone levels and their PBI and NPT assessments. They suggested that expensive tests be reserved for patients whom the psychiatrist and urologist disagree or cannot determine the diagnosis.

The pharmacological erection test is increasingly being used to assess penile vascular supply in erectile dysfunction. Vasodilating chemicals are injected into one of the cavernous sinuses of the subject's penis. Development of a rigid, well-sustained erection within 10 minutes indicates no major vascular abnormality and, as assessed by Rigiscan, a slow onset indicates some degree of arterial disease, and rapid detumescence, a venous leak (McMahon, 1994). The Rigiscan is a portable monitoring instrument which continuously records frequency, duration, and degree of penile tumescence using two strain gauge loops, one placed at the base of the penis and one immediately behind the glans. The loops tightened periodically, indenting the penis and providing a measure of turgidity. If the subject does not develop an adequate erection following the injection, he may do so if he views an erotic video or employs manual genital stimulation (McConaghy, in press). If vascular pathology is indicated by the pharmacological erection test, further investigations are necessary to determine its nature, generally commencing with evaluation of the cavernosal arteries by color Duplex Doppler ultrasonography. If the equipment is available this investigation is commonly carried out as part of the pharmacological erection test. Assessment of neurogenic factors producing erectile dysfunction is indicated if there is a need to establish the etiology and the patient has a history of diabetes, pelvic pathology, or radical prostatectomy, or if physical examination reveals the absence of the cremasteric, bulbocavernosal, or reduced lower limb reflexes. Because investigations of organic factors producing erectile dysfunction require more expensive equipment and considerable experience in interpretation, they are increasingly being taken over by urologists with an interest in the treatment of erectile disorder.

Apart from the need for gynecological examination when dyspareunia or symptoms indicative of atrophic vaginitis are present, physical and laboratory examination of women with sexual dysfunctions are rarely carried out. As in men, it is necessary to exclude illness, medication, or substances as responsible for reduced sexual interest or decreased ability to reach orgasm. However, the effects of neurological and vascular disease and of medications and drugs of abuse on the sexuality of women are much more poorly documented. Hormone studies are rarely considered in the absence of indications of hormonal imbalance such as excessive hirsutism.

Treatment

The mean age of subjects in studies reporting treatment of sexual dysfunctions is almost invariably in the 30s. It would seem that of subjects seeking treatment for sexual problems older women present mainly to general practitioners or gynecologists with physical rather than psychological symptoms, mainly attributable to menopausal changes, and men present with erectile difficulties to urologists or specialized clinics. Hormone replacement with estrogen is the usual treatment for hot flushes and symptoms of atrophic vaginitis, with the addition of a progestogen in nonhysterectomized women to prevent the increased risk of endometrial hyperplasia and adenocarcinoma. Walling and colleagues (1990) reviewed the various forms of administration of hormone replacement and concluded that androgens may be of value to enhance sexual desire when it has not responded to the estrogen-progesterone combination and that this may be more likely in women who have undergone oophorectomy.

Organic factors almost invariably contribute to the erectile dysfunction of older persons. It is not uncommon for men who present with this problem to a urologist or sex therapist to report having received testosterone from a general practitioner without having been investigated to determine that they were hormonally hypogonadal. LoPiccolo (1990) and Schwartz, Kolodny, and Masters (1980) considered it was generally agreed that use of testosterone administration for sexual dysfunctions in men with normal levels of testosterone is without value. In view of the finding of Salmimies and colleagues (1982) that testosterone administration increased frequency of erections and ejaculations in some men with serum testosterone levels of up to 4.5 ng/ml, it seems reasonable to use this level as a cutting point below which to give men with sexual dysfunctions (particularly reduced sexual interest) a trial of testosterone administration. In view of the evidence that reduction in total testosterone level at least to 30% of the subjects' previous levels reduces sexual desire but not erectile ability (McConaghy, 1993), administration of testosterone is likely to be of more than placebo value only in those few men with below-normal levels who complain of reduced sexual desire. Bruning, DeWolf, and Morgentaler (1995) considered that prostate needle biopsy should be mandatory prior to testosterone therapy in hypogonadal men older than 60 and strongly encouraged in men 50 to 59. Such biopsy revealed presence of cancer in 6 men aged greater than 60 years, among 33 hypogonadal men aged 45 to 70, all of whom had negative digital rectal examination and a normal age-adjusted prostate specific antigen (PSA) level. The authors speculated that the men's low androgen levels may have falsely lowered their PSA into the normal range.

In the absence of treatable medical conditions or a psychogenic etiology, men with erectile dysfunction are usually offered a choice of self-injecting a chemical vasodilator into one of the corpora cavernosa of the penis or using a vacuum constriction device prior to intercourse, or of having a penile implant. It would seem that the first is becoming the most widely accepted initial treatment, possibly because it was demonstrated in the assessment procedure to produce a satisfactory and persistent erection. Althof and colleagues (1991) followed up 42 men of mean age 54 years who commenced the procedure. The improvement in quality of erections with foreplay and intercourse, sexual satisfaction, frequency of intercourse, and coital orgasm reported at 1 month was stated to be still present 1 year, but this seems to have applied only to those who remained in treatment. Fifty-seven percent dropped out, with treatment ineffectiveness given as one reason. Comparable percentages of subjects dropping out have been reported by other workers. In a study of 110 men, 34 of the 76 men who opted not to initiate or who discontinued treatment did so because of loss of interest in sexual activity (Irwin & Kata, 1994). Althof and colleagues (1991) expressed surprise at the poor patient acceptance of an efficacious and relatively safe procedure, though pointing out that some subjects could not afford the cost of approximately $100 monthly. As to the chemical employed, prostaglandin E1 has been reported to produce a better erectile response (Siraj, Bomanji, & Akhtar, 1990) and a much lower rate of prolonged erection (Meuleman *et al.*, 1992) than papaverine. Pain at the injection site or during erection was the most frequent side effect, occurring in 17% of subjects according to the review by Linet and Neff (1994).

The vacuum constriction device (VCD) consists of an acrylic tube that the subject places over his penis and presses against his body to produce an airtight seal. He then evacuates air from the tube using an attached vacuum pump. The resulting erection is maintained by transferring an elastic band from the base of the acrylic tube to the base of the penis; the tube is then removed. Subjects are instructed not to leave the band on for more than 30 minutes; it has loops attached to facilitate its removal. Some subjects have difficulty learning to establish the essential airtight seal, some complain the procedure produces pain or numbness in the penis, and some find it unacceptable as its use cannot be concealed from the partner. L. A. Turner and colleagues (1991) followed up 45 men of mean age 60 years who had commenced its use a year previously. Six men ceased because the erections produced were of insufficient rigidity, 2 because of relationship difficulties, and 1 recovered. Using the VCD resulted in erections sufficient for intercourse on about 80% of occasions. The most frequent side effects were blocked ejaculation in 40% and discomfort in 33%. Improvement in quality of erections and sexual satisfaction were the most marked

responses reported by patients; subjective sexual desire and frequency of intercourse increased at 1 month but then returned to baseline. Single men often felt
uncomfortable using the VCD with a new partner; unlike self-injection, its use
could not be concealed. Althof and colleagues (1992) reported that partners reported equally good responses to both procedures when assessed at five periods
over a year. They felt more at ease in their relationships and characterized sex
as more leisurely, relaxed, and assured. Their negative reactions focused on the
lack of spontaneity and on hesitation about initiating sex. L. A. Turner and colleagues (1991) considered that the dropout rate of only 20% over a year of use
of the VCD compared very favorably with that following self-injection. However, review of other studies indicated that if the dropout rates of all men recommended use of VCDs or on whom it was tested are compared with the
dropout rates of all men who commenced self-injection programs, the rates are
approximately the same (McConaghy, 1996).

Men with erectile disorder not wishing or responding satisfactorily to use
of intracavernous injections or of VCDs may accept penile implantation of a
prosthesis. This can be a semirigid silastic rod which increases penile rigidity
but not its size, or a device which the subject can inflate by a pump placed in
the scrotum. Steege, Stout, and Carson (1986) concluded that about a quarter
of recipients had significant dissatisfaction with the procedure, complaining of
alterations in penile dimensions or in sensations during arousal or ejaculation.
There were no significant differences in relation to the type of implant and
90% would have the procedure again if confronted with the same therapeutic
choices.

Some men with erectile dysfunction of organic etiology who do not accept
self-injection, VCD, or penile implants can be helped by a cognitive-behavioral
psychotherapeutic approach emphasizing improved sexual communication
and employment of sexual activities not requiring a firm erection, possibly including "penile stuffing"; this can be easier if the man lies in the supine position. Counseling may be necessary for subjects with medical conditions that
impair their sexual functioning either through the associated anxiety or physical disability. Of men who received sexual counseling following myocardial infarction, 24% reported fear of resuming intercourse in the next 6 months
compared with 80% of men who were not counseled (Dhabuwala *et al.*, 1986).
The authors did not report whether there were differences in the number who
resumed intercourse. They stated that most of those counseled had been advised to resume sexual activity if they could climb one or two stairs without
symptoms. This is probably a misprint for one or two flights of stairs. Being able
to climb two flights of stairs was the criterion cited by Brecher (1984); those
who could not do so without suffering cardiac pain or shortness of breath were
advised to take their usual dose of nitroglycerine 15 to 30 minutes before engaging in sex, advice that would seem more appropriate for those who reacted
with pain.

Schiavi and colleagues (1990) pointed out that many older couples continued to engage in satisfying intercourse in the face of significant decrements in
erectile function and suggested that it may be as important to focus attention on
attitudinal factors and coping strategies as on the mechanisms involved in erectile capacity. Given the wealth of information concerning frequencies of sexual

activities in the elderly, it is disappointing that there is so little concerning the communication between sexual partners and how they deal with the problems connected with increase in frequency of men's erectile problems with age and dependence of women's sexual activity on the presence of an active partner. Evaluation of therapy aimed at reducing the dependence of men's self-esteem on their ability to maintain erections and increasing their acceptance of sexual activity not requiring this ability is also necessary. Althof and colleagues (1991) noted that, of men prior to their use of intracavernous injections when intercourse was not possible, it often led to sexual abstinence with a concomitant loss of affectionate holding and touching. They added that the couple commonly expressed frustration by saying: "Why bother trying when you can't do anything?" and that from the women's perspective restoration of potency led to more generalized changes in the men's self-esteem that made it easier to be with them. One woman was quoted as saying: "How the hell can a man feel when he can't have sex? He becomes cranky and mean." The relationship between comfort with sexual communication and marital happiness found by Brecher (1984) was referred to earlier. He quoted a 66-year-old husband as saying, "Most partners go through life playing a guessing game. By the time they really know what turns each other on, it's turn-off time" (p. 95).

SUMMARY

After middle age an increasing percentage of men and women cease partnered sexual activity with subsequent aging; the percentage of women doing so is considerably higher than that of men of the same age. In those who continue the activity, its frequency, duration, and enjoyment declines with age. Cessation of coitus in women is commonly due to absence or inability of their partner, and in men to their own inability. Married women 60 years or older are much more likely to be sexually active than unmarried women of the same age; the difference is much less in men, reflecting the much greater opportunity for unmarried older men than women to find a heterosexual partner. The evidence suggests that few men and women adopt nonpenetrative partnered sexual activity or solitary masturbation as substitutes for coitus; those masturbating, however, may be continuing an earlier practice The sexual interest and activity of socioeconomically and health advantaged subjects are greater than those of subjects of similar age representative of the total population. The level of sexual activity of elderly men and to a less consistent extent of elderly women has been found to be related to the level in their early adulthood, suggesting that a biological determinant may contribute. A weak relationship between older men's levels of sexual activity and of testosterone has been found; evidence is conflicting as to whether decline in testosterone levels with age found in representative population samples occurs in those selected for good health.

Studies of the prevalence of sexual dysfunctions in the elderly are limited and tend to use different diagnostic criteria. A representative Swedish town population sample reported a much lower prevalence of dysfunctions in women aged around 40 years than did a representative American population sample; presumably related to this difference the Swedish women showed a marked increase in prevalence of dysfunctions with subsequent age, whereas American women showed little increase and for some dysfunctions a decrease in their prevalence with age. Studies of less representative American samples generally showed increases in prevalence of dysfunctions with age. Subjects of superior health reported lower incidences than the less healthy of orgasmic difficulties and loss of sexual interest (particularly men), but not of erectile dysfunction or lack of vaginal lubrication. Sexual satisfaction was not related to presence of dysfunctions, consistent with the significant number of subjects with dysfunctions not wishing treatment. Sexual satisfaction was related to couples' marital adjustment and communication.

Studies of the etiology of erectile dysfunction of elderly men varied in percentages that showed the organic causes of vascular or neurological pathology, hormonal abnormalities, other illnesses, or medications. Dysfunctions of elderly women reported were mainly considered sequelae of menopause. Assessment of sexual problems in older men and women requires direct inquiry; without this they seldom report such problems to their health caregivers. Physical examination is usually required for both older men and older women with dysfunctions, but laboratory tests are carried out almost exclusively in men. Hormonal replacement therapy for women and men and the options of intracavernous injections, vacuum constriction devices, and penile implants for men with erectile dysfunction were discussed. Evaluation of attempts to encourage men not accepting these treatments to adopt nonpenetrative sexual activities with their partners is needed.

REFERENCES

Adams, C. G., & Turner, B. F. (1985). Reported changes in sexual activity from young adulthood to old age. *Journal of Sex Research, 21,* 126–141.

Althof, S. E., Turner, L. A., Levine, S. B., Risen, C., Bodner, D. Kursh, E. D., & Resnick, M. (1991). Sexual, psychological, and marital impact of self-injection of papaverine and phentolamine: A long-term prospective study. *Journal of Sex and Marital Therapy, 147,* 101–112.

Althof, S. E., Turner, L. A., Levine, S. B. Kursh, E. D., Bodner, D., & Resnick, M. (1992). Through the eyes of women—The sexual and psychological responses of women to their partner's treatment with self-injection or external vacuum therapy. *Journal of Urology, 147,* 1024–1027.

American Psychiatric Association. (1994). *Diagnostic and statistic manual of mental disorders* (4th ed.). Washington, DC: Author.

Bergstrom-Walan, M-B, & Nielsen, H. H. (1990). Sexual expression among 60–80-year-old men and women: A sample from Stockholm, Sweden. *Journal of Sex Research, 27,* 289–295.

Brecher, E. M. (1984). *Love, sex and aging.* Boston: Little, Brown.

Bretschneider, J. G., & McCoy, N. L. (1988). Sexual interest and behavior in healthy 80- to 102-year-olds. *Archives of Sexual Behavior, 17,* 109–129.

Bruning, C. O., III, DeWolf, W. C., & Morgentaler, A. (1995). Occult prostate cancer in hypogonadal men? *Urology Review, 3,* 1.

Chambers, K. C., & Phoenix, C. H. (1982). Sexual behavior in old male rhesus monkeys: Influence of familiarity and age of female partners. *Archives of Sexual Behavior, 11,* 299–308.

Christenson, C. V., & Gagnon, J. H. (1965). Sexual behavior in a group of older women. *Journal of Gerontology, 20,* 351–356.

Dhabuwala, C. B., Kumar, A., & Pierce, J. M. (1986). Myocardial infarction and its influence of male sexual function. *Archives of Sexual Behavior, 15,* 499–504.

George, L. K., & Weiler, S. J. (1981). Sexuality in middle and late life. *Archives of General Psychiatry, 38,* 919–923.

Gewertz, B. L., & Zarins, C. K. (1985). Vasculogenic impotence. In R. T. Segraves & H. W. Schoenberg (Eds.), *Diagnosis and treatment of erectile disturbances* (pp. 105–113). New York: Plenum.

Hallstrom, T. (1979). Sexuality of women in middle age: The Goteberg study. *Journal of Biosocial Science* (Supp. 6), 165–175.

Hallstrom, T., & Samuelsson, S. (1990). Changes in women's sexual desire in middle life: The longitudinal study of women in Gothenburg. *Archives of Sexual Behavior, 19,* 259–268.

Harrison, W. M, Rabkin, J. G., & Ehrhardt, A. A. (1986). Effects of antidepressant medication on sexual function: A controlled study. *Journal of Clinical Pharmacology, 6,* 144–149.

Hawton, K, Gath, D, & Day, A. (1994). Sexual function in a community sample of middle-aged women with partners: Effects of age, marital, socioeconomic, psychiatric, gynecological, and menopausal factors. *Archives of Sexual Behavior, 232,* 375–395.

Hegeler, S, & Mortensen, M. (1978). Sexuality and ageing. *British Journal of Sexual Medicine,* 16–19.

Hunt, M. (1974). *Sexual behavior in the 1970's.* New York: Dell.

Irwin, M. B., & Kata, E. J. (1994). High attrition rate with intracavernous injection of prostaglandin E1. *Urology, 43,* 84–87.

Johnson, A. M., Wadsworth, J., Wellings, K., Field, J., & Bradshaw, S. (1994). *Sexual attitudes and lifestyles.* Oxford: Blackwell.

Karacan, I. (1978). Advances in the psychophysiological evaluation of male erectile impotence. In J. LoPiccolo & L. LoPiccolo (Eds.), *Handbook of sex therapy* (pp. 137–145). New York: Plenum.

Kinsey, A. C., Pomeroy, W. B., & Martin, C. E. (1948). *Sexual behavior in the human male.* Philadelphia: Saunders.

Kinsey, A. C., Pomeroy, W. B., Martin, C. E., & Gebhard, P. H. (1953). *Sexual behavior in the human female.* Philadelphia: Saunders.

Korenman, S. G., Morley, J. E., Mooradian, A. D., Davis, S. S., Kaiser, F. E., Silver, A. J., Viosca, S. P., & Garza, D. (1990). Secondary hypogonadism in older men; Its relation to impotence. *Journal of Clinical Endocrinology and Metabolism, 71,* 963–968.

Laumann, E. O., Gagnon, J. H., Michael, R. T, & Michaels, S. (1994). *The social organization of sexuality.* Chicago: University of Chicago Press.

Leibman, S., Bachmann, G., Kemmann E., Colburn, D., & Swartzman, L. (1983). Vaginal atrophy in the postmenopausal woman. *Journal of the American Medical Association, 249,* 2195–2198.

Lewontin, R. C. (1995a, April 20). Sex, lies, and social science. *New York Review of Books,* pp. 24–29.

Lewontin, R. C. (1995b, August 10). "Sex, lies, and social science": Another exchange. *New York Review of Books,* p. 56.

Linet, O. I., & Neff, L. L. (1994). Intracavernous prostaglandin E(1) in erectile dysfunction. *Clinical Investigator, 72,* 139–149.

LoPiccolo, J (1990). Sexual dysfunction. In A. S. Bellack, M Hersen & A. E. Kazdin (Eds.), *International handbook of behavior therapy and modification* (2nd ed., pp. 547–564). New York: Plenum.

Marsiglio, W, & Donnelly, D. (1991). Sexual relations in later life: A national study of married persons. *Journal of Gerontology: Social Sciences, 46,* S338–S344.

Martin, C. E. (1981). Factors affecting sexual functioning in 60–79-year-old married males. *Archives of Sexual Behavior, 10,* 399–420.

McConaghy, N (1993). *Sexual behavior: Problems and management.* New York: Plenum.

McConaghy, N. (1996). Treatment of sexual dysfunctions. In V. B. Van Hasselt & M. Hersen (Eds.), *Source book of psychological treatment manuals for adult disorders* (pp. 333–373). New York: Plenum.

McConaghy, N. (in press). Assessment of sexual dysfunction and deviation. In A. S. Bellack & M. Hersen (Eds.), *Behavioral assessment: A practical handbook* (3rd ed.). Elmsford, New York: Pergamon.

McCoy, N., Cutler, W., & Davidson, J. M. (1985). Relationships among sexual behavior, hot flashes, and hormone levels in perimenopausal women. *Archives of Sexual Behavior, 14,* 385–394.

McCoy, N. L., & Davidson, J. M. (1985). A longitudinal study of the effects of menopause on sexuality. *Maturitas, 7,* 203–210.

McMahon, C. G. (1994). Management of impotence part II: Diagnosis. *General Practitioner, CME Files, 2,* 83–85.

Meuleman, E. J. H., Bemelmans, B. L. H, Doesburg, W. H., van Asten, W. N. J. C., Skotnicki, S. H., & Debruyne F. M. J., (1992). Penile pharmacological duplex ultrasonography: A dose-effect study comparing papaverine, papaverine/phentolamine and prostaglandin E1. *Journal of Urology, 148*, 63–66.

Mulligan, T., & Katz, P. G. (1989). Why aged men become impotent. *Archives of Internal Medicine, 149*, 1365–1366.

Mulligan, T, & Moss, C. R. (1991). Sexuality and aging in male veterans: A cross-sectional study of interest, ability, and activity. *Archives of Sexual Behavior, 20*, 17–25.

Myers, L. S., & Morokoff, P. J. (1986). Physiological and subjective sexual arousal in pre- and post-menopausal women and postmenopausal women taking replacement therapy. *Psychophysiology, 23*, 283–292.

Osborn, M., Hawton, K., & Gath, D. (1988). Sexual dysfunctions among middle-aged women in the community. *British Medical Journal, 296*, 959–962.

Patterson, R. L., & Dupree, L. W. (1994). Older adults. In M. Hersen & S. M. Turner (Eds.), *Diagnostic Interviewing* (2nd ed., pp. 373–397). New York: Plenum.

Persson, G., & Svanborg, A. (1992). Marital coital activity in men at the age of 75: Relation to somatic, psychiatric, and social factors at the age of 70. *Journal of the American Geriatrics Society, 40*, 439–444.

Pfeiffer, E., & Davis, G. C. (1972). Determinants of sexual behavior in middle and old age. *Journal of the American Geriatrics Society, 20*, 151–158.

Pfeiffer, E., Verwoerdt, A, & Davis, G. C. (1972). Sexual behavior in middle life. *American Journal of Psychiatry, 128*, 1262–1267.

Reiss, I. L. (1995). Is this the definitive sexual survey? *Journal of Sex Research, 32*, 77–85.

Riley, A. J., Steiner, J. A., Cooper, R., & McPherson, C. K. (1987). The prevalence of sexual dysfunction in male and female hypertensive patients. *Sexual and Marital Therapy, 2*, 131–138.

Salmimies, P., Kockott, G., Pirke, K. M., Vogt, H. J., & Schill, W. B (1982). Effects of testosterone replacement on sexual behavior in hypogonadal men. *Archives of Sexual Behavior, 11*, 345–353.

Saypol, D. C., Peterson, G. A., Howards, S. S., & Yazel, J. J. (1983). Impotence: Are the newer diagnostic methods a necessity? *Journal of Urology, 130*, 260–262.

Schiavi, R. C. (1992). Laboratory methods for evaluating erectile disorder. In R. C. Rosen & S. R. Leiblum (Eds.), *Erectile disorders assessment and treatment* (pp. 141–170). New York: Guilford.

Schiavi, R. C., Schreiner-Engel, P., Mandeli, J., Schanzer, H., & Cohen, E. (1990). Healthy aging and male sexual function. *American Journal of Psychiatry, 147*, 766–771.

Schwartz, M. F., Kolodny, R. C., & Masters, W. H. (1980). Plasma testosterone levels of sexually functional and dysfunctional men. *Archives of Sexual Behavior, 9*, 355–366.

Segraves, R. T., & Segraves, K. A. (1992). Aging and drug effects on male sexuality. In R. C. Rosen & S. R. Leiblum (Eds.), *Erectile disorders assessment and treatment* (pp. 96–138). New York: Guilford.

Seidman, S. N., & Rieder, R. O. (1994). A review of sexual behavior in the United States. *American Journal of Psychiatry, 151*, 330–341.

Sennett, R. (1995, May 25). "Sex, lies and social science": An exchange. *New York Review of Books*, p. 43.

Siraj, Q. H., Bomanji, J., & Akhtar, M. A. (1990). Quantitation of pharmacologically-induced penile erections: The value of radionuclide phallography in the objective evaluation of erectile haemodynamics. *Nuclear Medicine Communications, 11*, 445–458.

Slag, M. F., Morley, J. E., Elson, M. K., Trence, D. L., Nelson, C. J., Nelson, A. E., Kinlaw, W. B., Beyer, H. S., Nuttall, F. Q., & Shafer, R. B. (1983). Impotence in medical clinic outpatients. *Journal of the American Medical Association, 249*, 1736–1740.

Solstad, K., & Hertoft, P. (1993). Frequency of sexual problems and sexual dysfunction in middle-aged Danish men. *Archives of Sexual Behavior, 22*, 51–58.

Steege J. F., Stout, A. I., & Carson, C. C. (1986). Patient satisfaction in Scott and Small-Carrion penile implant recipients: A study of 52 patients. *Archives of Sexual Behavior, 15*, 393–399.

Tsitouras, P. D., Martin, C. E., & Harman, S. M. (1982). Relationship of serum testosterone to sexual activity in healthy elderly men. *Journal of Gerontology, 37*, 288–293.

Turner, B. F., & Adams, C. G. (1988). Reported change in preferred sexual activity over the adult years. *Journal of Sex Research, 25*, 299–303.

Turner, L. A., Althof, S. E., Levine, S. B., Bodner, D. R., Kursh, E. D., & Resnick, M. I. (1991). External vacuum devices in the treatment of erectile dysfunction: A one-year study of sexual and psychosocial impact. *Journal of Sex and Marital Therapy, 17*, 81–93.

von Sydow, K. (1995). Unconventional sexual relationships: Data about German women ages 50 to 91 years. *Archives of Sexual Behavior, 24*, 271–290.

Wabrek, A. J., & Burchell, R. C. (1980). Male sexual dysfunction associated with coronary artery disease. *Archives of Sexual Behavior, 9*, 69–75.

Walling, M., Andersen, B. L., & Johnson, S. R. (1990). Hormonal replacement therapy for postmenopausal women: A review of sexual outcomes and related gynecologic effects. *Archives of Sexual Behavior, 19*, 119–137.

Weizman, R., & Hart, J. (1987). Sexual behavior in healthy married elderly men. *Archives of Sexual Behavior, 16*, 39–44.

White, C. B. (1982). Sexual interest, attitudes, knowledge, and sexual history in relation to sexual behavior in the institutionalized aged. *Archives of Sexual Behavior, 11*, 11–21.

CHAPTER 13

Sleep Disturbances in Late Life

CHARLES M. MORIN, FRANCE C. BLAIS, AND VÉRONIQUE MIMEAULT

INTRODUCTION

Sleep disturbance is a prevalent problem in late life, affecting healthy seniors as well as medically ill and cognitively impaired individuals. In addition to normal age-related changes in sleep patterns, the increased incidence of health problems and medication use, combined with some inevitable stressful life events, place the older adult at increased risk for sleep disturbances. These problems can take many forms, including sleeping difficulties at night, excessive or undesired sleepiness during the day, and disruptive behaviors occurring during the sleep period (e.g., nocturnal wandering). Although not all changes in sleep patterns are noticeable or produce distress, severe and persistent sleep disturbances are associated with impaired daytime functioning, increased health care costs, and poorer quality of life for the affected individuals and their families.

Reports of daytime fatigue, memory and concentration problems, and dysphoria are much more common among poor sleepers than good sleepers (Gallup Organization, 1991). Although the magnitude of performance impairments are mild and selective (Hart, Morin, & Best, 1996), sleep disturbances are often associated with psychological distress and, when left untreated, they may increase the vulnerability to major depression (Ford & Kamerow, 1989). Poor sleepers use health-related services more frequently than good sleepers, both for sleep and other somatic problems (Mellinger, Balter, & Uhlenhuth, 1985). Nocturnal behavioral disturbances (e.g., wandering) among demented patients can cause a significant burden on caregivers, sometimes hastening placement of the impaired person in nursing care facilities (Pollak, Perlick, Linsner, Wenston, & Hsieh, 1990).

CHARLES M. MORIN, FRANCE C. BLAIS, AND VÉRONIQUE MIMEAULT • École de Psychologie, Université Laval, Cité Universitaire, Québec, Canada G1K 7P4

Handbook of Clinical Geropsychology, edited by Michel Hersen and Vincent B. Van Hasselt. Plenum Press, New York, 1998.

The higher incidence of sleep disturbances in elderly persons is paralleled by increased use of sedative-hypnotic drugs. Surveys indicate that 7.4% of the adult population, and 14% of those in the 69- to 79-year-old range, use either a prescribed hypnotic or over-the-counter sleeping aids during the course of a year (Mellinger *et al.*, 1985). These figures more than double in elderly patients attending general medical practices, where an estimated 26% of women and 6% of men older than 65 take prescribed hypnotics (Hohagen *et al.*, 1994). The large majority of long-term users (> 1 year) are older adults, particularly women, with one study reporting that 38% were aged between 50 and 64 years old and 33% were older than 65 (Mellinger *et al.*, 1985). Of a sample of community-dwelling subjects over 65, 11% reported using hypnotic drugs regularly for more than 1 year and an additional 4% for more than 10 years (Morgan, Dallosso, Ebrahim, Arie, & Fentem, 1988). These estimates nearly triple among institutionalized elders (Morgan, 1987). Overall, 39% of hypnotic drugs are prescribed for adults aged 65 or older, although they represent only 13% of the population.

Despite their increased incidence and debilitating effects in late life, sleep disturbances are often unrecognized by health care professionals and remain untreated (National Institutes of Health [NIH], 1991). This chapter describes the nature of sleep disturbances in late life, the main differential diagnostic issues and assessment procedures to consider in their evaluation, and effective treatment methods for their clinical management. In as much as insomnia is the most prevalent sleep complaint among elderly persons, and the problem most likely to be encountered by health care professionals, this chapter focuses primarily on this condition.

THE NATURE OF SLEEP DISTURBANCES IN LATE LIFE

The incidence of subjective sleep complaints increases across the life cycles. Among older adults, as many as 40% report some sleep problems, frequent awakenings, early morning awakenings, and undesired daytime sleepiness, and many more suffer from undiagnosed sleep disorders (Morgan, 1987). In this section, we describe some normal changes in sleep patterns and some of the most common forms of sleep disorders in late life.

Age-Related Changes in Sleep Patterns

Several age-related changes in sleep patterns occur even in normal aging. The amount of time spent awake or asleep and the proportion of time spent in NREM and REM sleep stages change over the course of the life span (D. L. Bliwise, 1993; Dement, Miles, & Carskadon, 1982; Webb, 1989). The most significant of these alterations involve a reduction of stages 3 and 4 (deep) sleep and a corresponding increase in stage 1 (light) sleep (Feinberg, Koresko, & Heller, 1967). These changes are accompanied by more frequent and longer nocturnal awakenings in older people (Webb & Campbell, 1980). Subjectively, they are ex-

perienced as lighter and more fragmented sleep, and may account for the increased prevalence of insomnia complaints in late life. The proportion of stage 2
sleep, which occupies about 50% of a night's sleep, remains fairly stable across
age groups. The amount of REM sleep is only slightly diminished in older age
relative to young and middle adulthood (20%–25%). The latency to the first
REM episode, which is used as a biological marker of depression, is shorter
among older than younger adults, and REM sleep is more evenly distributed
throughout the night (Reynolds, Kupfer, Taska, Hoch, Spiker, *et al.,* 1985).

Contrary to a common belief, total sleep time is not significantly reduced
from middle age to late life; however, older adults spend more time awake in
bed to achieve comparable sleep durations. Consequently, sleep efficiency (the
ratio of sleep time to time spent in bed), rather than sleep need per se, is diminished in late life. When sleep from daytime napping (a common practice in
the elderly) is added to nocturnal sleep, the total amount per 24-hour period
remains fairly stable in late life. Thus, the sleep of healthy older people is characterized by a reduction in sleep quality, not sleep duration. Sleep continuity is
impaired, as evidenced by more frequent and prolonged awakenings. Older
adults spend more time awake in bed, and sleep efficiency is correspondingly
diminished. Although it is important to distinguish between normative and
pathological changes in sleep patterns, insomnia is not an inevitable consequence of aging, and many elderly people suffer from sleep disruptions that exceed these developmental changes (Morin & Gramling, 1989).

Insomnia

Insomnia is the most common form of all sleep disturbances across the life
span. It can involve problems initiating sleep, trouble staying asleep through
the night (with frequent and prolonged nocturnal awakenings), or premature
awakenings in the morning with an inability to return to sleep (Morin, 1993).
Between 9% and 12% of the adult population report chronic and troublesome
insomnia during the course of a year, and for 12% to 25% of people age 65 or
older, sleep difficulties occur on a regular, chronic basis (Ford & Kamerow,
1989; Hohagen *et al.,* 1994; Mellinger *et al.,* 1985). The nature of sleep complaints changes with age. Older adults report primarily, although not exclusively, difficulty in maintaining sleep, whereas trouble initiating sleep is more
commonly reported by younger adults. Subjective sleep complaints are more
prevalent among women than among men. Paradoxically, sleep laboratory
recordings indicate more impaired sleep and a higher prevalence of such sleep
disorders as sleep apnea and periodic limb movements among noncomplaining
older men (Reynolds, Kupfer, Tascka, Hoch, Sewitch, & Spiker, 1985).

The clinical significance of insomnia complaints is sometimes difficult to
gauge. Although sleep disturbance increases with aging, this is not a universal
phenomenon, and some of the changes in sleep parameters do not necessarily
lead to the subjective complaint of insomnia. Some older adults are distressed
about changes in their sleep patterns, others notice but do not complain about
these changes, and still others do not report any changes in their sleep patterns.
Discrepancies between one's current sleep patterns and one's expectations may

also contribute to an insomnia complaint (Morin & Gramling, 1989). Further compounding this problem is the significant discrepancy between subjective and EEG sleep parameters; poor sleepers overestimate sleep latency and underestimate total sleep time.

The diagnosis of insomnia is made when there is a subjective complaint of difficulties initiating or maintaining sleep that is associated with marked distress and/or impairments of social or occupational functioning (American Psychiatric Association, 1994). These criteria are further operationalized in outcome research whereby insomnia is defined as a sleep onset latency or wake after sleep onset greater than 30 minutes, with a corresponding sleep efficiency lower than 85%; the problem must occur more than three times per week and last 6 months or longer (Lacks & Morin, 1992). Insomnia can be a primary problem or it can be associated with medical, psychiatric, alcohol and substance use, and other sleep disorders.

Other Sleep Disorders

Older adults are at increased risk for several sleep disorders other than insomnia. Obstructive *sleep apnea* is a breathing disorder characterized by a complete or partial cessation of airflow during sleep, lasting from a few seconds to a minute, followed by a brief awakening and a loud gasping for air (Guilleminault, 1989). These episodes may occur repeatedly through the night, causing severe sleep fragmentation. Older adults with central rather than obstructive sleep apnea may awake short of breath and develop secondary insomnia, as they become fearful of going back to sleep. Sleep apnea is associated with excessive daytime sleepiness and cognitive impairments and it may aggravate cardiovascular problems. *Restless legs syndrome* is a condition in which a person experiences an unpleasant, creeping sensation in the calves, and an irresistible urge to move the legs. Worse in the evening, this condition can significantly interfere with sleep onset. A related condition, *periodic limb movements,* consists of brief, stereotyped, and repetitive leg twitches or jerks during sleep (Montplaisir & Godbout, 1989). These movements may occur up to several hundred times a night, unknown to the sleeper. Some individuals with documented periodic limb movements are totally asymptomatic but, in severe cases, these movements cause severe sleep fragmentation and daytime somnolence. These three disorders can give rise to a subjective complaint of insomnia, excessive daytime somnolence, or both. Their incidence increases with aging (Ancoli-Israel, Kripke, Mason, & Messin, 1981), but patients are typically unaware of the underlying conditions. Some of our data suggest that about one third of older adults with a subjective complaint of insomnia are diagnosed with one of these disorders after undergoing a sleep laboratory evaluation.

REM sleep behavior disorder, a condition seen almost exclusively in middle-aged and older men, is characterized by violent behaviors (e.g., punching, kicking) while the person is asleep (Schenck, Bundlie, Patterson, & Mahowald, 1987). These behaviors arise from REM sleep, a period usually associated with muscle atonia; vivid dream recall is reported if the person is awakened from these episodes. Less prevalent than the other disorders just

described, little information is available on this condition. It may be drug induced or associated with neurological disorders. Psychopathology is generally not a contributing factor.

Sleep in Depression

Difficulties initiating and maintaining sleep are extremely common in affective disorders, with early morning awakening being one of the most classic
symptoms of major depression. The sleep of elderly depressive patients is also
characterized by REM sleep alterations, including a shortened latency to the
first REM sleep period, a longer first REM sleep period, an increase in percentage REM sleep, and more intense REM activity (i.e., frequency and intensity of
eye movements (Benca, Obermeyer, Thisted, & Gillin, 1992; Reynolds, Kupfer,
Taska, Hoch, Spiker, *et al.*, 1985). Although the specificity of these changes is
not always clear, some of them have been useful diagnostically to discriminate
depressed geriatric patients from demented and normal age-matched controls
(see the following discussion).

Sleep Disturbances in Dementia

The sleep patterns of patients with Alzheimer's disease (AD) are characterized by several impairments in sleep continuity and architecture (sleep stages;
D. L. Bliwise, 1993; Prinz *et al.*, 1982; Vitiello, Prinz, Williams, Frommlet, &
Ries, 1990). These include more interrupted sleep and time spent awake in bed,
resulting in a lower sleep efficiency; diminished stages 3 and 4 sleep (slow-
wave sleep) and increased stage 1 sleep. Sleep stages are also more difficult to
distinguish from one another as some of their distinctive EEG features become
less frequent and more blurred with the degenerative condition. These disturbances are similar to those seen in normal aging, but are significantly more pronounced in AD patients. As AD is a degenerative disease of the central nervous
system (CNS), sleep disturbances appear quite early and their severity increases
with progression of the illness. REM sleep is relatively unaffected in the early-
stage of AD. However, as the disease progresses, the percentage of REM sleep diminishes (Prinz *et al.*, 1982), and a general slowing of EEG activity is noted
during wakefulness, resulting in more daytime sleepiness (Coben, Chi, Snyder,
& Storandt, 1990; Prinz *et al.*, 1982).

With advancing severity of AD, the sleep-wake cycle becomes increasingly
desynchronized, resulting in significant amounts of sleep during the day and
wakefulness at night. AD patients spend nearly 40% of their nighttime hours
awake and considerable time asleep during the day (Prinz *et al.*, 1982). One
study of AD patients in a residential care facility found that every hour of the
day was characterized by some micro-sleep episodes and that every hour of the
night was perturbed by some wakefulness (Jacobs, Ancoli-Israel, Parker, &
Kripke, 1988). Daytime sleep is of poor quality, however, consisting almost exclusively of stages 1 and 2 sleep, and does not compensate for the nighttime
losses of slow-wave sleep (Vitiello, Bliwise, & Prinz, 1992).

About 20% of AD patients residing at home show some evidence of sundowning, a condition that is characterized by exacerbation of disruptive behaviors, agitation, confusion, and disorientation near the time of sunset or at night (D. L. Bliwise, Yesavage, & Tinklenberg, 1992). Typical behaviors reported by family members include wandering (often outside the house), turning on kitchen appliances, and watching television or listening to the radio at high volumes (D. L. Bliwise, 1993). Sundowning can be a very distressing feature of dementia and cause a significant burden for families and caregivers (Gallagher-Thompson, Brooks, Bliwise, Leader, & Yesavage, 1992); it may be the single most important factor precipitating institutionalization of demented patients (Pollak *et al.,* 1990; Rabins, Mace, & Lucas, 1982; Sanford, 1975). Families are usually able to manage and cope with the agitation, disorientation, incontinence, and other disruptive behaviors occurring during the daytime hours. However, when they cannot get some rest at night, the burden may simply be too intense for them to keep the older person at home.

Extensive research has been conducted with depressed and AD patients in the hope of identifying sleep abnormalities that might serve as early biological markers or provide indices for the differential diagnosis between dementia and depression in geriatric patients. Compared with normal aging, both conditions have impaired sleep continuity and reduced sleep efficiency. However, some features appear to discriminate between depressed and demented patients: sleep continuity (e.g., greater sleep fragmentation and early morning awakening in depressed than in AD patients), sleep architecture (e.g., greater proportion of REM sleep in depressed patients but greater loss of NREM transient stage 2 sleep features in demented patients), and first NREM-REM sleep cycle (e.g., shorter REM sleep latency in depressives) (Benca *et al.,* 1992; D. L. Bliwise *et al.,* 1989; Reynolds, Kupfer, Taska, Hoch, Spiker, *et al.,* 1985; Reynolds *et al.,* 1988; Vitiello *et al.,* 1990).

COMMON CAUSES OF SLEEP
DISTURBANCES IN OLDER PERSONS

Disturbed sleep can be a symptom of numerous conditions, including medical, psychiatric, and other sleep disorders. Older adults with sleep disturbances thus represent a very heterogeneous group. The following section outlines some important issues to consider in the evaluation and differential diagnosis of geriatric sleep disturbances.

Medical Factors

Two thirds of the elderly over age 65 suffer from one or more chronic medical conditions and many of those can interfere with sleep (Regenstein, 1980). Almost any condition producing pain (e.g., arthritis) or physical discomfort interferes with sleep, as does shortness of breath in congestive heart failures and respiratory diseases (e.g., chronic obstructive pulmonary disease [COPD]). All forms of degenerative neurological diseases, including the different dementias, disrupt the normal sleep-wake cycles. Several medications prescribed for health problems may disrupt sleep: bronchodilators (e.g., theodur), steroids (e.g., prednisone), and some antihypertensives (e.g., propanolol). Diuretics may cause frequent nocturia and sleep interruptions. Some psychotropic medications can also disrupt sleep. Among those are some of the SSRI antidepressants (e.g., fluoxetine) and the MAO inhibitors. Sedative-hypnotics can also produce a form of "iatrogenic insomnia." Caffeine and nicotine, both CNS stimulants, produce fragmented and lighter sleep. Alcohol, a CNS depressant, may facilitate sleep onset but it interferes with sleep maintenance.

Psychological Factors

There is a high rate of comorbidity between sleep and psychiatric disorders in the general population, with an estimated 35% to 44% of adults with a primary complaint of insomnia receiving a psychiatric diagnosis (mostly affective and anxiety disorders; Buysse *et al.,* 1994; Morin & Ware, 1996). The relationship of insomnia to psychopathology in late life is more equivocal. Some cross-sectional data suggest that insomnia is not as strongly associated with psychopathology in older adults as in younger people (N. G. Bliwise, Bliwise, & Dement, 1985; Roehrs, Lineback, Zorick, & Roth, 1982). Self-described older insomniacs tend to report higher levels of depression and anxiety symptomatology compared with good sleepers, but the severity of those symptoms does not necessarily reach clinical threshold (Morin & Gramling, 1989). Older adults are faced with some inevitable life events, such as retirement, deteriorating health, and the death of a spouse or friends, all of which can cause mood and sleep disturbances.

When insomnia is severe and persistent over time, it tends to be more strongly associated with depression (Ford & Kamerow, 1989; Hohagen *et al.,* 1994). In a longitudinal study of sleep and mood disturbances in 264 persons aged 62 to 90 years over a 3-year period (Rodin, McAvay, & Timko, 1988), depressed affect was positively correlated with sleep disturbances, even after controlling for age, gender, and health status. The probability of reporting moderate to severe sleep difficulties increased with the number of interviews at which a subject was categorized as depressed. Early morning awakening was the sleep problem most consistently related to depressed mood. A decrease in depressive symptomatology over time was associated with a corresponding reduction in early morning awakening. In a longitudinal study of late-life depression in 1,577 community-resident elderly persons (Kennedy, Kelman, & Thomas, 1991), subjects whose depressive symptoms persisted over a 2-year period ($n = 97$) were compared with those whose symptoms remitted over the same interval ($n = 114$). Subjects with persistent depressive symptoms tended to be older, experienced declining health, and reported more sleep disturbances, suggesting that persistent sleep disturbance may prevent or delay recovery from depression. Collectively, these findings suggest that the presence of insomnia at a given time is not a reliable indicator of psychopathology in elderly persons; however, severe and persistent sleep disturbance is more reliably associated with mood disturbances, particularly depression. There is not necessarily a direct cause-and-effect relationship, however, as mood disturbances may simply convey or represent a by-product of chronic insomnia rather than being its primary determinant.

Coexisting sleep and psychological disturbances may require separate therapeutic attention (Bootzin, Engle-Friedman, & Hazelwood, 1983).

Circadian Factors

The basic rest-activity cycle, along with sleep and wakefulness, is governed in large part by circadian principles. Their cyclic nature over the 24-hour period is regulated by both an endogenous biological clock and by environmental time markers. Of the several biological functions that are also regulated by circadian rhythms, body temperature is the one most closely linked to sleep and wakefulness. The periodicity, amplitude, and length of these circadian rhythms change with aging. For example, healthy older adults display an advanced phase and reduced amplitude in body temperature rhythm relative to younger adults (Czeisler *et al.*, 1992), resulting in an earlier bedtime in the evening and earlier arising time in the morning. Important timing cues regulating circadian rhythms in humans are daylight exposure, work schedules, meal times, and social interactions. With diminished activity levels and daily routines, many elderly have lost these important cues. Other behavioral factors, such as napping or resting in bed, may further desynchronize the natural circadian rhythms and interfere with nighttime sleep (Regenstein, 1980).

Behavioral and Lifestyle Factors

Behavioral and cognitive factors are also involved in late-life sleep disturbances, perhaps to a greater extent than at earlier ages. Aging and retirement are often associated with reduced activity level, decreased social rhythms, and increased daytime napping and time spent awake in bed. For instance, the amount of time spent awake in bed increases with aging, even among good sleepers. Older adults with sleep disturbances spend even more time awake in bed, in an attempt to compensate for poor nocturnal sleep. This pattern is further compounded by decreased physical activity associated with functional impairment, failure to readjust daily routines with retirement, and boredom or depression, in which the bed and bedroom may represent an escape for the older person. All these factors, and their interactions with circadian rhythms, may exacerbate an already fragmented sleep pattern in the elderly person. Dysfunctional sleep cognitions (e.g., unrealistic expectations) can also contribute to insomnia or transform otherwise normal age-related changes in sleep patterns into a clinical problem. These factors are discussed in the treatment section of this chapter.

ASSESSMENT

Because of the multifactorial etiology of sleep disturbances in late life, a comprehensive evaluation is required to make an accurate differential diagnosis. The following assessment procedures are recommended: a sleep history, psychological and physical examinations, sleep monitoring and, for some disorders, laboratory procedures.

Clinical History

A detailed sleep history is the most important diagnostic tool in the evaluation of sleep disorders. It should elicit the type of complaint, duration, chronology, and course; exacerbating and alleviating factors; and responses to previous treatments. It is important to inquire about life events, psychological and medical disorders, medication, and substance use to help establish a differential diagnosis. Two interviews are available to gather this information in a structured format: *The Structured Interview for Sleep Disorders* (Schramm *et al.*, 1993), designed according to *Diagnostic and Statistical Manual of Mental Disorders*, 3rd ed., rev. (*DSM-III-R;* American Psychiatric Association, 1987) criteria, is helpful to establish a diagnosis among the different sleep disorders, and the Structured Interview for Insomnia (Morin, 1993), is more specifically geared for patients with a suspected diagnosis of primary or secondary insomnia.

Determining the nature of the complaint is the first step for establishing a differential diagnosis. Difficulties falling asleep may suggest sleep-anticipatory or performance anxiety, pain, or restless legs syndrome, whereas difficulties maintaining sleep could be caused by nocturia, sleep apnea, periodic limb movements, or a variety of medical factors. At times, a sleep complaint paired with denial of affective symptoms may suggest a "masked depression." There may be less of a social stigma attached to sleep complaints than to depression or anxiety and some elderly persons will minimize psychological symptomatology and exclusively emphasize sleeplessness. Conversely, a subjective complaint of early morning awakening is not necessarily pathological or indicative of depression, as there is a phase advance in the circadian rhythms of older people, resulting in a natural tendency to feel sleepy earlier in the evening and to wake up earlier in the morning.

The duration and course of insomnia (acute, intermittent, chronic) can also have important implications for diagnosis and treatment planning. Transient insomnia may require an intervention that focuses directly on the precipitating conditions, whereas chronic insomnia will almost always require a treatment that also targets perpetuating factors (e.g., maladaptive sleep habits, dysfunctional cognitions). In light of the high comorbidity between sleep and psychiatric disorders, the history should identify relative onset and course of each condition in order to establish whether the sleep disorder is primary or secondary in nature.

A careful functional analysis of exacerbating and alleviating factors also can be quite useful for treatment planning. A detailed analysis of the following factors is crucial: activities leading up to bedtime; patient's cognitions at bedtime or in the middle of the night; sleep incompatible behaviors; perceived impact of sleep disruptions on mood, performance, and relationships; coping strategies; and secondary gains. Assessing the impact of disturbed sleep on mood and daytime functioning is important to determine the clinical significance of insomnia; inadequate or reduced sleep in the absence of residual effects or distress may not necessarily be pathological.

A medical evaluation is essential in clarifying the role of such factors as pain, anemia, thyroid functions, cardiovascular and respiratory problems. A detailed history of drugs, prescribed and over-the-counter, as well as alcohol use is necessary. Other important areas are the dietary (e.g., caffeine), smoking, and exercise habits and factors associated with the bedroom environment including room temperature, mattress comfort, sleep partners, and excessive noise and light. A review of the most common symptoms of other sleep disorders is essential to differentiate between primary insomnia and insomnia secondary to other sleep disorders. This should include a systematic review of symptoms of sleep apnea (e.g., loud snoring, pauses in breathing), restless legs and periodic limb movements (e.g., repetitive leg twitches during sleep), gastroesophageal reflux (e.g., heartburn), and parasomnias (e.g., sleep walking, violent behaviors). Interviewing the bed partner can yield most valuable diagnostic information as many patients may be unaware of their own snoring or breathing pauses in their sleep, and they may deny or underestimate their degree of daytime sleepiness.

Daily Self-Monitoring

Daily sleep diary monitoring is extremely useful for establishing a diagnosis of some sleep disorders, and especially for insomnia. A typical sleep diary includes entries for bedtime, arising time, sleep latency, number and duration of awakenings, sleep duration, naps, use of sleep aids, and various indices of sleep quality and daytime functioning (Morin, 1993). These data provide information about a patient's sleep habits and schedules, the type of sleep problem, and its frequency and intensity, all of which may vary considerably from the patient's global and retrospective report during a clinical interview. Despite some discrepancies between subjective and objective measurements of sleep parameters, daily morning estimates of specific sleep parameters represent a useful index of insomnia (Coates *et al.,* 1982). The sleep diary is a practical and economical assessment tool for tracking sleep patterns over long periods of time in the home environment. It is also helpful in establishing a baseline prior to treatment and in monitoring progress as the intervention unfolds. Due to extensive night-to-night variability in sleep patterns of insomniacs, baseline monitoring should last at least 1 or 2 weeks (Lacks & Morin, 1992).

Psychological Assessment

Psychological assessment should be an integral component in the evaluation of sleep disturbances. At the very least, a screening assessment is indicated because of the high rate of comorbidity between sleep and psychiatric disorders and, even when formal criteria for specific psychiatric disorders are not met, clinical features of anxiety or depression or both are extremely common among patients with sleep complaints. A cost-effective approach consists of using brief screening instruments that target specific psychological features (e.g., emotional distress, anxiety, depression) most commonly associated with sleep disturbance. Instruments such as the Brief Symptom Inventory, the Beck Depression Inventory, and the State-Trait Anxiety Inventory can yield valuable screening data. As for all self-report measures, these instruments are subject to bias resulting from denial or exaggeration of symptoms and should never be used in isolation to confirm a diagnosis. Psychometric screening should always be complemented by a more in-depth clinical interview.

Additional self-report measures tapping various dimensions of insomnia can also yield useful information. Some instruments are designed as a global measure of quality (Pittsburgh Sleep Quality Index; Buysse, Reynolds, Monk, Berman, & Kupfer, 1989), satisfaction (Coyle & Watts, 1991), or impairment of sleep (Morin, 1993). Other scales are helpful in evaluating mediating factors of insomnia, such as state (Pre-Sleep Arousal Scale; Nicassio, Mendlowitz, Fussel, & Petras, 1985) and trait arousal (Arousal Predisposition Scale; Coren, 1988), dysfunctional sleep cognitions (Beliefs and Attitudes About Sleep Scale; Morin, 1994), sleep-incompatible activities (Sleep-Behavior Self-Rating Scale; Kazarian, Howe, & Csapo, 1979, and sleep hygiene (Sleep Hygiene Awareness and Practice Scale; Lacks & Rotert, 1986). These measures are particularly useful for designing individually tailored insomnia interventions.

Behavioral Assessment Devices

Of several behavioral assessment devices available for estimating sleep-wake parameters, wrist actigraphy is increasingly being used in sleep research. This activity-based monitoring system uses a microprocessor to record and store wrist activity along with actual clock time. Data are processed through microcomputer software and an algorithm is used to estimate sleep and wake time based on wrist activity. Despite some limitations in assessing specific sleep parameters (e.g., sleep latency), wrist actigraphy is a useful tool for estimating sleep and wakefulness on a continuous basis throughout a 24-hour period.

Sleep Laboratory Evaluation

Nocturnal polysomnography (PSG) involves monitoring of the electroencephalogram (EEG), electro-oculogram (EOG), and electromyogram (EMG). These three parameters are sufficient to distinguish sleep from wake and to quantify the proportion of time spent in various stages of sleep. Several additional variables (respiration, EKG, oxygen saturation, and leg movements) are usually monitored to detect other sleep-related abnormalities (breathing pauses, leg twitches), not recognized by the sleeping person. Nocturnal PSG is essential for the diagnosis of sleep apnea, narcolepsy, and periodic limb movements. It can yield useful data to document the severity of insomnia, especially in light of the discrepancies between subjective complaints and objective findings. However, its clinical utility in the assessment and differential diagnosis of insomnia is more controversial.

When daytime alertness is compromised by a sleep disorder, a Multiple Sleep Latency Test (MSLT) is also recommended. The MSLT is a daytime assessment procedure in which a person is offered five 20-min nap opportunities at

2-hour intervals throughout the day. Latency to sleep onset provides an objective measure of physiological sleepiness. Individuals who are well rested and without sleep disorders take 10 min or more to fall asleep or do not fall asleep at all. A mean sleep latency of less than 5 min is considered pathological and is associated with increased risks of falling asleep at inappropriate times or places, such as while driving. The MSLT is performed almost exclusively on patients with a presenting complaint of excessive daytime sleepiness. Although insomnia patients may complain about daytime tiredness, typically they do not display pathological sleepiness on the MSLT.

Nocturnal PSG and daytime MSLT provides the most comprehensive assessment of a sleep disorder. These procedures are recognized as the "gold standards" in assessing sleep and its disorders, and are clinically indicated when the presenting complaint is excessive daytime sleepiness and when symptoms suggestive of breathing-related disorders and periodic limb movements are present. Although the cost-effectiveness of these procedures with insomnia patients is equivocal, in older adults with insomnia complaints a sleep study may still be particularly useful because this segment of the population is at increased risk for several other sleep pathologies (Edinger *et al.*, 1989). Coleman and colleagues (1982) reported that 37% of patients 60 years of age or older first diagnosed with a disorder of initiating and maintaining sleep were given a final diagnosis of periodic movements in sleep (27%) or sleep apnea syndrome (10%). Polysomnography is especially warranted to rule out any of these medical conditions.

TREATMENT

Much of the empirical evidence on the treatment of late-life sleep disturbances has been gathered in the past 10 years and focused predominantly on insomnia. In this section, we provide a brief description of treatment methods, summarize their efficacy, and discuss their clinical application with elderly patients. Table 13-1 outlines the main parameters of 15 outcome studies of nonpharmacological interventions for late-life insomnia.

Late-Life Insomnia

Education

Many individuals inadvertently engage in activities that are detrimental to sleep or refrain from simple activities that might improve sleep. Surveys indicate that poor sleepers are generally better informed about sleep hygiene; however, they also engage in more unhealthy practices than good sleepers (Lacks & Rotert, 1986). Educational interventions involve didactic teaching about lifestyles (e.g., diet, exercise) and environmental conditions (e.g., light, noise, temperature) that influence sleep. Education may also include information about normal age-related changes in sleep patterns, although this component is usually covered in cognitive therapy. A summary of sleep hygiene guidelines is provided in the following material and more extensive discussions of these recommendations are available elsewhere (Hauri, 1991; Morin, 1993).

Caffeine and nicotine are both stimulants that may interfere with sleep. Caffeine is contained in many products including coffee, tea, chocolate, and several over-the-counter preparations. Alcohol is a CNS depressant and, although it may facilitate sleep onset, it produces lighter and more fragmented sleep. Thus, all caffeine products and alcohol should be discontinued 4 to 6 hours prior to bedtime. There is little empirical evidence that any specific diet is helpful for sleep; however, liquid intake should be restricted in the evening to minimize sleep interruptions caused by nocturia, a problem that is more common among older adults. Exercising too close to bedtime should be avoided, but regular aerobic exercise scheduled in late afternoon or early evening may deepen and consolidate sleep. Because of the age-related reductions of deep sleep (stages 3 and 4) in older adults, aerobic exercise is a particularly appealing intervention awaiting controlled clinical trials. Excessive noise, light, and temperature should be minimized during the sleep period. The awakening threshold decreases with aging, and the noise factor can be especially problematic for institutionalized or hospitalized persons. The impact of environmental factors can be minimized by implementing simple changes such as wearing ear plugs, using window blinds, and using an electric blanket or air conditioner.

Treatment studies of late-life insomnia often integrate sleep hygiene education into multifaceted interventions (Edinger, Hoelscher, Marsh, Lipper, & Inonescu-Pioggia, 1992; Morin, Kowatch, Barry, & Walton, 1993). However, studies with both younger (Morin, Culbert, & Schwartz, 1994; Schoicket, Bertelson & Lacks, 1988) and older adults (Engle-Friedman, Bootzin, Hazlewood, & Tsao, 1992) indicate that sleep hygiene alone is unlikely to be effective for chronic and severe insomnia. Poor sleep hygiene may exacerbate insomnia but, in itself, it is rarely the primary cause of insomnia (Buysse & Reynolds, 1990). Nonetheless, sleep hygiene education provides a very sensible place to begin treatment to safeguard against interference from these factors, and clinicians would be negligent to ignore their potential influence (Lichstein & Riedel, 1994).

Stimulus Control

Stimulus control therapy (Bootzin, Epstein, & Wood, 1991) is designed to curtail sleep-incompatible behaviors and to regulate sleep-wake schedules. Insomnia is viewed as the result of maladaptive conditioning between temporal (e.g., bedtime) and environmental (e.g., bed) stimuli, which have been gradually associated with wakefulness, frustration, and arousal. Some older adults are more likely to engage in sleep-incompatible behaviors in the bedroom due to physical discomfort and restricted range of movement. Daytime napping is also common practice and, although it may not interfere with nighttime sleep in the elderly to the same extent as it does in young adults (Aber & Webb, 1986; Feinberg et al., 1985), multiple and long naps taken late in the day are likely to result in nighttime sleep that is light, restless, and subject to multiple awakenings.

Stimulus control therapy consists of the following instructions: (a) going to bed only when sleepy; (b) leaving the bed for another room when unable to fall

Table 13-1. Insomnia Treatment in Older Persons

Authors (year)	Format of treatment	Treatment duration (weeks/hours)	N (per condition)	Sex (% of female)	Age (group mean)	Diagnosis	Dependent sleep variables	Sleep medication
Alperson & Biglan (1979)	self-administered	4	N = 29 (RT, SC, MC)	48.0	55+	sleep-onset	SOL, TST	yes
Anderson et al. (1988)	individual	6/2.5	SRT = 8 SC = 8 WL = 4	70.0	63.8	mixed	TST, WASO, SE, SOL	no
Campbell, Dawson, & Anderson (1993)	individual	1.4/20	BLE = 8 MC = 8	56.3	70.4	advanced sleep phase syndrome	TST, SOL, SE, WASO	no
Davies, Lacks, Storandt, & Bertelson (1986)	group	4/4	CC = 22 WL = 12	47.1	58.6	maintenance	WASO	no
Edinger, Hoelscher, Marsh, Lipper, & Ionescu-Pioggia (1992)	individual	4/4	CBT & RT = 7	75.0	61.9	maintenance	SOL, WASO, TST, SE	no
Engle-Friedman, Bootzin, Hazelwood, & Tsao (1992)	individual	4/4	N = 53 (SH, RT, SC, MC)	66.3	59.6	mixed	SOL, WASO	no
Friedman, Bliwise, Yesavage, & Salom (1991)	individual	4/4	RT = 12 SRT = 10	63.6	69.2	mixed	TST, SE, SOL, WASO	yes
Hoelsher & Edinger (1988)	individual	4/4	MCT = 4	100.0	65.3	maintenance	WASO, SOL, TST, SE	no
Lichstein & Johnson (1993)	individual	2/3	MI = 19 NMI = 18 NI = 20	100.0	66.2	mixed	SOL, WASO, TST, SE	yes
Morin & Azrin (1987)	group	4/4	SC = 7 IT = 7 WL = 7	66.7	57.0	maintenance	WASO	no

Morin & Azrin (1988)	group	4/6	SC = 9 IT = 8 WL = 10	63.0	67.4	mixed	SOL, TST, WASO	yes
Morin, Colecchi, Stone, Sood, & Brink (1995)	group/individual	8/8	CBT = 18 PCT = 20 CBT + PCT = 20 PLA = 20	64.1	64.5	mixed	WASO, SOL, SE, TST, EMA, TWT, NA	yes
Morin, Kowatch, Barry, & Walton (1993)	group	8/12	CBT = 12 WL = 12	70.8	67.1	mixed	SOL, WASO, TST, SE	no
Puder, Lacks, Bertelson, & Storandt (1983)	group	4/4	SC = 9 WL = 7	81.3	67.1	sleep-onset	SOL	no
Riedel, Lichstein, & Dwyer (1995)	group	V = 30 min./2 V + G = 2/4	V + G NI = 25 V + G = 25 V NI = 25 V = 25 WL = 25	65.6	67.4	mixed	SOL, WASO, TST, SE	no

Note: SOL = Sleep Onset Latency, WASO = Wake After Sleep Onset, EMA = Early Morning Awakening, TWT = Total Wake Time, SE = Sleep Efficiency, TST = Total Sleep Time, NA = Number of Awakenings, SC = Stimulus Control, IT = Imagery Training, WL = Waiting List, RT = Relaxation Therapy, CBT = Cognitive Behavior Therapy, NI = Noninsomniacs, SH = Sleep Hygiene, MC = Measurement Control Group, CC = Countercontrol Treatment, BLE = Bright Light Exposure, SRT = Sleep Restriction Therapy, MCT = Multicomponent Treatment, PLA = Placebo, PCT = Pharmacotherapy, MI = Medicated Insomniacs, NMI = Nonmedicated Insomniacs, V = Video, G = Therapist Guidance.

asleep or return to sleep within 15 to 20 minutes, and returning to bed only when sleep is imminent; (c) repeating the previous instruction as often as necessary throughout the night; (d) arising at the same time every morning regardless of the amount of sleep obtained; (e) curtailing sleep-incompatible activities (e.g., reading, watching TV in the bedroom); the bed and bedroom are reserved for sleep and sexual activities; and (f) minimizing daytime napping. The main therapeutic goals are to strengthen the association between sleep and the conditions under which it typically occurs, and to consolidate a stronger sleep-wake rhythm.

Controlled studies with older adults indicate that stimulus control therapy, singly or combined with other interventions, is effective for both sleep-onset (Engle-Friedman *et al.*, 1992; Puder, Lacks, Bertelson, & Storandt, 1983) and sleep maintenance problems (Edinger *et al.*, 1992; Hoelscher & Edinger, 1988; Morin & Azrin, 1988; Morin, Kowatch, *et al.*, 1993). Improvement rates are comparable with those obtained with younger people (Lacks & Morin, 1992; Morin *et al.*, 1994), and therapeutic benefits are well maintained at long-term follow-ups. Substantial reduction of hypnotic usage has also been noted among medicated elderly patients (Morin & Azrin, 1988; Morin, Kowatch, *et al.*, 1993).

Although stimulus control therapy is a generally well accepted and credible treatment, adherence to these procedures is variable across individuals and for the different instructions. Some procedures (e.g., getting out of bed when unable to sleep) may be unpleasant, especially when they have to be implemented in the middle of the night. Countercontrol is a variation of the standard stimulus control instruction in that patients do not have to leave the bed. Rather, they are asked to stay in bed and engage in some worry-incompatible activity (e.g., reading) when unable to sleep. This technique has produced comparable results to the standard stimulus control instructions in one study (Davies, Lacks, Storand, & Bertelson, 1986). For older adults who are reluctant to comply with the standard stimulus control instructions, this can be a more acceptable alternative, although it is contrary to the basic principles of stimulus control procedures. Nonetheless, treatment adherence is a critical issue and the clinician must remain flexible to optimize outcome and prevent dropout or failures.

Sleep Restriction

Sleep restriction consists of curtailing the amount of time spent in bed to the actual sleep time (Spielman, Saskin, & Thorpy, 1987). The rationale behind this treatment is that insomniacs, especially older adults, spend excessive amounts of time in bed in a misguided effort to rest or sleep longer. However, excessive time spent in bed produces more fragmented sleep and may very well contribute to perpetuating insomnia. Restricting time in bed creates a mild sleep deprivation, which itself produces more consolidated and deeper sleep. Sleep-wake schedules are individualized according to estimated total subjective sleep time from a daily diary kept for 2 weeks. The amount of time allowed in bed is initially restricted to this average. For example, if a patient reports sleeping 6 hours per night but spends 8 hours in bed, the time allowed in bed (i.e., sleep window) would be 6 hours. Bedtimes and arising times are set at fixed hours. Weekly adjustments in the sleep window are made contingent on sleep efficiency (ratio of sleep time to time in bed multiplied by 100). Time in bed is increased by about 20 minutes when sleep efficiency exceeds 90%, decreased by the same amount when sleep efficiency is lower than 80%, and kept constant when sleep efficiency is between 80% and 90%. With the elderly, Glovinsky and Spielman (1991) recommend lowering the sleep efficiency criteria by 5%. These adjustments are made periodically, usually on a weekly basis, until an optimal sleep duration is reached. Time in bed should not be set below 4 to 5 hours per night, as it might cause excessive daytime sleepiness. A brief midday nap can counteract this effect without being detrimental to treatment. Daytime napping may be permissible early in treatment as long as it does not exceed 1 hour and is scheduled before midafternoon.

Sleep restriction is a relatively novel approach to treat insomnia; however, early studies suggest that it may be the best currently available intervention for late-life insomnia (Lichstein & Riedel, 1994). Only two studies have evaluated its efficacy when used alone with older adults (Anderson *et al.,* 1988; Friedman, Bliwise, Yesavage, & Salom, 1991), but several more have combined sleep restriction with stimulus control and cognitive restructuring procedures (Edinger *et al.,* 1992; Hoelscher & Edinger, 1988; Morin, Kowatch, *et al.,* 1993; Morin, Colecchi, Ling, & Sood, 1995). The main effect of sleep restriction is to improve sleep efficiency, which is reflected by a shorter time to fall asleep and by less frequent and shorter nocturnal awakenings. Although sleep duration is increased by a modest 30 to 60 minutes, patients are generally more satisfied with the quality of their sleep patterns. Therapeutic gains are also well maintained over time. Sleep restriction is a potentially useful treatment for the management of insomnia among elderly patients in institutions, an environment where excessive amounts of time spent in bed may be an important exacerbating factor of sleep disturbances.

Relaxation

Relaxation interventions are based on the premise that excessive arousal interferes with sleep. These methods seek to reduce somatic (e.g., progressive muscle relaxation, autogenic training) or cognitive arousal (e.g., imagery training, meditation). Relaxation-based interventions are the most widely used and studied nonpharmacological treatments for insomnia (Lichstein & Fisher, 1985). Although relaxation is helpful with younger adults, there is significantly more variability in outcome with advancing age (Edinger *et al.,* 1992; Friedman *et al.,* 1991). In a study comparing the efficacy of sleep restriction and relaxation in older adults, Friedman and colleagues (1991) reported significant benefits for both methods. However, improvement rate at the 3-month follow-up was twice as high in the sleep restriction condition compared with the relaxation group. Edinger and colleagues (1992) treated older adults sequentially with sleep restriction and relaxation and found that relaxation added little to the treatment effect of sleep restriction. When used alone, relaxation procedures may not be potent enough for chronic insomnia, especially in the elderly. Lichstein and Johnson (1993) obtained good results but only for nonmedicated insomniacs. They suggested that relaxation may be too physically demanding and complex with some older adults. Difficulties concentrating and sustaining attention for prolonged periods of time, as well as lower credibility for these procedures have also been reported (Morin & Azrin, 1988).

Cognitive Therapy

Older adults with chronic insomnia endorse more frequent and stronger dysfunctional beliefs and attitudes about sleep than self-defined good sleepers (Morin, Stone, Trinkle, Mercer, & Remsberg, 1993). Some entertain more unrealistic expectations regarding their sleep needs, whereas others believe that insomnia is an inevitable fact of aging. Still others are concerned about the fact that insomnia may have serious consequences for their physical health. Older persons are often unaware that age-related decreased nocturnal sleep time and quality do not necessarily produce daytime dysfunctions; consequently, they may struggle to maintain sleep patterns that are unrealistic for their age groups. For example, the belief that 8 hours of sleep is essential to maintain adequate daytime functioning is very common. If, because of lack of knowledge, seniors' sleep goals are not adjusted to conform with age-correlated sleep changes, the pursuit of superfluous sleep could ensue, a condition that Lichstein has labeled "insomnoid state" (Riedel, Lickstein, & Dwyer, 1995). Also, exclusive attribution of daytime fatigue, impaired performance, and mood disturbances to poor sleep is counterproductive and is likely to create performance anxiety. Faulty beliefs about sleep-promoting practices can also perpetuate sleep difficulties. For example, insomniacs often believe that the best way to get some sleep is to stay in bed and try harder, or that the best coping strategy to minimize the consequences of sleep loss is to take daytime naps.

Cognitive therapy seeks to alter dysfunctional beliefs and attitudes that are instrumental in exacerbating the vicious circle of insomnia, emotional arousal, fear of sleeplessness, and more sleep disturbances. Therapy relies on cognitive restructuring procedures similar to those used in the management of anxiety and affective disorders (e.g., reappraisal, reattribution, and decatastrophizing). Training and guidance is provided to identify dysfunctional sleep cognitions, challenge their validity, and replace them with more adaptive substitutes. The main issue is not to deny the presence of sleep difficulties or their impact on daytime functioning but to view insomnia from a more realistic perspective. Specific targets for intervention include (a) unrealistic sleep expectations, (b) misconceptions about the causes of insomnia, (c) misattributions or amplifications of its consequences, (d) performance anxiety resulting from excessive attempts at controlling the process of sleep, and (e) learned helplessness associated with the perceived unpredictability of sleep. The Dysfunctional Beliefs and Attitudes About Sleep Scale (Morin, 1993) is useful in identifying dysfunctional sleep cognitions and in selecting relevant targets for cognitive therapy. A more extensive discussion of cognitive therapy for insomnia is available elsewhere (Morin, 1993).

Cognitive therapy has been evaluated as a part of multicomponent treatment protocols with older adults (Edinger *et al.*, 1992; Morin, Kowatch, *et al.*, 1993; Morin, Colecchi, Ling, & Sood, 1995), but its efficacy as a single treatment modality has not yet been documented. Clinical evidence, however, suggests that cognitive therapy is a most important therapeutic component in the clinical management of insomnia and, perhaps, even more so in late life. It is particularly helpful in distinguishing pathological from normal changes in sleep patterns, which is useful in setting some realistic therapeutic goals, alleviating performance anxiety, and reinstating a sense of control over sleep. Cognitive therapy is also helpful in decatastrophizing the impact of insomnia and in preparing patients to cope more adaptively with some residual sleep difficulties that should be expected even after treatment completion.

Pharmacotherapy

Pharmacotherapy is the most frequently used method for treating sleep disturbances, and even more so among elderly patients. Several classes of drugs are used in the pharmacological management of insomnia: benzodiazepines (e.g., flurazepam, temazepam, triazolam) and related GABA-receptor agents (e.g., zolpidem and zopiclone), sedating antidepressants (e.g., amitriptyline, doxepin), antihistamines, and older drugs such as chloral hydrate and meprobamate. Neuroleptics are also used for the management of sleep disturbances associated with psychosis, dementia, and organic brain syndromes.

Benzodiazepine-receptor agents, the most commonly prescribed drugs for insomnia, are effective with short-term usage to reduce sleep latency and time awake after sleep onset, increase total sleep time, and improve sleep efficiency. However, most of these agents suppress slow-wave (stages 3 and 4) sleep, which is considered the most restorative sleep. Thus, although sleep continuity and duration are improved, sleep quality is usually worsened. All sedative-hypnotic drugs lead to tolerance and become ineffective with long-term usage. In addition, these drugs are especially hazardous to older people because of reduced metabolic functioning with aging and increased risk of interactions with other medications. Long-acting agents have residual effects that can impair cognitive functions, increase the risk of falls and hip fractures, and exacerbate the already higher incidence of sleep-related respiratory impairment. Other drawbacks include rebound anxiety and insomnia, withdrawal symptoms, drug and alcohol interactions, and the potential for dependency, which is often more psychological than physical in nature (Morin & Wooten, 1996). Although hypnotic medications can be useful in the short-term management of insomnia, these agents are not recommended for prolonged usage (NIH, 1991).

Combined Cognitive-Behavior Therapy and Pharmacotherapy

Only one study has been conducted to evaluate the efficacy of cognitive-behavior therapy and pharmacotherapy (temazepam), alone and in combination, for late-life insomnia (Morin, Colecchi, Stone, Sood, & Brink, 1995). The sample consisted of 78 older adults (mean age = 65 years) with primary and chronic insomnia, suffering predominantly from sleep-maintenance or mixed onset and maintenance difficulties. The findings showed that all three active treatments were more effective than drug-placebo at mid (4 weeks) and late treatment (8 weeks) on the two main outcome measures of time awake after sleep onset and sleep efficiency. Although there was a slight trend for the combined approach to yield better outcome, no statistically significant differences emerged among the active treatment conditions at posttreatment. These results were documented with both self-report data from daily sleep diaries and EEG-defined sleep measures from nocturnal polysomnography. Follow-up data obtained at 3, 12, and 24 months after treatment showed that subjects treated with cognitive-behavior therapy sustained their clinical gains, whereas those treated with drug therapy alone did not. Long-term effects of the combined intervention showed a significant loss of therapeutic benefits from posttreatment to follow-ups, although there was much variability across subjects in the combined condition and over the three follow-up periods.

Drug-Dependent Insomnia

Drug-dependent insomnia is recognized as a treatment-refractory health problem. Although controlled studies of psychological interventions for late-life insomnia have yielded promising results with unmedicated patients, only two studies have examined the efficacy of those treatment methods specifically for hypnotically medicated older adults. Lichstein and Johnson (1993) provided elderly community-dwelling women (hypnotically medicated insomniacs, non-hypnotically medicated insomniacs, and noninsomniacs) with three relaxation training sessions over a 2-week period. Medicated subjects reduced their medication by 47% from baseline to a 6-week follow-up without sleep deterioration. Modest improvements in sleep efficiency were obtained from baseline to posttreatment for either the medicated (62% to 70%) or drug-free (64% to 72%) insomniacs. In a pilot study (Morin, Colecchi, Ling, & Sood, 1995), five hypnotic-dependent insomnia patients were treated with cognitive-behavior therapy combined with a supervised medication tapering schedule. Four participants discontinued medication within 6 to 8 weeks and the fifth decreased drug intake by 90% over baseline. Sleep patterns initially deteriorated during the withdrawal period but tended to return toward normal values at follow-up. These findings, although very preliminary, suggest that psychological procedures, alone or combined with a supervised medication taper schedule, may facilitate reduction of hypnotic medications in older adults with insomnia. Additional research is needed to document long-term maintenance of therapeutic gains.

Management of Sleep Disturbances in Dementia

The management of sleep disturbances in dementia can be a challenging task for caregivers and clinicians alike. As for all other patients, sleep disturbances in demented patients can be caused or exacerbated by primary sleep disorders (e.g., sleep apnea) and by many other medical conditions (e.g., systemic diseases, drug toxicity, electrolyte imbalances). Thus, a careful diagnostic workup is necessary before initiating treatment.

Sedative-hypnotic drugs are prescribed three times more frequently among institutionalized than among community-dwelling elderly persons (Morgan, 1987). As for otherwise healthy insomniacs, short-term usage of sedative-hypnotics can be useful for acute sleep disturbances. However, these agents have minimal effects on nocturnal agitation accompanying dementia and, in some cases, may actually worsen the condition. Also, their long-term use often results in habituation, loss of efficacy, and drug-dependency. Adverse daytime effects on cognitive and psychomotor functioning can be more serious in the already more frail demented patients than in healthy individuals. Small doses of neuroleptic such as haloperidol and thioridazine are often used, but these potent drugs have important side effects and are always associated with risks of tardive dyskinesia.

With adequate family and nursing staff support, behavioral and environmental interventions can be of considerable help in minimizing nocturnal sleep and behavioral disturbances. The most important step is to maximize wakefulness during the daytime hours. Demented patients spend a good part of their days dozing and, given the inverse relationship between daytime wakefulness and nocturnal sleep (D. L. Bliwise, Bevier, Bliwise, Edgar, & Dement, 1990), it is essential for caregivers and nursing staff to keep patients awake during the day. This can be accomplished by scheduling a variety of social activities, restricting time spent in bed, and even by physical or manual stimulation. It is also important to incorporate light physical activity into the patient's daily routines. It may also be important for nursing home administrators to implement policies to enforce a regular arising time and to limit the amount of time patients are kept in bed, at least for those who are not bedridden. It is equally important to educate caregivers and nursing staff about the nature and extent of sleep disturbances to expect in demented patients. Even when daytime functioning may still be relatively adequate, it is certainly unrealistic to expect these patients to sleep uninterruptedly from 9:00 P.M. to 7:00 A.M.

The light-dark cycle is an important factor regulating the sleep-wake cycle in humans. Regular exposure to outdoor light is particularly important to older adults, as their circadian rhythms tend to become more disorganized. Several preliminary reports suggest that bright light exposure (i.e., phototherapy) may strengthen the circadian periodicity of the sleep-wake cycle and improve nighttime sleep in demented, as well as nondemented, elderly patients (Campbell, Dawson, & Anderson, 1993; Campbell, Kripke, Gillin, & Hrubovcak, 1988; Campbell, Satlin, Volicer, Ross, & Herz, 1991). Adequate intensity and duration of exposure to bright light are important factors in obtaining the desired effects. Light intensity should be above 2,000 lux (which is equivalent to outdoor exposure on at least a partially sunny day) for at least 2 to 3 hours. Simply leaving a patient near a window is unlikely to have any beneficial effect. Bright light therapy may also be helpful in alleviating some of the sleep disruptions and agitation in the sundown syndrome.

Nursing home patients are particularly at risk for environmentally induced sleep disturbances. Minimizing excessive noise and light and providing a comfortable mattress and adequate room temperature are essential. Routine medical procedures (e.g., vital signs) and drug administration should be scheduled, as much as possible, when the patient is already awake. Several environmental manipulations may also be helpful in minimizing disruptions and risk of injuries associated with nocturnal wandering. At home, it is important to have patients sleep on the first floor, to remove objects that may be dangerous, and even to install an alarm system to wake the caregiver if the patient attempts to leave the room. The use of nocturnal caregivers, modeled after the British "night-watchers" system, can provide some respite to family members and, in the institutional environment, nursing staff or occupational therapists might schedule supervised activities in the early morning hours to minimize disruptions for other patients.

IMPLICATIONS FOR CLINICAL PRACTICE AND FUTURE RESEARCH

Increased incidence of health problems, medication use, and stressful life events associated with aging may predispose older people to more frequent and more severe sleep disruptions. Sleep disturbances in later life are associated with significant medical and psychiatric comorbidity and can produce distress in the affected individuals, their families, and caregivers. In spite of their high incidence and debilitating effects, sleep disturbances are often unrecognized by health care professionals and, when treatment is initiated, it is too often limited to pharmacotherapy. This is unfortunate because significant advances have been made in the nonpharmacological management of sleep disturbances in the past few years and a wide variety of interventions have been successfully employed to treat this common problem in late life.

Behavioral, cognitive, and educational methods have produced substantial improvements on a number of sleep continuity parameters and have reduced emotional distress often associated with sleep disruptions. Sleep duration per se is only modestly improved, but treated patients are generally more satisfied with the quality of their sleep. Treatment effects have been documented with both subjective (daily sleep diaries) and objective measurements (polysomnography and mechanical devices). Although some early research suggested that older adults had a poorer prognosis (Alperson & Biglan, 1979), more recent findings indicate that once older patients are well screened for other sleep disorders (e.g., sleep apnea, periodic movements in sleep), their response to treatment is comparable with that of younger people. Sleep restriction and stimulus control procedures are the most effective single therapy components for late-life insomnia, with relaxation-based methods producing more variable outcomes. Cognitive therapy is a promising intervention, but has not been adequately evaluated as the sole treatment modality.

In light of the multifaceted nature of late-life sleep disturbances, clinicians do not have to (and should not) restrict their interventions to a single treatment modality. Multicomponent approaches that are specifically tailored to the changing needs and circumstances of the older adults should be considered to optimize therapeutic benefits. Despite the availability of effective treatment methods for the outpatient management of late-life insomnia, a number of barriers (e.g., cost, transportation) may prevent some elderly persons from accessing these resources. Group treatment not only reduces the cost, but has the distinct advantage of providing opportunities for social interactions with and support from peers experiencing similar problems. Although direct comparisons of individual and group therapies are needed with the elderly, these two treatment modalities have yielded comparable results with younger adults. Self-help treatment provided in the forms of written brochures and audio or video cassettes may also be a useful alternative to professionally guided treatment (Alperson & Biglan, 1979; Riedel *et al.*, 1995). This is an area for further study as many older adults do not have the financial resources or transportation to receive individual treatment provided by a professional therapist. Large-scale educational interventions targeting senior citizen groups could provide basic information about normal changes in sleep patterns with aging and specific recommendations for maintaining healthy sleep patterns in late life. This approach might prevent the development of clinical insomnia and minimize reliance on hypnotic medications. This is a particularly appealing avenue for future research as nonpharmacological interventions are generally perceived as more acceptable than pharmacotherapy (Morin, Gaulier, Barry, & Kowatch, 1992).

Much of the empirical evidence available on the treatment of late-life sleep disturbances has been obtained from healthy, medication-free, community-living older adults. The generalizability of the findings to medically ill, hypnotic-dependent, and to the more frail, institutionalized elderly patients is unknown. Although these patients may be more refractory to treatment, many of the procedures reviewed in this chapter may be of clinical benefit to those patients as well. For example, although some data suggest that hypnotic-dependent patients are not as responsive to treatment as drug-free patients are, preliminary findings indicate that combining cognitive-behavior therapy with a structured medication withdrawal program can facilitate discontinuation of hypnotic medications. Perhaps the greatest challenge for clinicians and researchers is to develop effective nonpharmacological interventions for demented and institutionalized patients. Sleep disturbances in demented patients are exceedingly difficult to manage, and it may be only through a judicious combination of behavioral, environmental, and pharmacological interventions that patients, caregivers, and nursing staff may obtain some relief.

REFERENCES

Aber, T., R., & Webb, W. B. (1986). Effects of a limited nap on night sleep in older subjects. *Psychology and Aging, 4,* 300–302.

Alperson, J., & Biglan, A. (1979). Self-administered treatment of sleep onset insomnia and the importance of age. *Behavior Therapy, 10,* 347–356.

American Psychiatric Association. (1987). *Diagnostic and statistical manual of mental disorders* (3rd ed., revised). Washington, DC: Author.

American Psychiatric Association. (1994). *Diagnostic and statistical manual of mental disorders* (4th ed.). Washington, DC: Author.

Ancoli-Israel, S., Kripke, D. F., Mason, W., & Messin, S. (1981). Sleep apnea and nocturnal myoclonus in senior population. *Sleep, 4,* 349–358.

Anderson, M. W., Zendeli, S. M., Rosa, D. P., Rubinstein, M. L., Herrera, C. O., Simons, O., Caruso, L., & Spielman, A. J. (1988). Comparison of sleep restriction therapy and stimulus control in older insomniacs: An update. *Sleep Research, 17,* 141.

Benca, R. M., Obermeyer, W. H., Thisted, R. A., & Gillin, J. C. (1992). Sleep and psychiatric disorders: A meta analysis. *Archives of General Psychiatry, 49,* 651–668.

Bliwise, D. L. (1993). Sleep in normal aging and dementia. *Sleep, 16,* 40–81.

Bliwise D. L., Tinklenberg, J., Yesavage, J. A., Davies, H., Pursley, A. M., Petta, D. E., Widrow, L., Guilleminault, C., Zarcone, V. P., & Dement, W. C. (1989). REM latency in Alzheimer's disease. *Biological Psychiatry, 25,* 320–328.

Bliwise, D. L., Bevier, W., Bliwise, N., Edgar, D., & Dement, W. C. (1990). Systematic 24-hr behavioral observations of sleep and wakefulness in a skilled care nursing facility. *Psychology and Aging, 5,* 16–24.

Bliwise, D. L., Yesavage, J., & Tinklenberg, J. (1992). Sundowning and rate of decline in mental function in Alzheimer's disease. *Dementia, 3,* 335–341.

Bliwise, N. G., Bliwise, D. L., & Dement, W. C. (1985). Age and psychopathology in insomnia. *Clinical Gerontologist, 4,* 3–9.

Bootzin, R., Engle-Friedman, M. E., & Hazelwood, L. (1983). Insomnia. In P. M. Lewinsohn & L. Teri (Eds.), *Clinical geropsychology: New directions in assessment and treatment* (pp. 81–115). Elmsford, NY: Pergamon.

Bootzin, R., Epstein, D., & Wood, J. M. (1991). Stimulus control instructions. In P. J. Hauri (Ed.), *Case studies in insomnia* (pp. 19–28). New York: Plenum.

Buysse, D. J., & Reynolds, C. F. (1990). Insomnia. In M. J. Thorpy (Ed.), *Handbook of sleep disorders* (pp. 395–433). New York: Dekker.

Buysse, D. J., Reynolds, C. F., Monk, T. H., Berman, S. R., & Kupfer, D. J. (1989). The Pittsburg Sleep Quality Index: A new instrument for psychiatric practice and research. *Psychiatry Research, 28,* 193–213.

Buysse, D. J., Reynolds, C. F., Kupfer, D. J., Thorpy, M. J. Bixler, E., Manfredi, R., Kales, A., Vgontzas, A., Stepanski, E., Roth, T., Hauri, P., & Mesiano, D. (1994). Clinical diagnoses in 216 patients using the international classification of sleep disorders (ICSD), DSM-IV and ICD-10 categories: A report from the APA/NIMH DSM-IV field trial. *Sleep, 17,* 630–637.

Campbell, S. S., Kripke, D. F., Gillin, J. C., & Hrubovcak, J. C. (1988). Exposure to light in healthy elderly subjects and Alzheimer's patients. *Physiology and Behavior, 42,* 141–144.

Campbell, S. S., Satlin, A., Volicer, L., Ross, V., & Herz, L. (1991). Management of behavioral and sleep disturbance in Alzheimer's patients using timed exposure to bright light. *Sleep Research, 20,* 446.

Campbell, S. S., Dawson, D. & Anderson, M. W. (1993). Alleviation of sleep maintenance insomnia with timed exposure to bright light. *Journal of the American Geriatrics Society, 41,* 829–836.

Coates, T. J., Killen, J. D., George, J., Marchine, E., Silverman, S., & Thoresen, C. (1982). Estimating sleep parameters: A multitrait multimethod analysis. *Journal of Consulting and Clinical Psychology, 50,* 345–352.

Coben, L. A., Chi, D., Snyder, A. Z., & Storandt, M. (1990). Replication of a study of frequency analysis of the resting awake EEG in mild probable Alzheimer's disease. *Electroencephalography Clinical Neurophysiology, 75,* 148–154.

Coleman, R. M., Roffwarg, H. P., Kennedy, S. J., Guilleminault, C., Cinque, J., Cohn, M. A., Karacan, I., Kupfer, D. J., Lemmi, H., Miles, L. E., Orr, W. C., Phillips, E. R., Roth, T., Sassin, J. F., Schmidt, H. S., Weitzman, E. D., & Dement, W. C. (1982). Sleep-wake disorders based on a polysomnographic diagnosis: A national cooperative study. *Journal of the American Medical Association, 247,* 997–1003.

Coren, S. (1988). Prediction of insomnia from arousabillty predisposition scores: Scale development and cross-validation. *Behaviour Research and Therapy, 26,* 415–420.

Coyle, K., & Watts, F. N. (1991). The factorial structure of sleep dissatisfaction. *Behaviour Research and Therapy, 29,* 513–520.

Czeisler, C. A., Dumont, M., Duffy, J. F., Steinberg, J. D., Richardson, G. S., Brown, E. N., Sanchez, R., Rios, C. D., & Ronda, J. M. (1992). Association of sleep-wake habits in older people with changes in output circadian pacemaker. *Lancet, 340,* 933–936.

Davies, R., Lacks, P., Storandt, M., & Bertelson, A. D. (1986). Counter–control treatment of sleep-maintenance insomnia in relation to age. *Psychology and Aging, 1,* 233–238.

Dement, W. C., Miles, L. E., & Carskadon, M. A. (1982). "White paper" on sleep and aging, *Journal of the American Geriatrics Society, 30,* 25–50.

Edinger, J. D., Hoelscher, T. J., Webb, M. D., Marsh, G. R., Radtke, R. A., & Erwin, C. W. (1989). Polysomnographic assessment of DIMS: Empirical evaluation of its diagnosis value. *Sleep, 12,* 315–322.

Edinger, J. D., Hoelscher, T. J., Marsh, G. R., Lipper, S., & Ionescu-Pioggia, M. (1992). A cognitive-behavioral therapy for sleep-maintenance insomnia in older adults. *Psychology and Aging, 7,* 282–289.

Engle-Friedman, M., Bootzin, R. R., Hazlewood, L., & Tsao, C. (1992). An evaluation of behavioral treatments for insomnia in the older adult. *Journal of Clinical Psychology, 48,* 77–90.

Feinberg, I., Koresko, R. L., & Heller, N. (1967). Sleep patterns as a function of normal and pathological aging in man. *Journal of Psychiatric Research, 5,* 107–144.

Feinberg, I., March, J. D., Floyd, T. C., Jimison, R., Bossom-Demitrach, L., & Katz, P. H. (1985). Homeostatic changes during postnap sleep maintain baseline levels of delta sleep EEG. *Electroencephalography and Clinical Neurophysiology, 61,* 134–137.

Ford, D. E., & Kamerow, D. B. (1989). Epidemiologic study of sleep disturbances and psychiatric disorders: An opportunity for prevention? *Journal of the American Medical Association, 262,* 1479–1484.

Friedman, L., Bliwise, D. L., Yesavage, J. A., & Salom, S. R. (1991). A preliminary study comparing sleep restriction and relaxation treatments for insomnia in older adults. *Journal of Gerontology, 46,* P1-8.

Gallagher-Thompson, D., Brooks, J. O., Bliwise, D. L., Leader, J., & Yesavage, J. A. (1992). The relations among caregiver stress, "sundowning" symptoms, and cognitive decline in Alzheimer's disease. *Journal of the American Geriatrics Society, 40,* 807–810.

Gallup Organization. (1991). *Sleep in America.* Princeton, NJ: Author.

Glovinsky, P. B., & Spielman, A. J. (1991). Sleep restriction therapy. In P. Hauri (Ed.), *Case studies in insomnia* (pp. 49–63). New York: Plenum.

Guilleminault, C. (1989). Clinical features and evaluation of obstructive sleep apnea. In M. H. Kryger, T. Roth, & W. C. Dement (Eds.), *Principles and practice of sleep medicine* (pp. 552–558). Philadelphia: Saunders.

Hart, R. P., Morin, C. M., & Best, A. M. (1995). Neuropsychological performance in elderly insomnia patients. *Aging and Cognition, 2*(4), 268–278.

Hauri, P. J. (1991). Sleep hygiene, relaxation therapy, and cognitive interventions. In P. J. Hauri (Ed.), *Case studies in insomnia* (pp. 65–84). New York: Plenum.

Hoelscher, T., & Edinger, J. E. (1988). Treatment of sleep-maintenance insomnia in older adults: Sleep period reduction, sleep education, and modified stimulus control. *Psychology and Aging, 3,* 258–263.

Hohagen, F., Kappler, C., Schramm, E., Rink, K., Weyerer, S. Riemann, D., & Berger, M. (1994). Prevalence of insomnia in elderly general practice attenders and the current treatment modalities. *Acta Psychiatrica Scandinavica, 90,* 102–108.

Jacobs, D., Ancoli-Israel, S., Parker, L., & Kripke, D. F. (1988). Sleep and wake over 24-hours in a nursing home population. *Sleep Research, 17,* 191.

Kazarian, S. S., Howe, M. G., & Csapo, K. G. (1979). Development of the sleep behavior self-rating scale. *Behavior Therapy, 10,* 412–417.

Kennedy, G. J., Kelman, H. R., & Thomas, C. (1991). Persistence and remission of depressive symptoms in late life. *American Journal of Psychiatry, 148,* 174–178.

Lacks, P., & Morin, C. M. (1992). Recent advances in the assessment and treatment of insomnia. *Journal of Consulting and Clinical Psychology, 60,* 586–594.

Lacks, P., & Rotert, M. (1986). Knowledge and practice of sleep hygiene techniques in insomniacs and poor sleepers. *Behaviour Research and Therapy, 24,* 365–368.

Lichstein, K. L., & Fisher, S. M. (1985). Insomnia. In M. Hersen & A. S. Bellack (Eds.), *Handbook of clinical behavior therapy with adults* (pp. 319–352). New York: Plenum.

Lichstein, K. L., & Johnson, R. S. (1993). Relaxation for insomnia and hypnotic use in older women. *Psychology and Aging, 8,* 103–111.

Lichstein, K. L., & Riedel, B. W. (1994). Behavioral assessment and treatment of insomnia: A review with an emphasis on clinical application. *Behavior Therapy, 25,* 659–688.

Mellinger, G. D., Balter, M. B., & Uhlenhuth, E. H. (1985). Insomnia and its treatment: Prevalence and correlates. *Archives of General Psychiatry, 42,* 225–232.

Montplaisir, J., & Godbout, R. (1989). Restless legs syndrome and periodic movements during sleep. In M. Kryger, T. Roth, & W. C. Dement (Eds.), *Principles and practice of sleep medicine* (pp. 402–409). Philadelphia: Saunders.

Morgan, K. (1987). *Sleep and aging: A research-based guide to sleep in later life.* Baltimore: Johns Hopkins University Press.

Morgan, K., Dallosso, H., Ebrahhn, S., Arie, T., & Fentem, P. H. (1988). Characteristics of subjective insomnia in elderly living at home. *Age and Aging, 17,* 1–7.

Morin, C. M. (1993). *Insomnia: Psychological assessment and management.* New York: Guilford.

Morin, C. M. (1994). Dysfunctional beliefs and attitudes about sleep: Preliminary scale development and description. *The Behavior Therapist, 17,* 163–164.

Morin, C. M., & Azrin, N. H. (1988). Behavioral and cognitive treatments of geriatric insomnia. *Journal of Consulting and Clinical Psychology, 56,* 748–753.

Morin, C. M., & Gramling, S. E. (1989). Sleep patterns and aging: Comparison of older adults with and without insomnia complaints. *Psychology and Aging, 4,* 290–294.

Morin, C. M., & Ware, J. C. (1996). Sleep and psychopathology. *Applied and Preventive Psychology, 5,* 211–224.

Morin, C. M., & Wooten, V. (1996). Psychological and pharmacological therapies for insomnia: Critical issues in assessing their separate and combined efficacy. *Clinical Psychology Review, 16,* 521–542.

Morin, C. M., Gaulier, B., Barry, T., & Kowatch, R. (1992). Patients' acceptance of psychological and pharmacological therapies for insomnia. *Sleep, 15,* 302–305.

Morin, C. M. Kowatch, R. A., Barry, T., & Walton, E. (1993). Cognitive behavior therapy for late-life insomnia. *Journal of Consulting and Clinical Psychology, 61,* 137–146.

Morin, C. M., Stone, I., Trinkle, D., Mercer, J., & Remsberg, S. (1993). Dysfunctional beliefs and attitudes about sleep among older adults with and without insomnia complaints. *Psychology and Aging, 8,* 463–467.

Morin, C. M., Culbert, J. P., & Schwartz, S. M. (1994). Nonpharmacological interventions for insomnia: A meta-analysis of treatment efficacy. *American Journal of Psychiatry, 151,* 1172–1180.

Morin, C. M., Colecchi, C. A., Ling, W. D., & Sood, R. K. (1995). Cognitive behavior therapy to facilitate benzodiazepine discontinuation among hypnotic-dependent patients with insomnia. *Behavior Therapy, 26,* 733–745.

Morin, C. M., Colecchi, C. A., Stone, J., Sood, R. K., & Brink, D. (1995). Cognitive-behavior therapy and pharmacotherapy for insomnia: Update of a placebo-controlled clinical trial. *Sleep Research, 24,* 303.

National Institutes of Health (NIH). (1991). Consensus development conference statement: The treatment of sleep disorders of older people. *Sleep, 14,* 169–177.

Nicassio, P. M., Mendlowitz, D. R., Fussel, J. J., & Petras, L. (1985). The phenomenology of the presleep state: The development of the pre-sleep arousal scale. *Behaviour Research and Therapy, 23,* 263–271.

Pollak, C. P., Perlick, D., Linsner, J. P., Wenston, J., & Hsieh, F. (1990). Sleep problems in the community elderly as predictors of death and nursing home placement. *Journal of Community Health 15,* 123–135.

Prinz, P. N., Vitaliano, P. P., Vitiello, M. V., Bokan, J., Raskind, M., Peskind, E., & Gerber, C. (1982). Sleep, EEG and mental function changes in senile dementia of the Alzheimer's type. *Neurobiology of Aging, 3,* 361–370.

Puder, R., Lacks, P., Bertelson, A. D., & Storandt, M. (1983). Short term stimulus control treatment of insomnia in older adults. *Behavior Therapy, 14,* 424–429.

Rabins, P. V., Mace, N. L., & Lucas, M. J. (1982). The impact of dementia on family. *Journal of the American Medical Association, 248,* 333–335.

Regenstein, Q. R. (1980). Insomnia and sleep disturbances in the aged: Sleep and insomnia in the elderly. *Journal of Geriatric Psychiatry, 13,* 153–171.

Reynolds, C. F., Kupfer, D. J., Taska, L. S., Hoch, C. C., Sewitch, D. W., & Spiker, D. G. (1985). The sleep of healthy seniors: A revisit. *Sleep, 8,* 20–29.

Reynolds, C. F., Kupfer, D. J., Taska, L. S., Hoch, C. C., Spiker, D. G., Sewitch, D. E., Zimmer, B., Marin, R. S., Nelson, J. P., Martin, D., & Morycz, R. (1985). EEG sleep in elderly depressed, demented, and healthy subjects. *Biological Psychiatry, 20,* 431–442.

Reynolds, C. F., Kuper, D. J., Houck, P. R., Hoch, C. C., Stack, J. A., Berman, S. R., & Zimmer, B. (1988). Reliable discrimination of elderly depressed and demented patients by electroencephalographic sleep data. *Archives of General Psychiatry, 45,* 258–264.

Riedel, B. W., Lichstein, K. L., & Dwyer, W. O. (1995). Sleep compression and sleep education for older insomniacs: Self-help versus therapist guidance. *Psychology and Aging, 10,* 54–63.

Rodin, I., McAvay, G., & Timko, C. (1988). A longitudinal study of depressed mood and sleep disturbances in elderly adults. *Journal of Gerontology, 43,* P45–P53.

Roehrs, T., Lineback, W., Zorick, F., & Roth, T. (1982). Relationship of psychopathology to insomnia in the elderly. *Journal of the American Geriatrics Society, 30,* 312–315.

Sanford, J. R. A. (1975). Tolerance of debility in elderly dependents by supporters at home: Its significance for hospital practice. *British Medicine Journal, 3,* 471–173.

Schenck, C. H., Bundlie, S. R., Patterson, A. L., & Mahowald, M. W. (1987). Rapid eye movement sleep behavior disorder: A treatable parasomnia affecting older adults. *Journal of the American Medical Association, 257,* 1786–1789.

Schoicket, S. L., Bertelson, A. D., & Lacks, P. (1988). Is sleep hygiene a sufficient treatment for sleep maintenance insomnia? *Behavior Therapy, 19,* 183–190.

Schramm, E., Hohagan, F., Grasshoff, U., Riemann, D., Hajak, G., Webb, H. G., & Berger, M. (1993). Test–retest reliability and validity of the structured interview for sleep disorders according to DSM-III-R. *American Journal of Psychiatry, 150,* 867–872.

Spielman, A. J., Saskin, P., & Thorpy, M. J. (1987). Treatment of chronic insomnia by restriction of time in bed. *Sleep, 10,* 45–56.

Vitiello, M. V., Prinz, P. P., Williams, D. E., Frommlet, M. S., & Ries, R. K. (1990). Sleep disturbances in patients with mild-stage Alzheimer's disease. *Journal of Gerontology, 45,* 131–138.

Vitiello, M. V., Bliwise, D. L., & Prinz, P. N. (1992). Sleep in Alzheimer's disease and the sundown syndrome. *Neurology, 42* (Suppl. 6), 83–93.

Webb, W. B. (1989). Age-related changes in sleep. *Clinical Geriatric Medicine 5,* 275–287.

Webb, W. B, & Campbell, S. S. (1980). Awakenings and the return to sleep in an older population. *Sleep, 3,* 41–46.

CHAPTER 14

Personality Disorders

Bunny Falk and Daniel L. Segal

INTRODUCTION

In this chapter we discuss personality disorders in older adults. After a brief look at the evolution of the *DSM* (*Diagnostic and Statistical Manual of Mental Disorders;* American Psychiatric Association) category Personality Disorders itself, and description of the disorders contained therein, our focus shifts to diagnosis and assessment of these Axis II disorders in older adults. Thereafter, we present viable treatment options available to the clinician. As we show, theoretical and research interest has varied greatly from disorder to disorder (Peterson, 1996), thus, treatment approaches for some disorders have a firmer empirical foundation than others.

OVERVIEW

Why Personality Disorders?

Why should we not refer to personality disorders as character or temperament disorders? Millon (1981) pointed out that these two words, character and temperament, are often used interchangeably with personality in the clinical as well as popular literature. He went on to cite the derivation of the word "character" from the Greek word for "engraving," and said it was originally used to "signify distinctive features that serve as the 'mark' of a person" (p. 7). Temperament, on the other hand, has come to mean the individual's "constitutional disposition" or biologically derived disposition to activity and emotionality (Millon, 1981). Allport (1937) declared the term "personality" to be "remarkably elastic" and "a perilous one for the psychologist to use." His concerns were

Bunny Falk • Center for Psychological Studies, Nova Southeastern University, Fort Lauderdale, Florida 33314. Daniel L. Segal • Department of Psychology, University of Colorado at Colorado Springs, Colorado Springs, Colorado 80933-7150.

Handbook of Clinical Geropsychology, edited by Michel Hersen and Vincent B. Van Hasselt. Plenum Press, New York, 1998.

aimed at the boundaries and principal features that the concept shares with others that are often seen as synonymous with personality.

Millon (1981) thoughtfully asked, "What then is personality?" (p. 8), and helpfully followed with the fact that it is derived from the Greek word "persona" for the masks used by dramatic actors. Although originally used to connote the hidden or "pretense of appearance," the word "persona" in time came to mean the real person, "his/her apparent, explicit, and manifest features" (p. 8). Contemporary use of the word "personality" has come to mean "a complex pattern of deeply imbedded psychological characteristics that are largely unconscious, cannot be eradicated easily, and express themselves automatically in almost every facet of functioning" (p. 8). As such, they arise from an idiosyncratic blend of biological dispositions and experiential learning to form the essence of the way a person perceives, thinks, feels, and behaves. *DSM-IV* (American Psychiatric Association, 1994) defines personality traits as "enduring patterns of perceiving, relating to, and thinking about the environment and oneself that are exhibited in a wide range of social and personal contexts." Personality Disorders are evidenced when these traits become "inflexible and maladaptive, and cause either significant functional impairment or significant distress" (p. 630).

Just as the terms normality and psychopathology represent arbitrary positions on the continuum of mental health, the particular personality disorders identified by the *DSM-IV* are somewhat arbitrary, both for what is included as well as what is not (Tyrer, 1988). Historically, limitations made sense. Over the past century, literally hundreds of personality disorders have been described on the basis of clinical observations, theoretical predictions, and empirical investigations (Peterson, 1996; Millon, 1981). To reduce these many personality disorders to a small number of the most useful, the American Psychiatric Association commissioned several committees (i.e., The Task Force on Nomenclature and Statistics) to facilitate formulation of Axis II–Personality Disorders of the *DSM-III* (American Psychiatric Association, 1980) and its successors (*DSM-III-R* and *DSM-IV*). What ensued was an obvious compromise (Pincus, Frances, Davis, First, & Widiger, 1992), not an overall vision of what it means to have a dysfunctional personality (Millon, 1990).

It was acknowledged by the task force that personality disorders represented syndromes that were "fuzzy around the edges"; on the one hand these disorders "shade imperceptibly into normal problems of everyday life," and on the other, "they have few clear and distinguishable symptoms that serve as identifying markers" (Task Force, 1976). According to Millon (1981), the task force had hoped to differentiate personality types along the dimension of severity. As yet, no such criteria for these distinctions have been developed. However, since *DSM-III*, personality disorders have been grouped into three clusters based on descriptive similarities. The *DSM-IV* includes ten Personality Disorders. Cluster A groups the disorders in which individuals often appear odd or eccentric: Paranoid, Schizoid, and Schizotypal Personality Disorders. Cluster B includes Antisocial, Borderline, Histrionic, and Narcissistic Personality Disorders, in which individuals appear to be dramatic, emotional, or erratic. Cluster C includes the disorders in which individuals often appear fearful or anxious: Avoidant, Dependent, and Obsessive-Compulsive Personality Disorders (American Psychiatric Association, 1994). Although the descriptive focus of each cluster remains intact, the disorders included have been amended somewhat as *DSM* has evolved. For example, in the *DSM-III,* the term "obsessive" was dropped in an effort to avoid confusion with the Axis I Obsessive-Compulsive Disorder. Also, Passive-Aggressive Personality Disorder, which has been reassigned for further study in the *DSM-IV,* was originally included in Cluster C in *DSM-III* and *DSM-III-R.* Interestingly, *DSM-IV* also has listed Depressive Personality Disorder as a condition requiring further study.

We will not replicate the diagnostic criteria presented within the pages of the *DSM-IV* here, but it will be helpful to define and present the clinical picture for each of the ten personality disorders included in the *DSM-IV* with one additional but often neglected feature (the clinical presentation seen in the older adult). Several researchers (Casey & Schrodt, 1989; Abrams, 1991) have suggested that the "clinical lore" that some personality disorders "burn out" with advancing age is unfounded. While it is true that markedly fewer older adults receive diagnoses of Axis II disorders as compared to younger patients, investigators have speculated that personality disorders may exist in altered form in this population, with different symptomatology, resulting in misdiagnosis when *DSM* criteria are applied (Casey & Schrodt, 1989). Kroessler (1990) noted that "diagnostic reliability is lower" using criteria in the *DSM-III* for Personality Disorders because they require more inferential judgment than those for the Axis I disorders. In an effort to improve reliability, the *DSM-III-R* included more behavioral descriptors in the personality disorder guidelines, and the *DSM-IV* elaborated on this behavioral emphasis by including narrative descriptions to clarify the contextual associations of behavior (Kroessler, 1990).

DSM-IV Personality Disorders

1. *Paranoid Personality Disorder*

The disorder manifests itself as a pervasive pattern of distrust and suspicion without any justification. Persons with the disorder tend not to confide in others, refuse to give personal information, and maintain the expectation that all others will do them harm. Suspiciousness and distrust occur in situations where others would be hard pressed to find justification for their beliefs. The pervasiveness of suspicion is such that even events that have nothing to do with them will be interpreted as personal attacks. In older adults, any decline in hearing, vision, or cognitive ability may incorrectly lead to ideas of reference that others are talking about them or threatening them in some way. Therefore, people with the disorder are often experienced as complaining, argumentative, or hostile.

2. *Schizoid Personality Disorder*

The hallmark of this disorder is a preference for isolation to a point of detachment from social relationships accompanied by a restricted range of emotional expression. Such people are often experienced as aloof, cold, or indifferent to others, but, most notably, they seem to have no desire for nor enjoyment of interpersonal relationships so that they seem immune to criticism or praise. Unlike the other two disorders included in cluster A, persons with Schizoid Personality Disorder do not have unusual thought processes that characterize Paranoid and Schizotypal Personality Disorders. In older adults, withdrawal from social relationships is often viewed as an accompaniment of a decline in physical stamina. If these clinical signs were a part of a pervasive behavioral style, this note should outweigh the assumption that what is being observed is due to normal aging.

3. Schizotypal Personality Disorder

Individuals with this disorder are described as odd, bizarre, or eccentric. Most often such persons experience extreme discomfort with interpersonal relationships; therefore, they tend to withdraw socially. Their speech and dress are often clearly unusual. "Ideas of reference" and "magical thinking" in the form of odd beliefs or possession of special powers such as clairvoyance or telepathic thinking are reported. Perceptual distortions are not as extreme as those reported by individuals with schizophrenia; people diagnosed as Schizotypal may report that they feel as though someone is in the room with them, but stop short of saying that they actually see the person. Even so, others often question their perceptions and this doubting fuels the formation of suspiciousness and paranoid thinking. In the absence of obvious organicity, an older adult who is unkempt, malodorous, experiences suspiciousness, paranoia, and ideas of reference, and has few friends could be diagnosed with Schizotypal Personality Disorder.

4. Antisocial Personality Disorder

The hallmark of the disorder is a lifelong pattern of disregard for, and failure to comply with, societal norms. Rights of others are never a consideration, and when these rights are violated, they experience no remorse. Such people are often perceived as aggressive because they take what they want, when they want it, with no regard for the impact their action will have on others. Lying, cheating, and stealing appear to be part of their nature. Several behavioral descriptors of the disorder, such as aggressiveness, impulsiveness, lawlessness, and physical fighting, clearly require physical activity (Kroessler, 1990). These behaviors may diminish in frequency as the person's stamina and strength decline with advancing age. However, Perry (1993) reported in his review of longitudinal studies of personality disorders that several researchers (Guze, 1976; Hoke, Livori, & Perry, 1992; Martin, Cloninger, & Guze, 1982) found that felons either incarcerated or on probation continued to meet criteria for Antisocial Personality Disorder 6 to 9 years after their arrest. This finding may demonstrate that even externally imposed physical limitations do not assure that the personality disorder will remit.

5. Borderline Personality Disorder

This disorder is highlighted by extreme instability in interpersonal relationships, self-image, mood, and affect. Also present is marked impulsivity, which usually results in poor judgment and engaging in high-risk behaviors such as substance abuse, sexual promiscuity, and self-injurious acts or suicide attempts (Widiger & Trull, 1993). People with this disorder often complain of being chronically "bored" and are experienced by others as extremely "needy" and demanding. Emotionally labile, they will sometimes be described as intense, shifting from anger to deep depression very quickly (Barlow & Durand, 1995). Snyder, Pitts, and Gustin (1983) reported that it is "uncommon to find patients over the age of 40 with the diagnosis of borderline personality disorder" (p. 271). Often, "older patients fulfill fewer *DSM-III* criteria for the disorder than they did when they were younger and receive other diagnoses as they reach middle age" (p. 271). The *DSM-III-R* (American Psychiatric Association, 1987) stated: "The manifestations of Personality Disorders are often recognized by adolescence or earlier and continue throughout most of adult life, though they often become less obvious in middle or old age" (p. 335). However, McCrea and Costa (1984) seemingly disagreed when they hypothesized that one's character is stable throughout the life course. Perhaps the lower incidence of the disorder in older adults "reflects more the lack of fit of our existing diagnostic yardsticks than the lack of borderline personality disorder in old age" (Rosowsky & Gurian, 1991).

6. *Histrionic Personality Disorder*

People diagnosed with this disorder tend to present themselves in an overstated, theatrical manner, engaging in excessive emotional displays, with the primary goal of remaining the center of attention. Their exaggerated sense of self often prohibits any sensitivity or compassion for others. Relationships typically are superficial. Grandiose self-descriptions are not uncommon and are usually accompanied by unreasonable expectations of special attention from everyone. Histrionic people tend to become outraged at the mere suggestion of a confrontation about their behavior (Beck & Freeman, 1990). In addition, they seek reassurance continuously and become very angry or upset when others do not give them their undivided attention. Older adults so disordered are often described by their adult children as "acting like spoiled little children." Such individuals, with their flirtatious and superficial style, tend to adjust poorly to the physical changes (wrinkles, gray hair) associated with normal aging (they do not like to look old!)

7. *Narcissistic Personality Disorder*

The main feature of this disorder is the exaggerated sense of self-importance a person demonstrates, to the point of being described as "grandiose" by others. Such persons also tend to be preoccupied with themselves, lack sensitivity and compassion for others, have a sense of entitlement, and express discomfort in situations in which they are not surrounded by people they perceive as being as special and privileged as they see themselves. People with the disorder also tend to take advantage of others to get what they want (Zimmerman, 1994). Older adults with the disorder are experienced by others as insensitive, demanding, boorish, and selfish. Alienation of family members is not uncommon after a lifetime of perceived callous disregard for, and purposeful manipulation of, others in their family.

8. Avoidant Personality Disorder

People diagnosed with this disorder have an extreme sensitivity to the opinion of others. Therefore, they avoid placing themselves in any social situation wherein they might be rejected. In essence, they reject others to avoid being rejected themselves. Such people have low self-esteem and feel inadequate to cope with the anxiety and fearfulness associated with social relationships. Such individuals typically are isolated across the life span.

9. Dependent Personality Disorder

For individuals with this disorder, the task of making any decision, whether it will impact their life or determine everyday activities, is relinquished to others. As a result, disordered people are left with an overwhelming fear of being abandoned. Although often characterized as submissive, passive, and timid, people with dependent personality disorder are not without their own opinions or beliefs. However, rather than risk rejection, they do not express their opinions and beliefs. Often after the death of their spouse, dependent older adults appear helpless, unable to perform the most mundane of functions after decades of relying on their partners to make all the decisions for the couple. Feeling lost and vulnerable, older adults then turn to their adult children to fill the void left by the decision maker. Such a situation is described as "role reversal," with adult children finding themselves acting "en loco parentis" for their elderly parents.

10. Obsessive-Compulsive Personality Disorder

People with this disorder are so preoccupied with details that it interferes with functioning in several areas of their life. They manifest a pervasively rigid and moralistic style that hinders forming interpersonal relationships. Often described by others as "workaholics," those with this personality disorder forgo leisure activities for the sake of productivity. Ironically, it is productivity that suffers because the point of many an activity is lost among the rules, regulations, lists, and schedules to which they scrupulously and overconscientiously adhere. Delegation of responsibility or work to others is unheard of, usually for fear that the task will not be completed in the "right way." Older men find it particularly difficult to modify their approach.

DIAGNOSIS AND ASSESSMENT

Overview

The *DSM-IV* (American Psychiatric Association, 1994) takes a view regarding the course of dysfunctional patterns of inner experience and behavior (i.e., personality disorders) that some disorders tend to "remit with age, whereas this appears to be less true for some other types [of disorders]" (p. 632). Recognition of the persistent course of at least some personality dysfunction into later life can be contrasted with the view proffered in the *DSM-III-R* (American Psychiatric Association, 1987), in which it was specifically noted that the personality disorders become less pronounced in middle or old age.

Epidemiological and prevalence data for Axis II disorders in older adults are scant. As noted by Spar and La Rue (1990), "Few data have been gathered on Axis II disorders in elderly patients, in part because most of the personality disorders in *DSM-III-R* have not been defined long enough for thorough studies to take place" (p. 180). Indeed, prior to *DSM-III,* personality disorders did not have well-operationalized or specific criteria for each type. Therefore, early investigations of character pathology in older adults used classification systems that are quite dissimilar from current *DSM-III-R* and *DSM-IV* conceptualizations (Kroessler, 1990), thus preventing meaningful comparison of current and prior data. Overall, it appears that prevalence rates for diagnosable personality disorders in the elderly community range from 2% to 11% from report to report (Cohen, 1990).

Rates are even more variable (and generally higher) when psychiatric samples are evaluated. Three retrospective studies (Casey & Schrodt, 1989; Fogel & Westlake, 1990; Mezzich, Fabrega, Coffman, & Gavin, 1987), and one descriptive study (Kunik *et al.*, 1993), although limited by their reliance on clinical judgment in assigning diagnosis and the absence of reliability checks, reported prevalence of personality disorders in older adults to range from 5.1% to 24%. Obviously, results are likely to vary depending on type of sample (i.e., inpatient, outpatient, medical patients), method of diagnosis (i.e., clinical judgment, structured interview, self-report), and type of design (descriptive, chart review, longitudinal). Despite gaps in the epidemiological research base, extant data suggest that personality disorders in the elderly are possibly more common than previously was thought, and that a significant number of older adults suffer from debilitating personality dysfunction.

Diagnosis

Diagnosis of personality disorder in the older population has been complicated by several factors. One is the widely held, long-lasting (albeit erroneous) belief that personality dysfunction either was not present or was not a serious difficulty in older individuals. Some misdiagnoses occur because personality disorders often produce symptoms that constitute Axis I disturbances, which are more easily recognized and accepted by both clients and service providers (Segal, Hersen, Van Hasselt, Silberman, & Roth, 1996). Manifestations of characterological difficulties may be viewed as signs of other psychiatric disorders, most notably depression and anxiety (Segal *et al.*, 1996). These symptoms may, in fact, be consequences of the pervasive social difficulties and distorted self-images experienced by those suffering from personality dysfunction. Also, some signs of personality disturbance (e.g., dependency, avoidance, social withdrawal, odd thinking, emotional liability) are erroneously attributed to "old age" or may be perceived as "normal" in the aged population. Unfortunately, diagnostic misconceptions can translate into confusion about the most appropriate form of intervention. Too often, applied interventions target solely the more recognized affective component of the disturbance, while the etiologically significant underlying personality disorder is ignored.

Another obstacle to accurate diagnosis of personality disorder in older adults is that *DSM-IV* criteria for some personality disorders have limited relevance or applicability to aged clients given their unique physical, cognitive, and social circumstances. The need to attend to age-related issues has been noted only recently. Just as somatic problems may confound diagnosis of Axis I disorders, Kroessler (1990) noted similar difficulties with the diagnosis of personality disorders in older individuals. He contends that personality disorders are most reliably described in behavioral terms and that normal aging can alter preexisting behaviors and produce new behaviors. Lawlessness, aggressiveness, impulsiveness, initiating physical fights, child-beating, and promiscuity require physical activity. Consequently, some criteria may not be applicable to older adults for biological reasons in terms of normal decreases in energy, strength, and mobility (Kroessler, 1990). Along these lines, Fogel and Westlake (1990) use the aging borderline personality disorder as an example, observing that "some forms of impulsive sexual and self-injurious behaviors may become less likely, despite the persistence of characteristic personality traits and psychodynamics" (p. 233). Similar age bias is likely to apply to other personality types as well.

A major requirement for the diagnosis of any personality disorder is the experience of clinically significant distress or impairment in social or occupational functioning (criterion C; *DSM-IV*; American Psychiatric Association, 1994). As some individuals age, they work less frequently and have fewer friends and social networks due to deaths, physical disabilities, and transportation problems. Thus, the requirement of social and occupational impairment may preclude accurate diagnosis of personality disorder in older adults whose social world is much different from that of their younger counterparts upon whom many taxonomies are based. As age-related behavior change may mask presence of personality disorder, several investigators (Kroessler, 1990; Segal *et al.*, 1996) argue for inclusion of age-associated criteria in the diagnostic guidelines.

Several additional factors have contributed to the lack of attention to Axis II disorders in older adults. First, there appears to be a lack of consensus concerning age-related manifestations of certain disorders, as researchers and clinicians have only recently been interested in psychopathology of older adults. Second, treatment providers may lack appropriate knowledge about how personality disorders manifest themselves in an older patient. Consequently, their initial assessment measures may fail to detect this component. Third, diverse service providers to older individuals may be biased against diagnosing personality disorders or defining problems as characterological (Rose, Soares, & Joseph, 1993). Rose and colleagues suggest that the inflexibility and resistance to intervention attributed to individuals carrying an Axis II diagnosis often make the client seem "hopeless" and service providers feel "helpless." Professionals may also feel angry, frustrated, and manipulated by personality disordered elders and they may react by withdrawing or blaming the client. Unfortunately, despite the discomfort of service providers and the bias against diagnosing Axis II disorders, older clients with personality disorders exist and are in need of support and intervention. Fourth, there may be inadequate case-finding strategies for personality-disordered elders who view their characteristic modes of thinking and behaving as ego-syntonic and do not recognize a problem. Consequently, many older adults with significant character pathology simply see little reason to seek mental health services.

Several case reports have appeared in the literature documenting the unique diagnostic and intervention challenges faced by mental health professionals. Siegel and Small (1986) document these challenges in a case description of borderline personality disorder. More recently, case examples of histrionic, borderline, and avoidant personality disorders in old age have been presented (Rose *et al.*, 1993). Systematic evaluation to develop profiles of the manifestations of each disorder in the aged has not yet evolved. Longitudinal studies following personality-disordered individuals into later life are needed. Such studies would enable investigators to assess changes over time in symptom patterns and personality characteristics.

Assessment

The original Minnesota Multiphasic Personality Inventory (MMPI; Hathaway & McKinley, 1983), its revision, the MMPI-2 (Hathaway, & McKinley, 1989), the Millon Clinical Multiaxial Inventory III (MCMI-III; Millon, 1994), and the Coolidge Axis II Inventory (CATI, Coolidge, 1993) are among the most commonly utilized objective methods for measuring personality styles, disorders, and clinical syndromes (Segal *et al.*, 1996). These instruments are discussed below.

Minnesota Multiphasic Personality Inventory (MMPI)

Description.   The MMPI was not designed or standardized to measure functioning in older adult populations (Segal *et al.*, 1996). In fact, individuals over age 65 were not included in the normative sample (Colligan & Offord, 1992). The restandardization process involved in constructing the MMPI-2 (Hathaway & McKinley, 1989) incorporated persons up to 85 years of age. However, norms for older adults are noticeably absent from resource books (Graham, 1990), although separate MMPI-2 norms for men and women are provided and an adolescent version of the instrument is available.

MMPI and Older Adults.   As the original MMPI did not include persons over 65 in the normative group, several investigators have examined its effectiveness in normal, nonpatient, older samples (e.g., Colligan & Offord, 1992; Colligan, Osborne, Swenson, & Offord, 1984; Greene, 1980; Harmatz & Shader, 1975; Leon, Gillum, Gillum, & Gouze, 1979). In their review of these studies, Taylor, Strassberg, and Turner (1989) identified several trends. They noted that nonpsychiatric older respondents generally displayed substantial elevations (approximately one standard deviation) on Scales 1 (Hypochondriasis), 2 (Depression), and 3 (Hysteria). Smaller elevations were reported for Scales K and 0 (Social Introversion) when compared to the standard adult MMPI norms.

Application of the MMPI has also been investigated in older psychiatric populations (e.g., Dye, Bohm, Anderten, & Cho, 1983; Pennington, Peterson, &

Barber, 1979; Rusk, Hyerstay, Calsyn, & Freemen, 1979; Weiss, 1973). Taylor and colleagues (1989) concluded from the collective findings that the most common elevations were obtained on Scales 1 and 2, a finding similar to the normal samples of older adults. In addition, elevations of $1^{1}/_{2}$ standard deviations were found on Scales 3 and 8 (Schizophrenia), while deviations of about +1 standard deviation were noted for Scales F, 4 (Psychopathic Deviate), 6 (Paranoia), and 7 (Psychasthenia). Taylor and colleagues (1989) caution, however, that most results were based on either extremely small samples or highly specific clinical groups, thus limiting generalizability. The purpose of their effort was to identify norms for a nonclinical elderly sample and to assess the discriminant validity of the MMPI (clinical versus community elderly). Results suggested that the MMPI discriminated well between the two groups with significant differences reported on 9 of 13 scales. Overall the MMPI was considered valid for use with older populations.

Clearly, utility of the MMPI and the MMPI-2 in older adult samples has yet to be unequivocally ascertained. For example, questions about interpretation of elevations on Scales 1, 2, and 3 have been raised in light of the confounding influences of biological maturation. Given the likelihood of an increase in physical problems in the elderly, several investigators urge caution when interpreting elevations in Scale 2 (Bolla-Wilson & Bleecker, 1989) and Scales 1 and 3 (Taylor *et al.,* 1989). No research specifically applying the MMPI to older inpatient groups or to groups with specific personality disorders has been located. In addition, the MMPI-2 has not been empirically validated specifically in the older population (Segal *et al.,* 1996). Finally, it should be pointed out that the MMPI scales employed in the studies cited are not measures of *DSM-III-R* or *DSM-IV* personality disorders, but rather of personality traits, symptom profiles, and Axis I disorders. Further, while personality scales have been derived from the MMPI (see Morey, Waugh, & Blashfield, 1985), validation studies specific to an older population are lacking.

Millon Clinical Multiaxial Inventory (MCMI)

Description.   The original MCMI (Millon, 1983) was revised and reintroduced as the MCMI-II (Millon, 1987) and most recently as the MCMI-III (Millon, 1994). The MCMI-III is a self-report inventory designed to assess and diagnose *DSM-IV*–related personality disorders. Widely used in clinical and research contexts, its taxonomy is more consistent with the *DSM* system than the original MCMI. The MCMI-III has 24 scales (14 personality pattern scales and 10 Axis I scales) and is constructed to distinguish between Axis I and Axis II diagnoses, as well as to assess level of severity of all syndromes (Millon, 1992).

MCMI and Older Adults.   Application of the MCMI to older psychiatrically impaired adults has been explored in only one study, and norms for this measure are unavailable for nonpsychiatric elders (Segal *et al.,* 1996). Hyer and Harrison (1986) administered the instrument to elderly psychiatric inpatients, and reported that incidence rates of dependent and avoidant personality disorders were highest in this older group. In contrast, histrionic, narcissistic, and antisocial personality disorders had the lowest rates. These investigators characterized the latter disorders as "higher intensity personality styles" and concluded that "with age, there appears to be a mellowing of higher energy personality types" (p. 408). The paucity of studies clarifying age differences between younger and older adults, and the lack of normative data for older adults, are problems to be addressed by future research.

Coolidge Axis II Inventory (CATI)

Description. The CATI (Coolidge, 1993) is a true–false, self-report inventory originally developed to assess personality disorders according to the diagnostic criteria of the *DSM-III-R*. It has since been updated to match *DSM-IV* criteria for all personality disorders. The inventory contains 14 personality disorder scales, including the sadistic and self-defeating personality disorders, with items from *DSM-III-R* designed to match all the unique criteria for personality disorder diagnosis detailed in the *DSM-IV*. The CATI also provides scores on several Axis I scales (e.g., Brain Dysfunction, Depression, Anxiety, and PTSD). Excellent test–retest reliability (.90) has been established for the CATI, as well as moderate internal consistency (.76). With regard to validity, a 50% concordance rate with clinical diagnoses for 24 personality disordered patients was reported (Coolidge & Merwin, 1992).

CATI and Older Adults. Coolidge, Burns, Nathan, and Mull (1992) administered the CATI to normal younger (mean age 24.0 years) and older (mean age 69.4 years) individuals and found that for Axis I syndromes, older adults were significantly less anxious and showed more signs of brain damage, while reporting no differences on the depression scale. As for Axis II, the older adults scored significantly lower on antisocial, borderline, histrionic, narcissistic, paranoid, passive-aggressive, schizotypal, sadistic, and self-defeating scales than their younger counterparts. By contrast, older adults were significantly more obsessive-compulsive and schizoid. No group differences were obtained for avoidant or dependent personality disorder scales. Coolidge and colleagues (1992) note that, in general, the older sample scored lower on items associated with impulsivity and endorsed items consistent with restricted affectivity. These investigators attributed the nonsignificant finding for depression to the lack of somatic items on that particular scale. As with the MCMI, investigations of age differences with clinical samples have been conducted infrequently. Also, normative data for an older adult population of psychiatric patients has not been collected or examined.

Comparisons of the MMPI, MCMI, and CATI

MMPI and MCMI. Several studies have compared the MMPI and MCMI for Axis I disorders (see Libb, Murray, Thurstin, & Alarcon, 1992; Patrick, 1988). With regard to the Axis II disorders, controversy surrounds the fact that the MCMI is derived from Millon's personality/psychopathology theory (Segal *et al.*, 1996). Initially, conceptual differences between Millon's theory of psychopathology and nosology and *DSM-III* typology called into question the validity of the MCMI as a measure of *DSM-III* personality disorders (see Widiger,

Williams, Spitzer, & Francis, 1985); however, with updates in the new MCMI-III, the convergence between Millon's taxonomy and the *DSM* is appreciably strong.

Concurrent validity investigations generally have shown a modest degree of convergence between the MCMI and personality scales derived from the MMPI (McCann, 1989; Morey & LeVine, 1988; Streiner & Miller, 1988). A recent validity study with the updated MCMI-II and MMPI personality disorder scales demonstrated that, relative to the original MCMI, the updated MCMI-II generated higher concordance rates for antisocial and passive-aggressive disorders, but still failed to reach significant convergence on the obsessive-compulsive scale (McCann, 1991). None of these studies, however, specifically targeted older adults; therefore, the concurrent validity of the MCMI and the MMPI is presently unknown for this population.

MCMI and CATI.   Coolidge and Merwin (1992) compared the CATI and the MCMI-II in a sample of psychiatric outpatients (mean age 38.0 years) clinically assessed by their therapists to have a personality disorder. Similar to a previous MCMI–MMPI validation study (McCann, 1991), correlations for the obsessive-compulsive personality disorder were extremely low. Based on a criterion analysis of this scale, the investigators suggested that diagnostic criteria coverage of the MCMI-II was incomplete as only five of the nine stated *DSM-III-R* criteria were addressed. Coolidge and Merwin (1992) concluded that the low correlation was due to lack of adherence of the MCMI to *DSM-III-R* criteria upon which the CATI is based. In contrast, for the disorders for which the MCMI-II's adherence to *DSM-III-R* criteria was high, correlations between the two inventories were stronger. Overall, the MCMI-II diagnosed more subjects as having personality disorders than did the CATI.

Other Assessment Instruments and Older Adults

Several additional devices also have been designed to assess *DSM-IV* personality disorders; an example is the Personality Diagnostic Questionnaire–4 (PDQ-4; Hyler, 1994), an 85-item self-administered, true/false inventory that taps the ten standard *DSM-IV* personality disorders. Several popular structured interviews that yield *DSM-IV* diagnoses include the Structured Clinical Interview for *DSM-IV* Axis II Personality Disorders (SCID-I; First, Gibbon, Spitzer, Williams, & Benjamin, 1997), the International Personality Disorder Examination (IPDE; Loranger *et al.,* 1994), and the Structured Interview for *DSM-IV* Personality (SIDP-IV; Pfohl, Blum & Zimmerman, 1995).

As is the case with instruments discussed earlier, application of the aforementioned measures to older individuals is sparse. In two studies (Abrams, Alexopoulos, & Young, 1987; Abrams, Rosendahl, Card, & Alexopoulos, 1994) the PDE was administered to small samples of older adults. The earlier study compared 15 normal controls to 21 recovered depressives and found that only two participants met criteria for a personality disorder, but no reliability estimates for the PDE were reported. The latter study used the PDE to assess 30 recovered depressed elders and reliability estimates between two raters were calculated. Results suggested a high level of interrater reliability (range .75 to 1.0; mean .94) for all personality disorders except histrionic (.23). Schneider,

Zemansky, Bender, and Sloane (1992) assessed personality traits using the SCID-II in a small sample of euthymic elders with a history of depression. To investigate the relationship between personality disorder and treatment outcome for late-life depression, Thompson, Gallagher, and Czirr (1989) obtained Axis II formulations by using the Structured Interview for *DSM-III* Personality (SIDP; Pfohl, Stangl, & Zimmerman, 1983) in a sample of 79 elders. While interrater reliability for comparisons across all twelve personality classifications was high (kappa = .79), individual estimates were not reported.

Comment

All of the frequently administered structured interviews for *DSM* personality disorders (SCID-II, IPDE, SIDP-IV) have been applied to older populations, but definitive comparisons have been difficult to make because of small sample sizes, variant settings, and limited reliability, not to mention the fact that these new versions have been published only recently. In the absence of empirical verification, it cannot be assumed that structured interviews for Axis II disorders have acceptable operating characteristics for this unique population. As for self-report devices, normative and reliability data are limited for the PDQ-R (Hyler & Reider, 1987). For the MMPI, several large-scale studies have provided normative data for older adults. Results have clearly shown that older individuals respond in ways substantially different from their younger counterparts. However, such clinically significant information has not been incorporated into standard use of the instrument, as has been done with norms for men, women, and adolescents. Despite availability of these data, clinicians employing the MMPI with older adults continue to rely on clinical intuition to determine significance of profile elevations. Moreover, although normative data for the MMPI exist, neither the MMPI-2 nor the MMPI personality disorder scales developed by L. C. Morey and colleagues (1985) have been adequately researched in the elderly.

The MCMI and CATI self-report personality instruments have been applied to older adults, albeit minimally. Hyer and Harrison (1986) administered the MCMI to a group of older inpatients and reported incidence rates, although comparisons to matched normal or younger patients were not included in their investigation. For the CATI, only one report examined age difference between normal younger and older respondents (Coolidge *et al.*, 1992).

Comparisons among widely employed measures to assess their concurrent validity with older adults have been undertaken only recently. A recent comparison between MCMI-II and MMPI personality disorder scales in an adult sample has yielded encouraging results (McCann, 1991). Investigating this relationship in an older sample should not be delayed. Two studies have explored the concurrent validity of MCMI-II with the CATI, with one specifically targeting older mentally ill inpatients (Silberman, Roth, Segal, & Burns, 1997). Median concordance (correlation between raw score sums) in this study was .55, with a range of −.13 (schizoid) to .88 (borderline). Results for the older sample were also generally poorer than those obtained in the younger group (Coolidge & Merwin, 1992). These findings point to the need for specific validation in older samples who seem to manifest character disorders differently from younger adults.

Little attention has been accorded to systematic exploration of the relationship between Axis I and Axis II disorders, specifically within the older population. As shown by Mavissakalian and colleagues (Mavissakalian & Hamann, 1986; Mavissakalian & Hamann, 1988; Mavissakalian, Hamann, & Jones, 1990; Mavissakalian, Hamann, Haidar, & de Groot, 1993), personality disorders and many Axis I disorders (e.g., generalized anxiety, panic/agoraphobia, and obsessive-compulsive) can be linked, providing important conceptual clarification of the Axis I conditions. While some of Mavissakalian's work included older subjects, data were not separated for older and younger groups. There is still an unmet need for understanding of the characterological component to Axis I presentations in older patients. Research is needed to shed more light on the relationships between Axis I and Axis II disorders so as to yield more effective treatment strategies.

TREATMENT

Overview

Overall, inadequate assessment and diagnosis are major barriers to the treatment phase for personality dysfunction in older adults. Elder-specific assessment measures have yet to be developed and validated; thus, knowledge as to how personality disorders in older adults are identified and dealt with by service providers is limited. Because of the unique characteristics and differing presentation of older individuals with personality dysfunction, clinicians must be cognizant of specific variables associated with aging, as well as correlates of personality disorders in the elderly. Some investigators, however, posit that those with personality disorders seem to respond poorly to most forms of therapy (Reich & Green, 1991; Shea *et al.,* 1990). In addition, because of imprecise and overlapping criteria used to describe these disorders (Blashfield & Breen, 1989; Nurnberg *et al.,* 1991; Oldham *et al.,* 1992), multiple diagnoses seem almost inevitable (e.g., Herbert, Hope, & Bellack, 1992; Kavoussi & Siever, 1992; Schneier, Spitzer, Gibbon, Fyer, & Leibowitz, 1991).

Treatment of the Specific Disorders

Paranoid Personality Disorder

Clinicians are offered little in the way of treatment proposals for this disorder (Adler, 1990) except that it is "virtually a given that such individuals do not fare well in therapy" (Peterson, 1996, p. 385). The therapist is sure to be viewed with the same suspicion as everyone else (Bullard, 1960), and therapeutic alliance is difficult to form. Lack of insight into the internal origins of their suspicions fosters the notion that it is others who have "the problem." Ellison and Adler (1990) report that psychotropic medications used to treat positive symptoms of schizophrenia offer a viable treatment option, in that they reduce levels of suspicion in some patients.

Schizoid Personality Disorder

Treatment options for this disorder "remain a puzzle because so few people who warrant the diagnosis enter the mental health system" (Peterson, 1996, p. 385). In older adults, entrée into the medical system is usually when pathology is first addressed. Thus, success is hardly expected by most caregivers, and the low expectations probably account for the paucity of investigations into effective treatment. Links with schizophrenia suggest, however, that behaviorally oriented social and life skills training offer the most likely treatment options.

Schizotypal Personality Disorder

The social awkwardness and anxiety that characterize this personality style should be considered when planning treatment for individuals so diagnosed. Although treatment protocols have not been systematically investigated (Mehlum *et al.,* 1991), the disorder's proposed relationship to schizophrenia highlights the need to limit the patient's exposure to stressful situations (Peterson, 1996). When older adults so diagnosed lose the ability to live independently, their "odd" or "eccentric" peculiarities are an unwelcome imposition on others. Caregivers may look to psychotropic medications that prove useful in treating prominent delusions or hallucinations to quiet (albeit unsuccessfully) these "strange" behaviors. Bellack and Hersen (1985) and others (e.g., O'Brien, Trestman, & Siever, 1993) have suggested social skills training as a means to improve socialization and reduce isolation.

Antisocial Personality Disorder

Early intervention with persons at risk for developing the disorder in adulthood is the most successful treatment approach. This means that children at risk need to be identified and interventions implemented before the disorder manifests itself in early adulthood. Clinicians are, for the most part, pessimistic about treatment for patients who do not perceive themselves as having any problems (Patterson, 1982), a trait prominent in individuals with Antisocial Personality Disorder. Lack of early intervention usually results in clinicians' deferring to incarceration as a means of limiting future antisocial behavior (Barlow & Durand, 1995).

Borderline Personality Disorder

Treatment with people diagnosed with this disorder would be problematic and challenging even if their dropout rate from therapy was not so high (Gunderson *et al.,* 1989). Several investigators (Aronson, 1989; Higgit & Fonagy, 1992) have reported that inability to achieve insight, as well as the inability to focus on the self and monitor how they think and feel, limits the effectiveness of insight-oriented approaches. Cognitive-behavioral treatment formulations (Beck & Freemen, 1990; Fleming & Pretzer, 1990) teach the borderline individual to identify troublesome thoughts and feelings and then gain mastery of them. Westin (1991) points out that a blend of cognitive-behavior and object-relations strategies produces an effective approach, "because what they do in effect is teach the adult individual what most children learn while growing up" (Peterson, 1996, p. 394).

Histrionic Personality Disorder

Disappointingly, there is a paucity of research into the effectiveness of proposed treatment approaches for this disorder (Dulit, Marin, & Frances, 1993; Quality Assurance Project, 1991). Treatment usually takes a dual track: supportive, to foster growth through nurturing the individual to trust and relate better to others, and behavioral, to instruct the individual in more appropriate ways to ask for their wants and needs (Beck & Freeman, 1990).

Narcissistic Personality Disorder

Millon (1981) reports that typically, narcissistic individuals do not seek out treatment for their dysfunctional attitudes and behaviors, which are ego-syntonic. However, many narcissistic individuals experience depressed mood; they view this as ego-dystonic and seek treatment. Much of the treatment literature comes from a psychodynamic perspective, but even here, there is disagreement as to the effectiveness of treatment (Aronson, 1989; Glasser, 1992). Of the object relations school, Kernberg (1975) takes the position that narcissism can be successfully treated psychoanalytically. Kohut (1971, 1977) disagrees and argues that psychoanalysis is of limited usefulness. Cognitive-behaviorists aim to improve individuals' ability to see themselves in a more complex and realistic way, as opposed to either inflated or diminished (Beck & Freeman, 1990).

Avoidant Personality Disorder

Treatment strategies aimed at placing avoidant individuals in more situations that will allow them to challenge negative associations with social interactions have been developed by behavioral and cognitive-behavioral theorists (Alden, 1989; Alden & Caperol, 1993; Heimberg & Barlow, 1991; Renneberg, Goldstein, Phillips, & Chambless, 1990). Proceeding carefully, the therapy focuses on changing individuals' thoughts about themselves and the world and identifying and gathering evidence to support these notions. Social skills training is an integral part of the treatment protocol (Stravynski, Lesage, Marcouiller, & Elie, 1989).

Dependent Personality Disorder

Cognitive-behavioral strategies that include social skills training, assertiveness training, and learning to challenge automatic thoughts about abandonment have been demonstrated as being effective (Beck & Freeman, 1990; Turkat & Carlson, 1984). However, Millon (1981) cautions that dependent individuals often appear agreeable to and compliant with every suggestion that the clinician makes. Reports of "great success" at times represent attempts to please the therapist, rather than representing accurate outcome data.

Obsessive-Compulsive Personality Disorder

Insight-oriented therapy has long targeted the fears that seem to underlie the need for orderliness (Peterson, 1996). In addition, behavioral interventions such as systematic desensitization, relaxation training, and distraction techniques (Ricciardi *et al.,* 1992; Steketee, Foa, & Grayson, 1982) increase the individual's tolerance for anxiety experienced while exploring these fears and compulsions.

SUMMARY

Only recently have psychologists recognized the importance of evaluating specific diagnostic, assessment, and treatment strategies for elders with significant personality dysfunction. Accurate diagnosis of character pathology has been hampered by numerous factors. Given the unique physical, cognitive, and social factors encountered by this segment of society, some *DSM-IV* criteria may be inadequate for older adults. The decline in prevalence of some disorders (e.g., borderline, histrionic) may *not* be due to a "mellowing" or maturation of the individuals, but rather the inability of the current system to identify age-related manifestations of the disorders. Future research must clarify the clinical presentations, develop profiles, and identify age-related criteria that many investigators have reported as lacking in older adults. Subsequent versions of the *DSM* must acknowledge the existing age bias and provide age-associated criteria to better fit clinical presentation of the disordered older adult. Also, longitudinal studies are needed to follow younger individuals with personality disorders into later life; such investigations represent the only strategy for directly assessing and clarifying intraindividual changes over time in these disorders that may hamper accurate diagnosis (Segal *et al.,* 1996). Treatment strategies derived from the clarified picture of the personality-disordered older adult obviously will result in more efficient and effective outcomes.

REFERENCES

Abrams, R. C. (1991). The aging personality. *International Journal of Geriatric Psychiatry, 6,* 1–3.

Abrams, R. C., Alexopoulos, G. S., & Young, R. C. (1987). Geriatric depression and DSM-III-R personality criteria. *Journal of the American Geriatrics Society, 35,* 383–386.

Abrams, R. C., Rosendahl, E., Card, C., & Alexopoulos, G. S. (1994). Personality disorder correlates of late and early onset depression. *Journal of the American Geriatrics Society, 42,* 727–731.

Adler, D. A. (1990). Personality disorders: Treatment of the nonpsychotic chronic patient. *New Direction for Mental Health Services, 47,* 3–15.

Alden, L. E. (1989). Short-term structured treatment for avoidant personality disorder. *Journal of Consulting and Clinical Psychology, 57,* 756–764.

Alden, L. E., & Caperol, M. J. (1993). Avoidant personality disorder: Interpersonal problems as predictors of treatment response. *Behavior Therapy, 24,* 357–376.

Allport, G. W. (1937). *Personality: A psychological interpretation.* New York: Holt.

American Psychiatric Association. (1980). *Diagnostic and statistical manual of mental disorders* (3rd ed.). Washington, DC: Author.

American Psychiatric Association. (1987). *Diagnostic and statistical manual of mental disorders* (3rd ed., rev.). Washington, DC: Author.

American Psychiatric Association. (1994). *Diagnostic and statistical manual of mental disorders* (4th ed.). Washington, DC: Author.

Aronson, T. A. (1989). A critical review of psychotherapeutic treatments of the borderline personality: Historical trends and future directions. *Journal of Nervous and Mental Disease, 177,* 511–528.

Barlow, D. H., & Durand, V. M. (1995). *Abnormal psychology: An integrative approach.* Pacific Grove, CA: Brooks/Cole.

Beck, A. T., & Freeman, A. (1990). *Cognitive therapy of personality disorders.* New York: Guilford.

Bellack, A. S., & Hersen, M. (Eds.). (1985). *Dictionary of behavior therapy techniques.* New York: Pergamon.

Blashfield, R. K., & Breen, M. J. (1989). Face validity of DSM-III-R personality disorders. *American Journal of Psychiatry, 146,* 1575–1579.

Bolla-Wilson, K., & Bleecker, M. L. (1989). Absence of depression in elderly adults. *Journal of Gerontology, 44,* 53–55.

Bullard, D. M. (1960). Psychotherapy of paranoid patients. *Archives of General Psychiatry, 2,* 137–141.

Casey, D. A., & Schrodt, C. J. (1989). Axis II diagnoses in geriatric inpatients. *Journal of Geriatric Psychiatry and Neurology, 2,* 87–88.

Cohen, G. D. (1990). Psychopathology and mental health in the mature and elderly adult. In J. E. Birren & K. W. Schaie (Eds.), *Handbook of the psychology of aging* (3rd ed., pp. 359–371). San Diego, CA: Academic.

Colligan, R. C., & Offord, K. P. (1992). Age, stage, and the MMPI: Changes in response patterns over an 85 year age span. *Journal of Clinical Psychology, 48,* 476–493.

Colligan, R. C., Osborne, D., Swenson, W. M., & Offord, K. P. (1984). The MMPI: Development of contemporary norms. *Journal of Clinical Psychology, 40,* 100–107.

Coolidge, F. L. (1993). Coolidge Axis II Inventory manual. Clermont, FL: Synergistic Office Solutions.

Coolidge, F. L., & Merwin, M. M. (1992). Reliability and validity of the Coolidge Axis II Inventory: A new inventory for the assessment of personality disorders. *Journal of Personality Assessment, 59,* 223–238.

Coolidge, F. L., Burns, E. M., Nathan, J. H., & Mull, C. E. (1992). Personality disorders in the elderly. *Clinical Gerontologist, 12,* 41–55.

Dulit, R. A., Marin, D. B., & Frances, A. J. (1993). Cluster B personality disorders. In D. L. Dunner (Ed.), *Current psychiatric therapy* (pp. 405–411). Philadelphia: Saunders.

Dye, C. J., Bohm, A., Anderten, P., & Cho, D. W. (1983). Age group differences in depression on MMPI-D scale. *Journal of Clinical Psychology, 39,* 227–234.

Ellison, J. M., & Adler, D. A. (1990). A strategy for the pharmacotherapy of personality disorders. *New Directions for Mental Health Services, 47,* 43–63.

First, M. B., Gibbon, M., Spitzer, R. L., Williams, J. B. W., & Benjamin, L. S. (1997). *Structured Clinical Interview for DSM-IV Axis II Personality Disorders (SCID-II),* Washington, DC: American Psychiatric Press.

Fleming, B., & Pretzer, J. L. (1990). Cognitive-behavioral approaches to personality disorders. *Progress in Behavior Modification, 25,* 119–151.

Fogel, B. S., & Westlake, R. (1990). Personality disorder diagnosis and age in inpatients with major depression. *Journal of Clinical Psychiatry, 51,* 232–235.

Glasser, M. (1992). Problems in the psychoanalysis of certain narcissistic disorders. *International Journal of Psychoanalysis, 73,* 493–503.

Graham, J. R. (1990). *MMPI-2: Assessing personality and psychopathology.* New York: Oxford University Press.

Greene, R. L. (1980). *The MMPI: An interpretive manual.* New York: Grune & Stratton.

Gunderson, J. G., Frank, A. F., Ronningstam, E. F., Wachter, S., Lynch, V. J., & Wolf, P. J. (1989). Early discontinuance of borderline patients from psychotherapy. *Journal of Nervous and Mental Disease, 177,* 38–42.

Guze, S. B. (1976). *Criminality and psychiatric disorders.* New York: Oxford University Press.

Harmatz, J. S., & Shader, R. E. (1975). Psychopharmacological investigations in healthy elderly volunteers: MMPI depression scale. *Journal of the American Geriatrics Society, 23,* 350–354.

Hathaway, S. R., & McKinley, J. C. (1983). *The Minnesota Multiphasic Personality Inventory manual*. New York: Psychological Corporation.

Hathaway, S. R., & McKinley, J. C. (1989). *MMPI-2: Minnesota Multiphasic Personality Inventory–2: Manual for administration and scoring*. Minneapolis: University of Minnesota Press.

Heimberg, R. G., & Barlow, D. H. (1991). New developments in cognitive-behavioral therapy for social phobia. *Journal of Clinical Psychology, 52*, 21–30.

Herbert, J. D., Hope, D. A., & Bellack, A. S. (1992). Validity of the distinction between generalized social phobia and avoidant personality disorder. *Journal of Abnormal Psychology, 101*, 332–339.

Higgitt, A., & Fonagy, P. (1992). Psychotherapy of borderline and narcissistic personality disorder. *British Journal of Psychiatry, 161*, 23–43.

Hoke, L. A., Livori, P. W., & Perry, J. C. (1992). Mood and global functioning in borderline personality disorder: Individual regression models for longitudinal measurements. *Journal of Psychiatric Research, 26*, 1–16.

Hyer, L., & Harrison, W. R. (1986). Later life personality model. *Clinical Gerontologist, 5*, 399–416.

Hyler, S. E. (1994). *Personality Diagnostic Questionnaire, 4th edition (PDQ-4)*. New York: New York State Psychiatric Institute.

Hyler, S. E., & Reider, R. O. (1987). *PDQ-R: Personality Diagnostic Questionnaire–Revised*. New York: New York State Psychiatric Institute.

Kavoussi, R. J., & Siever, L. J. (1992). Overlap between borderline and schizotypal personality disorders. *Comprehensive Psychiatry, 33*, 7–12.

Kernberg, O. (1975). *Borderline conditions and pathological narcissism*. New York: Jason Aronson.

Kohut, H. (1971). *The analysis of the self*. New York: International Universities Press.

Kohut, H. (1977). *The restoration of the self*. New York: International Universities Press.

Kroessler, D. (1990). Personality disorders in the elderly. *Hospital and Community Psychiatry, 41*, 1325–1329.

Kunik, M. E., Muisant, B. H., Rifai, A. H., Sweet, R. A., Pasternak, R., Rosen, J., & Zubenko, G. S. (1993). Personality disorders in elderly inpatients with major depression. *American Journal of Geriatric Psychiatry, 1*, 38–45.

Leon, G. R., Gillum, B., Gillum, R., & Gouze, M. (1979). Personality stability and change over a 30 year period middle age to old age. *Journal of Consulting and Clinical Psychology, 47*, 515–524.

Libb, J. W., Murray, J., Thurstin, H., & Alarcon, R. D. (1992). Concordance of the MCMI-II, the MMPI, and Axis I discharge diagnosis in psychiatric inpatients. *Journal of Personality Assessment, 58*, 580–590.

Loranger, A. W., Sartorius, N., Andreoli, A., Berger, P., Channabassavanna, S. M., Coid, B., Dahl, A., Diekstra, R. F. W., Fegeson, B., Jacobsberg, L. B., Mombour, W., Pull, C., Ono, Y., & Regier, D. (1994). The International Personality Disorder Examination: The World Health Organization/Alcohol, Drug Abuse, and Mental Health Administration international pilot study of personality disorders. *Archives of General Psychiatry, 51*, 215–224.

Loranger, A. W., Susman, V. L., Oldham, J. M., & Russakof, L. M. (1987). The Personality Disorder Examination: A preliminary report. *Journal of Personality Disorders, 1*, 1–13.

Martin, R. L., Cloninger, C. R., & Guze, S. B. (1982). The natural history of somatization and substance abuse in women criminals: A six year follow-up. *Comprehensive Psychiatry, 23*, 528–537.

Mavissakalian, M., & Hamann, M. S. (1986). Correlates of DSM-III personality disorder in agoraphobia. *Comprehensive Psychiatry, 27*, 471–479.

Mavissakalian, M., & Hamann, M. S. (1988). Correlates of personality disorders in panic disorder and agoraphobia. *Comprehensive Psychiatry, 29*, 535–544.

Mavissakalian, M., Hamann, M. S., & Jones, B. (1990). Correlates of DSM-III-R personality disorder in obsessive-compulsive disorder. *Comprehensive Psychiatry, 31*, 481–489.

Mavissakalian, M., Hamann, M. S., Haidar, S. A., & de Groot, C. M. (1993). DSM-III personality disorders in general anxiety, panic/agoraphobia, and obsessive-compulsive disorders. *Comprehensive Psychiatry, 34*, 243–248.

McCann, J. T., (1989). MMPI personality scales and the MCMI: Concurrent validity. *Journal of Clinical Psychology, 45*, 365–369.

McCann, J. T. (1991). Convergent and discriminant validity of the MCMI-II and MMPI personality disorder scales. *Psychological Assessment: A Journal of Consulting and Clinical Psychology, 3*, 9–18.

McCrae, R. R., & Costa, P. T. (1984). The search for growth or decline in personality. In R. R. Mc-
Crae & P. T. Costa (Eds.), *Emerging lives, ednduring dispositions: Personality in adulthood* (pp.
13–28). Boston: Little, Brown.

Mehlum, L., Friis, S., Irion, T., Johns, S., Karterud, S., Vaglum, P., & Vaglum, S. (1991). Personality
disorders 2–5 years after treatment: A prospective follow-up study. *Acta Scandinavica, 84,*
72–77.

Mezzich, T. E., Fabrega, H., Coffman, G. A., & Gavin, Y. (1987). Comprehensively diagnosing geriatric patients. *Comprehensive Psychiatry, 28,* 68–76.

Millon, T. (1981). *Disorders of Personality: DSM-III, Axis II.* New York: Wiley.

Millon, T. (1983). *Millon Clinical Multiaxial Inventory.* Minneapolis, MN: Interpretive Scoring Systems.

Millon, T. (1987). *Millon Clinical Multiaxial Inventory II (MCMI-II) manual.* Minneapolis, MN: National Computer Systems.

Millon, T. (1990). *Toward a new personology: An evolutionary model.* New York: Wiley-Inter-
science.

Millon, T. (1992). Millon Clinical Multiaxial Inventory: I & II. *Journal of Counseling and Development, 70,* 421–426.

Millon, T. (1994). *Millon Clinical Multiaxial Inventory III (MCMI III) manual.* Minneapolis, MN: National Computer Systems.

Morey, L. C., Waugh, M. H., & Blashfield, R. K. (1985). MMPI scales for DSM-III personality disorders: Their derivation and correlates. *Journal of Personality Assessment, 49,* 245–256.

Morey, L. C., & LeVine, D. J. (1988). A multi-trait, multimethod examination of Minnesota Multiphasic Personality Inventory (MMPI) and Millon Clinical Multiaxial Inventory (MCMI). *Journal of Psychopathology and Behavioral Assessment, 10,* 333–344.

Nurnberg, H. G., Raskin, M., Levine, P. E., Pollack, S., Siegel, O., & Prince, R. (1991). The comorbidity of borderline personality disorder and other DSM-III-R Axis II personality disorders.
American Journal of Psychiatry, 148, 1371–1377.

O'Brien, M. M., Trestman, R. L., & Siever, L. J. (1993). Cluster A personality disorders. In D. L. Dunner (Ed.), *Current psychiatric therapy* (pp. 399–404). Philadelphia: Saunders.

Oldham, J. M., Skodol, A. E., Rellman, A. D., Hyler, S. E., Rosnick, L., & Davis, M. (1992). Diagnosis
of DSM-III-R personality disorders by two structured interviews: Patterns of co-morbidity.
American Journal of Psychiatry, 149, 213–220.

Patrick, J. (1988). Concordance of the MCMI and the MMPI in the diagnosis of three DSM-III Axis I
disorders. *Journal of Clinical Psychology, 44,* 186–190.

Patterson, G. R. (1982). *Coercive family process.* Eugene, OR: Castalia.

Pennington, B. H., Peterson, L. P., & Barber, H. R. (1979). The diagnostic use of the MMPI in organic
brain dysfunction. *Journal of Clinical Psychology, 35,* 484–492.

Perry, J. C. (1993). Longitudinal studies of personality disorders. *Journal of Personality Disorders, 7,*
63–85.

Peterson, C. (1996). *Personality* (2nd ed.). San Diego, CA: Harcourt Brace Jovanovich.

Pfohl, B., Stangl, D., & Zimmerman, M. (1983). *Structured Interview for DSM-III Personality* (SIDP)
(2nd ed.). Iowa City: University of Iowa.

Pfohl, B., Blum, N., & Zimmerman, M. (1995). *Structured Interview for DSM-IV Personality SIDP IV.*
Iowa City: University of Iowa.

Pincus, H. A., Frances, A., Davis, W. W., First, M. B., & Widiger, T. A. (1992). DSM-IV and new diagnostic categories: Holding the line on proliferation. *American Journal of Psychiatry, 149,*
112–117.

Quality Assurance Project. (1991). Treatment outlines for paranoid, schizotypal, and schizoid personality disorders. *Australian and New Zealand Journal of Psychiatry, 24,* 339–350.

Reich, J. H., & Green, A. I. (1991). Effect of personality disorders on outcome of treatment. *Journal
of Nervous and Mental Disease, 179,* 74–82.

Renneberg, B., Goldstein, A. J., Phillips, D., & Chambless, D. L. (1990). Intensive behavioral group
treatment of avoidant personality disorder. *Behavior Therapy, 21,* 363–377.

Ricciardi, J. N., Baer, L., Jenike, M. A., Fischer, S. C., Sholtz, D., & Buttolph, M. L. (1992). Changes
in DSM-III-R Axis II diagnoses following treatment of obsessive-compulsive disorder. *American Journal of Psychiatry, 149,* 829–831.

Rose, M. K., Soares, H. H., & Joseph, C. (1993). Frail elderly clients with personality disorders: A
challenge for social work. *Journal of Gerontological Social Work, 19,* 153–165.

Rosowsky, E., & Gurian, B. (1991). Borderline personality disorder in late life. *International Psychogeriatrics, 3,* 39–52.

Rusk, R., Hyerstay, B. J., Calsyn, D. A., & Freeman, C. W. (1979). Comparison of the utility of two abbreviated forms of the MMPI for psychiatric screening of the elderly. *Journal of Clinical Psychology, 35,* 104–107.

Schneider, L. S., Zemansky, M. F., Bender, M., & Sloane, R. B. (1992). Personality in recovered depressed elderly. *International Psychogeriatrics, 4,* 177–185.

Schneier, F. R., Spitzer, R. L. Gibbon, M., Fyer, A. J., & Leibowitz, M. R. (1991). The relationship of social phobia subtypes to avoidant personality disorder. *Comprehensive Psychiatry, 32,* 496–502.

Segal, D. L., Hersen, M., Van Hasselt, V. B., Silberman, C. S., & Roth, L. (1996). Diagnosis and assessment of personality disorders in older adults: A critical review. *Journal of Personality Disorders.*

Shea, M. T., Pilkonis, P. A., Bechman, E., Collins, J. F., Elkin, I., Sotsky, S. M., & Docherty, J. P. (1990). Personality disorders and treatment outcome in the NIMH treatment of depression: Collaborative Research Program. *American Journal of Psychiatry, 147,* 711–718.

Siegel, D. J., & Small, G. W. (1986). Borderline personality disorder in the elderly: A case study. *Canadian Journal of Psychiatry, 31,* 859–860.

Silberman, C. S., Roth, L., Segal, D. L., & Burns, W. (1997). Relationship between the Millon Clinical Multiaxial Inventory-II and Collidge Axis II Inventory in chronically mentally ill older adults: A pilot study. *Journal of Clinical Psychology, 53,* 559–566.

Snyder, S., Pitts, W. M., & Gustin, Q. (1983). Absence of borderline personality disorder in later years. *American Journal of Psychiatry, 140,* 271–272.

Spar, J. E., & La Rue, A. (1990). *Concise guide to geriatric psychiatry.* Washington, DC: American Psychiatric Press.

Steketee, G., Foa, E. B., & Grayson, J. B. (1982). Recent advances in the behavioral treatment of obsessive-compulsives. *Archives of General Psychiatry, 39,* 1365–1371.

Stravynski, A., Lesage, A., Marcouiller, M., & Elie, R. (1989). A test of the therapeutic mechanism in social skill training with avoidant personality disorder. *Journal of Nervous and Mental Disease, 177,* 739–744.

Streiner, D. L. & Miller, H. R. (1988). Validity of the MMPI scales for DSM-III personality disorders: What are they measuring? *Journal of Personality Disorders, 2,* 238–242.

Task Force on Nomenclature and Statistics, American Psychiatric Association. (1976). *DSM-III in midstream: Conference publication.* Missouri Institute of Psychiatry.

Taylor, J. R., Strassberg, D. S., & Turner, C. W. (1989). Utility of the MMPI in geriatric populations. *Journal of Personality Assessment, 53,* 665–676.

Thompson, L. W., Gallagher, D., & Czirr, R. (1989). Personality disorder and outcome treatment of late life depression. *Journal of Geriatric Psychiatry, 21,* 133–146.

Turkat, I. D., & Carlson, C. R. (1984). Data-based versus symptomatic formulation of treatment: The case of a dependent personality. *Journal of Behavior Therapy and Experimental Psychiatry, 15,* 153–160.

Tyrer, P. (1988). What's wrong with the DSM-III personality disorders? *Journal of Personality Disorders, 2,* 289–291.

Weiss, J. M. (1973). The natural history of antisocial attitudes: What happens to psychopaths? *Journal of Geriatric Psychology, 2,* 236–242.

Westin, D. (1991). Cognitive-behavioral interventions in the psychoanalytic psychotherapy of borderline personality disorders. *Clinical Psychology Review, 11,* 211–230.

Widiger, T. A., & Trull, T. J. (1993). Personality and psychopathology: An application of the five-factor model. *Journal of Personality, 60,* 363–393.

Widiger, T. A., Williams, J. B., Spitzer, R. F., & Francis, A. (1985). The MCMI as a measure of DSM III. *Journal of Personality Assessment, 49,* 366–378.

Zimmerman, M. (1994). Diagnosis of personality disorders. *Archives of General Psychiatry, 51,* 225–244.

CHAPTER 15

Aging and Mental Retardation

Ellen M. Cotter and Louis D. Burgio

INTRODUCTION

With the recent growth in the population of older adults, there has been a concomitant increase in the visibility of "special populations" of elders. One "special population" consists of older adults with mental retardation and other developmental disabilities. Although estimates of the size of this population vary, it is expected that by the year 2025 there will be between 400,000 and one million people over the age of 65 with developmental disabilities living in the United States (see Anderson, 1993, for a review of other pertinent statistics). It is believed that older adults with mental retardation constitute a group with special needs beyond those of the general aged population (Newbern & Hargett, 1992). For example, older adults with mental retardation have fewer compensatory abilities than their nonretarded peers to adjust for age-associated declines in functioning (Jenkins, Hildreth, & Hildreth, 1993). As a result, there has been a recent effort by researchers, health care professionals, and other service providers to identify the pertinent characteristics and needs of this special population. This information would help to determine whether existing services for older adults and persons with mental retardation are adequate for meeting their needs.

The American Association on Mental Retardation (AAMR) put forth the following definition of mental retardation in 1992:

> *Mental retardation* refers to substantial limitations in present functioning. It is characterized by significantly subaverage intellectual functioning, existing concurrently with related limitations in two or more of the following applicable adaptive skill areas: communication, self-care, home living, social skills, community use, self-direction, health and safety, functional academics, leisure, and work. Mental retardation manifests before age 18. (p. 1)

Ellen M. Cotter and Louis D. Burgio • Center for Aging, Division of Gerontology and Geriatric Medicine, and Department of Psychology, University of Alabama at Birmingham, Birmingham, Alabama 35294-4410.

Handbook of Clinical Geropsychology, edited by Michel Hersen and Vincent B. Van Hasselt. Plenum Press, New York, 1998.

Mental retardation is portrayed commonly as the result of genetic or chromo-somal anomalies, as in the case of Down syndrome. However, mental retarda-tion can be caused by many other factors, such as environmental neglect, consumption of lead, anoxia at birth, or brain trauma following a head injury or serious illness. It is important to reiterate that onset of mental retardation oc-curs during childhood; events such as head injuries are considered to cause mental retardation only if they occur before the age of 18. Other conditions, such as epilepsy, cerebral palsy, mental illness, or sensory impairments, may coexist with mental retardation and may themselves change over the life span, along with changes in other areas of functioning experienced by the aging adult with mental retardation. In sum, persons with mental retardation constitute a heterogeneous population at any point during the life span, and the diversity of this population increases with age.

Until recently, individuals with mental retardation manifested a shorter life span than the nonretarded population, although improved medical technology has resulted in nearly equivalent life spans for both the retarded and general pop-ulations. Because of this history of shortened life expectancy, however, there re-mains a somewhat liberal definition regarding the age at which an adult with mental retardation can be considered to be "elderly." Furthermore, differential loss of function at a particular age between retarded and nonretarded older adults, as well as variability within the group of older adults with mental retardation, ren-der the description "elderly" problematic. The age of 65, which is one standard marker for senior citizenship in the general population, is now commonly at-tained by many adults with mild to moderate mental retardation. However, it has been suggested that adults with mental retardation who are as young as 55 can be classified as "elderly" (Eklund & Martz, 1993; M. M. Seltzer & Krauss, 1987), par-ticularly if other conditions such as Down syndrome are present or if the person has severe or profound mental retardation. Such lack of agreement on age stan-dardization presents an important challenge to service providers and researchers.

It is crucial that geropsychologists be aware of the special needs of their clients with mental retardation. Unlike other forms of psychopathology, such as anxiety disorders and depression, mental retardation itself is not treatable, al-though some specific aspects of mental retardation can be treated and allevi-ated. In addition, it is important that clinicians be sensitive not only to the age-related changes experienced by older adults with mental retardation but also to the inherent difficulties in assessing these changes with this population. The primary purpose of this chapter is to present a few of the more salient is-sues clinicians may face when providing services for aging retarded individu-als. Topics covered include diagnosis and assessment of aging-related changes, treatment of problem areas, special issues regarding aging persons with Down syndrome, caregiving, and service needs.

DIAGNOSIS AND ASSESSMENT

Although the diagnosis of mental retardation is generally formed in child-hood, it is possible that the condition may be undiagnosed until adulthood due to coexistence of other conditions, such as mental illness or a severe sensory impairment. However, even with individuals who are not diagnosed until later in life, regular assessment across the remaining life span is vital to effective service provision. Like their nondisabled peers, individuals with mental retardation continue to change throughout their lives, and regular assessment of abilities will ensure that needs are being met.

Because individuals with mental retardation constitute a diverse population, it should be expected that these individuals will display characteristics of aging variably. In particular, there appears to be a qualitative difference in the aging process for persons with Down syndrome when compared with individuals whose mental retardation was caused by other factors. Some of these differences will be addressed in a separate section on the relationship between Down syndrome and Alzheimer's disease. Other differences will be discussed as needed in this section.

Cognitive Functioning

Longitudinal research investigating aging-related cognitive changes in nondisabled adults has revealed that cognitive processes, particularly those requiring speed or perceptual abilities, decline with increasing age, but that this decline is less than was previously found in cross-sectional studies of cognitive function. A similar pattern has been found in individuals with mental retardation. In their now classic 1970 study, Fisher and Zeaman found that adults with mental retardation show relatively intact performance on verbal tasks throughout their lives, with a greater decline in performance-based tasks with increased age. Overall IQ scores were found to remain relatively stable until at least age 60. Eklund and Martz (1993), however, note that this and other studies have focused primarily on institutionalized persons and used post hoc evaluations of archival data.

In a cross-sectional examination of adults with mental retardation (age range 20–90 years) who did not have Down syndrome or profound mental retardation, Hewitt, Fenner, and Torpy (1986) found that mental age remained constant until around age 65, and then showed a slight decline. These findings are consistent with the work of Bell and Zubek (1960), who found no decline in IQ over a 5-year span in retarded adults over the age of 45 who did not have Down syndrome, and Harper and Wadsworth (1990), who found that chronological age was not related to IQ change in adults with mental retardation ranging in age from 35 to 79 years. In summary, it appears that among retarded adults without Down syndrome, cognitive ability remains stable until roughly age 65, after which slight and gradual declines are seen. It should be noted that persons with Down syndrome appear to display a different pattern of cognitive aging, and thus should be considered separately in studies of associated cognitive changes. In particular, data suggest that individuals with Down syndrome begin experiencing cognitive decline in their late 40s (e.g., Fenner, Hewitt, & Torpy, 1987; Hewitt, Carter, & Jancar, 1985).

Accurate assessment of cognitive ability in older adults with mental retardation is essential not only for determining current levels of functioning but also for documenting changes in cognitive ability over time. Unfortunately, selection of an appropriate assessment tool is problematic. Different intelligence tests, such as the Wechsler Adult Intelligence Scale–Revised (WAIS-R) and the Stanford-Binet Intelligence Scale: Fourth Edition, have been found to produce disparate IQ scores (Spitz, 1986). The Stanford-Binet does not have adequate standardization norms for older adults (Spruill, 1991), and the directions for administration of the Stanford-Binet may unfairly penalize examinees with mental retardation (Wersh & Thomas, 1990). Moreover, neither the WAIS-R nor the Stanford-Binet provides explicit instructions for use with persons who have severe language, physical, or sensory impairments. Proposed solutions to these problems include the use of "hybrid" assessments containing components from more than one instrument (e.g., Eklund & Martz, 1993) or a children's assessment battery adapted for adults (e.g., Hogg & Moss, 1993); however, these approaches are also problematic. It is not the purpose of this chapter to propose a particular cognitive assessment tool, but it is recommended that clinicians familiarize themselves with these issues and exercise caution when selecting or interpreting the results of an intelligence test.

Adaptive Behavior

The term "adaptive behavior" refers to a class of skills encompassing management of activities of daily living (ADLs), performance of instrumental activities of daily living (IADLs), and the ability to interact in socially appropriate ways (AAMR, 1992). As with assessment of cognitive ability, measuring adaptive behavior skills in elderly adults with mental retardation is complicated by lack of appropriate instruments. Two instruments are particularly worthy of discussion because of their common usage. Although the Vineland Adaptive Behavior Scale is a popular assessment tool, it has been noted that this instrument contains many items geared toward children. The scale also overemphasizes written communication in older examinees, and it does not provide standardization norms for older adults (Kerby, Wentworth, & Cotten, 1989).

The American Association on Mental Deficiency (AAMD) Adaptive Behavior Scale (Nihira, Foster, Shellhaas, & Leland, 1974), which assesses both adaptive behavior skills and the occurrence of maladaptive behaviors, includes appropriate norms for use with older adults. However, this instrument is difficult to score, was standardized on an institutional population, and includes a number of biased items. For example, self-care during menstruation is rated on a five-point scale, with a higher score denoting more independence. Male clients, for whom menstruation is irrelevant, are automatically given five points in scoring, regardless of their abilities in other aspects of self-care. An updated version of this scale, the AAMR Adaptive Behavior Scale (Nihira, Leland, & Lambert, 1993), alleviates some of these problems by eliminating some biased items and providing norms for both institutional and community-dwelling populations; unfortunately, this instrument is not yet widely used.

Although finding an appropriate instrument is problematic, measurement of adaptive behavior is central to the continuing habilitation of older adults with mental retardation. It has been noted that the client's functional ability is an important factor in guiding the allocation of services and achieving the least restrictive environment (Kerby *et al.*, 1989). In fact, when assessing the "goodness of fit" between elderly persons with mental retardation and their environments, adaptive skills are frequently targeted (G. B. Seltzer, Finaly, & Howell, 1988). In addition, documentation of adaptive behavior skills over time has been proposed as a valid way to assess the life-span development of persons with mental retardation. Longitudinal assessment of adaptive behavior skills has revealed that functional abilities of both institutionalized and community-dwelling adults with mild to moderate mental retardation plateau in early adulthood and remain relatively intact through age 64 (Eyman & Widaman, 1987). However, adaptive behavior of individuals with more severe impairments or levels of mental retardation flattens out in early childhood and tends to decline in the mid-40s (Eyman & Widaman, 1987). These results again highlight the heterogeneity of older individuals with mental retardation and suggest that different levels of impairment must he considered when examining longitudinal performance of adaptive behavior skills.

Longitudinal issues aside, the assessment of adaptive behavior skills has relevance for determining current service needs. Using a slightly modified version of the Katz Index of ADL (Katz, Ford, Moskowitz, Jackson, & Jaffe, 1963), Eklund and Martz (1993) conducted a 2-year study of 128 older adults with mental retardation, 64 of whom had Down syndrome and 87% of whom lived with their parents or in group homes. Results indicated that older adults with mental retardation were largely independent in terms of basic ADLs (e.g., bathing, dressing, and toileting) but required more assistance with IADLs (e.g., using money, preparing meals, traveling in the community). Eklund and Martz (1993) also suggest that a decline in IADL performance indicates the need for increased environmental supports, whereas a decrease in ADL independence may suggest the need for out-of-home placement.

Fine, Tangeman, and Woodard (1990) assessed postdeinstitutionalization changes in the adaptive functioning of older adults with mental retardation. The 32 residents in this study had lived in a state institution and had been transferred to a smaller, neighborhood-based facility. Residents ranged in age from 40 to 78 at the time of deinstitutionalization. In this study, deinstitutionalization was related to increases in both adaptive and maladaptive behaviors, similar to results obtained with younger samples of adults with mental retardation. Specific types of adaptive behaviors that showed improvement were economic, language, and domestic skills; the increase in maladaptive behaviors—specifically, antisocial behavior, untrustworthy behaviors, and unacceptable vocal habits—appeared to be related to increased interaction with other people. These results show that older adults with mental retardation can learn new ADL skills following a change to a less restrictive environment. The results also suggest that alerting facility staff of potential maladaptive behavior changes and training them in behavior management skills might make the residential transfer smoother for both clients and staff.

Physical Health

Knowledge of the health status and health needs of older adults with mental retardation is critical for effective service planning. It is important to determine not only how older adults with mental retardation compare to their nonretarded peers in their experience of certain health conditions, but also whether or not the health services currently available to older adults can accommodate mentally retarded individuals. Variations in life history, including such factors as institutionalization and prior health care availability, will affect the health status and needs of older adults with mental retardation. In addition, there is some evidence that differences in the severity of mental retardation or the presence of other disabling conditions or both also produce variability in aging-related health status and health care needs. These differences also need to be taken into account when planning services to address the health needs of these individuals.

Assessment of physical well-being in this population can be less problematic than the assessment of cognitive or functional abilities because medical professionals use a fairly standard set of techniques to assess, diagnose, and treat illness. Lack of appropriate age norms and poor psychometric properties are less relevant issues. However, older adults with mental retardation may have difficulty describing or expressing their symptoms; as a result, medical professionals must be attuned to nonverbal expressions of pain or illness. Moreover, family members may not be available to provide medical history or supervise treatment, and the frequent staff turnover in residential facilities may result in staff members' being unaware of a resident's medical history or needs.

As they age, adults with mental retardation face the same health issues as their nonretarded peers. For example, increased prevalence of age-related conditions such as arthritis, heart disease, and sensory impairments is common to all aging individuals. Problems related to medication use are also common in these two groups. Alterations in body metabolism affect the absorption and effectiveness of medications, onset of age-related health problems may result in the necessity for new medications, and lack of communication between patients and physicians may result in deleterious drug interactions. However, older adults with mental retardation may experience some age-related medication complications unique to this population. Many individuals with mental retardation take medication throughout their lives for the control of seizure disorders, behavioral disturbances, or mental illness. Some of these medications, such as antipsychotic drugs, can produce long-lasting negative side effects, such as tardive dyskinesia, if taken over long periods of time. It is also known that, as they age, individuals become more susceptible to the adverse side effects of antipsychotic drugs.

To date, much of the data on the health of older adults with mental retardation has been gathered through the National Nursing Home Survey (NNHS; National Center for Health Statistics, 1979, 1986). This database contains an abundance of information on both retarded and nonretarded nursing home residents. Results from this database suggest that older adults with mental retardation have better overall health than their nonretarded peers. More specifically, nursing home residents aged 65 and older with mental retardation typically have a lower incidence of health problems such as arthritis, respiratory disorders, Parkinson's disease, and circulatory system disorders than their nonretarded peers. However, epilepsy and other nervous system disorders are more common in nursing home residents with mental retardation (Anderson, 1989, 1993).

A longitudinal study conducted at the University of Minnesota Center for Residential and Community Services (CRCS; Anderson, Lakin, Bruininks, & Hill, 1987) has also provided valuable data on the characteristics of older adults with mental retardation residing in state-run residential facilities, including small group homes, foster homes, and large public and private institutions. Unlike the NNHS project, the CRCS study does not include data from nonretarded individuals. The CRCS sample of 370 adults was studied longitudinally over a 5-year period. During this time, overall incidence of heart disease and arthritis increased, a phenomenon not unexpected in this aging group. Paradoxically, there was a higher incidence of reported chronic diseases and muscle atrophy among individuals who had remained in their original residences during the study, compared with those who were transferred to a setting offering more functional and medical assistance. Anderson (1993) suggested that these seemingly incongruous results are caused by staff underreporting of various conditions. Whether this hypothesized underreporting is deliberate or accidental is unclear. However, as previously mentioned, high staff turnover rates in residential facilities may result in a lack of information about the medical histories and current health status of the residents. Although direct comparison of the CRCS and NNHS data sets is problematic because of differences in the methods of data collection, a cursory examination suggests that the overall prevalence of medical conditions in older adults with mental retardation who live in community residential facilities is similar to that of the retarded nursing home residents (Anderson, 1989, 1993).

It has been noted that diversity among older adults with mental retardation renders it difficult to discuss in general terms the physical aging of this population (e.g., Anderson, 1993). In particular, individuals with different degrees of mental retardation or other debilitating conditions or both may have different patterns of aging. Individuals with mild to moderate mental retardation appear to have a life expectancy similar to that of the general aging population. As these individuals age, they also experience many of the health problems common to their age group, such as sensory losses, incontinence, and confusion. As mentioned previously, diagnosis of these conditions can be difficult. For example, older adults with mild to moderate mental retardation may not be able to convey sensory losses or understand how these sensory losses affect their interactions with their environment and other people. Incontinence in a retarded individual may be viewed as a behavior problem and not as an outcome of an underlying medical condition. Also, confusion may not be easily detectable, particularly if the client has a history of mental illness or behavior problems (Anderson, 1993). All of these factors can affect the accurate diagnosis and treatment of common medical conditions in aging retarded individuals.

Greater levels of cognitive and functional impairment appear to be correlated with more frequent and serious health problems. Individuals with severe to profound mental retardation have a shortened life expectancy due to frequent presence of other complicating medical conditions, such as respiratory diseases (Anderson, 1993). They also have a higher incidence of non-age-related health conditions and sensory deficits and, consequently, are severely limited in their ability to report physical signs and symptoms. Furthermore, addition of a condition such as epilepsy or cerebral palsy to existing mental retardation, regardless of degree of cognitive impairment, may reduce life expectancy and introduce additional health complications (Anderson, 1993).

Finally, individuals with Down syndrome have a life expectancy of approximately 55 years (Eyman, Call, & White, 1989). This life expectancy is lower than that of other adults with mental retardation not caused by Down syndrome. People with Down syndrome are also more susceptible to congenital heart disease, middle ear infections (which eventually cause a conductive hearing loss), hypothyroidism, and premature aging of the immune system (Adlin, 1993). Consequently, it has been suggested that individuals with Down syndrome age faster than people without Down syndrome (Eklund & Martz, 1993); however, the mechanism by which such premature aging occurs is still unknown.

Behavior Problems

It is estimated that between 10% and 60% of individuals with mental retardation evince behavior problems (Davidson *et al.,* 1992). Examples of these behavior problems include physical aggression, noncompliance, running away, and self-injurious behaviors. These maladaptive behaviors have obvious potential consequences, such as damage to property and injury to the self and others. It is thought that maladaptive behaviors also cause difficulty in social relationships, lessen employment opportunities, and increase the risk of institutionalization (see McGrew, Ittenbach, Bruininks, & Hill, 1991, for a review). Indeed, behavioral disturbances are cited as a primary barrier to inclusion in the community for individuals with mental retardation (Davidson *et al.,* 1992).

Assessment of behavioral disorders in older adults with mental retardation can be conducted in many ways. The most useful for establishing the antecedents and consequences of maladaptive behavior is to record a behavioral disturbance as it occurs. Graphing the occurrence of behavioral disturbances over time can establish possible patterns of behavior, identify antecedents and consequences, and show the effectiveness of interventions. However, direct observation of behavioral disturbances can be time-consuming for caregivers and may not be feasible in some situations. More standardized measures of behavioral disturbances are also available. One section of the AAMD/AAMR Adaptive Behavior Scales (Nihira *et al.,* 1974, 1993) assesses occurrence of maladaptive behavior in 14 domains, including one domain that assesses use of medications. Behaviors are rated as occurring "occasionally" (one point) or "frequently" (two points). Point totals in different domains are then compared to standardized norms for different age groups. Although this method of assessing behavior problems is convenient and useful for comparing one client's behavior with that of other individuals, it is not as effective in documenting behavior patterns or behavior change. Furthermore, this method does not always differentiate the frequency of a behavior problem from its severity. A behavior problem, for example, disruptive vocalization, may occur frequently but may not be as troublesome as a less frequent problem, such as physical aggression that results in injury.

A frequently asked question is whether behavioral disturbances in mentally retarded individuals change with the aging process. The answer to this question depends on several factors. One is the accuracy of reporting the frequency, duration, and severity of these behaviors. Inaccurate reporting will, of course, result in inaccurate profiles of behavior over time. A second factor is the presence or absence of age-related disease conditions. People who develop respiratory or circulatory system disorders as they age may not have the strength to engage in behaviors such as trespass or physical aggression but may show an increase in verbal disruption and noncompliance. In addition, an older adult with mental retardation who develops a dementing illness may show a different pattern of behavioral disorders than had been present earlier in life; this change in behavior can be attributed to the dementia and not to aging per se. A third factor is related to changes in life events. Older adults with mental retardation may have difficulty adjusting to such life transitions as a change in residence, the death of a family member, or retirement from a work setting. Changes in behavioral disorders may occur for lack of other, more appropriate, coping mechanisms or methods of expression.

Davidson and colleagues (1992) conducted a cross-sectional study of aging effects on behavioral and psychiatric disorders in community-dwelling adults with mental retardation. Records of clients who had been referred for crisis intervention services due to the severity of their behavior problems were examined. With increasing age, number of referral problems increased. However, some of the referral problems included in this sample, such as caregiver illness or death, client abuse or neglect, and client illness, cannot be considered to be client behavior problems. When client behaviors such as aggression and noncompliance were examined separately from the larger list of referral problems, occurrence of aggression remained relatively constant with age, noncompliance increased with age, and prevalence of psychiatric symptoms declined. When older clients with mild and severe mental retardation were compared, different patterns of behavior problems emerged. Clients with mild mental retardation who were at least 50 years of age showed a marked increase in noncompliance and a marked decrease in physical aggression compared with adults with mild mental retardation who were 40 to 49 years of age. Specifically, the percentage of each group that engaged in aggressive behavior dropped from over 30% to zero, while the percentage of each age group that exhibited noncompliant behaviors increased from roughly 40% to 85%. Older adults with severe mental retardation, however, showed a different pattern of behavior. Compared to middle-aged adults with severe mental retardation, older adults showed a increase in noncompliance from none to 25% and an increase in aggression from 40% to approximately 60%. This interaction of "pattern of behavioral crisis" and severity of mental retardation suggests that different methods of assessment and intervention may be necessary for older adults with varying levels of mental retardation, although it is noted that "the role played by psychiatric factors in determining age-dependent patterns of severe behavioral disturbances is unclear" (p. 1).

In a more recent study, Davidson and colleagues (1994) have reported that in a sample of community-based adults with mental retardation (approximately 18% were aged 40 or above), aggressive behaviors did not decrease with age, and the proportion of the sample who engaged in aggressive behaviors remained constant across the life span. In contrast with results reported by McGrew and colleagues (1991), these clients did not display an increase in self-injurious behaviors with age; however, differences in sampling procedures and problem definition may be responsible for this discrepancy.

TREATMENT OF PROBLEM AREAS

Behavior Problems

As stated previously, behavior problems are common among individuals with mental retardation, and many of these problems are maintained into old age. Two common forms of treatment are the use of psychotropic medications and behavioral interventions.

Psychotropic Medication

Use of psychotropic medications to treat behavior disorders is common, although prevalence varies by residential setting. It is estimated that 30%–50% of adults with mental retardation who live in institutions receive major tranquilizers on a regular basis, but only 26%–36% of community-based clients take neuroleptic drugs (Anderson & Polister, 1993; Rinck & Calkins, 1989). Additional evidence of high use of psychotropic medications among individuals with mental retardation can be found in J. W. Jacobson (1988) and James (1986). The many risks associated with the use of psychotropic medications, particularly among older adults, are discussed elsewhere (Butler, Burgio, & Engel, 1987; Ray, Federspiel, & Schaffner, 1980) and will not be reiterated here.

Rinck and Caikins (1989) examined psychotropic medication use among older adults with mental retardation and found that nearly 31% of individuals over age 55 took at least one antipsychotic medication, compared with 23% of adults aged 25 to 54 and 8% of persons younger than age 21. Older adults with mental retardation were also more likely to take more than one antipsychotic medication. Similarly, approximately 8% of adults with mental retardation aged 75 and above took antianxiety medications, compared with approximately 4% of adults aged 25 to 54. In addition, the highest prevalence rates of antipsychotic drug use were found among older residents of skilled nursing homes and intermediate care facilities; residential setting, not occurrence of maladaptive behavior, was the primary predictor of psychotropic drug use in adults with mental retardation who were more than 65 years of age. Unfortunately, little is known about effectiveness of pharmacotherapy in older adults with mental retardation; however, based on data from research with nonretarded elders, there is little compelling evidence supporting the use of pharmacotherapy for treating geriatric behavioral disturbances. A recent metanalysis concluded that only one in five elderly patients appears to benefit from pharmacotherapy (Schneider, Pollock, & Lyness, 1990).

Behavioral Interventions

Use of behavioral interventions to manage maladaptive behaviors in older adults with mental retardation poses less risk than use of pharmacotherapy and has been recommended for geriatric populations (Burgio & Burgio, 1986; Carstensen, 1988; Jencks & Clausen, 1991). Behavior therapy has been used frequently to teach self-care skills to adults with mental retardation (e.g., Whitman, Scibak, & Reid, 1983) and to control behavior disturbances in children with mental retardation (e.g., Friman, Barnard, Altman, & Wolf, 1986). As a result, it would appear that behavior therapy techniques, such as differential reinforcement of incompatible behavior (DRI), would have utility for use with a geriatric population of individuals with mental retardation. However, creating a useful explanatory model to assess antecedents and consequences of some maladaptive behaviors, such as pica, may be difficult, and the cognitive and language limitations present in many persons with mental retardation will make some models and types of treatment infeasible (Matson & Gardner, 1991). Although research has demonstrated some utility of behavior therapy principles in treating the maladaptive behaviors of adults with mental retardation (Matson & Gardner, 1991; Peterson & Martens, 1995), older adults with mental retardation have not been extensively examined, and thus no definitive conclusions can be drawn at this time about the use of behavior therapy with this population.

One strategy of behavior therapy postulated to be effective in controlling behavior disturbances involves use of exercise to decrease maladaptive behavior. Participating in vigorous exercise may provide a socially acceptable outlet for agitated or aggressive behaviors. Furthermore, exercise or athletic activity provides a natural setting for ignoring maladaptive behaviors (e.g., throwing a ball can be deliberately misinterpreted as participation) and for the performance of behaviors incompatible with aggression or self-abuse. In their review of the available literature, Gabler-Halle, Halle, and Chung (1993) found a general trend for maladaptive behaviors in adults with mental retardation to improve following exercise; however, none of the studies reviewed included older adults among their samples. Elliott, Dobbin, Rose, and Soper (1994) compared vigorous aerobic exercise (e.g., jogging on a treadmill) to less vigorous exercise (e.g., riding an exercise bike, lifting light weights) and found that aerobic exercise effectively, though temporarily, reduced stereotypic and aggressive behaviors in adults with autism and mental retardation. While older adults were not specifically targeted, it was noted that the three oldest adults in the sample (mean age = 35 years) displayed the most significant reductions in maladaptive behaviors following exercise.

Mental Illness

Overview

It has been demonstrated that individuals with mental retardation have a higher probability of developing mental illnesses during their lives. The reasons for such increased risk have not been determined, although it has been hypothesized that impairments in communicative and information-processing abilities might result in a reduced ability to cope with stressful life situations (Menolascino & Potter, 1989). As in the general population, hereditary factors may also place the individual at increased risk for developing a mental illness. A particularly relevant risk factor for older adults with mental retardation is "the severe psychosocial deprivation" associated with institutional environments (Menolascino & Potter, 1989).

Foelker and Luke (1989) outlined some primary problems associated with the detection and accurate diagnosis of mental illness in individuals of any age with mental retardation. Because the primary duty of psychologists working in mental retardation settings is to assess cognitive and adaptive behavior skills, occurrence of mental illness in a client may be overlooked. Individuals with mental retardation may be unable to label or interpret their feelings and also may not know how to ask others for help in managing their feelings. Existing patterns of behavior may mask symptoms of a mental illness, particularly if the individual commonly exhibits maladaptive behaviors. In addition, symptoms of a mental illness may be interpreted by caregivers as a behavior problem that is related to environmental factors (Alford & Locke, 1984). The high staff turnover at residential facilities may result in a lack of information about clients' behavior patterns and mental health history. Finally, many psychometric tests used to diagnose psychopathology are written at the eighth-grade level and may not be understood by adults with mental retardation; moreover, the normative data for these instruments are not based on data from persons with mental retardation.

Types of Mental Illness

Depression. As recently as the 1970s, it was believed that people with mental retardation did not have the cognitive abilities necessary to experience depression (Winokur, 1974). This view is no longer widely held, although it is believed that the diagnosis of depression in individuals with mental retardation can include somewhat "nontraditional" depressive symptoms such as self-injury and aggression. However, self-reported feelings of depression and "traditional" signs of depression such as sad affect or withdrawal should also be considered when forming a depression diagnosis in these individuals (see Harper & Wadsworth, 1990).

Because of the types of life transitions common to aging retarded individuals, they are thought to have a high risk of developing depression. For example, older adults with mental retardation may experience depression following personal losses such as the death of a family member or friend, loss of a job due to retirement, or residential transitions due to declining health. Harper and Wadsworth (1990) investigated occurrence of depression in adults with moderate mental retardation who were at least 45 years of age. In this sample, there was a positive relationship between age and depression as measured by the Hamilton Rating Scale for Depression. However, occurrence of life events that may have produced depression was not examined. In a later study, Harper and Wadsworth (1993) examined the experience of grief in adults with mental retardation (including subjects in their 70s) and determined that the types of grief reactions (e.g., sadness, confusion, and anger) experienced by adults with moderate to severe mental retardation were similar to those experienced by nonretarded adults; however, differences in the manner in which these reactions were expressed and the intensity of the reactions were less clear.

Dementia. Dementia is a global term applied to a group of disorders character by progressive decline in cognitive and functional abilities. Dementias of certain etiologies, such as dementia caused by adverse drug interactions, are potentially reversible. However, as in the case of Alzheimer's disease, most dementias are irreversible. It is thought that adults with mental retardation are particularly susceptible to developing dementia as they age because of neurological vulnerability and the interaction of organic and psychiatric disease (Harper & Wadsworth, 1990). (Older adults with Down syndrome appear to be especially vulnerable to this condition; this phenomenon will be discussed later in this chapter.) A diagnosis of dementia is properly made following extensive medical and cognitive evaluations to rule out other causes of impairment. Memory loss is generally the first noticeable feature of dementia, but other symptoms (such as behavior changes, decline in ADLs, or loss of social skills) may also indicate the onset of a dementing illness.

Misdiagnosis of dementia can occur when a physical ailment or mental illness causes confusion, behavioral changes, or functional decline in a client. Older adults with mental retardation are particularly at risk for misdiagnosis of dementia because of the poor communicative skills of this group. The confusion or behavioral changes that can result from poor nutrition or that accompany physical ailments such as infections or endocrine disorders may resemble dementia and could be diagnosed as such if not differentially diagnosed by the clinician. One example is the case of delirium, a cognitive disorder characterized by a disturbance of attentive function and a decline in cognitive abilities which is frequently misdiagnosed as dementia. Delirium generally develops over a short period of time and is caused by a medical condition (e.g., head trauma or infections). Substance abuse, exposure to toxins, and medication side effects are also potential causes of delirium. If properly treated, delirium is usually reversible. However, misdiagnosis can result in unnecessary treatment for the supposed dementia and an absence of treatment for the underlying medical condition, which may worsen and could be fatal. Mental illnesses, particularly depression, sometimes manifest themselves as dementia-like symptoms in older adults (Adlin, 1993); this phenomenon is often referred to as "pseudodementia." The misdiagnosis of dementia can result in unnecessary nursing home placement and further deterioration of skills (Benson & Gambert, 1984). Therefore, careful evaluation and consideration of symptoms are necessary to avoid misdiagnosis.

With regard to the accurate assessment of dementia in older adults with mental retardation, Harper and Wadsworth (1990) state that variable cooperation, limitations in cognitive ability, and diminished senses and responsiveness resulting from old age and medication use complicate such an assessment. Lack of client education may also present assessment problems, as some dementia screening tools require reading, writing, or performing math calculations. Neuropsychologists or other professionals administering these tests may not be aware of these special considerations. Therefore, it is difficult to determine whether a low score on a dementia screening instrument actually reflects the presence of dementia or is merely the result of an educationally biased assessment tool, an undertrained evaluator, the limitations imposed by mental retardation, or some combination of these factors. Harper and Wadsworth (1990) advocate the use of multiple assessments to overcome these potential problems; however, neuropsychological batteries require a substantial length of time to administer, and the cognitive limitations of older adults with mental retardation would almost certainly require that testing be completed over several days.

It has been suggested that, at the very least, frequent ADL evaluations should be the minimum nonmedical evaluations performed to assess changes in skill level in older adults with severe or profound mental retardation (Janicki, Heller, Seltzer, & Hogg, 1995).

Other Mental Illnesses

Other forms of mental illness have been reported in older adults with mental retardation. Schizophrenia, bipolar affective disorder, brief reactive psychosis, personality disorders, anxiety disorders, and phobias have been documented in clinical and research literature (Foelker & Luke, 1989; Menolascino & Potter, 1989). The problems associated with the diagnosis of these conditions are similar to those associated with the diagnosis of dementia and depression. However, the more chronic psychological disorders (e.g., schizophrenia) may be harder to diagnose than disorders with a more sudden onset (e.g., brief reactive psychosis) because staff or clinicians are habituated to the client's symptoms. Mental illnesses that have delusions or hallucinations as part of their defining symptoms can present particular problems for individuals with communication difficulties, due to their inability to report these symptoms. Failure to diagnose a mental illness accurately can not only worsen the severity of an existing problem but also perpetuate the onset of additional disorders. For example, phobias or anxiety disorders may impair the individual's ability to establish relationships or be integrated into the community, thereby leading to social isolation and perhaps the occurrence of more problems.

Treatment

Treatment of mental illness in older adults with mental retardation frequently takes the form of pharmacotherapy. Theoretically, the primary reason for using medications is to reduce behavioral symptoms to a manageable level, at which time another therapeutic activity can be used (Menolascino & Potter, 1989). However, too often medication becomes the sole treatment, and the client is placed in a "chemical restraint" with potentially harmful side effects. In addition, using only pharmacological methods to treat mental illness does not permit the older adult with mental retardation to learn coping strategies or other, more effective means of dealing with his or her emotions.

Therapeutic practices such as psychotherapy or cognitive-behavioral therapy, although practiced commonly with nonretarded individuals, are rarely used as first-line treatments for mental illness in older adults with mental retardation. It may be assumed that mental illness is a normal part of aging in mentally retarded individuals, or that older adults with mental retardation will not benefit from psychotherapy; however, preliminary research has suggested that both of these beliefs may be inaccurate (see Foelker & Luke, 1989, for a more detailed review). In-service training for mental retardation professionals and paraprofessionals, as well as greater communication among the mental health and mental retardation service delivery systems, is needed to provide more information about the use of nonpharmacological methods of treating mental illness in older adults with mental retardation.

The treatment of dementia in older adults with mental retardation requires considerations different from the treatment of other types of psychological disorders. As dementia progresses, the treatment of coexisting medical disorders and mental illnesses intensifies, and new conditions develop which may also require treatment. When a diagnosis of dementia has been established, caregivers require education regarding the behavioral and cognitive changes that are likely to occur. If the client has the cognitive ability to understand his or her condition, he or she should also be told of the changes to come. Environmental supports that maximize familiarity and safety are crucial for maintenance of skills and prevention of behavior problems and accidents. With increasing cognitive deterioration, decisions regarding nursing home placement, guardianships, and advance directives become necessary. Family caregivers, residential staff, and clinicians must be trained to recognize the symptoms of dementia and to develop strategies to manage these symptoms in older adults with mental retardation (Janicki *et al.*, 1995).

Impairment in Physical or Motor Ability

Functional ability, commonly defined as the ability to perform ADLs, is essential to adequate quality of life and independent functioning. Functional ability is related to motor ability, for loss of motor ability impacts the performance of ADLs. Adults with mental retardation are thought to be particularly at risk for age-related declines in motor function (Pitetti & Campbell, 1991), not only because they may have preexisting physical limitations, but also because they tend to exercise less than nonretarded adults. One reason for this lack of exercise is that instructional programming provided to adults with mental retardation typically does not include exercise or physical fitness except for specific rehabilitative goals. A second reason is that older adults with mental retardation are likely to live in restrictive settings, which provide few opportunities for exercise. Third, older adults with mental retardation may be unable to comprehend or appreciate the long-term benefits of exercise, particularly when the short-term consequences can be aversive (Moon & Renzaglia, 1982; Neef, Bill-Harvey, Shade, Iezzi, & DeLorenzo, 1995).

The exercise participation of these individuals is particularly relevant in light of evidence indicating that adults with mental retardation are more likely to manifest problems in cardiovascular function, obesity, and muscular strength and endurance (see Fernhall, 1993). These three health aspects can greatly impact the physical and functional abilities of individuals with mental retardation (Shepard, 1987) and are particularly likely to worsen with age. Studies examining the effects of training on these areas have shown mixed results. Providing training in muscular strength and endurance does improve performance on activities such as sit-ups and pull-ups; however, improvement on clinical measures such as isokinetic tests has not yet been investigated. Similarly, cardiovascular function (measured by maximal oxygen uptakes) has been found to improve with training. However, effects of physical training on body composition (specifically, percentage of body fat) are still unknown (Fernhall, 1993); furthermore, information specific to older adults with mental retardation is lacking.

Because of the various factors working against older adults with mental retardation in their exercise participation, and because intact physical functioning is so critical for maintaining independence, improving the exercise
participation of older adults with mental retardation is an important goal. Several approaches have shown promise. Neef and colleagues (1995) used videotaped self-modeling of a therapeutic exercise routine to improve the gait and
balance of elderly women with mental retardation. In addition to producing increases in the independent exercise participation of these subjects, this intervention appeared to improve the women's ability to perform a balance board
walk test. Use of a system of fading prompts, similar to that used to teach vocational and self-care skills, has been effective with nonretarded individuals (see
Moon & Renzaglia, 1982, for a partial review), and it could be extended to practice with older adults with mental retardation. Finally, although not yet tested
with exercise, external aids such as picture cards or computer-provided cues
have been found to improve independent activity engagement in adults with
mental retardation (Lancioni, Brouwer, Bouter, & Coninx, 1993).

Down Syndrome and Alzheimer's Disease

The high prevalence of Alzheimer's disease among older adults with Down
syndrome is well documented and has even led to the suggestion that the condition of Trisomy 21 Down syndrome constitutes a risk factor for the development of Alzheimer's disease (Dalton & Crapper-McLachlan, 1986). Autopsy
studies have demonstrated that nearly 100% of individuals with Down syndrome who live past the age of 40 years have the cerebral neurofibrillary tangles
and neurotic plaques that are the defining features of Alzheimer's disease. However, it is estimated that only 40% of adults with Down syndrome over age 55
have the memory loss and behavioral symptoms characteristic of Alzheimer's
disease. Why some individuals with Down syndrome fail to develop the external
manifestations of Alzheimer's disease even though their brains show the neuropathological features of the disease is still unclear, although this discrepancy
does suggest the role of environmental or polygenetic factors in the expression of
Alzheimer's disease (Adlin, 1993; Dalton & Crapper-McLachlan, 1986).

Why might individuals with Down syndrome be at increased risk for
developing Alzheimer's disease? Because the likelihood of developing Alzheimer's disease increases with age, it is argued that Alzheimer's disease is an
age-related health condition. Individuals with Down syndrome also develop
other age-related health conditions, such as sensory impairments and osteoporosis, earlier in life than individuals without Down syndrome; thus, it has
been suggested that Down syndrome represents a condition of premature aging
(see Dalton, Seltzer, Adlin, & Wisniewski, 1993). Consequently, these individuals are predisposed to developing age-related diseases. This hypothesis would
also account for the data indicating that adults with Down syndrome develop
Alzheimer's disease at an earlier age and experience a more rapid progression
of symptoms than do adults without Down syndrome (Adlin, 1993). Many professionals hypothesize that there is a genetic link between Alzheimer's disease
and Down syndrome. It has been reported that specific markers located on chro-

mosome 21 are linked to the gene coding for beta amyloid precursor protein, which is thought to be involved in Alzheimer's disease neuropathology (e.g., Robakis *et al.,* 1987). Because chromosome 21 occurs in triplicate in individuals with Down syndrome, it is likely that individuals with Down syndrome are at increased risk for developing this neuropathology.

Difficulties associated with assessing Alzheimer's disease in the general population of older adults with mental retardation also apply to older adults with Down syndrome. Lack of appropriate assessment instruments (Dalton, 1992; Dalton & Wisniewski, 1990), problems imposed by limited intellectual and communicative abilities (Janicki *et al.,* 1995), and association of mental retardation with impaired physical development and limited opportunities for social development (Dalton *et al.,* 1993) all complicate the diagnosis of Alzheimer's disease in older adults with Down syndrome. These difficulties are compounded by the possibility that older adults with Down syndrome may exhibit a pattern of symptoms different from that of older adults whose mental retardation is not caused by Down syndrome. Memory loss is almost always the first symptom of dementia noted among older adults with mild to moderate mental retardation not caused by Down syndrome. However, in the early stages of Alzheimer's disease in older retarded adults with Down syndrome, symptoms such as personality changes, decline in ADLs, incontinence, and seizures are most commonly noted (Dalton & Crapper-McLachlan, 1986; McVicker, Shanks, & McClelland, 1994). These deviations highlight the need for thorough diagnostic procedures to determine the presence of Alzheimer's disease in individuals with Down syndrome.

CAREGIVING

The study of issues surrounding caregiving in older adults with mental retardation has received increasing attention in recent years. One reason for this recent attention is that the increased life expectancy of adults with mental retardation has prolonged the length of time that care must be provided to this population. Family caregivers provide care to their adult children with mental retardation during much of their lives. Although the probability of out-of-home residential placement increases with age (Meyers, Borthwick, & Eyman, 1985), it is estimated that 85% of individuals with mental retardation live with their families through adulthood (Fujiura & Braddock, 1992). Transition to an institutional setting or group home generally occurs following caregiver death or incapacitation, although factors such as the frequency of behavior problems and the severity of retardation are also highly associated with out-of-home placement (Blacher, Haneman, & Rousey, 1992; M. M. Seltzer & Krauss, 1984).

The bulk of caregiver research has focused on the caregivers of dementia patients. At this time, very little is known about the care or the caregivers of older adults with mental retardation. However, there is an increasing tendency in caregiving research to examine the caregiving relationship from a family systems perspective instead of focusing on one particular caregiver (e.g., M. M. Seltzer & Krauss, 1994; Smith, Fullmer, & Tobin, 1994). Thus, this section will review the research on so-called older families that include a co-residing adult with mental retardation. In keeping with the terminology used in the research literature, a co-residing adult with mental retardation will frequently be referred to as a "child," with the word "child" denoting the existence of a living parent (see M. M. Seltzer & Krauss, 1994) and not implying any perceptions of care receiver ability.

Older family caregivers of adults with mental retardation differ from other groups of family caregivers in several ways. First, providing direct care to an adult child is not generally perceived as a normative parental responsibility, whereas providing direct care to young children is seen as normative. Second, the caregiving responsibilities of parents of adult children with mental retardation tend to be lifelong in duration, whereas those families who care for non-retarded elders generally provide this care for a much shorter period of time (M. M. Seltzer & Krauss, 1989). Third, mental retardation is a chronic condition that manifests itself during childhood and is marked by relative stability of functioning over time, whereas other dependent conditions (e.g., mental illness) are characterized by a later age of onset and/or a more insidious decline in functioning (e.g., dementia). All of these factors are thought to affect the manner in which caregivers of adults with mental retardation cope with the demands of the caregiving situation.

Research examining characteristics of older families caring for adult children with mental retardation suggests that the heterogeneity of this population may lead to different degrees and sources of stressors for different groups of caregivers. For example, M. M. Seltzer, Krauss, and Tsunematsu (1993) compared the caregiving relationships in families whose adult children with mental retardation either had Down syndrome or did not have Down syndrome and found that aging mothers of adults with Down syndrome reported less caregiving stress and burden, less conflicted family environments, and more satisfaction with social supports than did mothers whose adult children's mental retardation had other causes. These results complement the findings of research conducted with families of young children with Down syndrome and mental retardation with other etiologies (e.g., Mink, Nihira, & Meyers, 1983). M. M. Seltzer and colleagues (1993) suggested that elderly caregivers' differences in reported stress and social supports may result from differential social expectations (not specified) placed on the two groups of adults with mental retardation. Alternatively, because people with Down syndrome are frequently thought to have "easier" temperaments, it is possible that group differences in temperament and/or behavior may influence caregiver stress. Another possibility is that the more definitive diagnosis of Down syndrome may give these two groups of caregivers different perspectives on their caregiving. Down syndrome is usually diagnosed at birth, whereas mental retardation of unknown etiology may not be diagnosed for several years, and then only after a great deal of parental frustration and uncertainty. Furthermore, more is known about the developmental trajectory of Down syndrome than of other types of mental retardation. Finally, parental support groups for families of children with Down syndrome are more common than support groups for families of children with other types of mental retardation (see M. M. Seltzer *et al.,* 1993). These factors may give parents of individuals with Down syndrome an "advantage" in terms of more predictability and social support.

Research examining older families caring for adults with mental retardation has frequently used as a comparison group families caring for adults with chronic mental illnesses. Greenberg, Seltzer, and Greenley (1993) found that aging mothers of adults with mental illness reported higher levels of subjective burden and poorer caregiving relationships than did aging mothers of adults with mental retardation. In addition, the maternal caregivers of adults with mental retardation had larger and more cohesive support networks, faced a smaller range of behavior problems in their adult children and, because the adults with mental retardation were more likely to attend job or day programs, received more respite during the day. Reporting of relatively low caregiver burden among caregivers of adults with mental retardation is a common thread throughout this research. It has been found that caregivers of adults with mental retardation report lower levels of caregiving-related burden than have been reported by caregivers of adults with mental illness (e.g., Greenberg *et al.,* 1993) and dementia (Zarit, Reever, & Bach-Peterson, 1980; Zarit, Todd, & Zarit, 1986), although to date no direct comparisons have been made between dementia and mental retardation caregiving relationships. Although the mothers of adults with mental retardation experienced more stress associated with providing more ADL assistance, this area was the only source of stress in which the mothers of the adults with mental retardation experienced more stress than did the mothers of adults with mental illness. Low levels of burden have been reported in both rural and urban caregivers of adults with mental retardation, including a recent survey conducted with Alabama caregivers (Baumhover, Gillum, LaGory, Burgio, & Beall, 1995). It is possible that this lower burden arises from the relative stability of a caregiving relationship involving mental retardation compared to the fluctuation and uncertainty found in a relationship where the care receiver has a dementing or psychiatric illness.

In a study with similar populations, M. M. Seltzer, Greenberg, and Krauss (1995) found that mothers of adults with mental illness used more "emotion-focused" coping strategies—considered to be less adaptive than "problem-focused" coping strategies—than did aging mothers of adults with mental retardation. Moreover, these between-group differences in use of emotion-focused coping strategies were accounted for by between-group differences in sources and amounts of caregiving-related stressors. As in the Greenberg and colleagues (1993) study, mothers of the adults with mental retardation reported providing more ADL assistance, whereas the mothers of the adults with mental illness reported a higher frequency of care receiver behavior problems. However, multiple regression analyses showed that providing more ADL assistance was a significant predictor of stress only in the caregivers of adults with mental illnesses, while higher frequency of behavior problems was a significant predictor of stress among the caregivers of adults with mental retardation. M. M. Seltzer and colleagues (1995) hypothesized that, although mothers of adults with mental retardation provide more ADL assistance than mothers of adults with mental illness, they may see it as a normative part of their caregiving duties, whereas mothers of adults with mental illness may regard ADL assistance as an unanticipated duty. Conversely, mothers of adults with mental illness may perceive behavior problems as being normative aspects of the caregiving relationship, even though these behavior problems may themselves be unpredictable, whereas mothers of adults with mental retardation may regard behavior problems as being incongruous with their adult children's condition.

In general, results of caregiving research highlight the importance of stability and predictability in determining caregiver well-being. As the mental and physical health of the caregiver ultimately impacts the care receiver, it is vital that these factors be carefully considered in the design and implementation of interventions for the management of caregiving-related stress and burden. In addition, attention must be paid to factors associated with the aging of the caregivers, as well as the aging of the care receiver. The aging caregivers of adults with mental retardation may require increased amounts of assistance and supports that are independent of their needs as caregivers. Finally, the heterogeneity of caregivers of adults with mental retardation, as well as variability among adults with mental retardation, must be taken into account when designing interventions to alleviate caregiver stress.

SERVICE DELIVERY ISSUES

Because individuals with mental retardation have traditionally died at younger ages than their nonretarded peers, developmental disabilities service systems until recently have paid little attention to the needs of older adults with mental retardation. However, it is now acknowledged that service delivery systems cannot meet the needs of this population without adequate preparation. The extent to which both aging and developmental disabilities service networks can provide for this population is considered to be of vital importance in determining the trajectory of service provision over the life span. In addition, the possibility of increased "cross-training"—i.e., interdisciplinary training and sharing of knowledge between the aging and developmental disabilities service systems (Kultgen & Rominger, 1993)—has recently been investigated as a means of providing more comprehensive and coordinated care to older adults with mental retardation. Studies of the service utilization patterns of older adults with mental retardation have revealed a trend toward continuation of existing developmental disabilities services into old age (Lakin, Anderson, Hill, Bruininks, & Wright, 1991) and a strong presence of older adults with mental retardation among the aging network services (M. M. Seltzer, Krauss, Litchfield, & Modlish, 1989). However, a 1988 study of service utilization patterns in Massachusetts noted that only about 5% of the services received by older adults with mental retardation in this state were age-specialized mental retardation services (M. M. Seltzer, 1988), suggesting that the aging and developmental disabilities service systems may currently be running in parallel rather than in tandem.

The difficulty in planning services for older adults with mental retardation, and the lack of widespread training in this area, may arise in part from philosophical differences between the aging and developmental disabilities service networks. In a 1992 survey of perceived "critical issues" and training needs, 31% of the aging and developmental disabilities "experts" expressed confusion regarding the application of treatment principles across the life span of this client population due to their differences in foci of treatment. The primary difference between the two service systems was perceived as a focus on skill building in the developmental disabilities services versus a focus on skill maintenance in the aging services. Of special concern was how to reconcile these different perspectives and plan appropriate services for these clients. Another relevant topic was whether the principle of active treatment could continue to be applied when clients with developmental disabilities reached old age (Gibson, Rabkin, & Munson, 1992).

Residential Services

The issue of treatment needs will have a profound impact on the residential options available to older adults with mental retardation. Medicaid-funded Intermediate Care Facilities for People with Mental Retardation (ICFs/MR), which provide a full-time habilitative treatment program, may not be wholly appropriate for older adults with declining health or functional abilities. Older clients with mental retardation may have difficulty maintaining participation in a rigorous schedule of active treatment. These declines in participation will then almost certainly result in lack of progress in treatment, which could cause the loss of Medicaid eligibility. Furthermore, one can question whether many of the self-care skills that are taught in ICF/MR programs are appropriate for older adults with mental retardation. These clients may instead require programming to help them regain or maintain, rather than acquire, self-care skills (Redjali & Radick, 1988). For example, a 70-year-old man who has participated in shoe-tying and time-telling programs may better spend his time on other activities, such as learning new leisure skills. Although one strategy for reaching these goals would be to move the older client with mental retardation to another type of facility, doing so may seriously disrupt the social supports available to that client (S. Jacobson & Kropf, 1993).

Another option involves modifying the existing facility to accommodate these new needs. Converting a residential facility to a level of care more compatible with geriatric needs, such as an ICF/General, requires consideration of multiple factors. The physical plant, staff composition, activities program, and records systems of the existing facility may all need modification to conform to federal Medicaid guidelines (Redjali & Radick, 1988). These modifications may be minor, as will probably be the case when changing from an ICF/MR to an ICF/General, but may be more substantial if the starting point is a somewhat less structured setting such as a foster care home.

When considering residential treatment options for older adults with mental retardation, it is important to consider the service objectives of a residential setting. Service professionals have stated that enhancing client independence, improving clients' daily functioning, and delaying or preventing institutionalization are considered to be among the most important service objectives (Coogle, Ansello, Wood, & Cotter, 1995). The social integration of retarded older adults, or the degree to which these individuals interact with nondisabled peers through participation in leisure activities, neighborhood relationships, and community services, has also been investigated. Not surprisingly, residents of more restrictive residential settings tend to be less integrated, as are residents with increased age and more severe levels of impairment. When resident characteristics such as age and level of impairment are controlled, the differences between residential facilities remain (Anderson, Lakin, Hill, & Chen, 1992), suggesting that the nature of the facility, rather than the age of its residents, is the most salient factor in determining social integration opportunities. However, because older adults with mental retardation are more likely to live in restrictive settings, further investigation of the opportunities available to the residents of these facilities, and the quality of life provided therein, is warranted.

Retirement

The issues of retirement and the options available after retirement are somewhat problematic when older adults with mental retardation are involved. Retirement is a life change that can affect social relationships, self-concept, and income; older adults with mental retardation are not immune to these changes. Adults with mental retardation may have their primary social contacts through their jobs and may have difficulty adjusting to the loss of this network of friends. A nonretarded retiree typically has other social roles, such as grandfather, caregiver, or wife, that compensate for the loss of the work role. An older adult with mental retardation may not be able to fall back on such roles to establish or maintain a self-concept and thus may experience even more keenly the loss of the worker role. Financial issues may also pose a problem. An adult who receives Supplemental Security Income (SSI) due to lifelong disability frequently uses this money to cover the cost of room and board at his or her place of residence; money received from working is generally the only money the client has to spend on incidentals. The loss of this income upon retirement is rarely replaced by a pension, nor do SSI benefits increase. As a result, the retiree with mental retardation may suddenly be unable to participate in activities such as outings that require the use of "discretionary monies." This, in turn, can result in social isolation and feelings of devaluation (Janicki, 1994).

Following retirement, there may be few activities options available to older adults with mental retardation. This client population may not have the knowledge of community services necessary for initiating meaningful postretirement activities and may not have considered previously how they would like to spend their retirement years. Moreover, it can be difficult for these individuals to maintain useful vocational and adaptive skills after retirement. Therapeutic recreation programming, including art-and-craft-related endeavors, has been suggested as a means of providing purposeful yet entertaining activities to older adults with mental retardation. These types of activities (e.g., tossing horseshoes, painting) are frequently flexible enough that all clients can participate at some level with some degree of prompting. Through careful task analysis and documentation of client participation and enjoyment, older adults with mental retardation can explore new outlets of self-expression, learn new skills and maintain old ones, and establish contacts with peers who have similar interests (Carter & Foret, 1990; Edelson, 1990).

Activities involving integration of older adults with mental retardation into the nondisabled elder community can widen the available network of services. The principle of normalization (Wolfensberger, 1972) suggests that older adults

with mental retardation should have access to the same services as their nonretarded, same-age peers, and that the presence of a disability should not be the
sole criterion for withholding opportunities from older adults (Wilhite, Keller,
& Nicholson, 1990). However, senior citizens' activities may be too complex
(e.g., book discussion groups) or understimulating (e.g., "activities" in adult day
care centers). Furthermore, the clients and staff in senior citizens' programs
may not be familiar with the special needs of older adults with mental retardation, potentially resulting in inadequate supervision of and discrimination
against these clients (Janicki, 1994). Adequate staff training, as well as client
education, will help ensure that older adults with mental retardation move
smoothly into integrated services.

SUMMARY

Although the increased population of older adults with mental retardation
has not remained unnoticed by researchers and service providers, relatively little is known about their needs, and even less is known about how best to meet
these needs. Collaboration of academic researchers and direct care providers is
crucial for achieving goals related to the care of the older adult with mental retardation. More information is needed on nearly every aspect of aging and mental retardation. At the most basic level, the area requires a clearer and more
standardized definition of what constitutes "old" for the general population and
various subpopulations of adults with mental retardation. Research is needed on
individual and group differences in cognitive ability, adaptive behavior skills,
physical health status, maladaptive behavior, psychological disturbances, and
service needs of individuals with mental retardation over the life span. Increased
knowledge regarding the accurate diagnosis of mental illness and dementia, the
effectiveness of pharmacological and behavioral treatments for psychological
and behavioral disorders, and the remediation of functional and physical losses
is of paramount importance in determining the quality of life for older individuals with mental retardation. Further investigation of the possible connections
between Down syndrome and Alzheimer's disease has the potential of providing
valuable information on the prevention of Alzheimer's disease not only among
individuals with Down syndrome but also in the population at large. Finally, the
opportunities for cooperation between the aging and developmental disabilities
service networks, and the extent to which client needs can best be met through
the collaboration of these networks, remain largely unexplored. Unfortunately,
the growth of our knowledge base has not kept pace with the growth of this population. We can only hope that this trend will reverse in time to avert a crisis of
care that, at this point, appears inevitable.

REFERENCES

Adlin, M. (1993). Health care issues. In E. Sutton, A. R. Factor, B. A. Hawkins, T. Heller, & G. B.
Seltzer (Eds.), *Older adults with developmental disabilities: Optimizing choice and change*
(pp. 49–60). Baltimore: Brookes.

Alford, J. D., & Locke, B. J. (1984). Clinical responses to psychopathology of mentally retarded persons. *American Journal of Mental Deficiency. 89*, 195–197.

American Association on Mental Retardation. (1992). *Mental retardation: Definition, classification, and systems of supports* (9th ed.). Washington, DC: Author.

Anderson, D. J. (1989). Healthy and institutionalized: Health and related conditions among older persons with developmental disabilities. *Journal of Applied Gerontology, 8*, 228–241.

Anderson, D. J. (1993). Health issues. In E. Sutton, A. R. Factor, B. A. Hawkins, T. Heller, & G. B. Seltzer (Eds.), *Older adults with developmental disabilities: Optimizing choice and change* (pp. 29–48). Baltimore: Brookes.

Anderson, D. J., & Polister, B. (1993). Psychotropic medication use among older adults with mental retardation. In E. Sutton, A. R. Factor, B. A. Hawkins, T. Heller, & G. B. Seltzer (Eds.), *Older adults with developmental disabilities: Optimizing choice and change* (pp. 61–75). Baltimore: Brookes.

Anderson, D. J., Lakin, K. C., Bruininks, R. H., & Hill, B. K. (1987). *A national study of residential and support services for elderly persons with mental retardation*. Minneapolis: University of Minnesota Press.

Anderson, D. J., Lakin, K. C., Hill, B. K., & Chen, T.-H. (1992). Social integration of older persons with mental retardation in residential facilities. *American Journal on Mental Retardation, 96*, 488–501.

Baumhover, L. A., Gillum, J. L., LaGory, M., Burgio, L., & Beall, S. C. (1995). A *statewide study to determine the status and needs of elderly types with developmental disabilities.* (Report available from the Alabama Developmental Disabilities Planning Council, RSA Union Building, 100 North Union Street, P.O. Box 301410, Montgomery, AL 36130-1410.)

Bell, A., & Zubek, J. (1960). The effect of age on the intellectual performance of mental defectives. *Journals of Gerontology, 15*, 285–295.

Benson, D., & Gambert, S. (1984). The impact of misdiagnosis on nursing home placement. *Psychiatric Medicine, 1*, 309–315.

Blacher, J. B., Hanneman, R. A., & Rousey, A. B. (1992). Out-of-home placement of children with severe handicaps: A comparison of approaches. *American Journal on Mental Retardation, 96*, 607–616.

Burgio, L. D., & Burgio, K. L. (1986). Behavioral gerontology: Application of behavioral methods to the problems of older adults. *Journal of Applied Behavior Analysis*, 321–328.

Butler, F., Burgio, L., & Engel, B. (1987). A behavioral analysis of geriatric nursing home patients receiving neuroleptic medication: A comparative study. *Journal of Gerontological Nursing, 13*, 15–19.

Carstensen, L. L. (1988). The emerging field of behavioral gerontology. *Behavior Therapy, 19*, 259–281.

Carter, M. J., & Foret, C. (1990). Therapeutic recreation programming for older adults with developmental disabilities. *Activities, Adaptation & Aging, 15*, 35–51.

Coogle, C. L., Ansello, E. F., Wood, J. B., & Cotter, J. J. (1995). Partners II—Serving older persons with developmental disabilities: Obstacles and inducements to collaboration among agencies. *Journal of Applied Gerontology, 14*, 275–288.

Dalton, A. J. (1992). Dementia in Down syndrome: Methods of evaluation. In L. Nadel & C. J. Epstein (Eds.), *Down syndrome and Alzheimer disease* (pp. 51–76). New York: Wiley-Liss.

Dalton, A. J., & Crapper-McLachlan, D. R. (1986). Clinical expression of Alzheimer's disease in Down syndrome. *Psychiatric Clinics of North America, 9*, 659–670.

Dalton, A. J., & Wisniewski, H. M. (1990). Down's Syndrome and the dementia of Alzheimer disease. *International Review of Psychiatry, 2*, 43–52.

Dalton, A. J., Seltzer, G. B., Adlin, M. S., & Wisniewski, H. M. (1993). Association between Alzheimer disease and Down syndrome: Clinical observations. In J. M. Berg, H. Karlinsky, & A. J. Holland (Eds.), *Alzheimer disease, Down syndrome, and their relationship* (pp. 53–69). Oxford, England: Oxford University Press.

Davidson, P. W., Cain, N. N., Sloane-Reeves, J., Kramer, B., Quijano, L., VanHeyningen, J., & Giesow, V. (1992, November). *Aging effects on severe behavior disorders in community-based clients with mental retardation*. Paper presented at the meeting of the Gerontological Society of America, Washington, DC.

Davidson, P. W., Cain, N. N., Sloane-Reeves, J. E., Van Speybroech, A., Segel, J., Gutkin, J., Quijano, L. E., Kramer, B. M., Porter, B., Shoham, I., & Goldstein, E. (1994). Characteristics of community-based individuals with mental retardation and aggressive behavioral disorders. *American Journal on Mental Retardation, 98,* 704–716.

Edelson, R. T. (1990). ART AND CRAFTS—Not "arts and crafts"—Alternative vocational day activities for adults who are older and mentally retarded. *Activities, Adaptation & Aging, 15,* 81–97.

Eklund, S. J., & Martz, W. L. (1993). Maintaining optimal functioning. In E. Sutton, A. R. Factor, B. A. Hawkins, T. Keller, & G. B. Seltzer (Eds.), *Older adults with developmental disabilities: Optimizing choice and change* (pp. 3–27). Baltimore: Brookes.

Elliott, R. O., Jr., Dobbin, M. A., Rose, G. D., & Soper, H. V. (1994). Vigorous, aerobic exercise versus general motor training activities: Effects on maladaptive and stereotypic behaviors of adults with both autism and mental retardation. *Journal of Autism and Developmental Disorders, 24,* 565–576.

Eyman, R. K., & Widaman, K. F. (1987). Life-span development of institutionalized and community-based mentally retarded persons, revisited. *American Journal of Mental Deficiency, 91,* 559–569.

Eyman, R. K., Call, T. L., & White, J. F. (1989). Mortality of elderly mentally retarded persons in California. *Journal of Applied Gerontology, 8,* 203–215.

Fenner, M. E., Hewitt, K. E., & Torpy, D. M. (1987). Down's syndrome: Intellectual and behavioural functioning during adulthood. *Journal of Mental Deficiency Research, 31,* 241–249.

Fernhall, B. (1993). Physical fitness and exercise training of individuals with mental retardation. *Medicine and Science in Sports and Exercise, 25,* 442–450.

Fine, M. A., Tangeman, P. J., & Woodard, J. (1990). Changes in adaptive behavior of older adults with mental retardation following deinstitutionalization. *American Journal on Mental Retardation, 94,* 661–668.

Fisher, M. A., & Zeaman, D. (1970). Growth and decline of retarded intelligence. *International Review of Research in Mental Retardation, 4,* 151–191.

Foelker, G. A., Jr., & Luke, E. A., Jr. (1989). Mental health issues for the aging mentally retarded population. *Journal of Applied Gerontology, 8,* 242–250.

Friman, P. C., Barnard, J. D., Altman, K., & Wolf, M. M. (1986). Parent and teacher use of DRO and DRI to reduce aggressive behavior. *Analysis and Intervention in Developmental Disabilities, 6,* 319–330.

Fujiura, G. T., & Braddock, D. (1992). Fiscal and demographic trends in mental retardation services: The emergence of the family. In L. Rowitz (Ed.), *Mental retardation in the year 2000* (pp. 316–338). New York: Springer.

Gabler-Halle, D., Halle, J. W., & Chung, Y. B. (1993). The effects of aerobic exercise on psychological and behavioral variables of individuals with developmental disabilities: A critical review. *Research in Developmental Disabilities, 14,* 359–386.

Gibson, J. W., Rabkin, J., & Munson, R. (1992). Critical issues in serving the developmentally disabled elderly. *Journal of Gerontological Social Work, 19,* 35–49.

Greenberg, J. S., Seltzer, M. M., & Greenley, J. R. (1993). Aging parents of adults with disabilities: The gratifications and frustrations of later-life caregiving. *Gerontologist, 33,* 542–550.

Harper, D. C., & Wadsworth, J. S. (1990). Dementia and depression in elders with mental retardation: A pilot study. *Research in Developmental Disabilities, 11,* 177–198.

Harper, D. C., & Wadsworth, J. S. (1993). Grief in adults with mental retardation: Preliminary findings. *Research in Developmental Disabilities, 14,* 313–330.

Hewitt, K. E., Carter, G., & Jancar, J. (1985). Ageing in Down's syndrome. *British Journal of Psychiatry, 147,* 58–62.

Hewitt, K. E., Fenner, M. E., & Torpy, D. (1986). Cognitive and behavioral profiles of the elderly mentally handicapped. *Journal of Mental Deficiency Research, 30,* 217–225.

Hogg, J., & Moss, S. (1993). The characteristics of older people with intellectual disabilities in England. *International Review of Research in Mental Retardation, 19,* 71–96.

Jacobson, J. W. (1988). Problem behavior and psychiatric impairment within a developmentally disabled population III: Psychotropic medication. *Research in Developmental Disabilities, 9,* 23–38.

Jacobson, S., & Kropf, N. P. (1993). Facilitating residential transitions of older adults with developmental disabilities. *Clinical Gerontologist, 14,* 79–93.

James, D. H. (1986). Psychiatric and behavioural disorders amongst older severely mentally handicapped inpatients. *Journal of Mental Deficiency Research, 30,* 341–345.

Janicki, M. P. (1994). Policies and supports for older persons with mental retardation. In M. M. Seltzer, M. W. Krauss, & M. P. Janicki (Eds.), *Life course perspectives on adulthood and old age* (pp. 143–165). Washington, DC: American Association on Mental Retardation.

Janicki, M. P., Heller, T., Seltzer, G., & Hogg, J. (1995). *Practice guidelines for the clinical assessment and care management of Alzheimer and other dementias among adults with mental retardation.* Washington, DC: American Association on Mental Retardation.

Jencks, S. F., & Clausen, S. B. (1991). Managing behavior problems in nursing homes. *Journal of the American Medical Association, 265,* 502–503.

Jenkins, E. L., Hildreth, B. L., & Hildreth, G. (1993). Elderly persons with mental retardation: An exceptional population with special needs. *International Journal of Aging and Human Development, 37,* 69–80.

Katz, S., Ford, B. S., Moskowitz, R. W., Jackson, B. A., & Jaffe, M. W. (1963). Studies of illness in the aged. The Index of ADL: A standardized measure of biological and psychosocial function. *Journal of the American Medical Association, 185* (12), 94–99.

Kerby, D. S., Wentworth, R., & Cotten, P. D. (1989). Measuring adaptive behavior in elderly developmentally disabled clients. *Journal of Applied Gerontology; 8,* 261–267.

Kultgen, P., & Rominger, R. (1993). Cross training within the aging and developmental disabilities service systems. In E. Sutton, A. R. Factor, B. A. Hawkins, T. Heller, & G. B. Seltzer (Eds.), *Older adults with developmental disabilities: Optimizing choice and change* (pp. 239–256). Baltimore: Brookes.

Lakin, K. C., Anderson, D. J., Hill, B. K., Bruininks, R. H., & Wright, E. A. (1991). Programs and services received by older persons with mental retardation. *Mental Retardation, 29,* 65–74.

Lancioni, G. E., Brouwer, J. A., Bouter, H. P., & Coninx, F. (1993). Simple technology to promote independent activity engagement in institutionalized people with mental handicap. *International Journal of Rehabilitation Research, 16,* 235–238.

Matson, J. L., & Gardner, W. I. (1991). Behavioral learning theory and current applications to severe behavior problems in persons with mental retardation. *Clinical Psychology Review, 11,* 175–183.

McGrew, K. S., Ittenbach, R. F., Bruininks, R. H., & Hill, B. K. (1991). Factor structure of maladaptive behavior across the lifespan of persons with mental retardation. *Research in Developmental Disabilities, 12,* 181–199.

McVicker, R. W., Shanks, O. E. P., & McClelland, R. J. (1994). Prevalence and associated features of epilepsy in adults with Down's syndrome. *British Journal of Psychiatry, 164,* 528–532.

Menolascino, F. J., & Potter, J. F. (1989). Mental illness in the elderly mentally retarded. *Journal of Applied Gerontology, 8,* 192–202.

Meyers, C. E., Borthwick, S. A., & Eyman, R. (1985). Place of residence by age, ethnicity, and level of retardation of the mentally retarded/developmentally disabled population of California. *American Journal of Mental Retardation, 90,* 266–270.

Mink, I. T., Nihira, K., & Meyers, C. E. (1983). Taxonomy of family life styles. I: Homes with TMR children. *American Journal of Mental Deficiency, 87,* 484–497.

Moon, M. S., & Renzaglia, A. (1982). Physical fitness and the mentally retarded: A critical review of the literature. *Journal of Special Education, 16,* 269–287.

National Center for Health Statistics. (1979). *The national nursing home survey: 1977 summary for the United States.* Washington, DC: United States Department of Health, Education, and Welfare.

National Center for Health Statistics, Public Health Services. (1986). Prevalence of selected chronic conditions, United States, 1979–1981. *Vital and Health Statistics,* Series 10, No. 155 (DHHS Publ. No. (PHS) 86-1583). Washington, DC: U.S. Government Printing Office.

Neef, N. A., Bill-Harvey, D., Shade, D., Iezzi, M., & DeLorenzo, T. (1995). Exercise participation with videotaped modeling: Effects on balance and gait in elderly residents of care facilities. *Behavior Therapy, 26,* 135–151.

Newbern, V. B., & Hargett, M. V. (1992). A gerontological nursing issue: The aged developmentally disabled/mentally retarded. *Holistic Nurse Practitioner, 7,* 70–77.

Nihira, K., Foster, R., Shellhaas, M., & Leland, H. (1974). *AAMD Adaptive Behavior Scale.* Washington, DC: American Association on Mental Deficiency.

Nihira, K., Leland, H., & Lambert, N. (1993). *Adaptive Behavior Scale—Residential and Community* (2nd ed.). Austin, TX: Pro-Ed.

Peterson, F. M., & Martens, B. K. (1995). A comparison of behavioral interventions reported in treatment studies and programs for adults with developmental disabilities. *Research in Developmental Disabilities, 16,* 27–41.

Pitetti, K. H., & Campbell, K. D. (1991). Mentally retarded individuals—A population at risk? *Medicine and Science in Sports and Exercise, 23,* 586–593.

Ray, W. A., Federspiel, C. F., & Schaffner, W. (1980). Antipsychotic drug use in nursing homes: Evidence of misuse. *American Journal of Public Health, 70,* 485–491.

Redjali, S. M., & Radick, J. R. (1988). ICF/General: An alternative for older ICF/MR residents with geriatric care needs. *Mental Retardation, 26,* 209–212.

Rinck, C., & Calkins, C. F. (1989). Patterns of psychotropic medication use among older persons with developmental disabilities. *Journal of Applied Gerontology, 8,* 216–227.

Robakis, N. K., Wisniewski, H. M., Jenkins, E. C., Devine-Gage, E. A., Houck, G. E., Yao, X. L., Ramakrishna, N., Wolfe, G., Silverman, W., & Brown, W. T. (1987). Chromosome 21q21 sublocalization of gene encoding beta amyloid peptide in cerebral vessels and neurotic (senile) plaques of people with Alzheimer's disease and Down syndrome. *Lancet, 1* (8529), 384–385.

Schneider, L. S., Pollock, V. E., & Lyness, S. A. (1990). A metaanalysis of controlled trials of neuroleptic treatment in dementia. *Journal of the American Geriatrics Society, 38,* 553–563.

Seltzer, G. B., Finaly, E., & Howell, M. (1988). Functional characteristics of elderly persons with mental retardation in community settings and nursing homes. *Mental Retardation, 26,* 213–217.

Seltzer, M. M. (1988). Structure and patterns of service utilization by elderly persons with mental retardation. *Mental Retardation, 26,* 181–185.

Seltzer, M. M., & Krauss, M. W. (1984). Family, community residence, and institutional placements of a sample of mentally retarded children. *American Journal of Mental Deficiency, 89,* 257–266.

Seltzer, M. M., & Krauss, M. W. (1987). *Aging and mental retardation: Extending the continuum* (Monograph No. 9). Washington, DC: American Association on Mental Retardation.

Seltzer, M. M., & Krauss, M. W. (1989). Aging parents with adult mentally retarded children: Family risk factors and sources of support. *American Journal on Mental Retardation, 94,* 303–312.

Seltzer, M. M., & Krauss, M. W. (1994). Aging parents with coresident adult children: The impact of lifelong caregiving. In M. M. Seltzer, M. W. Krauss, & M. P. Janicki (Eds.), *Life course perspectives on adulthood and old age* (pp. 3–18). Washington, DC: American Association on Mental Retardation.

Seltzer, M. M., Krauss, M. W., Litchfield, L. C., & Modlish, N. J. K. (1989). Utilization of aging network services by elderly persons with mental retardation. *Gerontologist, 29,* 234–238.

Seltzer, M. M., Krauss, M. W., & Tsunematsu, N. (1993). Adults with Down Syndrome and their mothers: Diagnostic group differences. *American Journal on Mental Retardation, 97,* 496–508.

Seltzer, M. M., Greenberg, J. S., & Krauss, M. W. (1995). A comparison of coping strategies of aging mothers of adults with mental illness versus mental retardation. *Psychology and Aging, 10,* 64–75.

Shepard, R. J. (1987). Human rights and the older worker: Changes in work capacity with age. *Medicine and Science in Sports and Exercise, 19,* 168–173.

Smith, G. C., Fullmer, E. M., & Tobin, S. S. (1994). Living outside the system: An exploration of older families who do not use day programs. In M. M. Seltzer, M. W. Krauss, & M. P. Janicki (Eds.), *Life course perspectives on adulthood and old age* (pp. 19–37). Washington, DC: American Association on Mental Retardation.

Spitz, H. H. (1986). Disparities in mentally retarded persons' IQs derived from different intelligence tests. *American Journal of Mental Deficiency, 90,* 588–591.

Spruill, J. (1991). A comparison of the Wechsler Adult Intelligence Scale–Revised with the Stanford-Binet Intelligence Scale (4th edition) for mentally retarded adults. *Psychological Assessment, 3,* 133–135.

Wersh, J., & Thomas, M. R. (1990). The Stanford-Binet Intelligence Scale: Fourth edition; Observations, comments, and concerns. *Canadian Psychology, 31,* 190–193.

Whitman, T. L., Scibak, J. W., & Reid, D. H. (1983). *Behavior modification with the severely and profoundly retarded: Research and application.* New York: Academic.

Wilhite, B., Keller, M. J., & Nicholson, L. (1990). Integrating older persons with developmental disabilities into community recreation: Theory to practice. *Activities, Adaptation & Aging, 15,* 111–129.

Winokur, B. (1974). Subnormality and its relation to psychiatry. *Lancet, 2,* 270–273.

Wolfensberger, W. (1972). *The principle of normalization in human services.* Toronto, Ontario, Canada: National Institute on Mental Retardation.

Zarit, S. H., Reever, K. E., & Bach-Peterson, J. (1980). Relatives of impaired elderly: Correlates of feelings of burden. *Gerontologist, 20,* 649–655.

Zarit, S. H., Todd, P. A., & Zarit, J. M. (1986). Subjective burden of husbands and wives as caregivers: A longitudinal study. *Gerontologist, 26,* 260–266.

CHAPTER 16

Behavioral Medicine Interventions with Older Adults

MARY J. GAGE AND ANTHONY J. GORECZNY

INTRODUCTION

Behavioral medicine is an area that has flourished since the 1960s. In large part, this is due to the fact that the primary conditions that have led to death and illness since then have involved significant psychosocial or biobehavioral risk factors (Goreczny, 1995b). Despite the growth in the area of behavioral medicine in general, until recently there had been only very scant references to behavioral medicine interventions with older adults. There may be several reasons for this. First, many health care professionals shy away from treating older adults. Second, some thought it difficult, if not impossible, to teach older adults the strategies often used in behavioral medicine interventions, including techniques such as biofeedback, relaxation training, and disease self-management. The view that older adults cannot learn these techniques was prevalent among health care professionals and prospective patients alike. Third, some initial research studies provided apparent proof that older adults could not benefit from behavioral medicine interventions. Thus, for quite some time, although researchers usually did not exclude older adults from studies, there was very little attempt to study this population independently of their younger cohorts. Studies that did include older adults usually statistically adjusted for demographic factors such as age rather than examining the effects of these factors outright.

With demographic data revealing that older adults comprise one of the largest growing segments of the population, there has been an increase in interest in conducting research with this population. Much of the research still confounds data from older and younger adults, thereby making it impossible to

MARY J. GAGE • Mellon Center, Cleveland Clinic, Cleveland, Ohio 44195 ANTHONY J. GORECZNY • Director of Clinical Training Program, Department of Psychology, University of Indianapolis, Indianapolis, Indiana 46227-3697.

Handbook of Clinical Geropsychology, edited by Michel Hersen and Vincent B. Van Hasselt. Plenum Press, New York, 1998.

delineate effects of interventions specifically on older adults. Nonetheless, some excellent studies have begun to isolate these effects. In this chapter, we review only those studies that permit a clear appraisal of intervention effects on older adults or that have significant implications for these individuals.

The field of behavioral medicine includes many areas; in this chapter, we address only a few. Some of the areas that might fall under the rubic of behavioral medicine appear elsewhere in this book: Chapter 12 deals with sexual dysfunction, Chapter 13 with sleep disorders, Chapter 18 with pain management, and Chapter 24 with physical activity. Therefore, we do not address those topics in this chapter. Instead, we focus our attention on issues related to stress, HIV/AIDS, health maintenance, and smoking, and on two issues of special importance to older adults, specifically, falls and tremors. In these areas, we have provided a brief overview of recent research regarding the topic. Because of the rapidly growing database, we focus almost exclusively on research published in the 1990s.

This chapter provides a primer for readers rather than a comprehensive review; it is intended to spark the interest of readers to further investigate this exciting area. Those who develop such as interest might want to consult the book by Goreczny (1995a), which deals comprehensively with a wide variety of behavioral medicine and health psychology topics but without the emphasis on older adults.

STRESS

The area of stress is an area that, in general, needs much work just to define the topics of study. What constitutes stress and how to measure stress are just two of the many questions that lack definitive answers. Nonetheless, stress remains one of the largest areas of research in the behavioral sciences. Since 1985, there have been more than 1,500 published articles each year that have become part of the PsycLit database (Goreczny, 1997). This represents more than 4% of all such articles each year. Fortunately, the area of stress as it pertains to older adults has also received significant attention. As will be clear from the literature review below, however, much work and many questions remain.

One of the first and most obvious questions to ask is whether the numbers and types of stressors are different among older and younger adults. Certainly, one would expect that the types of stressors older adults experience are different from the types of stressors experienced by younger cohorts. One of the stressors that older adults are more likely to experience than are younger adults is the death of a spouse or even of an adult child. One recent study revealed that, as one would expect, bereavement has significant stress effects on older adults who experience such losses (Arbuckle & de Vries, 1995). There is, however, little recent research that addresses the question as to differences in type of stressors among older and younger adults. There is also very little, if any, recent research that addresses the question of whether the number of stressors experienced by older adults differs from the number experienced by younger adults. Most of the recent research in older adults has focused on stress effects and coping. It is to this literature that we now turn our attention.

The effects of stress on health-related problems in the general population are quite clear, so much so that "stress management has become a universally accepted form of health intervention and has improved the quality of life for many individuals" (Brantley & Thomason, 1995, p. 286). There have been several studies that have looked specifically at the effects of stress on the health of older adults. In one study, Krause (1996) noted that the stress of living in deteriorated living environments and neighborhoods contributes to an increase in self-reported physical health problems among older adults, relative to older adults who live in neighborhoods that have not experienced significant deterioration. Krause noted that this relationship is present only for the extremely deteriorated neighborhoods, however, and attributed the stress–health connection in this case to a breakdown and weakening of friendships. Research by Kahana, Redmond, Hill, & Kircher (1995) is consistent with this attribution. In Kahana and colleagues' study, the authors obtained a variety of measures from 397 adults more than 54 years of age. One of the main conclusions from this study was that the effect of stressors on well-being in this population came via an indirect mechanism—satisfaction with various domains of the individuals' lives. In addition to overall self-rated health, studies have revealed likely stress effects on specific physiological functions of older adults, including potentiation of age-related decreases in testicular functioning among men (Vermeulen, 1994).

Additional research has attempted to examine effects of stress on normal activities of daily living among adults. For example, there has been some indication of deleterious stress effects on sleep. Friedman et al. (1995) found a positive association between amount of stress and amount of sleep difficulty among a group of older adults. This relationship, however, was present only in a group of poor sleepers and not in a group of good sleepers. Though there was this within-group relationship between number of stressors and amount of sleep, there was no difference between the group of good sleepers and the group of poor sleepers with regard to amount of stress. Thus, the specific role of stressors in problems of sleep among older adults remains unknown.

Still other researchers have attempted to implicate stressors as significant factors in the onset of late-life alcoholism as well as dementia. For example, although research by Liberto and Oslin (1995) suggested that late-onset alcoholics tend to have greater psychological stability than do early-onset alcoholics, this research has also suggested that late-life stress may be one factor contributing significantly to late-onset alcohol problems. However, Krause (1995b) also noted that alcohol use may serve a beneficial role among older adults: Alcohol may mitigate effects of minor stressors. Of importance, though, is that alcohol tends to increase effects of highly significant stressors among older adults. Some researchers have also attempted to implicate stress in the development of dementias (see Carpenter, Strauss, & Kennedy, 1995). However, there is evidence that stress experienced by patients suffering from dementia may be the result of disruption of their social lives as a consequence of the disorder rather than a contributing factor to development of the disorder (Ortell & Bebbington, 1995).

Interestingly, recent research has revealed that older adults appear to handle stressors better than do younger adults (Carmack *et al.*, 1995). In a recent study by Nussbaum and Goreczny (1995), one of the interesting findings was that there was a significant negative relationship between age and self-reported level of overall stress. Thus, older adults reported feeling less stressed in general than did younger adults. Other recent research is consistent with this finding. In a study by Talbert, Wagner, Braswell, and Husein (1995), older adults were the least susceptible age group with regard to experiencing stress symptoms in response to an emergency room visit. Also consistent with this is a recent study revealing that low-functioning fibromyalgia patients tended to be younger than their higher-functioning cohorts (Schoenfeld-Smith, Nicassio, Radojevic, & Patterson, 1995). Finally, Rose and West (1996) noted that among cardiac rehabilitation patients, younger patients presented with more depression than did older patients.

Several researchers have investigated the stress effects and coping strategies used by individuals suffering from chronic illnesses. One model frequently cited as explaining psychological adjustment to stressors is the stress and coping model proposed by Lazarus and Folkman (1984). One recent study revealed that such a stress and coping model appears to be applicable specifically to older adults as well as to the general population (Landreville, Dube, Lalande, & Alain, 1994). In this study, the authors found a positive relationship between amount of perceived stress among older adults suffering from mobility limitations and the amount of coping efforts they made. Interestingly, subjects who used coping strategies of taking on increased amounts of responsibility or attempting to escape or avoid stressors, or both, reported high levels of perceived stress and a large number of depressive symptoms.

Some other researchers have also attempted to investigate stress effects specifically among older adults with chronic illnesses. As one example, Melanson and Downe-Wamboldt (1995) noted that their sample of older adults suffering from rheumatoid arthritis identified several illness-related stressors associated with the condition. However, those subjects also reported utilizing active, confrontative types of strategies to help them cope with the identified stressors. Interestingly, in another study, the same investigators reported that higher socioeconomic status clients tended to utilize active, confrontative coping strategies more often than did lower socioeconomic status clients (Downe-Wamboldt & Melanson, 1995).

Life stressors frequently result in the manifestation of anxiety symptoms. On the other hand, anxiety symptoms may also be due to some specific illness or disease process. Given that with aging comes an increasing likelihood of developing an illness that has an identified physiological process, it is especially important to rule out specific organic pathology among older adults. Hocking and Koenig (1995) discuss the importance of proper diagnosis prior to implementing treatment for older adults who report anxiety symptoms. Treatment will then depend upon etiological considerations. If no identified physiological process appears to be contributing to the anxiety symptoms, assessment can progress along the lines of attempting to ascertain whether the symptoms represent an anxiety disorder, per se, or the response to life stressors. Treatment would proceed accordingly. However, assessment of anxiety among older adults represents a challenging endeavor because of the limited amount of data available for this population (Hersen, Van Hasselt, & Goreczny, 1993).

As is the case with anxiety, depressive symptoms in older adults may be due to stressors or to some other factor. Some investigators have posited a stress-diathesis model to account for depression among older adults and to emphasize the importance of taking into account the complex interaction of biological, social, and psychological factors (e.g., Carpenter et al., 1995; Rossen & Buschmann,

1995). This type of model addresses the potential role of both environmental and neurobiological variables in the etiological conceptualization of depression. Recent research has been largely consistent with this postulation. For example, one recent study revealed that mild depressive symptomatology in older adults may be due to stressors but that major depressive disorders are likely to be exacerbations of a long-term vulnerability to mood disturbances (Beekman, Deeg, van Tilburg, Smit, Hooijer, & van Tilburg, 1995). Thus, older clients with major depressive symptoms are likely to have suffered from depressive symptoms previously in their lives and new-onset depressive symptoms among patients who previously suffered from depression thus represent a pattern of mood fluctuations rather than a reaction to life stressors. It is wise, nonetheless, to conduct a full biopsychosocial assessment of older adults when new depressive symptoms recur, because of the possibility that such depressive symptoms may have resulted from recent psychosocial changes in that client's life or may be due to a new-onset illness or physiologically based disease process (e.g., cancer).

Thus, research on assessment of stress with older adults is largely consistent with the stress literature in general. Older adults tend to utilize a variety of coping strategies and experience reactions to stressors similar to those of younger adults. Similarly, research has revealed that, like younger adults, social support of older adults has an initial positive effect but that increased social support over prolonged periods of time may result in increased psychological difficulties (Krause, 1995a). Older adults appear to suffer from stress-related problems less than do younger adults. Research needs to identify the reasons for this difference. Possible explanations are that (a) older adults have learned which coping mechanisms work best for them and how to best implement those strategies; (b) older adults have learned how to selectively choose which challenges to accept and which challenges to reject, thereby experiencing fewer but more rewarding stress challenges than those of younger adults; (c) older adults, relative to their younger cohorts, have fewer stressors imposed upon them (e.g., less concern about children, more stable interpersonal relations); or (d) younger adults who coped with stress poorly died as a consequence of stress-related disease processes. In contrast to the self-report data, recent psychophysiological data indicate that older adults respond to stressors more strongly than do younger adults (Goreczny, Keen, & Walter, 1997). In conclusion, there is much research needed to identify the process of stress interpretation across the life span and to determine why older adults appear to report less stress and anxiety but evidence greater psychophysiological reactivity to stressors than do younger adults. Such information may help all age cohorts.

There is very little research on stress management or treatment of older adults. However, one recent and very promising study revealed that stress inoculation training tends to have positive short- and long-term effects on measures of cognitive functioning (Hayslip, Maloy, & Kohl, 1995). Additional research is necessary to verify these data. Also, although there is a fair amount of research on the stress of caring for older adults, including those with dementia or other problem areas; this remains an important area for additional research because of the aging population. Contributing to this is the fact that older adults with ill parents will likely experience more stress than younger adults with ill parents because of the need of the older adults to deal with their own physical problems. On the other hand, younger adults may have their families to raise, feel less financially secure, and have more tentative interpersonal relationships than do older adults. Thus, future research will need to address the many issues of caregiver stress that remain unknown.

HEALTH PROFMOTION AND HEALTH MAINTENANCE

Although there has been an increase of interest in helping older adults who are already suffering some type of physical malady, very few studies have investigated the effects of health promotion services to older adults. This is despite the fact that several studies have revealed significant relationships between age and health protective behaviors (e.g., Jones, Greaves, & Iliffe, 1992) and that there is a clear relationship between age and manifestation of disease (Brackstone, Delehunty, Mann, & Pain, 1995). Most important for health psychology is that specific lifestyle factors associated with survival differ based on age (Davis, Neuhaus, Moritz, Lein, Barclay, & Murphy, 1994).

A study by Ma and Chi (1995) evaluated health promotion services for older adults. The authors invited clients to participate in a health counseling service; as part of this service, clients attended small group meetings and individual counseling sessions. Group sessions were available for a variety of conditions, including hypertension, diabetes, obesity, and hypercholesteremia. Clients learned to take some control of their health by first monitoring and recording health-associated variables.

Unfortunately, as indicated previously, the literature contains very few recent references to health promotion efforts aimed at older adults. In the next few sections, we briefly review some of the relevant issues related to obesity, eating disorders, Type A behavior, and smoking. Of these, only smoking has any significant recent literature that pertains to older adults.

Obesity

A recent literature search revealed no studies that have evaluated obesity treatment programs specifically with older adults. This is surprising in light of recent data that indicate obesity is one of the risk factors for disability among older ambulatory women (Ensrud *et al.,* 1994). Other factors associated with disability in this cohort of women included physical inactivity, smoking, and alcohol abuse. Of particular note, the study examined only non-Black women; thus, the generalizability of these findings to the African American population remains unknown. Lack of data on obesity among older adults is especially surprising given that several studies have linked development of obesity to menopause in women (Abraham, Llewellyn-Jones, & Perz, 1994; Huerta, Mena, Malacara, & Diaz-de-Leon, 1995) and that obesity is one of the primary factors related to lipid levels in postmenopausal women (Laws, King, Haskell, & Reaven, 1993). These data indicate a need to address the issue of obesity in older adults.

Eating Disorders

Although incidence of eating disorders is likely to be very low among older adults, there have been some reported cases. In one case, Riemann, McNally, and Meier (1993) reported on the case of a 72-year-old man who had a 20-year history of an apparent eating disorder. Symptoms included chronic fears of becoming overweight, distorted body image, and very low weight (95 pounds). The authors had administered a battery of questionnaires to the patient, and his scores on these questionnaires were consistent with scores obtained from patients who have confirmed diagnoses of anorexia nervosa.

There have been several such cases in the recent literature (Fenley, Powers, Miller, & Rowland, 1990; Gowers & Crisp, 1990; Hall & Driscoll, 1993; Morley, 1993), and a question of whether eating disorders among older adults deserves recognition as a distinct diagnostic entity has arisen (Lee, 1992; Russell & Gilbert, 1992). This view is supported by some research that has implicated brain metabolism in the pathogenesis of anorexia among older adults (Martinez, Arnalich, Vazquez, & Hernanz, 1993). However, a recent literature review of the topic indicated that older adults with eating disorders share most all of the same features as their younger cohorts (Cosford & Arnold, 1992).

Given that there are clearly some cases of eating disorder among the older adult population, studies evaluating incidence of eating disorders in this population are warranted. It is possible that health care professionals overlook presence of eating disorders among older adults because of the presumed low base rates or because they attribute it to a specific disorder frequently found in later life rather than as a distinct problem. Some recent research has indicated that a large number of older adults admit to problems related to self-control of food intake (Miller, Morley, Rubenstein, & Pietroszka, 1991). These and related factors have led some investigators to question whether eating disorders are indeed more prevalent than previously considered (Cosford & Arnold, 1991).

Type A Behavior

Despite the large amount of work on the Type A behavior pattern and the effects of hostility on health, especially cardiac conditions (Smith, 1995), there exists very little work on Type A behavior with older adults. This is especially surprising given that some research has found increased hostility and competitiveness among Type As as they age (Carmelli, Dame, & Swan, 1992). Older adults who report that their middle-age environment was a Type A challenging form of environment are more likely than those who do not report such an environment to have diseases associated with advancing age (Kopac, 1990). Given these facts, it is remarkable that only a limited amount of current work on Type A behavior with older adults is available. The extant studies for the most part continue to support the notion of Type A behavior and hostility as contributing factors to physical problems. For example, in a study by Vitaliano, Russo, and Niaura (1995), Type A behavior and various forms of anger-related problems contributed significant variance to measures of triglycerides and both high- and low-density lipoproteins.

The role of expressed emotion in the physical factors of older adults may prove to be a fruitful avenue for future research. Some research has indicated that older adults tend to be more emotionally expressive than younger adults (Malatesta-Magai, Jonas, Shepard, & Culver, 1992) and tend to respond with greater cardiovascular responses to emotional tasks than to cognitive ones (Vitaliano, Russo, Bailey, Young, & McCann, 1993). Also, future research must focus on the interaction between stress and Type A behavior among older adults. For example, one study revealed that Type A individuals tend to experience more involuntary retirement than do non-Type As (Swan, Dame, & Carmelli, 1991). Given the stress of retirement and generally poorer adjustment to involuntary than voluntary retirement, it would be reasonable to hypothesize that Type As forced to retire would be at greatest risk for physical and psychosocial problems. Surprisingly, there appear to be only minimal physical and psychosocial differences between Type As who retire voluntarily and those who retire involuntarily (Swan *et al.,* 1991). Thus, it is clear that additional research needs to clarify the relationship among Type A behavior, stress, anger, physical problems, and psychosocial difficulties among older adults.

Smoking

Smoking is one of the leading risk factors contributing to death in the United States and Western European countries. Among older adults, it remains a risk factor or complicating factor for 9 of the 14 primary causes of death (Fincham, 1992). However, one paper notes that smoking is a risk factor for premature death among women but not men (Samuelsson, Hagberg, Dehlin, & Lindberg, 1994). Despite this inconsistency, it is clear that smoking remains a significant risk factor for health problems, and that this is the case for older adults as well as for the population in general.

In addition to the well-known risks associated with smoking, such as heart attack and stroke, one recent study (Nelson, Nevitt, Scott, Stone, & Cummings, 1994) revealed that older women smokers, relative to nonsmokers, tend to be weaker and have a number of physical or physiological difficulties; these difficulties, which may also contribute to the weakness, include neuromuscular performance impairment and poor balance. This study is consistent with earlier research studies, which have revealed an association between smoking and disability among older women (Ensrud *et al.,* 1994) and between smoking and measures of lung functioning among older men (Bosse, Sparrow, Garvey, Costa, Weiss, & Rowe, 1980). In addition, smoking is a significant predictor of lipid levels among postmenopausal women (Laws *et al.,* 1993), and increased lipid levels may place one at risk of heart attack. Fincham (1992) also confirmed that smoking affects many organ systems, including the respiratory and cerebrovascular systems. Thus, numerous research studies have confirmed a strong association between smoking and various physiological parameters.

In addition to direct physiological consequences associated with smoking, smoking may also affect health and health quality indirectly. For example, among older adults, smoking relates to an increased need for and use of medication as well as impaired quality of life (Jensen, Dehlin, Hagberg, Samuelsson, & Svenson, 1994). Smoking also relates to other health risk behaviors, such as lowered probability of adhering to health care providers' requests to have a mammogram (Taplin, Anderman, Grothaus, Curry, & Montano, 1994) and an increased likelihood of severe drinking problems (Nakamura, Molgaard, Stanford, Peddecord, Morton, Lockery, Zuniga, & Gardner, 1990). In one study that evaluated smoking behavior in a long-term care facility, the authors concluded that nearly 20% of smoking interactions involved behaviors that put people at risk (Barker, Mitteness, & Wolfsen, 1994). Foster (1992) found that among older African Americans there is an inverse relationship between number of cigarettes smoked and health promoting behaviors. Also, though the implications are unclear, a recent study revealed an association between smoking status and specific food and food supplement intake (Itoh & Suyama, 1995). Japanese smokers tended to have a lower intake of plant foods than did nonsmokers (Suyama & Itoh, 1992). Other studies have also shown that smoking status is a predictor of specific nutrient intake (Zipp & Holcomb, 1992) Finally, smokers tend to evidence more depression symptomatology than do nonsmokers (Colsher, Wallace, Pomrehn, La Croix, Coroni–Huntley, Blazer, Scherr, Berkman, & Hennekens, 1990; Salive & Blazer, 1993) and smoking is a risk factor for future development of depression among older adults (Green, Copeland, Dewey, Sharma, Saunders, Davidson, Sullivan, & McWilliam, 1992).

The studies just cited make implications of smoking among older adults quite clear. One important question to address is the rate of smoking among older adults versus that of younger adults. The literature suggests that older adults tend to be less likely to smoke than younger adults (Maxwell & Kirdes, 1993). Consistent with this, a recent study revealed that among Chinese men aged 15 to 65, rates of smoking reached a peak among the group of men in the 36–45 age range and then began to decline (Wei, Young, Lingiang, Shuiyuan, Jian, Hanshu, Zhunghong, Xiouying, & Xudong, 1995). Unfortunately, the authors did not evaluate rates of smoking beyond age 65. Though these data provide some good news regarding smoking among older adults, not all information is positive. For example, although physicians have a lower rate of smoking than the general population, older physicians are more likely than younger physicians to be current or former smokers (Hensrud & Sprafka, 1993). In addition, among older adults who smoke, there is a high rate of nicotine addiction (Orleans *et al.,* 1991). Also, in Orleans and colleagues' study, older adults reported a variety of concerns as barriers to quit attempts; these concerns centered around loss of pleasure associated with cigarette smoking, likelihood of cigarette cravings, and increased nervousness or irritability. As with younger adults, prior and recent attempts at quitting related to quit contemplations.

Thus, these studies indicate that there is a significant need to investigate factors related to smoking cessation among older adults. The literature contains many examples of studies that have addressed smoking cessation attempts and factors related to these attempts specifically among older adults. For example, a recent study of older rural adults receiving Medicare benefits provided several interesting and informative conclusions (Lave, Ives, Traven, & Kuller, 1995). Most interesting is that the study revealed that rural, older adults will take advantage of opportunities to participate in health promotion activities and that the likelihood of doing so increases if they receive encouragement to do so by their physicians. This study also revealed that there is a positive relationship between participation in health prevention services and education level. A second study indicated findings similar to those of Lave and colleagues. In this second study, older adults who received only minimal preventive health care showed a higher rate of smoking cessation as compared with a control group who received nothing other than usual care. However, this difference in quit rates was not statistically significant (Burton, Paglia, German, Shapiro, & Damiano, 1995). Notably, Fincham (1992) indicated that many treatments used by the general population also tend to have positive effects among older adults. Thus, smoking cessation attempts must remain a priority for older adults as well as for younger adults.

Recent research has attempted to determine whether age is a factor associated with quit attempts and successes. For example, one group of authors found that among patients hospitalized for nonterminal and nonpregnancy reasons older smokers were more likely than younger smokers to quit smoking and remain free from smoking upon follow-up (Glasgow, Stevens, Vogt, & Mullooly, 1991). Consistent with this study is a large telephone survey (13,031 subjects), in which Pierce, Giovino, Hatzindreu, and Shopland (1989) found that older smokers (> 65 years of age) were more likely than younger adult smokers to attempt to quit and remain abstinent. Interestingly and somewhat inconsistently, younger women appear more willing to make smoking cessation attempts than do older women. In large-scale population-based surveys, it is clear that most older men are former or current smokers while most older women never smoked (Colsher *et al.*, 1990). Among older adults with smoking histories, men are more likely than women to have quit (Colsher *et al.*, 1990). Finally, a study by Lichtenstein and Hollis (1992) found that older smokers who smoked a relatively large amount were more likely than other patients seen by their primary care provider to attend a group smoking cessation program. Thus, it is clear that age and sex do play a role in smoking cessation attempts. In general, most research shows that older smokers are more likely than younger smokers to attempt to quit and that men are more likely to have been smokers than older women. This latter finding is probably due to prevailing societal norms 40 to 50 years ago, when these subjects would likely have begun smoking.

The relationship of age to smoking cessation attempts is quite interesting. Part of the reason for younger adult smokers to make fewer attempts to quit and have less success than older smokers is that younger smokers tend to have a greater denial of average risk of developing a smoking-related disease than do older smokers (Lee, 1989). This helps explain why African American older adults with cardiovascular disease tend to report behavior modification attempts related to stopping smoking (Hamm, Bazargan, & Barbre, 1993). When faced with occurrence of a smoking-related disorder, it is hard for denial to remain intact. With denial broken down, patients must face the likelihood that their smoking may be harmful. Another interesting finding, however, is that the factors (e.g., education level) that predict smoking cessation at various stages of change differ depending upon the age of participants (Kviz, Clark, Crittenden, Warneeke, & Freels, 1995). The implication of this is that producing successful smoking cessation programs may require inclusion of different components based not just on stage of change but also on participants' ages. Several studies have provided support for this notion by showing that motivation for smoking differs between younger and older adult smokers (Oei, Tilley, & Gow, 1991; Zaimov, Fertcheva, & Vanev, 1994). Similarly, reasons for participating in a smoking cessation program differ between older and younger adults (O'Hara & Portser, 1994). Older adults who receive self-help materials tailored specifically to them rate those materials relatively high, and the use of these materials may enhance quit rates (Rimer, Orleans, Fleisher, & Cristinzio, 1994). Unlike their younger counterparts, older men who quit smoking tend to lose weight whereas younger men who quit smoking tend to gain weight (Bosse, Garvey, & Costa, 1980).

A recent study revealed that people who successfully quit smoking tend to learn about self-help programs at work (Lefebvre, Cobb, Goreczny, & Carleton, 1990). One of the possible reasons for the success of workplace programs is that workers may find support systems to aid in their attempts. Because most older adults are obviously more likely to have retired from work than are younger adults, older adults may have to seek out support systems not in place at the worksite. Also problematic is that among smokers joining a community-wide contest to quit smoking, contestants are likely to be younger rather than older (Cummings, Kelly, Sciandra, & De Loughry, 1990). However, older adults who enlist the assistance of a buddy to provide support in their attempt to quit tend to be twice as likely to quit as do those patients who do not enlist this type of support (Kviz, Crittenden, Clark, & Madura, 1994). Thus, these studies suggest that in order for older adults to obtain the support they need to begin and maintain a smoking cessation program, future clinical research efforts will need to address ways of building in social support mechanisms that will encourage smoking cessation among older adults.

It is also clear that psychological factors play a role in smoking behavior among older adults. For instance, there is an inverse relationship between self-efficacy and health risk among older adults (Grembowski, Patrick, Diehr, Durham, Beresford, Kay, & Hecht, 1993). In particular, high self-efficacy among older adults, relative to low self-efficacy among this population, relates to a greater likelihood of contemplating quitting smoking (Orleans *et al.*, 1991). Also, older women with high depressive symptomatology are nearly four times as likely as older women without depression to quit smoking (Salive & Blazer, 1993). These studies indicate a need to examine how psychological factors and disorders influence smoking behavior among older adults.

Other Areas

One area within the broad area of health promotion that has not received sufficient attention in the literature is behavioral treatment of hypertension in older adults. In a national survey, Tuthill (1989) found that age was the primary variable related to development of hypertension, with social variables showing no or only weak relationships to hypertension. Tuthill concluded that social stress may have little effect on development of hypertension. This conclusion is inconsistent with much of the literature (Pickering, 1995). Thus, research must focus on identifying factors that may be contributing to the inconsistent results and on evaluating the use of behavioral treatments (e.g., relaxation, biofeedback) with older adults who have hypertension. These treatments may be effective for newly diagnosed cases but ineffective for patients in whom long histories of hypertension have led to permanent physiological changes or damage resulting from long-term high pressures on the arteries.

Another area that may prove promising is the area of health risk assessment among older adults. Of particular interest is the recent development of the Seniors' Life-style Inventory (Schwirian, 1991–1992). The scale consists of 26 items that measure health behaviors, and initial reliability data appear satisfactory. However, additional research on the reliability and validity of this instrument is necessary before its utility is certain.

HIV/AIDS

There has been little focus on HIV infection among older adults because of the perception that AIDS is a disease of younger adults. One presumption is that older adults are less sexually active than younger adults and they, therefore, have less risk of contracting HIV. Recent data from a national survey of 2,058 adults suggest that older adults do indeed tend to be less sexually active than their younger cohorts (Leigh, Temple, & Trocki, 1993). However, data also indicate that approximately 10% of patients diagnosed with AIDS are 50 years of age or older (Gutheil & Chichin, 1991). Some investigators have actually argued that older adults may be at equal or increased risk, relative to their younger cohorts, for contracting HIV infection (e.g., Whipple & Scura, 1989). Such a view argues for specific attention to focus on HIV among older adults. One reason to do this is that age serves as a predictor of progression of the infection and survival among patients undergoing zidovudine therapy (Vella, Giuliano, Floridia, Chiesi, Tomino, Speber, Bacherini, Bucciardini, & Mariotti, 1995). Linsk (1994) also discusses the importance of screening HIV serostatus of older adults. The rationale for such use is the increasing number of older adults who have developed HIV infections. Linsk also addresses several other issues in relation to this matter that are typical for HIV infection in the general population. These issues include pretest and posttest counseling, prevention and treatment issues, and the importance of family support. Therefore, it is indeed important to assess HIV infection among older adults as well as to assess the effect of age on treatment outcomes.

Because of a recognition of the importance of addressing HIV and AIDS among older adults, several groups of investigators have noted how essential it is that we begin developing policies and prevention strategies aimed specifically at this population (Adamchak, Wilson, Nyanguru, & Hampson, 1991; Benjamin, 1988; Talashek, Tichy, & Epping, 1990). Lloyd (1989) raised the concern that, with research monies becoming increasingly difficult to obtain, older adults and younger patients with HIV infection may compete for research monies and other resources. Lloyd argued that older adults, having grown up in conservative times, may have difficulty being sympathetic to those affected by AIDS, whereas younger adults (those typically affected by AIDS) are likely to view older adults with less respect than they view those from their own age group. This sets the stage for a possible competition for resources between two groups that are both in need of increased clinical and research priorities. However, this is not consistent with data indicating that older adults may, in fact, be more sensitive to issues surrounding AIDS than are younger adults (B. E. Robinson, Walters, & Skeen, 1989).

Independent of the funding issues just discussed, one important component of research with HIV is the assessment of risk behaviors. One aspect of addressing HIV risk requires that patients answer questions about their sexual behavior and other potential risk factors. Despite some concerns that older adults might be less open to questions about sexual behavior than are younger adults, a recent study refuted this concern (Wiederman, Weis, & Allgeier, 1994). However, there is only one recent study that has addressed identification of risk factors associated with HIV infection specifically among older adults. This study focused on drinking behavior. Results indicated that heavy drinkers of all ages are more likely than nonheavy drinkers to report engaging in high-risk sexual behaviors, and regardless of drinking behavior, younger subjects are more likely than older subjects to engage in high-risk sexual behaviors (Shillington, Cottler, Compton, & Spitznagel, 1995). Thus, this study adds evidence that younger adults are more likely than older adults to engage in behaviors that risk contracting HIV. However, it is still important to identify those older adults who place themselves at risk and to attempt to intervene so as to decrease their chances of contracting HIV. Part of the problem is that younger adults appear to have more knowledge than do older adults regarding AIDS preventive measures (Dekker & Mootz, 1992). However, older adults appear more likely than younger adults to change their lifestyles with regard to sexual behavior (Vincke, Mak, Bolton, & Jurica, 1993). Thus, intervention to reduce risk of infection may be more successful with older adults than it has been with younger adults but this intervention requires education to help older adults learn about preventive measures.

Beside the usual problems associated with HIV infection, age brings an additional factor that highlights the need to work with older adults who have contracted HIV. A recent study (Piette, Wachtel, Mor, & Mayer, 1995) revealed that older adults with HIV score lower than younger adults with HIV on a variety of quality of life domains, including health perception, mental health, and several functioning domains (i.e., physical function, role function, and social function). After controlling for CD4 lymphocyte count, all variables except role function and mental health remained statistically significant. Surprisingly, older subjects reported feeling less pain than did the younger subjects in the study. Also, somewhat inconsistent with results from Piette and colleagues's study, are data that indicate that older age relates to lower levels of depression (Vincke & Bolton, 1994). Whether this is a real effect or an effect based on difficulties measuring depression among older adults remains unknown.

An important issue related to HIV infection among older adults is the development of cognitive difficulties. Younger adults with HIV encephalopathy and older adults without diagnosed neurological disease have similar patterns of results on neuropsychological tests. There are several studies that have highlighted the effect of age on cognitive functioning of individuals infected with HIV. One of these (Van Gorp, Miller, Marcotte, Dixon, Paz, Selnes, Wesch, Becker, Hinkin, & Mitrushina, 1994) primarily evaluated measures of reaction time along with some other timed neuropsychological tests. A recent study compared performance of individuals with various types of dementias on neuropsychological test performance and found that subjects who were in the early stages of AIDS dementia primarily evidenced difficulties in the areas of storage and retrieval, a pattern of results that is consistent with the pattern of test results typical for older adults who are aging without significant neurological impairment (Mitrushina *et al.*, 1994). These data and those of Hinkin et al. (1990), Kernutt, Price, Judd, & Burrows, (1993), and Van Gorp, Wilifred,

Mitrushina, Cummings, & Satz (1989) are consistent with AIDS dementia as representing a subcortical dementia. This is an important issue because assessment of AIDS among older adults may be difficult due to similarity of many of the symptoms with those symptoms associated with dementia and other disorders of later life (Rosenzweig & Fillit, 1992; Scura & Whipple, 1990). Patients with AIDS or who are HIV positive may simply be exhibiting the neurological signs associated with the disorder, and bias among health care professionals may limit the ability of these professionals to consider HIV infection among older adults. Fortunately, emergence of single photon emission tomography (SPET) technology has the potential to significantly improve the assessment and diagnosis of AIDS dementia (Beats, Burns, & Levy, 1991).

ISSUES OF PRIMARY RELEVANCE
TO OLDER ADULTS

Tremors

Tremors represent a problem primarily associated with older age and with disorders that develop with advancing age. One study (Moghal, Rajput, Meleth, D'Arcy, & Rajput, 1995) revealed that nearly 20% of institutionalized elderly suffer from some form of tremor (i.e., essential tremor, Parkinson's disease, drug-induced Parkinsonism), and Marti-Masso and Poza (1992) conducted an epidemiological study that revealed that nearly 7% of the population older than 65 has some form of tremor-type disorder. Another recent study (Jeste, Caligiuri, Paulsen, Heaton, Lacro, Harris, Bailey, Fell, & McAdams, 1995) revealed that in a sample of 266 patients receiving treatment with neuroleptics, incidence of those suffering from tardive dyskinesia doubled in just 3 years. Finally, another study revealed significant psychosocial effects associated with essential tremor and physical and psychosocial effects associated with Parkinsonism (Busenbark, Nash, Nash, Hobble, & Keller, 1991). Thus, tremors are relatively common among older adults and, when present, may result in significant physical and psychosocial difficulties.

In an effort to help ameliorate tremors, some investigators have developed treatment programs based on behavioral medicine applications. One group of investigators has incorporated relaxation training and coping skills training into a biobehavioral rehabilitation treatment program for tremors (Chung, Poppen, & Lundervold, 1995; Lundervold & Poppen, 1995). As part of the program, subjects also undergo a medical and neurologic assessment as well as a functional analysis of behavior. In addition to relaxation and coping skills training, participants receive education regarding neuromuscular functioning. In one of the studies (Chung et al, 1995) the investigators reported results for two older men (ages 63 and 86), with outcome measures including tremor severity ratings (both clinical and self-rated), ratings from informants, and forearm EMG. Results indicated improvements on all of these measures. Given that the most common tremors occur in the arms and hands (Zimmerman, Deuschl, Hornig, Schulze-Mouting, Fuchs, & Lucking, 1994), it make sense to utilize a measure of arm muscle tension (i.e., forearm EMG). In another examination of treatment for tremors, results from a case study of a 76-year-old man who treated his Parkinsonian tremors with self-hypnosis revealed that this technique may have some potential (Wain, Amen, & Jabbari, 1990).

Despite the early success and hopeful findings from these two studies, significant work remains before we can recognize behavioral medicine interventions as effective in the treatment of tremors. Some issues for future investigation include replication of the studies and use of appropriate control groups. The issue of psychogenic tremors (Koller, Lang, Vetere-Overfield, Cleeves, Factor, Singe, & Weiner, 1989) also remains an area for future investigation. Finally, there is the question of how these types of treatment programs compare with medication and how a combined protocol might work.

Falls

Falls are a major problem among older adults. With the older adult population growing rapidly in the United States, this is likely to become an area of ever greater importance. This is especially true because the old-old group (over 80 years of age) is among the fastest growing segments of the population, and balance problems are one of the main factors that distinguishes the old-old group from those in the younger (65 to 75) age range (Kaye, Oken, Howieson, Howieson, Holm, & Dennison, 1994).

A thorough review of the literature on falls among older adults is not possible. Interested readers may wish to refer to an excellent article by Steinmetz and Hobson (1994), which details issues related to falls among older adults living in the community. Some of the research conducted on balance and falls has attempted to ascertain what defect is responsible for the problem. Some recent information suggests that falls among older adults may be due to decreased sensitivity of tactile information from the toes (Tanaka, Hashimoto, Noriyasu, Ino, Itokube, & Mizumoto, 1995). This is consistent with much of the other evidence that points to the importance of involvement of the kinesthetic system and necessity of proprioceptive information in balance among older adults (Bergin, Bronstein, Murray, Sancoric, & Zeppenfeld, 1995; Elliot, Patta, Flanagan, Spaulding, Rietdyk, Strong, & Brown, 1995).

Another important etiological factor in falls among older adults involves pharmacologic treatments (Monfort, 1995). This is especially problematic among older adults because health care professionals may fail to recognize falls as a side effect of medication but may instead interpret falls as additional evidence of declining mobility. Several medications may produce falls as a side effect. Of significance to mental health professionals is a recent study by Liu, Topper, Reeves, Gryfe, & Maki (1995), which revealed that use of antidepressant medications has predictive value in determining who falls. Other medications implicated in producing falls as one side effect among older adults include clozapine (Pitner, Mintzner, Pennypacker, & Jackson, 1995), clomipramine (Leo & Kim, 1995), and benzodiazepines (Cooper, 1994). The study by Cooper also revealed that longer-acting benzodiazepines produce more falls among older adults than do shorter-acting benzodiazepines.

Attempts have also proceeded to identify other risk factors associated with falls. One recent study (Tinetti, Doucette, Claus, & Marottoli, 1995) identified several factors associated with what the authors defined as serious fall injuries;

the risk factors identified in this study included cognitive impairment, female gender, and low body mass index. Balance and gait disturbances, as one would expect, were also significant risk factors. Another study identified age, psychoactive drug use, and number of illnesses as primary predictors of falls among older adults (Sheahan, Coons, Robbins, Martin, Hendricks, & Latimer, 1995). However, in Sheahan and colleagues' study, frequency of alcohol use and living alone did not serve as good predictors of falls. In addition, unlike Tinetti and colleagues' study, gender had no predictive value. Other research (Nelson *et al.*, 1994) has implicated smoking as another predictor of poor balance.

An interesting study by Salgado, Lord, Packer, and Ehrlich (1994) attempted to identify predictors to classify fallers from nonfallers among older hospitalized adults. These authors obtained impressive results, correctly classifying 80% of their subjects. Variables that contributed to this classification included impaired orientation, psychoactive medication use, evidence of prior cerebrovascular accident, and poor scores on a test called the get-up-and-go test.

From these studies, it is clear that many studies have identified cognitive impairment as a significant predictor of falls among older adults; some of the studies identify inability to avoid obstacles that are in the intended path as one of the significant problems. With regard to this latter concern, one recent study (Persad, Giordani, Chen, Aston-Milles, Alexander, Wilson, Berent, Guire, & Schultz, 1995) attempted to assess neuropsychological variables associated with deficits in avoidance ability. This study revealed that measures of memory and visuo-spatial discrimination were not helpful in predicting avoidance deficits among older adults. Measures that did predict avoidance difficulties involved problem-solving abilities, general anxiety, assessment of response inhibition, and evaluation of sustained attention.

Given the large amount of data that implicates cognitive impairment in falls, one would suspect that patients who suffer from neurological disorders are likely to have difficulties with falling. Recent research shows this to be true for both patient's with Alzheimer's disease and patients who have suffered from cerebrovascular accidents. A recent study by Alexander, Mollo, Giordani, Ashton-Miller, Schultz, Grunawalt, & Foster, (1995) indicated that the problem with falling among Alzheimer's patients is likely due to balance difficulties in new situations and in situations where obstacles are blocking their intended paths. Interestingly, in this study, patients with Alzheimer's were able to maintain balance in situations that were essentially similar, but they walked significantly more slowly than one might consider normal. As for falls related to cerebrovascular accidents, it appears to depend upon the site of the cerebrovascular accident. For example, patients with hemispatial deficits, as measured by the Complex Figure Test or Letter Cancellation Test, may evidence some difficulties falling (Rapport, Dutra, Webster, & Charter, 1995).

One of the main problems associated with falling is, of course, the potential for harm. Another problem is that approximately 25% of patients who experience a fall sufficient for admission to a hospital indicate a fear of falling again (Liddle & Gilleard, 1995). This fear may lead to decreased walking and subsequently decreased independence, as they restrict their activities in an unnecessary preventative effort. However, the Liddles and Gilleard study indicated that the fear of falling appears to have little or no effect on outcome of patients' rehabilitation efforts. Recurrent falls, nonetheless, do affect life satisfaction (Ho *et al.*, 1995), and even one fall can affect patients' confidence in their ability to arise from a fall. This is an important factor because such confidence relates to patients' willingness to learn how to arise from falls (Simpson & Mandelstam, 1995). One factor that appears related to fear of falling among older adults is dizziness (Burker, Wong, Sloane, Mattingly, Preister, & Mitchell, 1995).

Clinical investigators have attempted to devise programs to help people who fall and to help prevent falls. Treatment programs aimed at increasing mobility have yielded positive results. One recent study showed that a low-intensity 6-week exercise program was successful in decreasing amount of time and number of steps the older adults in this study used to traverse a measured course, and that patients who continued to participate in regular exercise were able to maintain their gains at an 18-week follow-up (Hickey, Wolf, Robins, & Wagner, 1995). In addition, as is consistent with similar literature, the exercise program led to improved optimism as measured at the 18-week follow-up. In another recent study, Lord, Ward, Williams, and Strudwick (1995) evaluated efficacy of a 12-month program of twice weekly, hour-long exercise sessions on a variety of measures. Results from this study indicated that subjects who participated in the exercise program evidenced improved neuromuscular control, increased lower limb muscle strength, and decreased reaction time. A control group that did not participate in the exercise program did not evidence these changes. The main problem with this type of study is that adherence to exercise programs over a 12-month period of time is generally quite low.

In an effort to address this issue, one set of investigators utilized a videotaped modeling paradigm to improve exercise performance among five women aged 56 to 70, who also suffered from mental retardation (Neef, Bill-Harvey, Shade, Iezzi, & DeLorenzo, 1995). Subjects would utilize the videotape to guide performance of the exercises, thereby enabling the subjects to perform exercises independently. Results from this study indicated high levels of independent exercise with noted improvements in balance. Also of importance, however, is that several studies have noted the importance of continued social activity and support as well as continued physical activity in the prevention of falls among older adults (Cwikel, Fried, Galinsky, & Ring, 1995; Seeman, Berkman, Charpeutier, Blazer, Albert, & Tinetti, 1995).

Adherence

Because older adults are more likely than younger adults to develop many chronic conditions that require long-term treatment, there is a definite need to develop methods that will improve adherence among older adults. The treatment regimen of older adults is likely to be more complicated than that of younger adults because older adults are likely to have more medications prescribed than younger adults. When patients have multiple medications to take along with finite resources (e.g., money) to obtain the prescriptions, nonadherance is likely to occur. Nonadherence to medication treatment can occur in many forms, including decreasing frequency of prescribed dosage to make a prescription last longer than intended by the physician or failing to get prescriptions filled or refilled. However, even when resources are scarce, patients often find ways to obtain prescribed medications, such as via borrowed money, pharmacy credit, and physician samples (Chubon, Schulz, Lingler, & Foster-Schulz, 1994). Unfortunately, older adults inappropriately discontinue prescription use for as many as 40% of prescribing situations (Salzman, 1995). One major problem with this is that such a discontinuation may itself lead to complications and even death. In addition to decreased use or none use of medication, nonadherence includes overuse and abuse, as well as medication other than for the intended use, or by a person other than the one for whom the physician prescribed the medication.

Unfortunately, as with younger adults, education alone as to importance of adhering to treatments and avoiding risks does not typically change older adults' behaviors (El-Faizy & Reinsch, 1994; Herman, Speroff, & Cebul, 1994). As with younger adults, however, physicians do play a significant role in patient adherence among older adults. A recent study by Bula, Afessi, Aronow, Yubas, Gold, Niesenbaum, Beck, & Rubenstein (1995) revealed a correlation between physician cooperation with a Health Promotion Program for older adults and patient adherence to recommendations from the program. This is consistent with data that show that among older adults, authoritarian beliefs relate to utilization of health care services (Ditto, Moore, Hilton, & Kalish, 1995). Thus, one way to improve adherence may involve improving physician–patient communications (Salzman, 1995). Weinberger, Samsa, Schmader, & Greenberg (1994) found that in an outpatient geriatric sample with substantial limitations in the areas of activities of daily living, patients adhered to only 67% of the recommendations made. Number of recommendations made was 5.9 per patient, which may represent part of the problem. Patients may have felt overwhelmed by number of issues to address and may therefore have attended only to the most salient recommendations. Interestingly, the authors noted that patient adherence to medical and social recommendations was similar, and no predictors of adherence were found. Consistent with results from this study are those from a study by Chubon and colleagues (1994), in which the researchers interviewed subjects on Medicaid who had more than the three prescriptions per month that needed to be filled. These authors found that patients made their choices based primarily on three factors: (1) what they believed to be the most important medications or the seriousness of the problem for which they had the prescription, (2) symptoms that were present at the time, and (3) cost of the medication. Thus, both the Weinberger and colleagues (1994) and Chubon and colleagues (1994) studies indicate that older patients often make decisions about their own care after having received recommendations from their physicians. The decisions they make may not be in their best interest, and one wonders whether these patients ever inform their health care provider of such decisions.

Provision of health care services may improve if physicians and other health care providers take additional time to understand their patients' circumstances and aid in the decision-making process. Patients who disagree with treatment recommendations are unlikely to adhere to those recommendations (Devor, Wang, Renvall, Feigal, & Ramsdell, 1994). Unfortunately, the current health care climate makes longer time for appointments with physicians unlikely at present (Goreczny & O'Halloran, 1995).

Salzman (1995) did note, however, that in addition to improving physician–patient communication, another method of improving medication adherence among older adults is to simplify drug treatment regimens, especially complex regimens that include multiple medications. In such cases, involving pharmacists as consultants may increase patients' knowledge about their medications and also increase adherence. Lipton and Bird (1994) found that this was indeed the case in their sample of 706 hospitalized older adults. The investigators also noted that consultation with pharmacists resulted in patients' being able to take fewer medications and be on less complex regimens than a sample of control patients.

An obvious but often forgotten concern is to take into account patients' medical problems as a possible reason for nonadherence. A study by Nussbaum, Allender, and Copeland (1995) found that adults with compromised cardiovascular functioning evidenced significant difficulties learning verbal material. Thus, the well-documented increase in cardiovascular problems associated with aging increases likelihood that older adults will have problems understanding and remembering medication instructions. This seems especially likely for adults with medical difficulties that might further compromise the cardiovascular system, and these would be the patients most in need of the ability to learn and remember complex medication regimens. A recent study by Fitten, Coleman, Siembieda, Yu, & Ganzell (1995) confirms that older adults with medical problems have difficulties learning or remembering medication regimens. Consistent with this is a study by Ensrud and colleagues (1994) that evaluated cognitive functioning of older, non-Black women and found that deterioration in cognitive functioning appears related to several medical conditions.

A recent study compared various methods of improving memory for medication schedules among older adults (D. G. Morrow, Leirer, & Andrassy, 1996). In this study, the authors asserted that use of a timeline icon may prove helpful but would require training. Older adults in this study were better able to understand and remember schedules provided to them via text than via icons. Another study investigating improvement of medication adherence among older adults found that older adults prefer lists of medications as compared to paragraph instructions (D. Morrow, Leirer, & Altieri, 1995). Patients expressed preference for a categorized list but were better able to recall information from a simple listing than from a categorized listing.

Treatment adherence applies not only to medication but also to other therapeutic regimens, and adherence to treatments varies based on type of recommendation made. For example, Devor and colleagues (1994) noted that older adult outpatients were most likely to adhere to recommendations regarding prior health directives (81% adherence), but least likely to comply with recommendations to make changes in living situations (37%); surprisingly, only 57.5% of patients adhered to recommendations to wear a medic alert bracelet. Also, when patients have choices between two different procedures to correct for the same problem, age differences often influence that choice (Liddell, Pollett, & MacKenzie, 1995).

A patient factor that health care providers must consider when working with older adults is onset of dementia. At the beginning of a dementia, signs of cognitive difficulties may be subtle and unrecognizable by the patient, family members, and even health care providers. Poor insight into presence of such difficulties and compromised reasoning abilities associated with dementia may decrease adherence (Rees, Bayer, & Phillips, 1995). Depression may also decrease adherence to treatment protocols (Carney, Freedland, Eisen, Rich, & Jaffe, 1995). Because depression rates are likely to increase over the years, it is especially important to develop mechanisms to improve adherence to depression treatments. For example, Reynolds, Frank, Perel, Mazumdar, & Kupfer (1995) note that a major challenge for treating depression among older adults includes compliance with recommendations. In addition, Schneider and Olin (1995) found that arranging for a regular evaluation of the client's compliance with recommendations is one necessary component in effectively treating depression in older adults. Fortunately, when primary care physicians suggest use of cognitive-behavioral techniques to patients suffering from depression, likelihood of adhering to use of those techniques increased. However, physicians tend to suggest use of cognitive-behavioral techniques to older adults less than they do to younger adults (P. Robinson, Bush, Von Koroff, Katon, Lin, Simon, & Walker, 1995).

Another patient factor that health care providers must consider involves cultural traditions and expectations (Natow, 1994; Parry, Mobley, & Allen, 1996), in addition to issues of personal preference. For example, Cameron and Quine (1994), in their study of older women who could have benefited from use of external hip protectors, noted that primary reasons for not wearing these devices were discomfort. These older women believed that the device was not necessary because they did not perceive that they had a high-risk condition that would warrant use of the device. The researchers also noted other factors associated with lack of adherence, but these were not as prominent as the two just mentioned. Nonetheless, by identifying patient-perceived impediments to specific treatments, it may be possible to increase adherence to those treatments. Another factor associated with nonadherence may be time of day. Leirer, Tanke, and Morrow (1994) found that adherence tends to be higher in the morning than at midday, with no further decrement beyond midday.

Efforts to increase adherence have extended beyond that of medication regimen. For example, King, Ross, Seag, & Balshem (1995) attempted to increase mammography rates of women who had failed to obtain a mammogram within the year prior to the study. The authors found that telephone counseling about mammography improved adherence rates from 13% for a control group to 27% for the counseling group. In addition to counseling, the authors noted that factors that significantly correlated with adherence to obtaining mammography included prior mammography use, ability to access the mammography equipment or placement easily, and whether or not the person had a friend or relative who had breast cancer. Additionally, the authors noted that specific beliefs about breast cancer and mammography significantly predicted mammography use.

Adherence to exercise programs is essential (Dubert & Stetson, 1995). In addition to playing a significant health promotion role, exercise also serves an important rehabilitative role among patients with chronic obstructive pulmonary disease (Carter & Nicotra, 1996). The factors that contribute to exercise adherence among the elderly may be different from those for younger adults. In an effort to assess factors associated with adherence among older adults, Williams and Lord (1995) evaluated many variables among 102 older women, 69 of whom completed a 12-month exercise trial and 54 of whom continued their participation for at least 6 months after completion of the program. The authors found that there was a difference between the factors that predicted exercise adherence during training and factors associated with continued participation after completion of the training. Muscle strength was a factor in adherence to both measures, but reaction time and psychoactive drug use were significant factors only for adherence during the trial. Conversely, the only factors associated with adherence after completion of the trial included reasoning ability, depression, and a subject's own rating of strength improvement. Thus, physiological factors appear to play a substantial role in short-term adherence, but longer-term adherence also involves presence and degree of depression and self-perceptions of program efficacy in producing desired or expected changes.

Finally, in addition to assessments and interventions occurring at the level of patient interaction, interventions can occur at the multidisciplinary treatment team or organizational level. Although few studies have specifically evaluated such interventions with teams that primarily treat older adults, one study that did so showed that administrative interventions may indeed have an impact on adherence (Wright, Lunt, Harris, & Wallace, 1995). For more information on how to implement administrative interventions, see Corrigan and McCracken (1997).

Other Areas

Another area for investigation is work with older spinal cord injury survivors. Although the number of people who sustain spinal cord injuries resulting in permanent disability is relatively low, technological and medical care advances in the past two decades have substantially decreased morbidity and mortality rates in this group (Heinemann, 1995). Thus, number of spinal cord injury survivors is likely to continue to increase, and combined with the aging population, this suggests that the number of older adults who have a permanent disability due to spinal cord injury will also increase. This is especially important because of research that indicates that age is one factor related to health complications and cognitive difficulties among patients with spinal cord injuries (Herrick, Elliot, & Crow, 1994). Herrick and colleagues also noted that increased age was related to decreased adherence to routine follow-up health care in this population. Although this study included no subjects over the age of 66, the implications for adults over age 66 are clear. It is also clear that there is a need for study of older adults who have suffered from spinal cord injuries.

Health care providers also need to be aware that unexplained symptoms may be indicative of systemic lupus erythematosus. A recent paper (M. Dennis, 1994) indicated that systemic lupus erythematosus (SLE) may actually be more common among older adults than previous research had indicated. In an earlier paper, M. S. Dennis, Byrne, Hopkinson, and Bendall (1992) reported on five patients ranging in ages from 75 to 93 who all presented with symptoms later diagnosed as lupus.

SUMMARY

The current chapter reviewed several areas within the field of health psychology and behavioral medicine as they applied specifically to older adults. Although research in the area of health psychology with older adults has generally, lagged behind other research the last few years have witnessed increased attention to this population. Despite the advances in recent years, much work remains. For instance, there is relatively little work with helping to meet the social needs of older, visually impaired adults (Hersen, Van Hasselt, & Segal, 1995), yet this population is a growing exponentially.

Future studies must begin to examine psychometric properties of instruments administered to older adults. Most of the test instruments developed for clinical use in psychology have only limited data on their applicability to older adults because the standardization and norms do not adequately apply to older adults. Recent studies have attempted to correct this problem (e.g., Hersen, Van Hasselt, & Segal, 1995; Laatsch, 1996), but much work remains in this area.

There exist very few treatment studies on older adults with regard to behavioral medicine interventions. Also, there is still a need to investigate the differential effects of medication on younger and older adults. This is especially true for the old-old population. Medications may have differential effects due to decreasing body functioning, differential rates of adherence, or a variety of other factors (Andersson, Antonsson, Corin, Swahn, & Fridlund, 1995). Additional research into factors affecting adherence is also necessary. For example, too many recommendations from health care providers may result in patients ignoring some of the recommendations and choosing on their own which to implement. Research will also need to further determine the effect of cognitive difficulties on adherence. Research into health beliefs among older adults may also prove to be helpful in improving adherence. The Cognitive Orientation Model (Kreitler & Kreitler, in press) may prove helpful in this regard. In the area of cognitive impairment, some recent studies have begun showing that cognitive retraining for patients with dementias may prove helpful. Programs that seem to have the most benefit, however, are those that have focused on implicit memory skills as opposed to explicit memory skills (Ford, 1996); this presents a potentially very fruitful area of clinical research. Exercise also appears to have some benefit on cognitive functioning (Van Sickle, Hersen, Simco, Melton, & Van Hasselt, 1996).

Thus, the area of older adult health psychology is a burgeoning field. In more ways than other fields, it brings together the full continuum of health care providers, both for prevention and rehabilitation. The range of health problems experienced by older adults and the sheer number of problems they experience along with the growing proportion of this segment of the population makes this a promising arena for future research.

REFERENCES

Abraham, S., Llewellyn-Jones, D., & Perz, J. (1994). Changes in Australian women's perception of the menopause and menopausal symptoms before and after the climacteric. *Maturitas, 20,* 121–128.

Adamchak, D. J., Wilson, A. O., Nyanguru, A., & Hampson, J. (1991). Elderly support and intergenerational transfer in Zimbabwe: An analysis by gender, marital status, and place of residence. *Gerontologist, 31,* 505–513.

Alexander, N. B., Mollo, J. M., Giordani, B., Ashton-Miller, J. A., Schultz, A. B., Grunawalt, J. A., & Foster, N. L. (1995). Maintenance of balance, gait patterns, and obstacle clearance in Alzheimer's disease. *Neurology, 45,* 908–914.

Andersson, E., Antonsson, M., Corin, B., Swahn, B., & Fridlund, B. (1995). The preventive effect of lithium therapy on bipolar disorder patients, with special reference to gender and age. *International Journal of Rehabilitation and Health, 1,* 203–210.

Arbuckle, N. W., & de Vries, B. (1995). The long-term effects of later life spousal and parental bereavement on personal functioning. *Gerontologist, 35*, 637–647.

Barker, J. C., Mitteness, L. S., & Wolfsen, C. R. (1994). Smoking and adulthood: Risky business in a nursing home. *Journal of Aging Studies, 8*, 309–326.

Beats, B., Burns, A., & Levy, R. (1991). Single photon emission tomography in dementia. *International Journal of Geriatric Psychiatry, 6*, 57–62.

Beekman, A. T. F., Deeg, D. J., van Tilburg, T., Smit, J. H., Hooijer, C., & van Tilburg, W. (1995). Major and minor depression in later life: A study of prevalence and risk factors. *Journal of Affective Disorders, 36*, 65–75.

Benjamin, A. E. (1988). Long-term care and AIDS: Perspectives from experience with the elderly. *Milbank Quarterly, 66*, 415–443.

Bergin, P. S., Bronstein, A. M., Murray, N. M., Sancovic, S., & Zeppenfeld, D. K. (1995). Body sway and vibration perception thresholds in normal aging and in patients with polyneuropathy. *Journal of Neurology, Neurosurgery, and Psychiatry, 58*, 335–340.

Bosse, R., Garvey, A. J., & Costa, P. T. (1980). Predictors of weight change following smoking cessation. *International Journal of the Addictions, 15*, 969–991.

Bosse, R., Sparrow, D., Garrey, A. J., Costa, P. T., Jr., Weiss, S. T., & Rowe, J. W. (1980). Cigarette smoking, aging, and decline in pulmonary function: A longitudinal study. *Archives of Environmental Health, 35*, 247–252.

Brackstone, M. J., Delehanty, R., Mann, B., & Pain, K. (1995). The nature and severity of distress among rehabilitation hospital patients. *International Journal of Rehabilitation and Health, 1*, 37–48.

Brantley, P. J., & Thomason, B. T. (1995). Stress and stress management. In A. J. Goreczny (Ed.), *Handbook of health and rehabilitation psychology* (pp. 275–289). New York: Plenum.

Bula, C., Alessi, C. A., Aronow, H. V., Yubas, K., Gold, M., Niesenbaum, R. Beck, J. C., & Rubenstein, L. Z. (1995). Community physicians' cooperation with a program of in-home comprehensive geriatric assessment. *Journal of the American Geriatrics Society, 43*, 1016–1020.

Burker, E. J., Wong, H., Sloane, P. D., Mattingly, D., Preisser, J., & Mitchell, C. M. (1995). Predictors of fear of falling in dizzy and nondizzy elderly. *Psychology and Aging, 10*, 104–110.

Burton, L. C. Paglia. M. J. German, P. S., Shapiro, S., & Damiano, A. M. (1995). The effect among older persons of general preventive visit on three behaviors: Smoking, excessive alcohol drinking, and sedentary lifestyle. The Medicare Preventive Services Research Team. *Preventive Medicine: An International Journal Devoted to Practice and Theory, 24*, 492–497.

Busenbark, K. L., Nash, J., Nash, S., Hubble, J. P., & Koller, W. C. (1991). Is essential tremor benign? *Neurology, 41*, 1982–1983.

Cameron, I. D., & Quine, S. (1994). External hip protectors: Likely non-compliance among high risk elderly people living in the community. *Archives of Gerontology and Geriatrics, 19*, 273–281.

Carmack, C. L., Amaral-Melendez, M., Boudreaux, E., Brantley, P. J., Jones, G. N., Franks, B. D., & McKnight, G. T. (1995). Exercise as a component of the physical and psychological rehabilitation of hemodialysis patients. *Journal of Rehabilitation and Health, 1*, 13–24.

Carmelli, D., Dame, A., & Swan, G. E. (1992). Age-related changes in behavioral components in relation to changes in global Type A behavior. *Journal of Behavioral Medicine, 15*, 143–154.

Carney, R. M., Freedland, K. E., Eisen, S. A., Rich, M. W., & Jaffe, A. S. (1995). Major depression and medication adherence in elderly patients with coronary artery disease. *Health Psychology, 14*, 88–90.

Carpenter, B. D., Strauss, M. E., & Kennedy, J. S. (1995). Personal history of depression and its appearance in Alzheimer's disease. *International Journal of Geriatric Psychiatry, 10*, 669–678.

Carter, R., & Nicotra, B. (1996). The effect of exercise training and rehabilitation on functional status in patients with chronic obstructive pulmonary disease (COPD). *International Journal of Rehabilitation and Health, 2*, 143–167.

Chrischilles, E. A., Lemke, J. H., Wallace, R. B., & Drube, G. A. (1990). Prevalence and characteristics of multiple analgesic drug use in an elderly study group. *Journal of the American Geriatrics Society, 38*, 979–984.

Chubon, S. J., Schulz, R. M., Lingle, E. W., & Coster-Schulz, M. A. (1994). Too many medications, too little money: How do patients cope? *Public Health Nursing, 11*, 412–415.

Chung, W., Poppen, R., & Lundervold, D. A. (1995). Behavioral relaxation training for tremor disorders in older adults. *Biofeedback and Self-Regulation, 20*, 123–135.

Colsher, P. L., Wallace, R. B., Pomrehn, P. R., LaCroix, A. Z., Cornoni-Huntley, J., Blazer, D., Scherr, P. A. Berkman, L., Hennekens, C. (1990). Demographic and health characteristics of elderly smokers: Results from established populations for epidemiolgic studies of the elderly. *American Journal of Preventive Medicine, 6*, 61–70.

Cooper, J. W. (1994). Falls and fractures in nursing home patients receiving psychotropic drugs. *International Journal of Geriactric Psychiatry, 9*, 975–980.

Corrignan, P., & McCracken, S. (1997) Interactive staff training: Rehabilitation teams that work. New York: Plenum.

Cosford, P., & Arnold, E. (1991). Anorexia nervosa in the elderly. *British Journal of Psychiatry, 159*, 296–297.

Cosford, P. A., & Arnold, E. (1992). Eating disorders in later life: A review. *International Journal of Geriatric Psychiatry, 7*, 491–498.

Cummings, K. M., Kelly, J., Sciandra, R., & DeLoughry, T. (1990). Impact of a community-wide stop smoking contest. *American Journal of Health Promotion, 4*, 429–434.

Cwikel, J., Fried, A., Galinsky, D., & Ring, H. (1995). Gait and activity in the elderly: Implications for community falls-prevention and treatment programmes. *Disability and Rehabilitation: An International Multidisciplinary Journal, 17*, 277–280.

Davis, M. A. Neuhaus, J. M., Moritz, D. J., Lein, D., Barclay, J. D., & Murphy, S. P. (1994). Health behaviors and survival among middle-aged and older men and women in the NHANES I Epidemiological Follow-up Study. *Preventive Medicine: An International Journal Devoted to Practice and Theory, 23*, 369–376.

Dekker, P., & Mootz, M. (1992). AIDS as threat, AIDS as stigma: Correlates of AIDS beliefs among the Dutch general public. *Psychology and Health, 6*, 347–365.

Dennis, M. (1994). Neuropsychiatric lupus erythematosus and the elderly. *International Journal of Geriatric Psychiatry, 9*, 97–106.

Dennis, M. S., Byrne, E. J., Hopkinson, N., & Bendall, P. (1992). Neuropsychiatric systemic lupus erythematosus in elderly people: A case series. *Journal of Neurology, Neurosurgery and Psychiatry, 55*, 1157–1161.

Devor, M., Wang, A., Renvall, M., Feigal, D., & Ramsdell, J. (1994). Compliance with social and safety recommendations in an outpatient comprehensive geriatric assessment program. *Journals of Gerontology, 49*, M168–M173.

Ditto, P. H., Moore, K. A., Hilton, J. L., & Kalish, J. R. (1995). Beliefs about physicians: Their role in health care utilization, satisfaction, and compliance. *Basic and Applied Social Psychology, 17*, 23–48.

Downe-Wambodlt, B. L., & Melanson, P. M. (1995). Emotions, coping, and psychological well-being in elderly people with arthritis. *Western Journal of Nursing Research, 17*, 250–265.

Dubert, P. M., & Stetson, B. A. (1995). Exercise and physical activity. In A. J. Goreczny (Ed.), *Handbook of health and rehabilitation psychology* (pp. 255–274). New York: Plenum.

El-Faizy, M., & Reinsch, S. (1994). Home safety intervention for the prevention of falls. *Physical and Occupational Therapy in Geriatrics, 12*, 33–49.

Elliot, D. B., Patla, A. E., Flanagan, J. G., Spaulding, S., Rietdyk, S., Strong, G., & Brown, S. (1995). The Waterloo vision and mobility study: Postural control strategies in subjects with ARM. *Ophthalmic and Physiological Optics, 15*, 553–559.

Ensrud, K. E., Nevitt, M. C., Yunis, C., Cauley, J. A., Seeley, D. G., Fox, K. M., & Cummings, S. R. (1994). Correlates of impaired function in older women. *Journal of the American Geriatrics Society, 42*, 481–489.

Fenley, J., Powers, P. S., Miller, J., & Rowland, M. (1990). Untreated anorexia nervosa. A case study of the medical consequences. *General Hospital Psychiatry, 12*, 264–270.

Fincham, J. E. (1992). The etiology and pathogenesis of detrimental health effects in elderly smokers. *Journal of Geriatric Drug Therapy; 7*, 5–21.

Fishbein, M. Chan, D. K., O'Reilly, K., & Schnell, D. (1993). Factors influencing gay men's attitudes, subjective norms, and intentions with respect to performing sexual behaviors. *Journal of Applied Social Psychology, 23*, 417–438.

Fitten, L. J., Coleman, L., Siembieda, D. W., Yu, M., & Ganzell, S. (1995). Assessment of capacity to comply with medication regimens in older patients. *Journal of the American Geriatrics Society, 43*, 361–367.

Ford, S. (1996). Cognitive rehabilitation of patients with dementia: A review of the effectiveness of learning mnemonics. *International Journal of Rehabilitation and Health, 2*, 277–283.

Foster, M. F. (1992). Health promotion and life satisfaction in elderly Black adults. *Western Journal of Nursing Research, 14*, 444–463.

Friedman, L. Brooks, J. O. 3rd, Bliwise, D. L., Yesavage, J. A., & Wicks, D.S. (1995). Perceptions of life stress and chronic insomnia in older adults. *Psychology and Aging, 10*, 352–357.

Glasgow, R. E., Stevens, V. J., Vogt, J. M., & Mullooly, J. P. (1991). Changes in smoking associated with hospitalization: Quit rates, predictive variables, and intervention implications. *American Journal of Health Promotion, 6*, 24–29.

Goreczny, A. J. (1995a). *Handbook of health and rehabilitation psychology.* New York: Plenum.

Goreczny, A. J. (1995b). Introductory statement—Forging ahead into the 21st century: Issues in rehabilitation. *International Journal of Rehabilitation and Health, 1*, 1–3.

Goreczny, A. J. (1997). *The stress of being a stress researcher.* Manuscript submitted for publication.

Goreczny, A. J., & O'Halloran, C. M. (1995). The future of psychology in health care. In A. J. Goreczny (Ed.), *Handbook of health and rehabilitation psychology* (pp. 663–676). New York: Plenum.

Goreczny, A. J., Keen, A., & Walter, K. (1997). Psychophysiological responding among older versus younger adults. Manuscript in preparation.

Cosford, P. A., & Arnold, E. (1992). Eating disorders in later life: A review. *International Journal of Geriatric Psychiatry, 7*, 491–498.

Gowers, S. G., & Crisp, A. H. (1990). Anorexia nervosa in an 80-year-old woman. *British Journal of Psychiatry, 157*, 754–757.

Green, B. H., Copeland, J. R., Dewey, M. E., Sharma, V., Saunders, P. A., Davidson, I. A., Sullivan, C., McWilliam, C. (1992). Risk factors for depression in the elderly: A prospective study. *Acta Psychiatrica Scandinavica, 86*, 213–217.

Grembowski, D., Patrick D., Diehr, P., Durham, M., Beresford, S., Kay, E., & Hecht, J. (1993). Self-efficacy and health behavior among older adults. *Journal of Health and Social Behavior, 34*, 89–104.

Gutheil, I. A., & Chichin, E. R. (1991). AIDS, older people, and social work. *Health and Social Work, 16*, 237–244.

Hall, P., & Driscoll, R. (1993). Anorexia in the elderly—an annotation. *International Journal of Eating Disorders, 14*, 497–499.

Hamm, V. P., Bazargan, M., & Barbre, A. R. (1993). Life-style and cardiovascular health among urban Black elderly. *Journal of Applied Gerontology, 12*, 155–169.

Hayslip, B., Maloy, R. M., & Kohl, R. (1995). Long-term efficacy of fluid ability interventions with older adults. *Journals of Gerontology Series B—Psychological Sciences and Social Sciences, 50B*, P141–P149.

Heinemann, A. W. (1995). In A. J. Goreczny (Ed.), *Handbook of health and rehabilitation psychology* (pp. 341–360). New York: Plenum.

Helzlsouer, K. J., Ford, D. E., Hayward, R. S., Midzenski, M., & Perry, H. (1994). Perceived risk of cancer and practice of cancer prevention behaviors among employees in an oncology center. *Preventive Medicine: An International Journal Devoted to Practice and Theory, 23*, 302–308.

Hensrud, D. D., & Sprafka, J. M. (1993). The smoking habits of Minnesota physicians. *American Journal of Public Health, 83*, 415–417.

Herman, C. J., Speroff, T., & Cebul, R. D. (1994). Improving compliance with immunization in the older adults: Results of a randomized cohort study. *Journal of the American Geriatrics Society, 42*, 1154–1159.

Herrick, S., Elliot, T. R., & Crow, F. (1994). Social support and the prediction of health complications among persons with spinal cord injuries. *Rehabilitation Psychology, 39*, 231–250.

Hersen, M., Van Hasselt, V. B., & Goreczny, A. J. (1993). Behavioral assessment of anxiety in older adults. *Behavior Modification, 17*, 99–112.

Hersen, M., Kabacoff, R. I., Ryan, C. F., Null, J. A., Melton, M. A., Pagan, V., Segal, D. L., & Van Hasselt, V. B. (1995). Psychometric properties of the Wolpe-Lazarus Assertiveness Scale for older visually impaired adults. *International Journal of Rehabilitation and Health, 1*, 179–188.

Hersen, M., Van Hasselt, V. B., & Segal, D. L. (1995). Social adaptation in older visually impaired adults: Some comments. *International Journal of Rehabilitation and Health, 1*, 49–60.

Hickey, T., Wolf, F. M., Robins, L. S., & Wagner, M. B. (1995). Physical activity training for functional mobility in older persons. *Journal of Applied Gerontology, 14*, 357–371.

Hinkin, C., Cummings, J. L., Van Gorp, W. G., & Satz, P. (1990). Frontal/subcortical features of normal aging: An empirical analysis. *Canadian Journal on Aging, 9*, 104–119.

Ho, S. C., Woo, J., Lau, J., Chan, S. G., Yuen, Y. K., Chan, Y. K., & Chi, I. (1995). Life satisfaction and associated factors in older Hong Kong Chinese. *Journal of the American Geriatrics Society, 43*, 252–255.

Hocking, L. B., & Koenig, H. G. (1995). Anxiety in medically ill older patients: A review and update. *International Journal of Psychiatry and Medicine, 25,* 221–238.

Huerta, R., Mena, A., Malacara, J.-M., & Diaz-de-Leon, J. (1995). Symptoms at the menopausal and premenopausal years: Their relationship with insulin, glucose, cortisol, FSH, prolactin, obesity and attitudes towards sexuality. *Psychoneuroendocrinology, 20,* 851–864.

Itoh, R., & Suyama, Y. (1995). Sociodemographic factors and life-styles affecting micronutrient status in an apparently healthy elderly Japanese population. *Journal of Nutrition for the Elderly, 14,* 39–54.

Jensen, E., Dehlin, O., Hayberg, B., Samuelsson, G., & Svensson, T. (1994). Medical, psychological, and sociological aspects of drug treatment in 80-year-olds. *Zeitschrift für Gerontologie, 27,* 140–144.

Jeste, D. V., Caligiuri, M. P., Paulsen, J. S., Heaton, R. K., Lacro, J. P. Harris, M. J., Bailey, A., Fell, R. L., & McAdams, L. A. (1995). Risk of tardive dyskinesia in older patients: A prospective longitudinal study of 266 outpatients. *Archives of General Psychiatry, 52,* 756–765.

Jones, A., Greaves, K., & Iliffe, S. (1992). Health protective behaviour and knowledge of coronary heart disease risk factors in a general practice population. *Medical Science Research, 20,* 71–73.

Kahana, E., Redmond, C., Hill, G. J., & Kercher, K. (1995). The effects of stress, vulnerability, and appraisals on the psychological well-being of the elderly. *Research on Aging, 17,* 459–489.

Kaye, J. A., Oken, B. S., Howieson, D. B., Howieson, J., Holm, L. A., & Dennison, K. (1994). Neurologic evaluation of the optimally healthy oldest old. *Archives of Neurology, 51,* 1205–1211.

Kernutt, G. J., Price, A. J., Judd, F. K., & Burrows, G. D. (1993). Human immunodeficiency virus infection, dementia and the older patient. *Australian and New Zealand Journal of Psychiatry, 27,* 9–19.

King, E. S., Ross, E., Seay, J., & Balshem, A. (1995). Mammography interventions for 65- to 74-year-old HMO women: Program effectiveness and predictors of use. *Journal of Aging and Health, 7,* 529–551.

Koller, W., Lang, A., Vetere-Overfield, B., Findley, L., Cleeves, L., Factor, S., Singer, C., & Weiner, W. (1989). Psychogenic tremors. *Neurology, 39,* 1094–1099.

Kopac, C. A. (1990). The environment and its relationship to the Type A behavior pattern in middle and old age: A pilot study. *Psychological Reports, 66,* 768–770.

Krause, N. (1995a). Assessing stress-buffering effects: A cautionary note. *Psychology and Aging, 10,* 518–526.

Krause, N. (1995b). Stress, alcohol use, and depressive symptoms in later life. *Gerontologist, 35,* 296–307.

Krause, N. (1996). Neighborhood deterioration and self-rated health in later life. *Psychology and Aging, 11,* 342–352.

Kreitler, S., & Kreitler, H. (1997). Cognitive orientation and health-protective behaviors. *International Journal of Rehabilitation and Health, 3,* 1–24.

Kviz, F. Crittenden, K. S., Clark, M. A., & Madura, K. J. (1994). Buddy support among older smokers in a smoking cessation programa. *Journal of Aging and Health, 6,* 229–254.

Kviz, F. J., Clark, M. A., Crittenden, K. S., Warnecke, R. B., & Freels, S. (1995). Age and smoking cessation behaviors. *Preventive Medicine: An International Journal Devoted to Practice and Theory, 24,* 297–307.

Laatch, L. (1996). Use of stratified norms for the Mattis Dementia Rating Scale in an urban rehabilitation sample. *International Journal of Rehabilitation and Health, 2,* 199–207.

Landreville, P., Dube, M., Lalande, G., & Alain, M. (1994). *Journal of Social Behavior and Personality, 9,* 269–286.

Lave, J. R., Ives, D. G., Traven, N. D., & Kuller, L. H. (1995). Participation in health promotion programs by rural elderly. *American Journal of Preventive Medicine, 11,* 46–53.

Laws, A., King, A. C., Haskell, W. L., & Reaven, G. M. (1993). Metabolic and behavioral covariates of high-density lipoprotein cholesterol and triglyceride concentrations in postmenopausal women. *Journal of the American Geriatrics Society, 41,* 1289–1294.

Lazarus, R. S., & Folkman, S. (1984). *Stress, appraisal, and coping.* New York: Springer.

Lee, C. (1989). Perceptions of immunity to disease in adult smokers. *Journal of Behavioral Medicine, 12,* 267–277.

Lee, S. (1992). The clinical validity of tardive anorexia nervosa. *Australian and New Zealand Journal of Psychiatry, 26,* 686–688.

Lefebvre, R. C., Cobb, G. D., Goreczny, A. J., & Carleton, R. A. (1990). Efficacy of an incentive-based community smoking cessation program. *Addictive Behaviors, 15,* 403–411.

Leigh, B. C., Temple, M. T., & Trocki, K. F. (1993). The sexual behavior of US adults: Results from a national survey. *American Journal of Public Health, 83*, 1400–1408.

Leirer, V. O., Tanke, E. D., & Morrow, D. G. (1994). Time of day and naturalistic prospective memory. *Experimental Aging Research, 20*, 127–134.

Leo, R. J., & Kim, K. Y. (1995). Clomipramine treatment of paraphilias in elderly demented patients. *Journal of Geriatric Psychiatry and Neurology, 8*, 123–124.

Liberto, J. G., & Oslin, D. W. (1995). Early versus late onset of alcoholism in the elderly. Drugs and the elderly: Use and misuse of drugs, medicines, alcohol, and tobacco [Special issue]. *International Journal of the Addictions, 30*, 1799–1818.

Lichtenstein, E., & Hollis, J. (1992). Patient referral to a smoking cessation program: Who follows through? *Journal of Family Practice, 34*, 739–744.

Liddell, A., Pollett, W. G., & MacKenzie, D. S. (1995). Comparison of postoperative satisfaction between ulcerative colitis patients who chose to undergo either a pouch or an ileostomy operation. *International Journal of Rehabilitation and Health, 1*, 89–96.

Liddle, J., & Gilleard, C. (1995). The emotional consequences of falls for older people and their families. *Clinical Rehabilitation, 9*, 110–114.

Linsk, N. L. (1994). HIV and the elderly. *Families in Society, 75*, 362–372.

Lipton, H. L., & Bird, J. A. (1994). The impact of clinical pharmacists' consultations on geriatric patients' compliance and medical care use: A randomized controlled trial. *Gerontologist, 34*, 307–315.

Liu, B. A., Topper, A. K., Reeves, R. A., Gryfe, C., & Maki, B. E. (1995). Falls among older people: Relationship to medication use and orthostatic hypotension. *Journal of the American Geriatrics Society, 43*, 1141–1145.

Lloyd, G. A. (1989). AIDS & elders: Advocacy, activism, & coalitions. *Generations, 13*, 32–35.

Lord, S. R., Ward, J. A., Williams, P., & Strudwick, M. (1995). The effect of a 12-month exercise trial on balance, strength, and falls in older women: A randomized controlled trial. *Journal of the American Geriatrics Society, 43*, 1198–1206.

Lundervold, D. A., & Poppen, R. (1995). Biobehavioral rehabilitation for older adults with essential tremor. *Gerontologist, 35*, 556–559.

Ma, S. S. Y., & Chi, I. (1995). Health counseling for older people in Hong Kong. Learning to live at all ages [Special Issue]. *Educational Gerontology, 21*, 515–528.

Malatesta-Magai, C., Jonas, R., Shepard, B., & Culver, L. C. (1992). Type A behavior pattern and emotion expression in younger and older adults. *Psychology and Aging, 7*, 551–561.

Marti-Masso, J. F. & Poza, J. J. (1992). A new type of epidemiological study: Questionnaire administered by medical personnel. *Neuroepidemiology, 11*, 296–298.

Martinez, M., Arnalich, F., Vazquez, J. J., & Hernanz, A. (1993). Altered cerebrospinal fluid amino acid pattern in the anorexia of aging: Relationship with biogenic amine metabolism. *Life Sciences, 53*, 1643–1650.

Maxwell, C. J., & Hirdes, J. P. (1993). The prevalence of smoking and implications for quality of life among the community-based elderly. *American Journal of Preventive Medicine, 9*, 338–345.

Melanson, P. M., & Downe-Wamboldt, B. (1995). The stress of life with rheumatoid arthritis as perceived by older adults. *Activities, Adaptation and Aging, 19*, 33–47.

Miller, D. K., Morley, J. E., Rubenstein, L. Z., & Pietruszka, F. M. (1991). Abnormal eating attitudes and body image in older undernourished individuals. *Journal of the American Geriatrics Society, 39*, 462–466.

Mitrushina, M., Satz, P., Drebing, C., Van Gorp, W., Mathews, A., Harker, J., & Chervinsky, A. (1994). The differential pattern of memory deficit in normal aging and dementias of different etiology. *Journal of Clinical Psychology, 50*, 246–252.

Moghal, S., Rajput, A. H., Meleth, R., D'Arcy, C., & Rajput, R. (1995). Prevalence of movement disorders in institutionalized elderly. *Neuroepidemiology, 14*, 297–300.

Monfort, J. C. (1995). The difficult elderly patient: Curable hostile depression or personality disorder. *International Psychogeriatrics, 7* (Suppl.), 95–111.

Morley, J. E. (1993). The strange case of an older woman who was cured by being allowed to refuse therapy. *Journal of American Geriatrics Society, 41*, 1012–1013.

Morrow, D., Leirer, V., & Altieri, P. (1995). List formats to improve medication instructions for older adults. *Educational Gerontology, 21*, 151–166.

Morrow, D. G., Leirer, V. O., & Andrassy, J. M. (1996). Using icons to convey medication schedule information. *Applied Ergonomics, 27*, 267–275.

Nakamura, C. M., Molgaard, C. A., Stanford, E. P. Peddecord, K. M., Morton, D. J., Lockery, S. A., Zuniga, M., & Gardner, L. (1990). A discriminant analysis of severe alcohol consumption among older persons. *Alcohol and Alcoholism, 25,* 75–80.

Natow, S. J. (1994). Cross-cultural counseling. *Journal of Nutrition for the Elderly, 14,* 23–31.

Neef, N. A., Bill-Harvey, D., Shade, D., Iezzi, M., & DeLorenzo, T. (1995). Exercise participation with videotaped modeling: Effects on balance and gait in elderly residents of care facilities. *Behavior Therapy, 26,* 135–151.

Nelson, H. D., Neritt, M. C., Scott, J. C., Stone, K. L., & Cummings, S. R. (1994). Smoking, alcohol, and neuromuscular and physical function of older women: *Journal of the American Medical Association, 272,* 1825–1831.

Nussbaum, P. D., & Goreczny, A. J. (1995). Self-appraisal of stress level and related psychopathology. *Journal of Anxiety Disorders, 9,* 463–472.

Nussbaum, P. D., Allender, J., & Copeland, J. (1995). Verbal learning in cardiac transplant candidates: A preliminary report. *International Journal of Rehabilitation and Health, 1,* 5–12.

Oei, T. P. S., Tilley, D., & Gow, K. (1991). Differences in reasons for smoking between younger and older smokers. *Drug and Alcohol Review, 10,* 323–329.

O'Hara, P., & Portser, S. A. (1994). A comparison of younger-aged and older-aged women in a behavioral self-control smoking program. *Patient Education and Counseling, 23,* 91–96.

Orleans, C. T., Rimer, B. K., Cristinzio, S., Keintz, M. K., & Fleisher, L. (1991). A national survey of older smokers: Treatment needs of a growing population. *Health Psychology, 10,* 343–351.

Orrell, M., & Bebbington, P. (1995). Life events and senile dementia. I: Admission, deterioration and social environment change. *Psychological Medicine, 25,* 373–386.

Parry, K. K., Mobley, T., & Allen, O. (1996). Use of folk treatments for diabetic plantar ulcers among African Americans with Type II diabetes. *International Journal of Rehabilitation and Health, 2,* 265–283.

Persad, C. C., Giordani, B., Chen, H. C., Ashton-Miller, J. A., Alexander, N. B., Wilson, C. S., Berent, S., Guire, K., & Schultz, A. B. (1995). Neuropsychological predictors of complex obstacle avoidance in healthy older adults. *Journals of Gerontology. Series B—Psychological Sciences and Social Sciences, 50,* P272–P277.

Pickering T. G. (1995). Hypertension. In A. J. Goreczny (Ed.), *Handbook of Health and Rehabilitation Psychology.* New York: Plenum.

Pierce, J., Giovino, G., Hatziandreu, E., & Shopland, D. (1989). National age and sex differences in quitting smoking. *Journal of Psychoactive Drugs, 21,* 293–298.

Piette, J., Wachtel, T. J., Mor, V., & Mayer, K. (1995). The impact of age on the quality of life in persons with HIV infection. *Journal of Aging and Health, 7,* 163–178.

Pitner, J. K., Mintzer, J. E., Pennypacker, L. C., & Jackson, C. W. (1995). Efficacy and adverse effects of clozapine in four elderly psychotic patients. *Journal of Clinical Psychiatry, 56,* 180–185.

Rapport, L. J., Dutra, R. L., Webster, J. S., & Charter, R. (1995). Hemispatial deficits on the Rey-Osterrieth complex figure drawing. *Clinical Neuropsychologist, 9,* 169–179.

Rees, J., Bayer, A., & Phillips, G. (1995). Assessment and management of the dementing driver. *Journal of Mental Health UK, 4,* 165–176.

Reynolds, C. F., Frank, E., Perel, J. M., Mazumdar, S., & Kupfer, D. J. (1995). Maintenance therapies for late-life recurrent major depression: Research and review circa 1995. *International Psychogeriatrics, 7,* 27–39.

Riemann, B. C., McNally, R. J., & Meier, A. (1993). Anorexia nervosa in an elderly man. *International Journal of Eating Disorders, 14,* 501–504.

Rimer, B. K., Orleans, C. T., Fleisher, L., & Cristinzio, S. (1994). Does tailoring matter? The impact of a tailored guide on ratings and short-term smoking-related outcomes for older smokers. *Health Education Research, 9,* 69–84.

Robinson, B. E., Walters, L. H., & Skeen, P. (1989). Response of parents to learning that their child is homosexual and concern over AIDS: A national study. *Journal of Homosexuality, 18,* 59–80.

Robinson, P., Bush, T., Von Korff, M., Katon, W., Lin, E., Simon, G. E., & Walker, E. (1995). Primary care physician use of cognitive behavioral techniques with depressed patients. *Journal of Family Practice, 40,* 352–357.

Rose, M. S., & West, M. (1996). Attachment problems and depressive symptomatology in cardiac rehabilitation patients. *International Journal of Rehabilitation and Health, 2,* 113–124.

Rosenzweig, R., & Fillit, H. (1992). Probable heterosexual transmission of AIDS in an aged woman. *Journal of the American Geriatrics Society, 40,* 1261–1264.

Rossen, E. K., & Buschmann, M. T. (1995). Mental illness in later life: The neurobiology of depression. *Archives of Psychiatric Nursing, 9,* 130–136.

Russell, J., & Gilbert, M. (1992). Is tardive anorexia a discrete diagnostic entity? *Australian and New Zealand Journal of Psychiatry, 26,* 429–435.

Salgado, R., Lord, S. R., Packer, J., & Ehrlich, F. (1994). Factors associated with falling in elderly hospital patients. *Gerontology, 40,* 325–331.

Salive, M. E., & Blazer, D. G. (1993). Depression and smoking cessation in older adults: A longitudinal study. *Journal of the American Geriatrics Society, 41,* 1313–1316.

Salzman, C. (1995). Medication compliance in the elderly. *Journal of Clinical Psychiatry, 56,* 18–23.

Samuelsson, G., Hagberg, B., Dehlin, O., & Lindberg, B. (1994). Medical, social and psychological factors as predictors of survival: A follow-up from 67 to 87 years of age. *Archives of Gerontology and Geriatrics, 18,* 25–41.

Schneider, L. S., & Olin, J. T. (1995). Efficacy of acute treatment for geriatric depression. *International Psychogeriatrics, 7,* 7–25.

Schoenfeld-Smith, K., Nicassio, P. M., Radojevic, V., & Patterson, T. L. (1995). Multiaxial taxonomy of fibromyalgia syndrome patients. *Journal of Clinical Psychology in Medical Settings, 2,* 149–166.

Schwirian, P. M. (1991–1992). The Seniors' Life-style Inventory: Assessing health behaviors in older adults. *Behavior, Health, and Aging, 2,* 43–55.

Scura, K. W., & Whipple, B. (1990). Older adults as an HIV-positive risk group. *Journal of Gerontological Nursing, 16,* 6–10.

Seeman, T. E., Berkman, L. F., Charpentier, P. A., Blazer, D. G., Albert, M. S., & Tinetti, M. E. (1995). Behavioral and psychosocial predictors of physical performance: MacArthur studies of successful aging. *Journals of Gerontology. Series A—Biological Sciences and Medical Sciences, 50,* M177–M183.

Sheahan, S. L., Coons, S. J., Robbins, C. A., Martin, S. S., Hendricks, J., & Latimer, M. (1995). Psychoactive medication, alcohol use, and falls among older adults. *Journal of Behavioral Medicine, 18,* 127–140.

Shillington, A. M., Cottler, L. B., Compton, W. M., & Spitznagel, E. L. (1995). Is there a relationship between "heavy drinking" and HIV high risk sexual behaviors among general population subjects? *International Journal of the Addictions, 30,* 1453–1478.

Simpson, J. M., & Mandelstam, H. (1995). Elderly people at risk of falling: Do they want to be taught how to get up again? *Clinical Rehabilitation, 9,* 65–69.

Smith, T. W. (1995). Assessment and modification of coronary-prone behavior: A transactional view of the person in social context. In A. J. Goreczny (Ed.), *Handbook of Health and Rehabilitation Psychology.* New York: Plenum.

Steinmetz, H. M., & Hobson, S. J. G. (1994). Prevention of falls among the community-dwelling elderly: An overview. *Physical and Occupational Therapy in Geriatrics, 12,* 13–29.

Suyama, Y, & Itoh, R. (1992). Multivariatc analysis of dietary habits in 931 elderly Japanese males: Smoking, food frequency and food preference. *Journal of Nutrition for the Elderly, 12,* 1–12.

Swan, G. E., Dame, A., & Carmelli, D. (1991). Involuntary retirement, Type A behavior, and current functioning in elderly men: 27-year follow-up of the Western Collaborative Group Study. *Psychology and Aging, 6,* 384–391.

Talashek, M. L., Tichy, A. M., & Epping, H. (1990). Sexually transmitted diseases in the elderly: Issues and recommendations. *Journal of Gerontological Nursing, 16,* 33–40.

Talbert, F. S., Wagner, P. J., Braswell, L. C., & Husein, S. (1995). Analysis of long-term stress reactions in emergency room patients: An initial study. *Journal of Clinical Psychology in Medical Settings, 2,* 133–148.

Tanaka, T., Hashimoto, N., Noriyasu, S., Ino, S., Ifukube, T., & Mizumoto, Z. (1995). Aging and postural stability: Change in sensorimotor function. *Physical and Occupational Therapy in Geriatrics, 13,* 1–16.

Taplin, S. H., Anderman, C., Grothaus, L., Curry, S., & Montano, D. (1994). Using physician correspondence and postcard reminders to promote mammography use. *American Journal of Public Health, 84,* 571–574.

Tinetti, M. E., Doucette, J., Claus, E., & Marottoli, R. (1995). Risk factors for serious injury during falls by older persons in the community. *Journal of the American Geriatrics Society, 43,* 1214–1221.

Tuthill, S. B. (1989). Physical and social factors affecting hypertension. *Journal of Human Behavior and Learning, 6*, 1–10.

Van Gorp, W. G., Wilfred, G., Mitrushina, M., Cummings, J. L., & Satz, P. (1989). Normal aging and the subcortical encephalopathy of AIDS: A neuropsychological comparison. *Neuropsychiatry, Neuropsychology, and Behavioral Neurology, 2*, 5–20.

Van Gorp, W. G., Miller, E. N., Marcotte, T. D., Dixon, W., Paz, D., Selnes, O., Wesch, J., Becker, J. T., Hinkin, C.D, & Mitrushina, M. (1994). The relationship between age and cognitive impairment in HIV-I infection: Findings from the Multicenter AIDS Cohort Study and a clinical cohort. *Neurology, 44*, 929–935.

Van Sickle, T. D., Hersen, M., Simco, E. R., Melton, M. A., & Van Hasselt, V. B. (1996). Effects of physical exercise on cognitive functioning in the elderly. *International Journal of Rehabilitation and Health, 2*, 67–100.

Vella, S., Giuliano, M., Floridia, M. Chiesi, A., Tomino, C., Seeber, A., Barcherini, S., Bucciardini, R., & Mariotti, S. (1995). Effect of sex, age and transmission category on the progression to AIDS and survival of zidovudine-treated symptomatic patients. *AIDS, 9*, 51–56.

Vermeulen, A. (1994). Clinical problems in reproductive neuroendocrinology of men. *Neurobiology of Aging, 15*, 489–493.

Vincke, J., & Bolton, R. (1994). Social support, depression, and self-acceptance among gay men. *Human Relations, 47*, 1049–1062.

Vincke, J., Mak, R., Bolton, R., & Jurica, P. (1993). Factors affecting AIDS-related sexual behavior change among Flemish gay men. *Human Organization, 52*, 260–268.

Vitaliano, P. P., Russo, J., Bailey, S. L., Young, H. M., & McCann, B. S. (1993). Psychosocial factors associated with cardiovascular reactivity in older adults. *Psychosomatic Medicine, 55*, 164–177.

Vitaliano, P. P., Russo, J., & Niaura, R. (1995). Plasma lipids and their relationships with psychosocial factors in older adults. *Journals of Gerontology Series B Psychological Sciences and Social Sciences, 50B*, P18–P24.

Wain, H. J., Amen, D., & Jabbari, B. (1990). The effects of hypnosis on a Parkinsonian tremor: Case report with polygraph/EEG recordings. *American Journal of Clinical Hypnosis, 33*, 94–98.

Wei, H., Young, D., Lingiang, L., Shuiyuan, X., Jian, T., Hanshu, S., Zhunghong, Y., Xiouying, Xudong, W. (1995). Psychoactive substance use in three sites in China: Gender differences and related factors. *Addiction, 90*, 1503–1515.

Weinberger, M., Samsa, G. P., Schmader, K., & Greenberg, S. M. (1994). Compliance with recommendations from an outpatient geriatric consultation team. *Journal of Applied Gerontology, 13*, 455–467.

Whipple, B., & Scura, K. W. (1989). HIV and the older adult: Taking the necessary precautions. *Journal of Gerontological Nursing, 15*, 15–19.

Wiederman, M. W., Weis, D. L., & Allgeier, E. R. (1994). The effect of question preface on response rates to a telephone survey of sexual experience. *Archives of Sexual Behavior, 23*, 203–215.

Williams, P., & Lord, S. R. (1995). Predictors of adherence to a structured exercise program for older women. *Psychology and Aging, 10*, 617–624.

Wright, B. D., Lunt, B., Harris, S. J., & Wallace, D. (1995). A prospective study in three psychogeriatric day hospitals using administrative interventions to improve non-attendance. *International Journal of Geriatric Psychiatry, 10*, 55–61.

Zaimov, K. A., Fertcheva, A., & Vanev, P. I. (1994). Motives of smoking and inborn behavioral preprogram of the personality. *International Journal of the Addictions, 29*, 957–970.

Zimmermann, R., Deuschl, G., Hornig, A., Schulte-Monting, J.; Fuchs, G., & Lucking, C. H. (1994). Tremors in Parkinson's disease: Symptom analysis and rating. *Clinical Neuropharmacology, 17*, 303–314.

Zipp, A., & Holcomb, C. A. (1992). Living arrangements and nutrient intakes of healthy women age 65 and older: A study in Manhattan, Kansas. *Journal of Nutrition for the Elderly, 11*, 1–18.

PART III

SPECIAL ISSUES

CHAPTER 17

Health and Well-Being in Retirement

A Summary of Theories and Their Implications

WILLIAM S. SHAW, THOMAS L. PATTERSON,
SHIRLEY SEMPLE, AND IGOR GRANT

INTRODUCTION

To consider the topic of retirement as a special clinical issue in this book along-side the comparatively severe stressors of chronic pain, elder abuse, caregiving, and bereavement may seem unwarranted to some. Retirement is now a normative process for most older workers, and available pension and savings plans have greatly eased the financial burdens of retirement. Yet, for many individuals, retirement may represent the single largest lifestyle transition since early adulthood. Therefore, this period of social development and its mental and physical health implications have continued to be a subject of theoretical speculation and empirical study. Retirement may alter family dynamics and social networks, challenge one's sense of self-worth and accomplishment, and prompt reprioritization of personal values and interests. The decision to retire may also be influenced by a complex set of variables, including physical health, occupational attitudes, personal values, and secular trends. By studying the antecedents and consequences of retirement, social scientists have sought to identify factors that contribute to a successful and healthful retirement process.

Retirement, like other experiences of later life, occurs among a tremendously diverse aging population. Health, occupational circumstances, socio-cultural factors, and other demographic indicators contribute to both retirement

WILLIAM S. SHAW, THOMAS L. PATTERSON, SHIRLEY SEMPLE, AND IGOR GRANT • Department of Psychiatry, School of Medicine, University of California, San Diego, La Jolla, California 92063-0680.

Handbook of Clinical Geropsychology, edited by Michel Hersen and Vincent B. Van Hasselt. Plenum Press, New York, 1998.

lifestyle and attitudes about the retirement process. For example, variables consistently associated with retirement satisfaction among male retirees (health, wealth, and work history) appear to be unrelated to satisfaction among female retirees (George, Fillenbaum, & Palmore, 1984). Another example is the difference in retirement predictors based on vocational status. Job dissatisfaction is the strongest predictor of retirement among older blue-collar workers (Goudy, Powers, & Keith, 1975), whereas self-perceptions of youthfulness and work effectiveness are the most salient variables for older executives (Eden & Jacobson, 1976). Also, the retirement process itself is changing as demographic shifts and technological innovations make flexible employment conditions more feasible. In this chapter, we explore factors that may delineate theoretically relevant subsets of retirees, and we review and contrast the psychological and sociological theories that have been advanced to explain retirement and its impacts.

A second focus of this chapter is to explore the complex relationships between physical health and retirement. Despite a widely held notion that retirement is responsible for declining health, we review studies that provide very little support for this belief. We also discuss the role of health in the decision to retire and whether this influences retirement outcomes. Although postretirement activities can be compromised by poor health, retirement may provide opportunities for improving health behaviors and directing more attention to treating physical health conditions. In our review of theoretical models, we examine in particular the applicability of retirement theories to describe the complex interaction of health and retirement.

DEFINING RETIREMENT AS A PROCESS

In the most basic sense of the word, retirement represents cessation of regular employment, regardless of circumstances, volition, or consequences. As a psychological construct, however, retirement represents a much broader concept—it may trigger a series of financial, social, and intrapsychic processes over an extended transitional period. In a review of gerontological studies of retirement, Quinn and Burkhauser (1990) noted a variety of operational definitions for categorizing individuals as retired: (1) retirement based on self-appraisal of perceived retirement status; (2) retirement predicated on receipt of retirement income or Social Security income; and (3) retirement based on a criterion degree of labor force participation. To remedy these definitional issues, Atchley (1991) has proposed that retirement occurs at the time at which an individual's primary financial source shifts from wage earnings to a pension income.

The stereotypical retirement is one of a quick and long-anticipated departure from full-time employment, and this event is often marked by a retirement party and the good wishes of fellow workers. This stereotype is accurate for most workers. The median pattern is to retire from full-time work at age 65 and permanently leave the work force (Quinn & Burkhauser, 1990). However, increased flexibility in employer retirement policies and diversification of pension programs have allowed many workers to make gradual retirement transitions over several years. This provides employers with part-time access to an experienced and knowledgeable labor force during peak periods without the burden of paying full-time employee benefits. For the older worker, part-time employment helps to ease the transition to retirement and provides a supplemental income source. Given these mutual benefits, it is surprising that phased retirement programs have not been more popular among older workers. Although 60% to 80% of workers of all ages favor a phased retirement (Jondrow, Breehling, & Marcus, 1987), fewer than one-third eventually chooses part-time retirement transitions (Gustman & Steinmeier, 1985).

The numerous possible patterns and phases of the retirement transition have led many researchers to conceptualize retirement as a process rather than a discrete event. The most influential description of this process has been Atchley's (1974) eight phases of retirement: (1) *preretirement,* in which anticipatory attitudes are formed; (2) *retirement event,* marked by a celebratory gesture; (3) *honeymoon phase,* marked by vacations and new interests; (4) *rest and relaxation phase,* a period of brief respite from the obligations of work; (5) *immediate retirement routine,* an immediate readjustment of schedules to maintain activity; (6) *disenchantment,* a perceived "letdown" following the honeymoon phase or as the result of negative circumstances; (7) *reorientation,* in which adjustments are made to accommodate realistic lifestyle goals; and (8) *retirement routine,* a stable period in which a satisfying retirement lifestyle is maintained. Although Atchley (1974) cautions that these stages do not occur in an orderly and consistent fashion for all individuals, they help to characterize the retirement experiences voiced by many older workers. Empirical studies have shown support for at least some of these phases of the retirement transition (Antonovsky & Sagy, 1990; Ekerdt, Bosse, & Mogey, 1980; Ekerdt, Bosse, & Levkoff, 1985; Evans, Ekerdt, & Bossee, 1985)

Three principal stages of the retirement process can be consolidated from the eight stages proposed by Atchley (1974): the retirement planning process, the retirement decision process, and adaptation to retirement. *Retirement planning* typically begins in early adulthood, when a variety of retirement pension plans are first offered and expectations about life after retirement begin to evolve. The *retirement decision* process includes contemplation and actions immediately preceding the decision to retire. *Adaptation to retirement* encompasses whatever actions are taken to reach a comfortable and satisfying lifestyle after retirement. Psychological and sociological theories of retirement have addressed these three stages of the retirement process with varying success. Later in this chapter, we use these three stages as a context for theory comparison.

Another aspect of retirement that favors a process approach is its voluntary nature. In the 1950s and 1960s, prior to the 1967 enactment of the Age Discrimination in Employment Act (ADEA), many employers enforced mandatory retirement, sometimes as early as age 45 (Schulz, 1988). Involuntary or coerced retirement has been linked to negative attitudes and maladjustment (Schulz, 1988) among retirees (Crowley, 1986; Hardy & Quadagno, 1995) . Since its enactment, the ADEA has been amended (most recently in 1986) to abolish mandatory retirement in America with the exception of a few selected occupations. Today, retirement is for most a self-guided process that is intimately connected with subjective perceptions of life circumstances.

A BRIEF HISTORY OF RETIREMENT

The ambivalence with which many older workers approach retirement may be a reflection of the confusing historical origins of retirement in America. Although touted as a benefit for older workers, retirement was clearly instituted to benefit younger workers. At the turn of the century, retirement as it exists today was unknown. By mid-century, the industrial revolution had reduced demand for poorly skilled older workers whose primary training and experience was inconsistent with technological advances. At the same time, life expectancy was increasing rapidly from 46 years in 1900 to 66 years in 1950 (Manheimer, 1994), and this resulted in a glut of older workers who were perceived as limiting the aspirations of younger, more promising candidates. Although retirement today is often considered a positive reward for a lifetime of hard work, the historical fact remains that retirement was first conceived to limit, not extend, opportunitites for older workers.

Since the Social Security Act was first passed by Congress in August 1935, thousands of minor (and some major) adjustments have been made to U.S. federal government policies concerning retirement programs and pensions. Today, unraveling the complexities of social security, pension plans, savings plans, and health care coverage can be a time-consuming and often aggravating process for many older Americans. Labor force participation rates among older Americans have steadily declined in response to increasing retirement benefits (see Figure 17-1). In 1950, 46% of men over the age of 65 were employed, compared with 16% in 1992. Employment rates among women over the age of 65

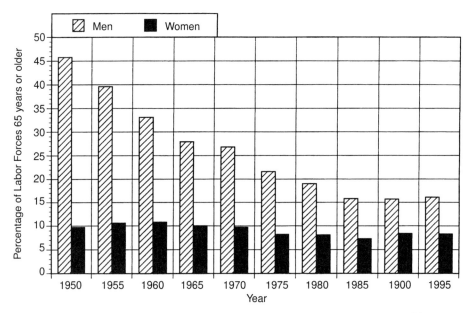

Figure 17-1. Civilian labor force rates among men and women 65 years or older. From *Older Americans Almanac* (p. 215), edited by J. Manhelmer, 1994, Washington, DC: Gale Research. Copyright 1994 by Gale Research Inc.

have remained surprisingly stable (about 10%) over this period, because the tendency for women to retire earlier was offset by a growing presence of women in the workplace in all age groups. Over the past decade, employment rates among older Americans have remained relatively stable, reflecting a newly established balance between the competing influences of labor demands and retirement benefits.

As the baby-boom generation (those born between 1942 and 1963) approaches retirement age, the demographic factors that originally precipitated the need for a uniform retirement policy may require adjustment. In 1930, only 5.4% of the population was over age 65; today, about 12% are over 65; and by the year 2010, approximately 20% of the population will be older than 65. As this demographic shift continues, it will become increasingly difficult for a shrinking younger workforce to support the entitlements of a burgeoning group of retirees. Economic principles of supply and demand within the workforce may lead employers to encourage delayed retirement among older workers. Recent legislative changes have already begun to reflect this pattern. For example, the minimum age to begin collecting Social Security has been raised for future workers (effective in 2010). Also, income tax laws have been changed to provide for taxation of the Social Security benefits of upper-income individuals. In the future, these policies should result in later retirement ages among future cohorts of retirees.

DIVERSITY IN RETIREMENT

One of the difficulties in establishing a single explanatory model of the retirement process is the degree to which circumstances may vary among retirees. For example, a "stress and coping" model of the retirement process that assumes retirement to be a stressor may be inaccurate for individuals who view retirement as a long-awaited escape from a stressful, physically demanding, or dissatisfying occupation. Similarly, theories that view retirement as a normative disengagement from society are inaccurate for those who choose to augment physical and social activities after retirement. Very few older workers retire because they are discouraged with work or are forced to retire by their employer (see Figure 17-2). Six variables of circumstance have been repeatedly shown to influence the nature of retirement. These are gender, health, wealth, job satisfaction, occupational type, and whether retirement is voluntary or involuntary (see Table 17-1). Examination of these variables is essential before assuming an accurate theoretical orientation to explain retirement processes.

Given the experiential diversity of retirement, we have chosen a typology of retirement that specifies four possible retirement possibilities: retirement as a *life stressor;* retirement as a *relief from employment;* retirement as a *marker for disability;* and retirement as a *developmental task*. These can be shown in a decision logic diagram (Figure 17-3) in which presence or absence of several factors determines which type of retirement experience is likely to occur. This typology specifies that if retirement is either involuntary or not preceded by adequate financial planning, retirement may be best characterized as a stressor. If neither of these conditions is met, but employment was either dissatisfying or physically demanding, retirement may be best characterized as a reward and a relief. If none

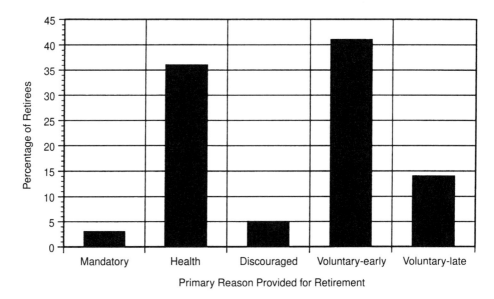

Figure 17-2. Primary reasons given for retirement among American men retired in 1981. From "Longitudinal Effects of Retirement on Men's Well-Being and Health," by J. E. Crowley, 1986, *Journal of Business and Psychology, 1,* p. 101.

of these four conditions is met, but retirement was related to disability or declining health, then retirement merely serves as a behavioral marker for poor health. If none of these circumstances apply, then retirement is best characterized as a developmental task requiring interpersonal and intrapsychic adjustments. This reduction of retirees into experiential subsets provides more homogeneous groups in which to understand the retirement process and explain empirical findings.

Gender

Empirical studies of retirement in the past have focused on traditional careers (auto workers, college professors, and medical and health professionals, for example) and have focused almost exclusively on men. The growing labor force participation rates of women warrants increased attention to the role and impacts of retirement among older female workers. Keith (1985) has identified formerly married women as a special group at risk for poor retirement outcomes because of reduced savings and less employment tenure at retirement. Other research suggests that although retirement outcomes are similar for men and women, the factors that account for retirement satisfaction are different. George and colleagues (1984) found that health, income, and work history were predictive of retirement satisfaction for men, but not for women. One explanation for this difference may be that women today have a narrower range of variability on measures of health, income, and work history; therefore, correlations with retirement satisfaction tend to be much lower. Another explanation is that married women's retirement decisions may be highly impacted by their husbands' re-

Table 17-1. Studies Investigating Variables Related to Retirement Satisfaction

Reference	Methods	Explanatory variables
Glamser (1976)	Investigated predictors of retirement attitude among 70 Pennsylvania factory workers.	Preparedness Financial future rating Life situation rating Number of close friends Times unemployed
Dorfman (1989)	Investigated predictors of retirement satisfaction among 451 rural retirees.	Health Financial adequacy Occupational prestige Retirement planning
Belgrave & Haug (1995)	Investigated predictors of retirement adaptation among 428 men and women.	Health Family income Work commitment Unemployment history
Gregory (1983)	Investigated predictors of life satisfaction among 79 retirees in Richmond, Virginia.	Amount of activity Enjoyment of activity Occupational behavior Meaningfulness of activity

tirement decisions. Husbands are more likely to have a higher income, longer tenure in their employment, and more physical health problems. Studies are needed to further explore the retirement decision process among women.

Another shortcoming of the retirement literature has been its exclusive focus on the health and well-being of the retiree without examining impacts as to other family members or family support structures. Although men and women generally report improved relationships after retirement (Vinick & Ekerdt, 1989), longitudinal studies of well-being and marital satisfaction fail to show improvements for men or women after retirement. In fact, retirement of married men may have some negative impacts on the well-being of their wives (Lee & Shehan, 1989). This may be the result of changes in the division of household labor that lead to interpersonal conflicts after retirement. Although one might predict that retirement would lead to improved marital relationships because more available time could be spent together, this hypothesis has not been supported. Retirement may follow a long phase of the marital relationship in which stability is achieved within the context of active employment. After retirement, a balance in the relationship must be reestablished based on a new set of routines and patterns of communication. Based on the tentative conclusions regarding women and retirement, we have not made any predictions in our decision-logic diagram (Figure 17-3) about the influence of gender on retirement characterization.

Compulsory Retirement

Compulsory retirement, although highly restricted by recent changes to U.S. employment laws, still affects some older workers. College professors, police officers, prison guards, and fire fighters were the last occupations in which

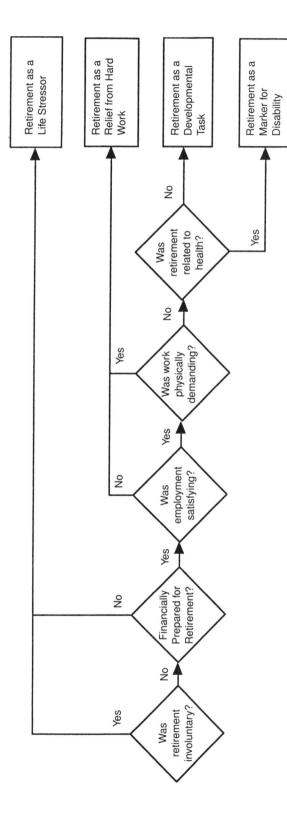

Figure 17-3. A decision logic diagram for identifying differences in retirement experiences among population subsets.

compulsory retirement was officially abolished in 1993. However, employees of small businesses and several other exempted groups may still encounter a compulsory retirement age. The percentage of older male workers facing compulsory retirement has decreased from approximately 50% in the 1960s to less than seven percent in 1985 (3% for older female workers) (Sherman, 1985). For those few workers still facing compulsory retirement, a mismatch may exist between the designated mandatory retirement age and the age at which an older worker feels "ready" to make the retirement transition. Voluntary retirees report greater well-being and life satisfaction after retirement than either mandatory retirees or those continuing to work (Crowley, 1986). Therefore, mandatory retirement may represent a life stressor that produces negative feelings about the retirement transition.

Today, although few workers face outright compulsory retirement based on age, many older workers may be coerced or induced to retire, either through financial incentives or by subtle attempts to convince older workers that their capabilities are reduced or skills outdated. Others may be forced to leave their employment during corporate downsizing and reorganization. Among older workers who lose their jobs, 28% are reemployed, 10% remain unemployed, and 62% decide to leave the labor force by retiring early (Manheimer, 1994). In a study of early retirees from the auto industry, Hardy and Quadagno (1995) found that both dissatisfaction with retirement and feelings of having "retired too early" were associated with the experience of undesired transfers and plant closings. Therefore, retirement may still be perceived by retirees as involuntary if coercive tactics are used to force an early retirement.

Financial Preparation

For many older workers, economic factors represent the largest single change associated with the retirement process. During this time, wage earnings are replaced by social security benefits and other asset and pension sources (see Figure 17-4). Preretirement income and financial losses associated with retirement have been shown to be related to the decision to retire (George et al., 1984) as well as to satisfaction with retirement (Dorfman, 1989; Palmore, Fillenbaum, & George, 1984). For most older workers, however, retirement today does not have the catastrophic financial implications that it held only several decades ago. On the average, retirees today experience an average reduction in income of only 25%, from $8,500 to $6,400 (Dorfman, 1989; Palmore et al., 1984). Such income is usually comprised of some combination of social security, pension plans, retirement savings plans, or entitlements for special or disabled groups. Although these programs appear to provide most retirees with a satisfactory retirement, poor financial planning may make the retirement process stressful for some. Of the 30% of retirees who find retirement stressful, poor family finances is one of the primary correlates (Bosse, Aldwin, Levenson, & Workman-Daniels, 1991). For this subset of retirees, models that characterize retirement as a potential stressor may be most appropriate.

The wide range of financial situations found among retirees has created dramatic diversity in retirement experiences. This has not always been the case.

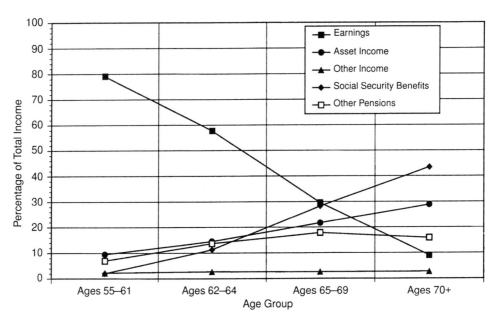

Figure 17-4. Sources of income by percentage among older Americans in 1986. From *A Generation of Change: A Profile of America's Older Population* (p. 490), by J. S. Siegel, 1993, New York: Russel Sage Foundation. Copyright 1993 by Russell Sage Foundation.

In the 1950s, more than a third of older adults had incomes that fell below the poverty line. This proportion has decreased dramatically with installment of social security, increasing availability of retirement pension plans, and increasing popularity of retirement savings plans. In 1984, only 12% of retirees fell below the poverty line (Crystal, 1986). Still, certain groups among older individuals continue to experience financial difficulties after retirement, particularly formerly married women (Keith, 1985), members of minorities (Crystal, 1986), and the very old (Crystal, 1986). As a group, however, there is reliable evidence to suggest that risk of becoming poor is no greater for older adults than it is for younger individuals (Crystal, 1982, 1986; Danzieger, van der Gaag, Smolensky, & Taussig, 1984). Among retirees, financial preparedness has been shown to be a strong predictor of life satisfaction after retirement (Glamser, 1976).

Recognizing the importance of financial security after retirement, researchers have begun to look at the success of employer-sponsored retirement preparation programs. Although currently offered by only a few of the largest employers, these programs have been well received by workers and appear to improve workers' attitudes about retirement. Abel and Hayslip (1987) found that workers participating in six weekly 2-hour retirement planning classes maintained more positive attitudes about retirement and a higher locus of control for making retirement plans. This study, however, included only one 2-week follow-up after the 6-week intervention. In a rural sample, Dorfman (1989) found that retirement preparedness was related to later retirement satisfaction. Retirement preparation programs, however, remain most popular among work-

ers needing help the least. In a study of older workers volunteering to participate in retirement preparation programs, Campione (1988) found that participants tended to be married with children, had no major health problems, and
were of higher occupational status. Future work is needed to develop methods
for recruiting in these programs groups of older workers who are at higher risk
for financial difficulties.

Occupational Characteristics and Employment Satisfaction

A high level of intrinsic job satisfaction may delay the decision to retire. In
cross-sectional studies, older workers show a higher degree of commitment to
their work (Hedges, 1983), and this difference can be explained by the greater
occupational prestige and job satisfaction attained by older workers (Hanlon,
1986). An inverse relationship between job attitudes and retirement attitudes
has been suggested for older workers (Johnson & Strother, 1962), although this
hypothesis has received only marginal support (Eden & Jacobson, 1976; Goudy
et al., 1975). The importance of job satisfaction in the decision to retire has been
supported by an apparent preretirement process: as older workers approach retirement, they tend to view their employment as more burdensome and less rewarding, regardless of age, health, or income (Ekerdt & DeViney, 1993).

For those in extremely stressful or dissatisfying work environments, retirement may represent an escape from the burden of work and an opportunity to
engage in more favorable leisure activities and interests. This subset of retirees
has received little research attention because few workers remain in high-stress
professions as they approach retirement. In addition, dissatisfied employees
have been excluded from research studies because they tend not to participate
in employer-sponsored research protocols. With increased seniority and cre-
dentials, older workers tend to gravitate away from, or be promoted away from,
the most psychologically stressful or least satisfying assignments unless these
come with great financial rewards. Paramedics, air traffic controllers, and urban
police officers are known to transfer to less stressful positions, develop second
careers, or retire early as they build seniority. Still, a sizable percentage of older
workers report that their work makes them nervous or tired (Ekerdt & DeViney,
1993). For these individuals, retirement may be an opportunity to improve
health and well-being.

Another subset of retirees consists of those who find their work satisfying
and rewarding, although the work is physically demanding and involves substantial risks for injury. For these older workers, muscle strain or chronic conditions may be aggravated by physical aging processes. Retirement offers a relief
from severe physical demands and may provide opportunities for increasing
medical attention to chronic conditions and improving muscle conditioning.
Among blue-collar workers, Jacobson (1972) found that fatigue-producing factors of employment led to a greater desire to find relief through retirement. Retirees from these occupations experience improved health after retirement
(Ekerdt, Bosse, & LoCastro, 1983), and few continue to engage in activities requiring heavy physical exertion (Kelly, Steinkamp, & Kelly, 1986). Therefore,
retirement may be qualitatively different for workers of physically demanding

occupations than for others. This is one illustration of the impacts of health on the retirement process. Because health has been frequently cited as both an antecedent and consequence of retirement, we dedicate the next session to exploring this complex interaction.

HEALTH AND RETIREMENT

A long-standing myth is that retirement signals the onset of a spiraling pattern of health decline among retirees. This is based on the belief that the health of older individuals depends on "keeping busy" and that reductions in activity may compromise intellectual and physical functioning. Although retirees as a group report slightly diminished health after retirement (Fillenbaum, George, & Palmore, 1985), this effect is probably spurious, reflecting the inclusion of the few individuals who leave work as a result of failing health. In other words, retirement is merely a marker for the poor health that led some individuals to retire. As an illustration of this common misattribution, Ekerdt (1987) presents the well-known case of college football coach Paul "Bear" Bryant, who suffered heart failure and died 37 days after his retirement from coaching. In response to his death, casual observers were quick to acknowledge that "the Bear should never have retired," attributing his death to retirement from football. However, a more detailed reporting of events would later reveal that Coach Bryant retired as a result of a 3-year illness that eventually took his life. The best-controlled studies of health and retirement have indicated that retirement does not increase the risk of either death or health deterioration (Ekerdt et al, 1983; Fillenbaum *et al.*, 1985; Kasl, 1980; Minkler, 1981; Palmore *et al.*, 1984).

The popular belief that retirement leads to poor health continues to proliferate despite contrary research evidence. Ekerdt (1987) provides several explanations for this myth. First, he cites the work of Brim and Ryff (1980), who reported that "most people, in thinking about life events and their effects on behavior, tend to attribute causality to a single, large, vivid, and recent event." Retirement easily meets these criteria. Second, Ekerdt (1987) points out that popular theories about aging and retirement (reviewed later in this chapter) implicitly suggest that poor health is a logical outcome of retirement, noting both life event stress models and activity theory models. Third, Ekerdt reasons that "negative views of retirement are consistent with the cultural ideology that celebrates work as the source of self-worth, self-esteem, identity, and personal fulfillment." With these strong influences on the development of scientific hypotheses, the question of whether retirement causes poor health is likely to remain open to debate.

Although retirement seems to have little direct influence on health, health may be a major factor in the decision to retire. From 25% to 30% of older workers retire because of their failing health (Sherman, 1985). After chronological age, self-reported health is the strongest single predictor of the decision to retire (Monahan & Greene, 1987; Taylor & McFarlane-Shore, 1995). However, little is known about which aspects of health provide the greatest influence on the retirement decision and whether a health rationale for retirement can, in fact, be justified. We have proposed a biopsychosocial model that incorporates various aspects of objective and subjective health measures to describe the influence of health on the older worker's decision to retire (see Figure 17-5). In this model, health is divided into four constructs: (1) *functional health status,* an objective measure of disability, (2) *perceived vitality,* the subjective component of health assessment, (3) *medical regimen,* encompassing patterns of health care use, specific diagnoses made, and medical treatments prescribed; and (4) *health behavior,* including diet, exercise, and risk behaviors that influence health status. To some degree, each of these aspects of health is determined by an individual's subjective interpretation of symptoms, health attitudes, and health knowledge. We have included this health mediator in the model as *psychological response* to physical signs and symptoms. *Psychosocial moderators* (e.g., social support, coping resources, personality factors) may further attenuate the influence of health on the retirement decision.

Health has repeatedly been shown to correlate with life satisfaction after retirement (Belgrave & Haug, 1995; Dorfman, 1989). Because most retirement studies have examined health using a global self-assessment, discrete models like the biopsychosocial model just presented are difficult to support from empirical evidence. A few studies, however, have suggested that some components of health may influence retirement differentially. For example, Antonovosky and Sagy (1990) suggested that retirement is coincident with an increased sense of health maintenance and epidemiological data (Karp, 1988; Siegel, 1993) support this hypothesis (see Figure 17-6). Therefore, the salience of health to individuals may be more important in their decision to retire than their health per se. Another study showed that perceptions of youthfulness were predictive of

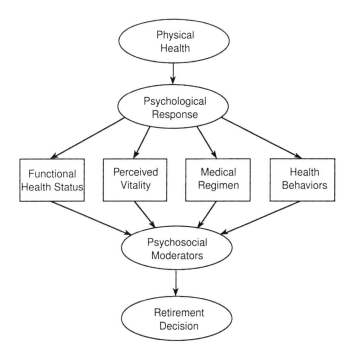

Figure 17-5. Aspects of health related to the retirement decision.

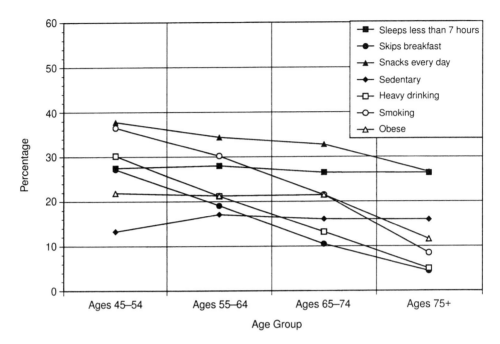

Figure 17-6. Percentage of older Americans with selected health practices. From *A Generation of Change: A Profile of America's Older Population* (p. 294), by J. S. Siegel, 1993, New York: Russell Sage Foundation. Copyright 1993 by Russell Sage Foundation.

retirement age among older executives (Eden & Jacobson, 1976). This finding highlights the importance of perceived vitality (or, conversely, frailty) in the decision to retire.

Older workers who retire for health reasons may be at increased risk for poor retirement outcomes. These individuals report less satisfaction with retirement (Crowley, 1986; Dorfman, 1989), report retirement to be more stressful (Bosse *et al.,* 1991), and possess greatest risk for poor health after retirement (Crowley, 1986). Unfortunately, those who retire for health reasons are also less likely to have engaged in financial planning for retirement (Campione, 1988; McPherson & Guppy, 1979), and this further complicates affordability of required health care services after retirement. Again, it is unclear whether the retirement event itself has any tendency to aggravate chronic health conditions. As discussed earlier, empirical studies have not supported this hypothesis. However, older workers with serious health concerns have not been studied as a separate subset. For this group, the opposite effect may actually exist. Retirement may result in improved health as a result of refocusing one's lifestyle to accommodate health concerns (e.g., smoking cessation, exercise, dietary improvements). In support of this hypothesis, 43% of retirees report improvements in health after retirement (Schnore, 1985).

The myth that retirement leads to health decline has been fueled by the stereotype that individuals become physically and socially inactive after retirement. This is the primary rationale for the disengagement theory of retirement that we discuss in the next sections. In fact, inactivity after retirement is rare

(Kelly *et al.,* 1986; Marino-Schorn, 1986). Instead, activity levels after retirement tend to mirror those experienced throughout the life span. Therefore, intraindividual differences in activity levels after retirement are minute in comparison with interindividual differences across the life span.

THEORIES OF RETIREMENT

In 1961, the first theory of social behavior in late adulthood described the disengagement of older Americans from social participation as a normative developmental process (Cumming & Henry, 1961). This influential yet controversial "disengagement theory" sparked several competing theories of normal aging, and these have further guided our exploration of retirement and other aging phenomena. The following review includes a hybrid list of both retirement-specific and more general theories of aging. Unlike previous reviews (Burbank, 1986; Jonsson, 1993; L. W. Smith, Patterson, & Grant, 1992) ours focuses on the application of the various theories to unique phases and circumstances of retirement and the overt or implied incorporation of health considerations into the theories.

One word of caution is necessary before we proceed with a review of psychological theories of retirement. Although theories of aging are often labeled *developmental* theories, this terminology implies both a universality and a biological determinism that are not empirically supported among older individuals. Whereas stages of infant development can be predicted with reasonable accuracy, developmental stages among older individuals can be extremely divergent and uncertain. Therefore, we prefer to characterize these theoretical models as probabilistic psychosocial theories of adult behavior that fall within the social and physiological contexts of aging. Although this argument may seem purely semantic, it highlights the need to address diversity among older individuals and avoid ageist beliefs related to reduced capacities.

Disengagement Theory

Disengagement theory proposes that the normative aging process involves a gradual and mutual withdrawal from individuals and society in the years preceding death. This theory (Cumming & Henry, 1961) is based on the declining rates of physical and social activity commonly observed among older individuals. Although this observation is factual, the disengagement theory provides few explanatory mechanisms. Presumably, the underlying purpose of social disengagement is that there be less disruption in social networks at the time of death. This theory has received little empirical support and has been criticized as untestable (Hochschild, 1975) and supporting negative stereotypes (Havinghurst, Neugarten, & Tobin, 1968). Moreover, this theory is contrary to the evidence that social support is related to increased life satisfaction at all ages (Neugarten, 1976). Nevertheless, this theory was influential in highlighting the need for further psychological study of lifestyle changes in late life. Disengagement theory characterized retirement as a step toward reduced status among peers and termination of collegial relationships.

Earlier in this chapter, we divided the retirement process into three separate stages: retirement planning, retirement decision, and retirement adaptation. Table 17-2 summarizes each of the major retirement theories and their ability to describe each of these three stages. The disengagement theory provides a framework for the decision to retire, but not for either retirement planning or retirement adaptation. The disengagement theory would predict that efforts to retain social standing and increase interaction (to "reengage") after retirement would be maladaptive, opposing empirical findings to the contrary. Similarly, financial planning for an active retirement would seem to counter the belief that retirement should be a period of reduced activity and social withdrawal. Therefore, disengagement theory provides a partial but unsupported explanation of the reasons people retire. The theory does not, however, attempt to describe the full range of behaviors and activities associated with the retirement process. Earlier in this chapter, we proposed that the nature of retirement varies depending on life circumstances (see Figure 17-3). We hypothesized that retirement may represent a life stressor for some, a relief from hard work for others, or a marker for poor health for still others. If none of these circumstances apply, then retirement might be best characterized as a normal developmental task of adulthood. Because disengagement theory assumes the latter characterization of retirement as a developmental task, it ignores the special circumstances of retirement that may warrant alternative conceptualizations.

Although health is not specifically included as a factor in the theory of disengagement, it may be the prevalence of poor health among older individuals that actually spawned this theory of aging. Older Americans report more physical health symptoms, receive more medical attention, and have more chronic health conditions than any other age group (*Older Americans Almanac;* Manheimer, 1994). Therefore, one might be tempted to conclude categorically that older individuals as a group are less equipped to maintain high levels of social interaction and physical activity. Disengagement theorists may have considered that social withdrawal would be health adaptive, in that less activity would reduce risks for stress and injury. This conclusion is contrary to the belief that social support may buffer the impacts of poor health. It also fails to address the majority of older individuals who, by and large, are in good health and have no physical disabilities.

Activity Theory

In opposition to disengagement theory, Havinghurst and colleagues (1968) developed a conceptualization of aging that promoted increased physical and social activity in later life. Referred to as *activity theory* by Atchley (1976), this theory suggests that retirement creates a void in peoples' lives that must be replaced by other activities. Four primary principles are associated with retirement: (1) retirement from work results in a sense of loss; (2) the focus of this sense of loss may vary between individuals; (3) satisfactory adjustment to retirement involves substituting something to replace the loss; and (4) the substi-

Table 17-2. A Comparison of Psychological Theories of Retirement

Theory	Description	Process best described			Characterization of retirement				Implied predictors of poor outcome
		Planning	Event	Adapting	Stressor	Relief	Task	Health	
Disengagement	Inevitable and mutual social withdrawal is normative and adaptive.		X				X	X	Failure to disengage from social activities and work relationships.
Activity	Postretirement social activities are necessary to replace sense of loss.			X	X			X	Failure to replace work activities with leisure activities after retirement.
Continuity	Lifestyle stability is the key to maintain well-being.	X		X	X			X	Failure to minimize lifestyle impacts of retirement.
Congruence	Personally meaningful activities must be maintained to ensure well-being.			X	X	X			Mismatch between normative retirement activities and personal values and goals.
Developmental	Retirement involves successful completion and advancement through developmental stages.	X	X	X			X		Failure to advance through normative stages of the retirement process.
Stress/coping	Coping strategies are key to managing the stress of retirement.			X	X				Failure to cope correctly with the stressors of the retirement transition.
Personality	Personality traits can predict successful adaptation to retirement.			X	X				Possessing strong personality traits of introversion and neuroticism.

tution typically involves replacing one set of activities for another. The activity theory is empirically supported by the frequent finding that social activities are positively correlated with adjustment among postretirement samples (e.g., Gregory, 1983; Havinghurst, Munnicks, Neugarten, & Thomas, 1969; Maddox, 1963). Activity theory also predicts that individuals who expect to experience the greatest sense of loss after retirement might delay its onset, and this has been shown among white-collar workers (Mitchell, Levine, & Pozzebon, 1988). However, the empirical evidence for an actual substitution of activities after retirement is much weaker (Beck & Page, 1988) and increased activities after retirement have been linked to negative as well as positive moods and attitudes (Reich, Zautra, & Hill, 1987). The activity theory also ignores the possibility that increased activities are a reflection, not a determinant, of positive adjustment after retirement.

Activity theory is primarily a model for adaptation to retirement (see Table 17-2). It suggests that poor adjustment to retirement results from a failure to replace work-related activities. This belief has achieved widespread popular support, and community programs for older Americans frequently promote increased social activity. In recent years, however, social researchers have begun to scrutinize more closely the causal relationships between social support and improved well-being and health. Metanalyses have indicated that social activity is only modestly correlated with subjective well-being (Okun, Stock, Haring & Witter, 1984) and is unrelated to recovery from illness (Reifman, 1995; C. E. Smith, Fernengel, Holcroft, Gerald, & Marien, 1994). Also, physical illness may have a tendency to mobilize greater support, further complicating the causal relationship between social support and health (Grant, Patterson, & Yager, 1988). Therefore, the primary thesis of the activity theory, that a consistent level of social activity is necessary for maintaining well-being after retirement, is becoming more suspect. Studies that are better equipped to dissect the bidirectional influences between social activity and well-being after retirement are needed.

An activity theory of retirement assumes that retirement is either a health marker (in the case of voluntary retirement) or a potential stressor (if retirement is involuntary). One shortfall of the activity theory is that, with the exception of poor health, it provides no explanation of the reasons for retirement. If maximizing activity levels is the key to well-being, why should a worker choose retirement over continued service? Perhaps the decision to retire is driven principally by the social influence of secular trends. Another explanation might be that retirement marks the time at which leisure activities become more desirable than work activities. As originally proposed, however, the activity theory does not specify the types of activities that are more helpful to alleviate the sense of loss experienced after retirement.

Because activity theory is primarily a theory about social behavior, physical health behavior was not included in its inception. Perhaps this is because physical and social activities are less distinguishable among older individuals. Nevertheless, physical health may be the spurious variable driving the correlations between activity and well-being after retirement that form the basis for this theory. Depressed mood and reduced social activity in postretirement years may be independent responses to deteriorating health. Both have been linked to poor health in older individuals with chronic health conditions (Grant *et al.*, 1988). Therefore, activity levels may reflect physical limitations, rather than volitional responses to a sense of loss after retirement. This is particularly likely given the apparent importance of health in the decision to retire (Fillenbaum *et al.*, 1985; McPherson & Guppy, 1979; Taylor & McFarlane-Shore, 1995).

Continuity Theory

Rosow (1963) observed that well-adjusted adults in their peak years (early to middle 50s) appeared to experience few life changes. Individuals from this age group were typically past stages of rapid career advancement, relocations, responsibilities of child rearing, and other lifestyle transitions. From this he concluded that life satisfaction is negatively correlated with change. Empirical support comes from retrospective studies that report more successful retirement adjustment among those experiencing the fewest lifestyle changes in retirement (Long, 1987). These studies have focused primarily on white-collar workers, and measurements of lifestyle change have not been objectively validated. Like the disengagement and activity theories, the continuity theory of retirement lacks specificity. By labeling change as an agent of maladjustment, the benefits of positive lifestyle changes are ignored.

In a study of leisure activities among older workers, only those activities characterized as "core" activities seemed to maintain continuity over time (Kelly *et al.*, 1986). These included family, social, and home-based activities. In contrast, recreational activities, exercise, and travel showed consistent reductions with age. This provides some support for the continuity theory over the activity theory, in that meaningful activities appeared constant over time, and no increase in leisure activities was observed after retirement. The activity theory, on the other hand, would predict that leisure activities should increase after retirement in order to fill the void left by reduced work-related activities. The continuity theory also predicts that workers should be weary of the lifestyle and social transitions of retirement. This appears to be true for many older workers. Retirees are often hesitant to retire, and their estimated retirement age increases as they approach their original estimated departure date (Ekerdt *et al.*, 1980). However, the continuity theory also predicts that retirees should welcome opportunities to engage in part-time work and this is not the case. Only 20% of retirees are interested in part-time employment after retirement (Toughill, Mason, Beck, & Christopher, 1993).

Like activity theory, continuity theory is better at predicting adaptation to retirement than explaining why older workers retire. However, the continuity theory also provides an explanation for why workers engage in retirement planning: to attenuate the lifestyle impacts of retirement. Early investments in retirement savings plans, for example, help to offset the financial losses of retirement and thereby increase lifestyle continuity. Successful retirement planning may prevent lifestyle changes such as relocating, giving up club memberships, or reducing social functions after retirement. Continuity theory, then, may help explain the desire to minimize the financial impacts of retirement. Like activity theory, continuity theory assumes retirement to be either a stressor (in the case of involuntary retirement) or a marker for poor health (when retirement is voluntary). It is also similar to the activity theory in that it provides no explanation for why individuals should choose to retire.

Congruence Theories

We have chosen to use a single heading, congruence theory, to describe a number of theories of retirement that emphasize the subjective interpretation of meaningful activity. Like the activity and continuity theories, congruence theories focus on activity as the key to successful retirement adaptation. Congruence theories, however, go one step further by attaching personal salience ratings to individual activities. These theories have included accommodation theory (Shanas, 1972), adjustment theory (Atchley, 1976), and the model of human occupation (Jonsson, 1993). Each of these theories seeks to group activities based on their subjective meaningfulness to individuals. For example, adjustment theory (Atchley, 1976) states that internal compromises are made in retirement that produce changes in one's hierarchy of personal goals. These value adjustments result in the changes in desired activities that constitute retirement. Similarly, the accommodation theory (Shanas, 1972) claims that changes in behavior after retirement occur because of changes in perceived needs or self-concept. The model of human occupation (Jonsson, 1993) predicts that postretirement activities involve a balance between work, rest, and leisure and that chosen activities are based on ratings of personal meaningfulness.

The goal of congruence theories was to incorporate specificity with regard to activities and to explain their differential relationships with life satisfaction after retirement. Each theory has received some empirical support. However, differences in terminology and psychological constructs have prevented attempts to consolidate these ideas into a single cohesive model of retirement. Like the activity and continuity theories, congruence theories describe primarily adaptation to retirement. Because congruence theories depend on subjective interpretations of activities, retirement might be characterized as either a stressor or a relief, depending on the perceived meaningfulness of work activities prior to retirement. Unlike the activity or continuity theories, congruence theories of retirement provide an explanation of the reasons for retirement: people are responding to a set of revamped values, personal goals, or life meaning.

If retirement is part of an age-related shift in personal goals and interests as the congruence theories suggest, then changing attitudes about health may also be a part of this transitional period. At retirement age, individuals are more likely to acknowledge their own mortality and perceive their physical conditions as potentially life threatening. If we return to our biopsychosocial model of health and retirement (Figure 17-5), the congruence theory might predict that the psychological response to physical health is amplified in later life and that this results in heightened perceptions of disability, frailty, medical needs, and health risks. These changes in health perceptions may partially influence the decision to retire; the conclusion is supported by the relationships between health and retirement (Fillenbaum *et al.,* 1985; McPherson & Guppy, 1979; Taylor & McFarlane-Shore, 1995). However, the importance of other factors in the decision to retire may sometimes overshadow the role of health perceptions (Belgrave & Haug, 1995).

Developmental Theory

The developmental theory of retirement is sometimes referred to as the salutogenic model or the sense of coherence model. This theory (Antonovsky, 1979; Antonovsky & Sagy, 1990) describes the retirement transition as a series of developmental tasks that lead to positive well-being and increased life satisfaction. Although very similar to congruence theories of retirement, the developmental theory is the first to represent retirement as both voluntary and process-based. In this theory, based loosely on the last two stages of Erikson's well-known life-cycle model, social reintegration and disintegration occurs as a process involving four factors: active involvement, reevaluation of life satisfaction, reevaluation of world outlook, and the sense of health maintenance. Active involvement describes challenges throughout the life span, but especially after retirement, to reorganize activities in response to changes in personal goals or societal expectations. Reevaluation of life satisfaction is the challenge for older adults to provide meaning and direction in their lives based on reflecting on and consolidating past accomplishments. Reevaluation of world outlook is the challenge to integrate knowledge and experiences into coherent and global attitudes about social order, science, religion, and the role of mankind. The fourth factor, sense of health maintenance, occurs as a result of increases in morbidity and mortality rates after age 55. Because the developmental theory does not characterize retirement as a single event, it is flexible enough to provide explanations for retirement preparation, the retirement event, and adaptation to retirement (see Table 17-2). For example, reevaluation of world outlook may begin to occur long before the actual date of retirement. Life experience and the evolution of both professional and social roles may foster changes in attitudes throughout the life span, and retirement may be just one by-product of this attitudinal process. After retirement, world outlook may continue to change in response to the shift from a work setting to other roles. The developmental theory suggests that the retirement event is merely a milestone for life-span changes in each of the four factors. The developmental theory is empirically supported by evidence for a preretirement process (Ekerdt & DeViney, 1993; Evans *et al.*, 1985), changes in preferred retirement ages over time (Ekerdt *et al.*, 1980; Ekerdt, Vinick & Bosse, 1989), and phased changes in satisfaction after retirement (Ekerdt *et al.*, 1985).

The developmental theory of retirement is the only psychological model that incorporates health as a component to the retirement transition. Its fourth factor, sense of health maintenance, recognizes the changing attitudes about health that seem to co-occur with retirement (Fries & Crapo, 1981). If we consider our biopsychosocial model for the impacts of health on the decision to retire (Figure 17-5), the sense of health maintenance factor from the developmental theory is consistent with our recognition that both health behaviors and perceived vitality may impact the decision to retire. As age-equivalent peers begin to experience more disabling or life-threatening illnesses, an individual, by social comparison, is more likely to feel vulnerable. Thus, more time might be spent in health contemplation, health-promoting activities, or grieving losses in physical vitality. More detailed studies of the changing health philosophies of older adults are needed.

Stress and Coping Theory

In the stress model, an individual's reaction to retirement depends on the degree to which retirement is perceived as stressful or threatening (Lazarus & Folkman, 1984). A number of variables, including the effectiveness of one's coping responses and the abundance and quality of social support available, may mediate the relationship between retirement and adjustment. George (1980) differentiates between coping responses, which consist of behavioral and intrapsychic reactions, and other moderating and mediating variables, including demographics, situational factors, or personality characteristics. Stress and coping models have been more descriptive than explanatory, including multiple variables and many potential relationships between variables (L. W. Smith *et al.,* 1992).

Stress and coping models of retirement have viewed retirement as a life event occurring within the context of personal meaning, threat appraisal, and contextual variables (Grant *et al.,* 1988; L. W. Smith *et al.,* 1992). Coping responses—the behavioral and cognitive reactions intended to reduce stress—may be more or less appropriate for specific stressors. This belief has spawned attempts to grade the appropriateness of particular coping strategies for specific types of stressors (L. W. Smith *et al.,* 1992). Stress and coping models have predominated in the study of aging and health. Symptoms of chronic illness, death of a spouse, and other life events have been characterized as stressors that require the use of coping skills to attenuate negative emotional impacts of these events. Retirement, for some, may have similar qualities. As we have indicated earlier (see Figure 17-3), retirement may be a stressor only under special circumstances; for example, when retirement is involuntary or coerced, or when individuals are financially ill prepared for their retirement years. Therefore, stress and coping models of retirement may be applicable only for those who experience unfortunate circumstances linked to their retirement transition.

In other applications, the primary outcome of stress and coping models has been diminished mental health or physical health or both. Although several underlying mechanisms have been proposed to link stressors to poor health outcomes, the primary paths have been via depressed mood or other symptoms of depression. Depression is strongly correlated with physical health symptoms, presumably because depression leads to reduced immunity or reductions in healthy behaviors. Others have speculated that depression may be simply an early reflection, rather than an agent, of physical health symptoms. In studies of retirement, the primary outcome has been life satisfaction, not depressive symptoms. However, these two variables appear to be strongly correlated as well. Therefore, for those individuals who are at risk for depression, dissatisfaction with life after retirement may contribute to depressive symptoms which, in turn, may lead to increased symptoms of physical illness. The stress and coping model of retirement may provide a useful theoretical framework in which to study the effects of retirement among a depression-prone subgroup, for example, a group of older workers with histories of affective disorders. For many other retirees, the stress and coping model appears to be inconsistent with empirical data that suggests only minor fluctuations in life satisfaction at the time of retirement.

Personality Theories

One recent addition to retirement theories has been the incorporation of personality traits as moderators of retirement outcomes. We include this brief addition as a separate theoretical category because conventional psychological variables such as personality traits have been noticeably absent from theories of retirement. As early as 1979, researchers noted that personality variables such as Type A behavior, orientation toward planning, and inner-directedness may be important to retirement adaptation (Atchley, 1976). Yet, few studies have investigated this possibility. Recently, Reis and Pushkar-Gold (1993) have suggested that successful adaptation to retirement may be related to the personality traits of hardiness, neuroticism, attachment, introversion, and personal flexibility. Although empirical studies have yet to test these hypotheses, the significant influence of personality on many other aspects of behavior would suggest a probable role in retirement. It is doubtful, however, that personality variables alone would provide the best model for understanding retirement preparation, the retirement decision, and adaptation to retirement for most older workers.

As we have suggested with previous theoretical frameworks, personality traits might be used to identify subgroups of older workers at high risk for poor retirement outcomes. Broader psychological theories of personality and psychopathology provide some support for this hypothesis. Attachment theory, for example, might predict that because retirement involves the dissolution of interpersonal relationships, it may result in feelings of loss or hostility in those who are insecurely or anxiously attached to their coworkers. For older workers who have some tendencies to be socially introverted, eccentric, or dysthymic, retirement may represent a difficult social transition. No empirical studies have examined the impacts of retirement to these at-risk populations of older workers.

SUMMARY

Implications of Theories

What do the aforementioned theories suggest about the nature of retirement? Although most of these theories describe retirement as a discrete event, we suggest that the developmental theory, which describes retirement as part of a long-term developmental process, may be more accurate. Three theories (stress and coping theory, activity theory, and continuity theory) portray retirement as an externally controlled event that requires adjustment and adaptation by the individual. In contrast, the remaining four theories provide for the role of the individual in planning for and scheduling their own retirement. The latter theories seem more relevant today, given the voluntary nature of retirement for most older workers. The congruence and developmental theories are the most dynamic of the theories because they accent the underlying importance of changing attitudes and interests during the retirement process. A personality theory of retirement is helpful to highlight the contribution of psychological characteristics, not just demographic characteristics, to the retirement process.

Empirical tests of the various theories of retirement have been few, and these studies have focused on limited professional and demographic subgroups. In general, the disengagement theory has received the least support, and the activity theory has received the most. Variables frequently cited to impact retirement satisfaction are health, wealth, retirement preparation, activity levels, and vocational type (see Table 17-1 for a partial listing of empirical studies). Studies of large, inclusive samples have demonstrated only slight variations in life satisfaction, health, and emotional distress during the retirement transition. Few studies, however, have identified population subgroups that may be more susceptible to maladjustment during the retirement transition. Special at-risk groups might include individuals facing mandatory retirement, those with greatly diminished income after retirement, those with high-risk personality features or psychiatric histories, those who retire due to ill health or caregiving, or those who are experiencing concurrent life stressors (e.g., relocation, bereavement).

Why is a theoretical framework necessary to study the phenomenon of retirement? The goal of retirement research is to understand what factors might lead to improved quality of life after the traditional "working years." Theories help to provide hypothesized causal links that can be empirically supported or rejected. They also help to narrow the focus of studies to only the most salient features responsible for causal influences. Theory development has recast retirement as a process rather than an event. It has also led us to consider variables that might increase the risks for poor retirement outcomes. As we have suggested here, it is not likely that a single theory will be sufficient to describe the retirement process for all older workers. Instead, a number of theories may be applicable depending on the circumstances of retirement, individual personality traits and values, and life history. More theory-based empirical studies of retirement are necessary in order to determine the most important factors contributing to satisfying retirement processes among special groups.

The Changing Face of Retirement

Why should retirement remain an important field of study in clinical geropsychology? Past evidence suggests only slight fluctuations in most outcome variables throughout the retirement transition, at least when heterogeneous and inclusive samples of retirees are studied. Nevertheless, future demographic and workplace changes may raise new questions about retirement. The "aging of America" as baby boomers reach retirement age with increased life expectancies will continue to generate interest in issues of aging such as retirement. Also, it appears that the normative age for retirement may gradually increase over the next fifty years. As this occurs, the psychological and health impacts of "nonretirement" may become a concern for those who would rather be retired.

Continuing changes in employment policies may also change the nature of retirement. During the past decade, the percentage of employees entitled to retirement benefits has begun to drop off, and the number of subcontracted employees has continued to grow. These employees must save (e.g., 402b) for their own retirements. Social Security benefits have been reduced and the definitions for receiving benefits have become more stringent. These forces suggest that new patterns of retirement and its meaning should emerge in the next 20 to 30 years. Finally, interest in retirement is fueled by a recognition that older individuals have been ignored in many areas of psychological study, and this has resulted in a shift from studying human development as a childhood process to studying it as a life-span process. There are probably fewer studies of retirement today than there are of the effects of school transfers among children, yet retirement affects a much larger population. For these reasons, increased interest in the psychological developmental processes of aging and probable changes in retirement itself are likely to fuel continued interest in retirement, its antecedents, and its consequences.

REFERENCES

Abel, B. J., & Hayslip, B. (1987). Locus of control and retirement preparation. *Journals of Gerontology, 42*, 165–167.

Antonovsky, A. (1979). *Health, stress and coping.* San Francisco: Jossey-Bass.

Antonovsky, A., & Sagy, S. (1990). Confronting developmental tasks in the retirement transition. *Gerontologist, 30*, 362–368.

Atchley, R. C. (1974). The meaning of retirement. *Journal of Communications, 24*, 97–101.

Atchley, R. C. (1976). *The sociology of retirement:* Schenkman.

Atchley, R. C. (1991). *Social forces and aging* (6th ed.). Belmont, CA: Wadsworth.

Beck, S. H., & Page, J. W. (1988). Involvement in activities and the psychological well-being of retired men. *Activities, Adaptation & Aging, 11*, 31–47.

Belgrave, L. L., & Haug, M. R. (1995). Retirement transition and adaptation: Are health and finances losing their effects? *Journal of Clinical Geropsychology, 1*, 43–66.

Bosse, R., Aldwin, C. M., Levenson, M. R., & Workman-Daniels, K. (1991). How stressful is retirement? Findings from the Normative Aging Study. *Journals of Gerontology, 46*, P9–P14.

Brim, O. G., & Ryff, C. D. (1980). On the properties of life events. In P. B. Baltes & O. G. Brim (Eds.), *Life-span development and behavior* (Vol. 3, pp. 368–388). New York: Academic.

Burbank, P. M. (1986). Psychosocial theories of aging: A critical evaluation. *Advances in Nursing Science, 9*, 73–86.

Campione, W. A. (1988). Predicting participation in retirement preparation programs. *Journals of Gerontology, 43*, S91–S95.

Crowley, J. E. (1986). Longitudinal effects of retirement on men's well-being and health. *Journal of Business and Psychology, 1*, 95–113.

Crystal, S. (1982). *America's old age crisis: Public policy and two worlds of aging.* New York: Basic Books.

Crystal, S. (1986). Measuring income and inequality among the elderly. *Gerontologist, 26*, 56–59.

Cumming, E., & Henry, W. H. (1961). *Growing old: The process of disengagement.* New York: Basic Books.

Danzieger, S., van der Gaag, J., Smolensky, E., & Taussig, M. (1984). Implications for the relative economic status of the elderly for transfer policy. In H. Aaron & G. Burtless (Eds.), *Retirement and economics behavior* (pp. 175–196). Washington, DC: Brookings Institution.

Dorfman, L. T. (1989). Retirement preparation and retirement satisfaction in the rural elderly. *Journal of Applied Gerontology, 8,* 432–450.

Eden, D., & Jacobson, D. (1976). Propensity to retire among older executives. *Journal of Vocational Behavior, 8,* 145–154.

Ekerdt, D. J. (1987). Why the notion persists that retirement harms health. *Gerontologist, 27,* 454–457.

Ekerdt, D. J., & DeViney, S. (1993). Evidence for a preretirement process among older male workers. *Journals of Gerontology, 48,* S35–S43.

Ekerdt, D. J., Bosse, R., & Mogey, J. M. (1980). Concurrent change in planned and preferred age of retirement. *Journals of Gerontology, 35,* 232–240.

Ekerdt, D. J., Bosse, R., & LoCastro, J. S. (1983). Claims that retirement improves health. *Journals of Gerontology, 38,* 231–236.

Ekerdt, D. J., Bosse, R., & Levkoff, S. (1985). An empirical test for phases of retirement: Findings from the Normative Aging Study. *Journals of Gerontology, 40,* 95–101.

Ekerdt, D. J., Vinick, B. H., & Bosse, R. (1989). Orderly endings: Do men know when they will retire? *Journals of Gerontology, 44,* S28–S35.

Evans, L., Ekerdt, D. J., & Bosse, R. (1985). Proximity to retirement and anticipatory involvement: Findings from the Normative Aging Study. *Journals of Gerontology, 40,* 368–374.

Fillenbaum, G. G., George, L. K., & Palmore, E. B. (1985). Determinants and consequences of retirement among men of different races and economic levels. *Journals of Gerontology, 40,* 85–94.

Fries, J. F., & Crapo, L. M. (1981). *Vitality and aging.* New York: Freeman.

George, L. K. (1980). *Role transition in later life.* Monterey: Brooks/Cole.

George, L. K., Fillenbaum, G. G., & Palmore, E. (1984). Sex differences in the antecedents and consequences of retirement. *Journals of Gerontology, 39,* 364–371.

Glamser, F. D. (1976). Determinants of a positive attitude toward retirement. *Journals of Gerontology, 31,* 104–107.

Goudy, W. J., Powers, E. A., & Keith, P. (1975). Work and retirement: A test of attitudinal relationships. *Journals of Gerontology, 30,* 193–198.

Grant, I., Patterson, T. L., & Yager, J. (1988). Social supports in relation to physical health and symptoms of depression in the elderly. *American Journal of Psychiatry, 145,* 1254–1258.

Gregory, M. D. (1983). Occupational behavior and life satisfaction among retirees. *American Journal of Occupational Therapy, 37,* 548–553.

Gustman, A. L., & Steinmeier, T. L. (1985). The effects of partial retirement on wage profiles of older workers. *Industrial Relations, 24,* 257–265.

Hanlon, M. D. (1986). Age and commitment to work. *Research on Aging, 8,* 289–316.

Hardy, M. A., & Quandagno, J. (1995). Satisfaction with early retirement: Making choices in the auto industry. *Journals of Gerontology, 50,* S217–S228.

Havinghurst, R. J., Neugarten, B. L., & Tobin, S. S. (1968). Disengagement and patterns of aging. In B. L. Neugarten (Ed.), *Middle age and aging: A reader in social psychology* (pp. 223–237). Chicago: University of Chicago Press.

Havinghurst, R. J., Munnicks, J. M., Neugarten, B. L., & Thomas, H. (1969). *Adjustment to retirement: A cross-sectional study.* New York: Humanities.

Hedges, J. N. (1983). Job commitment in America: Is it waxing or waning? *Monthly Labor Review, 106,* 17–24.

Hochschild, A. R. (1975). Disengagement theory: A critique and proposal. *American Sociological Review, 4,* 553–569.

Jacobson, D. (1972). Fatigue-producing factors in industrial work and preretirement attitudes. *Occupational Psychology, 46,* 193–200.

Johnson, J., & Strother, G. B. (1962). Job expectations and retirement planning. *Journals of Gerontology, 17,* 418–423.

Jondrow, J., Breehling, F., & Marcus, A. (1987). Older workers in the market for part-time employment. In S. H. Sandell (Ed.), *The problem isn't age: Work and older Americans* (pp. 81–98). New York: Praeger.

Jonsson, H. (1993). The retirement process in an occupational perspective: A review of literature and theories. *Physical & Occupational Therapy in Geriatrics, 11,* 15–34.

Karp, D. A. (1988). A decade of reminders: Changing age consciousness between fifty and sixty years old. *Gerontologist, 28,* 727–738.

Kasl, S. V. (1980). The impact of retirement. In C. L. Cooper & R. Payne (Eds.), *Current concerns in occupational stress* (pp. 171–193). New York: Praeger.

Keith, P. M. (1985). Work, retirement, and well-being among unmarried men and women. *Geron-tologist, 25*, 410–416.

Kelly, J. R., Steinkamp, M. W., & Kelly, J. R. (1986). Later life leisure: How they play in Peoria. *Gerontologist, 26*, 531–537.

Lazarus, R. S., & Folkman, S. (1984). *Stress, appraisal, and coping.* New York: Springer.

Lee, G. R., & Shehan, C. L. (1989). Retirement and marital satisfaction. *Journals of Gerontology, 44*, S226–S230.

Long, J. (1987). Continuity as a basis for change: leisure and male retirement. *Leisure Studies, 6*, 55–70.

Maddox, G. L. (1963). Activity and morale: A longitudinal study of selected elderly subjects. *Social Forces, 42*, 195–204.

Manheimer, R. J. (Ed.). (1994). *Older Americans almanac.* Detroit: Gale Research.

Marino-Schorn, J. A. (1986). Morale, work and leisure in retirement. *Physical & Occupational Therapy in Geriatrics, 4*, 49–59.

McPherson, B., & Guppy, N. (1979). Pre-retirement life-style and the degree of planning of retirement. *Journals of Gerontology, 34*, 254–263.

Minkler, M. (1981). Research on the effects of retirement: An uncertain legacy. *Journal of Health and Social Behavior, 22*, 117–130.

Mitchell, O. S., Levine, P. B., & Pozzebon, S. (1988). Retirement differences by industry and occupation. *Gerontologist, 28*, 545–551.

Monahan, D. J., & Greene, V. L. (1987). Predictors of early retirement among university faculty. *Gerontologist, 27*, 46–52.

Neugarten, B. L. (1976). Adaptation and the life cycle. *Geriatric Psychiatry, 6*, 16–20.

Okun, M. A., Stock, W. A., Haring, M. J., & Witter, R. A. (1984). The social activity/subjective well-being relation: A quantitative synthesis. *Research on Aging, 6*, 45–65.

Palmore, E. B., Fillenbaum, G. G., & George, L. K. (1984). Consequences of retirement. *Journals of Gerontology, 39* (1), 109–116.

Quinn, J. F., & Burkhauser, R. V. (1990). Work and retirement. In R. H. Binstock & L. K. George (Eds.), *Handbook of aging and the social sciences* (pp. 263–281). San Diego, CA: Academic.

Reich, J. W., Zautra, A. J., & Hill, J. (1987). Activity, event transactions, and quality of life in older adults. *Psychology and Aging, 2*, 116–124.

Reifman, A. (1995). Social relationships, recovery from illness and survival: A literature review. *Annals of Behavioral Medicine, 17*, 124–131.

Reis, M., & Pushkar-Gold, D.P. (1993). Retirement, personality, and life satisfaction: A review and two models. *Journal of Applied Gerontology, 12*, 124–131.

Rosow, H. (1963). Adjustment of the normal aged. In R. H. Williams, C. Tibbits, & W. Donahue (Eds.), *Processes of aging* (Vol. 2, pp. 195–223). New York: Atherton.

Schnore, M. (1985). *Retirement: Bane or blessing?* Toronto, Ontario, Canada: Wiffird Laurier University Press.

Schulz, J. H. (1988). *The economics of aging* (4th ed.). Dover, MA: Auburn House.

Shanas, E. (1972). Adjustment to retirement: substitution or accommodation? In F. M. Carp (Ed.), *Retirement* (pp. 219–243). New York: Behavioral Publications.

Sherman, S. R. (1985). Reported reasons retired workers left their last job: Findings from the New Beneficiary Survey, *Social Security Bulletin, 48*, 22–30.

Siegel, J. S. (1993). *A generation of change: A profile of America's older population.* New York: Russell Sage Foundation.

Smith, C. E., Fernengel, K., Holcroft, C., Gerald, K., & Marien, L. (1994). Meta-analysis of the associations between social support and health outcomes. *Annals of Behavioral Medicine, 16*, 352–362.

Smith, L. W., Patterson, T. L., & Grant, I. (1992). Work, retirement, and activity: Coping challenges for the elderly. In M. Herson (Ed.), *Handbook of social development: A life-span perspective* (pp. 475–502). New York: Plenum.

Taylor, M. A., & McFarlane-Shore, L. (1995). Predictors of planned retirement age: An application of Beehr's model. *Psychology and Aging, 10*, 76–83.

Toughill, E., Mason, D. J., Beck, T. L., & Christopher, M. A. (1993). Health, income, and postretirement employment of older adults. *Public Health Nursing, 10*, 100–107.

Vinick, B. H., & Ekerdt, D. J. (1989). Retirement: What happens to husband–wife relationships? *Journal of Geriatric Psychiatry, 24*, 23–40.

CHAPTER 18

Pain Management

Debra S. Morley and David I. Mostofsky

INTRODUCTION

Despite the increased interest in understanding age-related changes, and in developing service delivery systems for the expanding aging and elderly populations, there is a paucity of effort directed toward the effective utilization of behavioral theory and technologies in the analysis and remediation of pain problems in older adults. The accelerating nationwide increase in the elderly population, combined with the many behavior problems and deficits associated with their increased longevity, has contributed to the emergence of behavioral gerontology as an identified specialty, although there remains a relative lack of interest and research activity in the larger community of behavioral researchers concerning the problems of older individuals (Wisocki & Mosher, 1982). The need for an understanding of these problems is critical if we are to establish the basis for training and education of professional and other health specialists versed in the psychosocial aspects of comprehensive geriatric and gerontological management.

The elderly population is increasing. Older people are living longer, even when struck by catastrophic events (e.g., after experiencing strokes) and their vulnerability to pain leads to deterioration of the quality of life. Retrospective reports from surviving significant others of 200 deceased older community residents indicate that pain increased over the final year; 1 month before death, 66% experienced pain frequently or all the time. This was much higher than a matched comparison group of living persons (24%). Not surprisingly, these reports made clear that pain contributed significantly to a decrease in happiness and to depression (Moss, Lawton, & Glicksman, 1991).

Changes in health and mortality rates at later ages are important considerations for pain management. For example the 1960–1990 U.S. annual stroke

Debra S. Morley • Department of Psychology, Boston University, Boston, Massachusetts 02215.
David I. Mostofsky • Laboratory for Experimental Behavioral Medicine, Department of Psychology, Boston University, Boston, Massachusetts 02115.

Handbook of Clinical Geropsychology, edited by Michel Hersen and Vincent B. Van Hasselt. Plenum Press, New York, 1998.

411

mortality rate dropped 65.2%; for ages 85 and over, stroke mortality rates dropped 55.6%. The decline in total mortality for the entire U.S. population from 1960 to 1990 was 31.7%. For those 85 and over, the total mortality rate was 22.8% (Manton, 1997). Mortality rates for some deaths increased; for example, U.S. cancer mortality rates increased, including those for prostate cancer and female breast cancer. Relevant for our consideration is that the terminal stages of these cancer conditions are very painful and hard to manage.

With the dramatic changes taking place in medical health care organizations, and with an emphasis on the need to reduce the costs of hospital and drug charges (not to mention the likelihood of the attending iatrogenic complications that too frequently result from polypharmacy, especially in the elderly), use of behavioral protocols as primary or adjunctive interventions for pain control deserves serious consideration. Apart from economic pressures, programs and protocols must be developed that foster optimal conditions for extending independent living and an improved quality of living for the competent elderly. Pain left unattended is a major impediment to these goals. The prevalent medical or illness model of treatment is affected, in part, by cultural and professional ageism, and governed by the assumption of the inevitability of the aging process. This model tends to assign "sick roles" to older persons and postulates the irreversibility of problem behaviors. The most common treatment method for these behaviors and problems (especially when accompanied by dementia) relies on medication to the exclusion of any behavioral alternatives.

Depression and Pain

There are clear and powerful implications for pain management in both institutionalized or independent resident older persons; there is a compelling need to address issues of depression as an adjunctive if not primary factor in the etiology, modulation, and maintenance of pain associated with global discomfort. Psychological states such as depression have the potential to confound the treatment and assessment of pain. Depression can be masked by pain, and vice versa. Further, the *intensity* of existing depression or of a chronic pain condition may be aggravated by the presence of the other. The relationship between depression and pain may be intensified because older adults are at risk for an increased prevalence of both pain-producing ailments and depression (Kwentus, Harkins, Lignon, & Silverman, 1985). The association between depression and pain appears to vary as a function of age (Turk, Okifuji, & Scharff, 1995). Turk and colleagues studied 100 chronic pain patients divided into a group of younger patients (≤ 69 years of age) and another group of older patients (≥ 70 years of age). In the younger patient group, there was a low and nonsignificant association between pain severity and depression, whereas there was a significant association between pain and depression in the older patient group. An opposing view is represented by Gagliese and Melzack (1997), who reviewed a number of studies that have shown no age differences in the severity of depressive symptoms experienced by chronic pain patients, including Gagliese and Melzack (1995), Herr, Mobily, and Smith (1993), McCracken, Mosley, Plaud, Gross, and Penzien (1993), Middaugh, Levin, Kee, Barchiesi, and Roberts (1988),

Sorkin, Rudy, Hanlon, Turk, and Stieg (1990). In a study examining depression among chronic back pain sufferers, Herr and colleages (1993) failed to find any significant differences in the relationship of age and depressed mood between an elderly and a nonelderly group. The only significant finding about the relationship of age and depressed mood was that the elderly experienced fewer total hours per day in pain.

The neurotransmitter serotonin is common to both depression and pain, and this may account for the effectiveness of antidepressants in combating pain. Because depression and pain is more prevalent in the elderly, but most research on pain and psychological function has been done with younger populations, research applicability to aged populations is tenuous.

Part of the confounding nature of depression in older adults is that with failing health people experience more pain. In a study of 224 elderly subjects, subjective measures of physical health, such as pain and attitudes about one's own health, had a stronger association with depression than did more objective measures such as chronic diseases and functional limitations (Beekman, Kriegsman, Deeg, & van Tilburg, 1995). Crook, Rideout, and Browne (1984) reported that age-specific morbidity rates for persistent pain increased with age in a large epidemiological study of 500 randomly selected patients from a family practice. Depression appears to be closely linked with physical health. According to Bruce, Seeman, Merrill, and Blazer (1994), findings from the MacArthur Study of Successful Aging imply that depression and ill health influence each other. Poor physical health is a risk factor for depression in the elderly and depression may increase the risk of poor physical health. In a survey of 204 sufferers of chronic pain, depression was noted as one of the worst problems as a result of the chronic pain (Hitchcock, Ferrell, & McCaffery, 1994). Research findings of this kind require us to consider "wellness" programs for the elderly in which exercise and exposure to physical training are incorporated as part of the regular prophylactic and interventional programming for pain management. Such physical activities will likely go far in offsetting other age-related medical hazards whether or not they are causally linked to eventual pain and discomfort. The removal of confounding health problems implies the concurrent removal of potential added medication programs and sources of depression over failing health status.

Strong associations between pain and depression among elderly persons exist among those living in nursing homes as well as those living independently. For example, Cohen-Mansfield and Marx (1993) found, in a study of 408 nursing home residents with differing levels of cognitive impairment, that those who were depressed were more likely to be experiencing pain. Similarly, Parmelee, Katz, and Lawton (1991) obtained a significant relationship between pain and depression in a study of 598 nursing home and congregate apartment residents. Those with greater pain reported more depressive symptoms. G. M. Williamson and Schulz (1992) noted that pain and depression were correlated in a sample of community-residing elderly outpatients. Williams and Schulz (1988) found a direct relationship between depression and pain severity. That depressed elderly are more sensitive to pain than nondepressed elderly may be seen in Parmelee and colleagues' study, which found that those with possible major depression reported a greater amount of intense pain and had more pain complaints than did those with minor depression. Functional complaints were not more common among depressed than nondepressed. Rather, the depressed had a tendency to overstate pain complaints when there was a recognized health problem. Pain was studied in a group of 51 depressed elderly inpatients and 71 control subjects (Magni, Schifano, & DeLeo, 1985). They found that those patients suffering from dysthymia and atypical depression had the highest pain scores. Those patients suffering from major depression and adjustment disorder with depressive mood had lower scores. Pain is an often neglected area of research in the nursing home as may be seen from a study by Ferrell, Ferrell, and Osterweil (1990) who evaluated 97 patients from a 411-bed multilevel nursing home and found that 71% of the residents had at least one pain complaint, 34% with constant pain and 66% with intermittent pain.

Pain may function to conceal functional deficits (McIntosh, 1990) or as a means for getting attention, and as a result depression may be understated. For example, McCullough (1991) states that depression may be masked as pseudodementia, somatization, or anxiety, or it may be an underlying factor in pain or alcohol abuse. According to J. Williamson (1978), some elderly might mask depression with complaints of physical symptoms, such as pain, in an effort to avoid seeking help for or admitting to emotional issues. In contrast, others found no support for pain as a symptom of masked depression (Parmelee et al., 1991; Williams & Schulz, 1988). One must be cautious about surveys of depression and even diagnoses of depression. In a large study of 1,048 elderly subjects, Stewart and colleagues (1991) found that between 1% and 5% have major depression. They concluded that depression is underdiagnosed in older patients and that the best indicators of depression in older patients are multiple somatic complaints.

Anxiety and Pain

The relationship between anxiety and pain is not as well researched or understood as the association between depression and pain. The level of anxiety reported by older chronic pain patients appears to be lower than that reported for younger patients (Corran, Helme, & Gibson, 1993; McCracken et al., 1993). One study with a small number of subjects found no age difference (Middaugh et al., 1988) but another (Garron & Leavitt, 1979) found a small positive relationship of anxiety to pain although a correlation of depression with pain was not found. Casten, Parmelee, Kleban, Lawton, and Katz (1995) investigated the relationship between depression, anxiety, and pain in institutionalized elderly. Utilizing *Diagnostic and Statistical Manual of Mental Disorders,* 3rd edition, revised (*DSM-III-R*; American Psychiatric Association, 1987) criteria, the Profile of Mood States (POM), and the number of pain complaints and intensity, they concluded that anxiety, compared with depression, is more significantly related to pain.

Treatment Outcomes

Geriatric patients benefit from pain center treatment as much as younger patients (Cutler, Fishbain, Rosomoff, & Rosomoff, 1994). In one study, chronic pain patients were placed in three groups: geriatric, middle-aged, and younger. After pain center treatment, the geriatric group demonstrated a significant and meaningful improvement. Geriatric patients showed as great an improvement as the middle-aged and younger groups in the majority of measures utilized. Middaugh and colleagues (1988) found that geriatric patients profit just as much as, if not more than, than younger patients from chronic pain rehabilitation programs.

With rare exceptions, the concern with pain as it relates to the specific considerations of aging has been poorly documented. Despite the increased life incidence of pain associated with the elderly suffering from chronic and acute illnesses, there is often a neglected appreciation that proper pain management can ameliorate depression and vice versa. Admittedly, much has been written on the general subject of pain. Yet, a cautious observation seems justified: that inferences about pain from younger populations may not hold true for older persons, given the possible confounding presence of dementia, cognitive changes and decline, and an altered physiology (e.g., slower metabolism).

Psychophysics of Pain

Concerns with assessment issues, which have long plagued the scientific progress in the area of pain, present added problems when dealing with older adults. For example, it appears that, perhaps because of a long history with prior pain, older persons perceive more pain (chronic and acute) than younger persons (Closs, 1994), and may actually have different thresholds compared to younger groups (Yehuda & Carasso, 1997), although there are conflicting findings regarding pain threshold in the elderly (Collins & Stone, 1966; Harkins, Price, & Martelli, 1986; Sherman & Robillard, 1960). Chapman (1978), Sherman and Robillard (1964), and Schludermann and Zubek (1962) all report an increase in the pain threshold in older persons, whereas Procacci and colleagues (1974) report a decrease in sensitivity to pain in elderly. Others have found no change in pain threshold as a function of age (Birren, Shapiro, & Miller, 1959; Hardy, Wolff, & Goodell., 1943; Harkins & Chapman, 1976, 1977a; Mumford, 1965; Notermans, 1966; Schumacher, Goodell, Hardy, & Wolff, 1940). There also appear to be differences between young and old with regard to tolerance or threshold (or both) of pain *level*. A consensus in the research literature shows a decrease in pain tolerance in older persons; it appears that older persons are less able to cope with the pain (Collins & Stone, 1966; Harkins & Chapman, 1977b; Woodrow, Friedman, Siegalaub, & Collen, 1972). According to Zoob (1978), pain is a function of age. As a person ages, there appears to a decrease in sensitivity to pain. Fordyce (1976), on the other hand, states that older persons *complain* more of pain. Clark and Mehl (1973) try to bridge these contradictory results by proposing that the elderly just report more pain, and that this does not necessarily imply a greater *sensitivity* to pain. This would deny that altered physiology, psychological attitudes, and a reluctance to confirm the presence of pain may all contribute to raise the pain threshold. Indeed, for many elderly, pain is believed to be a normal part of aging (Ferrell *et al.*, 1990) and, therefore, they may not seek help and not infrequently may then go on to develop clinical depression as a result.

Chronic pain, which may be defined as the persistence of pain in the absence of any biological predisposing cause or significance, is considered to be more widespread in older persons than younger persons. Pain in the presence of pathology might be reported less often; however, in contrast to the situation with younger patients, chronic pain may have a greater impact on psychological, social, and physical function of older adults (Gibson, Katz, Corran, Farrell, & Helme, 1994).

ASSESSMENT ISSUES

Proper assessment of pain is needed for effective management. Too often, however, chronic pain goes undetected even in nursing homes where it is a familiar problem. This is a problem with both noncommunicative and communicative patients. In a study by Sengstaken and King (1993), physicians failed to detect pain in 34% of residents and, overall, pain was assessed less frequently among noncommunicative residents. The authors concluded that direct questioning at frequent intervals should be undertaken and that new assessment tools need to be created for the noncommunicative resident.

There are essentially two types of psychometric tools for use in the assessment of pain: (1) unidimensional instruments that are suitable for determining pain intensity, and (2) multidimensional instruments for measuring qualitative features of the pain experience (Melzack & Katz, 1992). These tools were designed for application with younger persons and there are potential problems if they are to be uncritically used with elderly populations. Caution must be used when interpreting results from traditional psychometric tools. If such tests must be used, it is advisable to ensure that the elderly patient clearly understands the directions and has the cognitive capacity to undertake such testing. Currently, there are no pain assessment measures specifically developed for use with older adults. An example of a frequently used unidimensional tool is the Visual Analog Scale (VAS; Huskisson, 1974). Patients are asked to place a mark on a line that represents the continuum from "no pain" to "worst pain possible." Kremer, Atkinson, and Ignelzi (1981) suggest that older individuals who have a deficit in abstract reasoning may have a problem with using such a scale. The McGill Pain Questionnaire (MPQ; Melzack, 1975) is an example of a multidimensional pain inventory; it consists of 20 sets of adjectives describing sensory, affective, evaluative, and miscellaneous aspects of pain. Herr and Mobily (1991) conclude that the MPQ may be too complicated and may take too much time to complete for use by older adults. A less complex assessment tool that might be preferable to use with older persons is the short form of the MPQ (SF-MPQ; Melzack, 1987). The SF-MPQ consists of 15 descriptors from the MPQ; pain intensity is measured on a VAS.

TREATMENT

Pharmacological Control

A thorough discussion of pharmacological management of pain and its relevance to older persons is beyond the scope of this chapter. Although pharmacology is the initial treatment of choice for elderly patients experiencing chronic or acute pain, care must be taken when dispensing medication for older adults because they have an increased sensitivity to and reduced metabolism for many drugs (Kaiko, Wallenstein, Rogers, Grabinski, & Houde, 1982). The interested reader will find numerous reports and monographs, including a recent critical review by Cherny and Popp (1997). We examine the essential elements that govern the judicious use of medicinal treatments.

For what may be considered "routine aches and pains" accompanying old age, the conventional medical wisdom is to prescribe nonprescription medication beginning with as low a dose as may be clinically effective. The rationale behind such a plan is to guard against contraindications with other more necessary medications and to prevent interference with proper nutritional intake, sleep, or optimal neuromuscular and cognitive functioning. When pain becomes severe enough to interfere with normal activities, and when the quality of life begins to seriously deteriorate, stronger and more effective medicants become justified. This is especially true for the management of pain associated with cancer. The WHO "Three Step Analgesic Ladder" (nonopioid, opioid, and adjuvant analgesics) provides basic guidance for undertaking drug therapy for cancer pain (Agency for Health Care Policy and Research, 1994). Analgesic treatment can be classified into three broad categories: nonopioid analgesics, opioid analgesics, and adjuvant analgesics.

Nonopioid Analgesics

For mild to moderate pain, nonopioid analgesics are preferred. Even for more severe pain they can be used in combination with opioid drugs. Included in this category are acetaminophen, aspirin, and other nonsteroidal anti-inflammatory drugs (NSAIDS). Acetaminophen is included in this category, even though it does not have much anti-inflammatory effect (Ferrell, 1991). A "ceiling effect" wherein increasing dosages beyond a certain level no longer increases the analgesic effects is associated with these drugs (Kanter, 1984). It must be recognized that there are risks with using NSAIDS drugs in older persons; adverse reactions include gastrointestinal bleeding (Alexander, Veitch, & Wood, 1985), peptic ulcer disease (Butt, Barthel, & Moore, 1988), and renal insufficiency (Maniglia, Schwartz, & Moriber-Katz, 1988).

Opioid Analgesics

Opioid therapy is preferred for moderate to severe pain such as cancer pain (Portenoy, Foley, & Inturrisi, 1990). This category includes propoxyphene, codeine, and morphine, among others. There are no "ceiling effects" with these drugs. Side effects with older persons can include opioid-induced constipation (Sykes, 1991), nausea (Campora *et al.*, 1991), cognitive disturbance, respiratory depression, and habituation (Ferrell, 1991).

Adjuvant Analgesics

Adjuvant analgesics do not have their own analgesic properties, but are helpful in treating some types of chronic pain (Ferrell, 1991). Included in this group are antidepressants, anticonvulsants, sedatives, and corticosteroids.

Corticosteroids are widely used as an all-purpose adjuvant analgesic (Ettinger & Portenoy, 1988). Amitriptyline is the most effective tricyclic adjuvant analgesic and is especially useful when the neuropathy is of a burning or dysaesthetic quality (Onghena & Van Houdenhove, 1992). Tricyclics have anticholinergic side effects such as constipation, urinary retention, hypotension, and confusion (Schuster & Goetz, 1994). Benzodiazepines might be effective against insomnia and anxiety associated with pain, but might lead to daytime sedation, falls, and confusion. Adjuvant analgesics have the benefit of simultaneously treating concurrent symptoms of depression and anxiety.

Behavioral Coping: Behavioral Intervention Techniques for Pain Management

Behavior modification, cognitive treatment, relaxation training, exercise, biofeedback, imagery, diaphragmatic breathing, and hypnosis are all techniques that can help manage pain in older persons. Some are utilized and more adaptable than others for the older patient. Certain techniques, such as behavior modification and cognitive therapy, might be more intense and take more time and practice, and although biofeedback might not be cost-effective, exercise, relaxation training, and imagery are all easy to complete for most elderly patients. Hypnosis might be a more difficult procedure and some patients might be resistant to it.

Techniques such as body positioning can offer pain relief. Nelson, Taylor, Adams, and Parker (1990) found that older adults with hip fractures found some pain relief when their legs were supported by pillows while in bed. Also, older persons who received back massages experienced a reduction in level of anxiety (Fraser & Kerr, 1993).

Unfortunately, many older adults, especially those living in long-term residential care facilities, have become resigned to pain, and they have become ambivalent regarding any changes in their pain status (Yates, Dewar, & Fentiman, 1995). Many studies have investigated behavioral treatments for pain, but only a few studies have incorporated geriatric patients in their research.

It is important to keep in mind that older patients might appreciate the benefits of certain pain management techniques differently from younger patients. Differences were found between older patients (65 to 82) and younger patients (25 to 63) with rheumatoid arthritis or osteoarthritis with regard to their ability to employ and to benefit from combined treatment approaches (Davis, Cortex, & Rubin, 1990). Davis and colleagues found that medication, rest, heat, distraction, and talking to others were most often used by the older patients with medication, rest, and heat being most helpful. Younger patients, on the other hand, participated in more combined methods and found relaxation techniques as being a significantly more beneficial procedure. Portenoy and Farkash (1988) suggested that older people might not be good candidates for psychological treatments aimed at alleviation of pain. They further state that older adults are rarely given opportunities to utilize psychological treatments that are already available. There are some older people, those with hearing or memory problems, for whom psychological treatment might not be effective; however, the majority of elderly, given the chance, can be expected to benefit greatly from psychological interventions.

Behavior Modification

There are not many studies on the efficacy of behavior modification specifically designed for elderly pain patients. Nevertheless, Fordyce (1986) states that chronic pain patients of all age groups can benefit from behavior modification techniques. Behavior change problems basically consist of (1) behavior that is not occurring often enough and needs to be increased or strengthened, (2) behavior that is occurring too much and needs to be diminished or eliminated, (3) behavior is missing that is needed and should be learned or acquired, or a combination of (1), (2), and (3) (Fordyce, 1976). The interested reader is advised to consult Fordyce and colleagues (1973) for a more detailed and complete description of various behavior modification techniques.

Contingency management is a behavior modification procedure based on principles of operant conditioning. Operant conditioning and behavior analysis may help explain to varying degrees the pain exhibited by chronic pain patients. If in fact such pains result from a history of reinforced "learning trials," learning theory principles may be applied to diminish that pain. The goal of contingency management for chronic pain is to help the patient change pain behaviors. The probability or frequency of limping, asking for medications, grimacing, moaning, complaining of pain, or not exercising often can be changed by following contingency management programs. Pain behaviors can become reinforced by contingencies in the environment and then become learned or habitual, regardless of whether the contingencies are obvious to the patient. We may consider an example of a pain patient who has incorporated in the repertoire of pain behaviors a profound limp. Regardless of how the behavior began it is now a learned behavior; one that has been reinforced by environmental contingencies. One form of treatment might be repeated walking practice. This is the behavior that needs to be increased, with limping as the targeted pain behavior to be decreased or diminished. The reinforcers used to increase the walking activity could be rest and therapist approval (or any number of other desirable consequences). That is, walking a certain distance leads to rest and therapist approval. However, it is important that the patient be reinforced only when he or she walks *without* limping. If the patient walks while limping, limping as a pain behavior will become strengthened. The patient might be instructed to initially walk two steps and then be allowed to limp. After two steps without limping, a brief rest period is allowed and therapist approval is given (see illustration in Fordyce, 1976).

Cognitive-Behavioral Techniques

Cognitive treatment for pain, which retains many features of the classical contingency management programs to which have been added "behaviors" or "stimuli" that might be in the realm of thought or imagery, also addresses depression and personality problems. Many chronic pain patients exhibit maladaptive thinking, which in turn, leads to increased subjective levels of pain

(Turk & Meichenbaum, 1994). Cognitive treatment would then be directed toward influencing patient's maladaptive and distorted patterns of thinking and toward helping them change to more productive and positive ways of coping with pain. Cognitive treatment encourages patients to take more control of their situations and to better understand the connections between emotions, thinking, and the experiences of pain. Most studies utilizing cognitive-behavioral techniques have utilized younger patients, although there is no reason to believe that older patients cannot benefit just as well.

Stress-Inoculation Therapy

Stress inoculation combines cognitive methods with positive self-statements and behavior management skills and usually consists of three phases: (1) education, (2) coping, and (3) application (Masters, Burish, Hollon, & Rimm, 1987). The education phase includes a "conceptualization of pain that stresses sensory, affective and cognitive components of the pain experience" (Turk, cited in Meichenbaum, 1977). In the coping phase, the patient may be taught to properly engage relaxation strategies to reduce tension and stress associated with the pain (although goal-directed imagery and distraction can also be utilized). In the final phase of the "application," patients can be subjected to the actual pain and be able to put to use the techniques they have mastered for pain control. In a study with 69 chronic pain outpatients who underwent a 10-week cognitive-behavioral stress inoculation group therapy program (mean age 53, with 22 patients over age 60), treatment had limited and little effect on perceived intensity of pain, however, there was an increase in the capability to cope with pain and a decrease in medication usage (Puder, 1988).

Relaxation Techniques

Relaxation techniques include progressive muscle relaxation, imagery, and controlled breathing that can be used separately or in combination. Relaxation training is a cost-effective way for any age group to manage pain, and relaxation training has been helpful in reducing medication usage (Arena, Hightower, & Chong, 1988). It is believed that relaxation training is helpful as a pain management tool because of its effect on sympathetic nervous system activity (Houston, 1993). Diaphragmatic or controlled breathing or both can help with pain management. As with relaxation training, this is a variation that often employs progressive and imaginal relaxation training, which have proven effective in decreasing anxiety levels in elderly patients (Scogin, Rickard, Keith, Wilson, & McElreath, 1992). This important study found that older persons who imagined muscle tension release benefited as much as those who employed actual tension release, even at 1-month follow up. This is a significant benefit for those older persons who have physical problems that might otherwise preclude them from actually tensing and releasing muscles. Similarly, modified progressive muscle relaxation has been found to be helpful with elderly tension headache suffers (Arena, et al., 1988). Their study evaluated an 8-week modified progressive muscle relaxation protocol administered to 10 elderly subjects with tension headaches. At 3-month follow-up, significant reductions in headache activity (50% or greater) were found in 7 patients. Significant reductions were also found in the number of headache-free days, peak headache activity, and medication usage.

According to Wisocki and Powers (1997), three clinical case studies have been reported in which older persons benefited from relaxation techniques. A male 89-year-old nursing home resident used taped relaxation instruction with background music that proved helpful in reducing headache pain (Linoff & West, 1982). An elderly female patient utilized relaxation techniques with success to help cope with the emotional side effects from chemotherapy long after chemotherapy treatment had terminated (Hamburger, 1982). After 7 weeks of treatment with relaxation and imagery, an elderly male with severe rheumatoid arthritis and moderate depression reported a 50% decrease in pain and a significant improvement in mood (Czirr & Gallagher, 1983).

Exercise

Regrettably, although even those at advanced age can benefit from exercise (Fiatarone *et al.*, 1990), compliance rates for home exercise and self-pain management is low (Bradley, 1989). The success of such programs depends on a number of factors, not least of which is the consideration that exercise programs for elderly pain patients may need to begin at a less strenuous level than might be advisable for younger pain patients. Exercise programs for older adults can range from nonstrenuous yoga techniques (Bender, 1992) to more strenuous water exercise programs (Meyer & Hawley, 1994). Results of such programs have generally been encouraging. Representative findings include studies in which participation in a water exercise decreased the pain and increased the strength of older persons with rheumatic disease when compared with a control group of patients (Meyer & Hawley, 1994). In another investigation, yoga exercises were significantly beneficial for relief of pain in the hands of patients with osteoarthritis compared with a control group (Garfinkel, Schumacher, Husain, Levy, & Reshetar, 1994).

Elderly myocardial infarction patients who engaged in regular aerobic exercise reported less chest pain 6 to 12 months after the myocardial infarction (Fridlund, Hogstedt, Lidell, & Larson, 1991) and improved rehabilitation efforts after the myocardial infarction (Dixhoorn, Duivenvoorden, Pool, & Verhage, 1990). In a study with mixed ages of MI patients, those in the exercise group had less anginal pain in 6- to 12-month follow-up compared to the control group (Stern, Gorman, & Kaslow, 1983). Perhaps such outcomes can modify the reluctance of physicians to prescribe exercise for treatment; currently less than half of all older post-MI and bypass patients (62 to 92) are so advised (Ades, Waldmann, McCann, & Weaver, 1992). Examples of specific exercise programs that take into consideration a variety of conditions can be found elsewhere (Bender, 1992; Biegel, 1984; Flatten, Wilhite & Reyes-Watson, 1988; Herning, 1993; Kerlan, 1991; Lehr & Swanson, 1990; Saxon & Etten, 1984)

Biofeedback

A derivative of learning-based therapy, biofeedback, which is based on the knowledge of results of biological states and events, has been successful in pain control. Strong criticism of biofeedback is that it is not cost-effective and that less costly techniques, such as relaxation and imagery, might provide the same results (Achterberg, Kenner, & Lewis, 1988). Biofeedback is not extensively employed with older patients, but some studies provide empirical support for its continued use. For example, a 69-year-old male who had a 37-year history of chronic cluster headaches realized an almost 100% reduction in PRN medicine as well as a decrease in reports of pain following treatment with thermal biofeedback and a spouse contingency program (King & Arena, 1984). These decreases were maintained at a 15-month follow-up. Electromyographic biofeedback training with elderly tension headache patients has also been shown to be effective (Arena, Hannah, Bruno, & Meador, 1991). Eight patients above the age of 62 participated in a 12-session frontal EMG training. At 3-month follow-up, four patients had significantly decreased their headache activity by at least 50%, and three patients decreased headache activity by 35% to 45%. There was also a reduction in headache-free days, peak headache activity, and use of medication. Biofeedback successfully reduced pain and stiffness in an 80-year-old osteoarthritic pain patient; the patient was taught to maintain proper blood flow by not contracting the muscles around the joints, thus alleviating pain (Boczkoski, 1984).

Age alone certainly should not constitute any constraint or limitation for employing such procedures. Middaugh, Woods, Kee, Harden, and Peters (1991) did not find any age differences in the use of biofeedback and relaxation techniques for patients with chronic musculoskeletal pain. Older patients (55 to 78 years old) were able to learn physiological self-regulation techniques, such as relaxation training, diaphragmatic breathing, and EMG biofeedback, just as well as younger patients (29 to 48 years old). The age groups had similar deficiencies and complaints on initial evaluation and both groups achieved the same level of improvement with training.

Hypnosis

Modern-day applications of hypnosis in pain control has been utilized in various medical conditions, such as helping burn patients better tolerate debridement (Patterson, Everett, Burns, & Marvin, 1992) and dressing changes (Van der Does, Van Dyck, & Spijker, 1988), as anaesthesia for pain control for colonoscopy patients (Cadranel *et al.*, 1994), and as an alternative to the use of intravenous sedation in interventional radiology (Lang & Hamilton, 1994). Compared to controls, hypnotized patients were better able to tolerate angioplasty longer and required less additional narcotic pain medication (Weinstein & Au, 1991). Hypnotic suggestions were used to aid in the motor movement recovery of left arm function in a 66-year-old woman (Holroyd & Hill, 1989). Patients with refractory fibromyalgia found hypnosis to be more effective in relieving symptoms than physical therapy (Haanen *et al.*, 1991). Forty patients were randomly to either hypnotherapy treatment or physical therapy treatment for 12 weeks with follow-up at 24 weeks. Significant improvement was noted in the hypnotherapy group with regard to pain experience, fatigue on awakening, sleep pattern, and global assessment at 12 and 24 weeks.

Several studies have investigated the biochemical correlates of hypoanalgesia (Domangue, Margolis, Lieberman, & Kaji, 1985), although the connection between the analgesic effects of hypnosis and its neurochemical correlates is still poorly understood (DeBenedittis, Panerai, & Villamira, 1989). In a sample of 19 arthritic pain patients, plasma levels of beta-endorphin, epinephrine, norepinephrine, dopamine, and serotonin were measured pre- and posthypnotic suggestion and decreases in pain, anxiety, and depression were noted following hypnotherapy, accompanied by an increase in beta-endorphin-like immunoreactive material (Domangue *et al.,* 1985)

Hypnosis is a tool that has great potential to alleviate pain, especially in the older population and especially for those who might not be able to tolerate certain medications. As with any application, when electing hypnosis for pain management, attention should be given to the degree of hypnotizability, attitudes, expectations, and beliefs of the patient in modulating the pain experience (Chaves, 1994).

Transcutaneous Electrical Nerve Stimulation (TENS)

The analgesic properties of Transcutaneous Electrical Nerve Stimulation (TENS) are attributed to its ability to stimulate neural pathways and to impede transmission of pain information to higher levels of the nervous system (Portenoy & Farkash, 1988). TENS can be used as part of a larger pain management program and has been particularly successful with cases of chronic neuropathy, postfractures, cancer pain, low-back pain, postherpetic neuralgia, myofascial pain, and phantom-limb pain (Thorsteinsson, 1987). Johnson, Ashton, and Thompson (1992) found TENS to be an effective analgesic treatment for a wide range of pain problems in 58.6% of 1,582 patients who attended their pain clinic over a period of 10 years, with a number of patients using this treatment for many years. They concluded that TENS can be utilized as a simple, safe and reusable first line treatment for many pain conditions. Deyo, Walsh, Martin, Schoenfield, and Ramamurthy (1990) evaluated TENS, stretching exercises, and a combination of the two for treatment of lower-back pain and concluded that TENS was no more effective than placebo. They further stated that TENS treatment did not add any advantage to the treatment of exercise alone. A study with 107 chronic pain patients (Johnson, Ashton, & Thompson, 1991) demonstrated that 47% of patients using TENS decreased their pain by more than half. There has been some controversy regarding the use of TENS with patients who have pacemakers, although Rasmussen, Hayes, Vlietstra, and Thorsteinsson (1988) consider it safe for most patients who have permanent cardiac pacemakers.

SUMMARY

This chapter provided an overview of the essential considerations in the generation, maintenance, and potential psychological processes for control of pain in the aging population. No single volume (and certainly no single chapter) is able to embrace all of the details that are necessary for effective design or utilization of a treatment intervention. Some sense of the complexity of the interrelatedness of the issues is represented in Figure 18-1. A useful summary of the principles for programs with elders has been provided by Melding (1997) in the following guidelines.

- Accept pain as "real"
- Stabilize health status
- Use appropriate analgesia as necessary
- Treat depression vigorously
- Enlist social and family support especially if behavior modification is needed
- Use cognitive behavioral approaches
- Build self-efficacy by experiential methods rather than didactic teaching
- Pace programs at client's speed
- Keep sessions short, one major concept at a time
- Give plentiful information, keep it simple and use large print fonts
- Set goals with individual, monitor progress with charts, instruments, review frequently
- Reduce catastrophic thinking

There is a real need for health professionals of all disciplines to recognize (1) the need to address pain management in the older patient and (2) the vast armamentarium of behaviorally-based interventions that is already available.

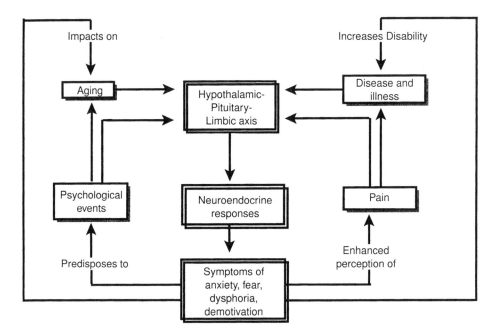

Figure 18.1. A summary of the essential and converging elements that affect pain in the aging. From "Psychiatric Aspects of Chronic Pain" (p. 197), by P. S. Melding, in Chronic Pain in Old Age: An Integrated Psychosocial Perspective, edited by R. Roy, 1995, Toronto: University of Toronto Press. Adapted by permission.

REFERENCES

Achterberg, J., Kenner, C., & Lewis, G. (1988). Severe burn injury: A comparison of relaxation, imagery, and biofeedback for pain management. *Journal of Mental Imagery, 12,* 71–87.

Ades, P. A., Waldmann, M. L., McCann, W. J., & Weaver, S. O. (1992). Predictors of cardiac rehabilitation participation in older coronary patients. *Archives of Internal Medicine, 152,* 1033–1035.

Agency for Health Care Policy and Research. (1994). *Cancer pain management panel. Management of cancer pain.* Clinical Practice Guideline Number 9. Washington, DC: U.S. Department of Health and Human Services.

Alexander, A. M., Veitch, G. B., & Wood, J. B. (1985). Anti-rheumatic and analgesic drug usage and acute gastro-intestinal bleeding in elderly patients. *Journal of Clinical and Hospital Pharmacy, 10,* 89–93.

American Psychiatric Association (1987). *Diagnostic and statistical manual of mental disorders* (3rd ed. rev.). Washington, DC: Author.

Arena, J. G., Hightower, N. E., & Chong, G. C. (1988). Relaxation therapy for tension headache in the elderly: A prospective study. *Psychology and Aging, 3,* 96–98.

Arena, J. G., Hannah, S. L., Bruno, G. M., & Meador, K. J. (1991). Electromyographic biofeedback training for tension headache in the elderly: A prospective study. *Biofeedback and Self Regulation, 16,* 379–390.

Beekman, A. T., Kriegsman, D. M., Deeg, D. J., & van Tilburg, W. (1995). The association of physical health and depressive symptoms in the older population: Age and sex differences. *Social Psychiatry and Psychiatric Epidemiology, 30,* 32–38.

Bender, R. (1992). Yoga exercises and gentle movements for the elderly. In S. Harris, R. Harris, & W. S. Harris (Eds.), *Physical activity and sports: Practice, program and policy* (Vol. II, pp. 344–371) Albany, NY: Center for the Study of Aging.

Biegel, L. (Ed.). (1984). *Physical fitness and the older person: A guide to exercise for health care professionals.* Rockville, MD: Aspen.

Birren, J. E., Shapiro, H. B., & Miller, H. H. (1959). The effect of salicylate upon pain sensitivity. *Journal of Pharmacology and Experimental Therapeutics, 100,* 67–71.

Boczkowski, J. (1984). Biofeedback training for the treatment of chronic pain in an elderly arthritic female. *Clinical Gerontology, 2,* 39–46.

Bradley, L. A. (1989). Adherence with treatment regiments among adult rheumatoid arthritis patients: Current status and future directions. *Arthritis Care and Research, 2,* 533–539.

Bruce, M. L., Seeman, T. E., Merrill, S. S., & Blazer, D. G. (1994). The impact of depressive symptomatology on physical disability: MacArthur studies of successful aging. *American Journal of Public Health, 84,* 1796–1799.

Butt, J. H, Barthel, J. S., & Moore, R. A. (1988). Clinical spectrum of the upper gastrointestinal effects of nonsteroidal anti-inflammatory drugs: Natural history, symptomatology and significance. *American Journal of Medicine, 84,* 5–14.

Cadranel, J. F., Benhamou, Y., Zylberberg, P., Novello, P., Luciani, F., Valla, D., & Opolon, P. (1994). Hypnotic relaxation: A new sedative tool for colonoscopy? *Journal of Clinical Gastroenterology, 18,* 127–129.

Campora, E., Merlini, L., Pace, M., Bruzzone, M., Luzzani, M., Gottlieb, A., & Rosso, R. (1991). The incidence of narcotic induced emesis. *Journal of Pain and Symptom Management, 6,* 428–430.

Casten, R. J., Parmelee, P. A., Kleban, M. H., Lawton, M P., & Katz, I. R. (1995). The relationship among anxiety, depression, and pain in a geriatric institutionalized sample. *Pain, 61,* 271–276.

Chapman, C. R. (1978). Pain: The perception of noxious events. In R. A. Sternbach (Ed.), *The psychology of pain* (pp. 169–202). New York: Raven.

Chaves, J. F. (1994). Recent advances in the application of hypnosis to pain management. *American Journal of Clinical Hypnosis, 37,* 117–129.

Cherny, N. I., & Popp, B. (1997). The management of cancer pain in elderly patients. In J. Lomranz & D. I. Mostofsky (Eds.), *Handbook of pain and aging* (pp. 267–308). New York: Plenum.

Clark, W. C., & Mehl, L. (1973). Signal detection theory procedures are not equivalent when thermal stimuli are judged. *Journal of Experimental Psychology, 97,* 48–53.

Closs, S. J. (1994). Pain in elderly patients: A neglected phenomenon? *Journal of Advanced Nursing, 19,* 1072–1081.

Cohen-Mansfield, J., & Marx, M. S. (1993). Pain and depression in the nursing home: Corroborating results. *Journal of Gerontology: Psychological Sciences, 48,* 96–97.

Collins, G., & Stone, L. A. (1966). Pain sensitivity, age and activity level in chronic schizophrenics and in normals. *British Journal of Psychiatry, 112,* 33–35.

Corran, T. M., Helme, R. D., & Gibson, S. J. (1993, August). *Comparison of chronic pain experience in young and elderly patients.* Paper presented at the 7th World Congress on Pain, Paris.

Crook, J., Rideout, E., & Browne, G. (1984). The prevalence of pain complaints in a general population. *Pain, 18,* 299–314.

Cutler, R. B., Fishbain, D. A., Rosomoff, R. S., & Rosomoff, H. L. (1994). Outcomes in treatment of pain in geriatric and younger age groups. *Archives of Physical Medicine and Rehabilitation, 75,* 457–464.

Czirr, R., & Gallagher, D. (1983). Case report: Behavioral treatment of depression and somatic complaints in rheumatoid arthritis. *Clinical Gerontology, 2,* 63–66.

Davis, G. C., Cortex, C., & Rubin, B. R. (1990). Pain management in the older adult with rheumatoid arthritis or osteoarthritis. *Arthritis Care and Research, 3,* 127–131.

DeBenedittis, G., Panerai, A. A., & Villamira, M. A. (1989). Effects of hypnotic analgesia and hypnotizability on experimental ischemic pain. *International Journal of Clinical Hypnosis, 37,* 55–69.

Deyo, R. A., Walsh, N. E., Martin, D. C., Schoenfield, L. S., & Ramamurthy, S. (1990). A controlled trial of transcutaneous electrical nerve stimulation (TENS) and exercise for chronic low back pain. *New England Journal of Medicine, 322,* 1627–1634.

Dixhoorn, J. V., Duivenvoorden, H. J., Pool, J., & Verhage, F. (1990). Psychic effects of physical training and relaxation therapy after myocardial infarction. *Journal of Psychosomatic Research, 34,* 327–337.

Domangue, B. B., Margolis, C. G., Lieberman, D., Kaji, H. (1985). Biochemical correlates of hypnoanalgesia in arthritic pain patients. *Journal of Clinical Psychiatry, 46,* 235–238.

Ettinger, A. B., & Portenoy, R. K. (1988). The use of corticosteroids in the treatment of symptoms associated with cancer. *Journal of Pain and Symptom Management, 3,* 99–103.

Ferrell, B. A. (1991). Pain management in elderly people. *Journal of the American Geriatrics Society, 39,* 64–73.

Ferrell, B. A., Ferrell, B. R., & Osterweil, D. (1990). Pain in the nursing home. *Journal of the American Geriatrics Society, 38,* 409–414.

Fiatarone, M. A., Marks, E. C., Ryan, N. D., Meredith, C. N., Lipsitz, L. A., & Evans, W. J. (1990). High-intensity strength training in nonagenarians. *Journal of the American Medical Association, 263,* 3029–3034.

Flatten, K., Wilhite, B., & Reyes-Watson, E. (1988). *Exercise activities for the elderly.* New York: Springer.

Fordyce, W. E. (1976). *Behavioral methods for chronic pain and illness.* St. Louis, MO: Mosby.

Fordyce, W. E. (1986). Learning processes in pain. In R. A. Steinbach (Ed.), *The psychology of pain* (2nd ed., pp. 49–65). New York: Raven.

Fordyce, W. E., Fowler, R., Lehmann, J., DeLateur, B., Sand P., & Trieschamann, R. (1973). Operant conditioning in the treatment of chronic pain. *Archives of Physical Medicine, 54,* 399–408.

Fraser, J., & Kerr, J. R. (1993). Psychophysiological effects of back massage on elderly institutional patients. *Journal of Advanced Nursing, 18,* 238–245.

Fridlund, B., Hogstedt, B., Lidell, E., & Larson, P. (1991). Recovery after myocardial infarction: Effects of a caring rehabilitation program. *Scandinavian Journal of Caring Sciences, 5,* 23–32.

Gagliese, L., & Melzack, R. (1995, May). *Age differences in the quality but not intensity of chronic pain.* Paper presented at the annual meeting of the Canadian Pain Society, Ottawa, Ontario, Canada.

Gagliese, L., & Melzack, R. (1997). The assessment of pain in the elderly. In J. Lomranz & D. I. Mostofsky (Eds.), *Handbook of pain and aging* (pp. 69–96). New York: Plenum.

Garfinkel, M. S., Schumacher, H. R. Jr., Husain, A., Levy, M., & Reshetar, R. A. (1994). Evaluation of a yoga based regimen for treatment of osteoarthritis of the hands. *Journal of Rheumatology, 21,* 2341–2343.

Garron, D. C., & Leavitt, F. (1979). Demographic and affective covariates of pain. *Psychosomatic Medicine, 41*, 525–535.

Gibson, S. J., Katz, B., Corran, T. M., Farrell, M. J., & Helme, R. D. (1994). Pain in older persons. *Disability and Rehabilitation, 16*, 127–139.

Haanen, H. C., Hoenderdos, H. T., van Romunde, L. K., Hop, W. C., Mallee, C., Terwiel, J. P., & Hekster, G. B. (1991). Controlled trail of hypnotherapy in the treatment of refractory fibromyalgia. *Journal of Rheumatology, 18*, 72–75.

Hamburger, L. (1982). Reduction of generalized aversive responding in a post-treatment cancer patient: Relaxation as an active coping skill. *Journal of Behavior Therapy and Experimental Psychiatry, 12*, 241–247.

Hardy, J. D., Wolff, H. G., & Goodell, H. (1943). The pain threshold in man. *American Journal of Psychiatry, 99*, 744–751.

Harkins, S. W., & Chapman, C. R. (1976). Detection and decision factors in pain perception in young and elderly men. *Pain, 2*, 253–264.

Harkins, S. W., & Chapman, C. R. (1977a). Age and sex differences in pain perception. In D. J. Anderson & B. Mathews (Eds.), *Pain in the trigeminal region* (pp. 435–441). Amsterdam: Elsevier.

Harkins, S. W., & Chapman, C. R. (1977b). The perception of induced dental pain in young and elderly women. *Journal of Gerontology, 32*, 428–435.

Harkins, S. W., Price, D. D., & Martelli, M. (1986). Effects of age on pain perception: Thermonociception. *Journal of Gerontology, 41*, 58–63.

Herning, M. M. (1993). Posture improvement in the frail elderly. In H. M. Perry, III, J. E. Morley, & R. M. Coe (Eds.), *Aging and musculoskeletal disorders: Concepts, diagnosis and treatment* (pp. 334–353). New York: Springer.

Herr, K. A., & Mobily, P. R. (1991). Complexities of pain assessment in the elderly. Clinical considerations. *Journal of Gerontological Nursing, 17*, 12–19.

Herr, K. A., Mobily, P. R., & Smith, C. (1993). Depression and the experience of chronic back pain: A study of related variables and age differences. *Clinical Journal of Pain, 9*, 104–114.

Hitchcock, L. S., Ferrell, B. R., & McCaffery, M. (1994). The experience of chronic nonmalignant pain. *Journal of Pain and Symptom Management, 9*, 312–318.

Holroyd, J., & Hill, A. (1989). Pushing the limits of recovery: Hypnotherapy with a stroke patient. *International Journal of Clinical and Experimental Hypnosis, 37*, 120–128.

Houston, K. (1993). An investigation of rocking as relaxation for the elderly. *Geriatric Nursing, 14*, 186–189.

Huskisson, E. C. (1974). Measurement of pain. *Lancet, 2*, 1127–1131.

Johnson, M. I., Ashton, C. H., & Thompson, J.W. (1991). An in-depth study of long-term users of transcutaneous electrical nerve stimulation (TENS). Implications for clinical use of TENS. *Pain, 44*, 221–229.

Johnson, M. I., Ashton, C. H., & Thompson, J.W. (1992). Long term use of transcutaneous electrical nerve stimulation at Newcastle Pain Relief Clinic. *Journal of the Royal Society of Medicine, 85*, 267–268.

Kaiko, R. F., Wallenstein, S. L., Rogers, A. G., Grabinski, P. Y., & Houde, R. W. (1982). Narcotics in the elderly. *Medical Clinics of North America, 66*, 1079–1089.

Kanter, T. G. (1984). Peripherally-acting analgesics. In M. Kuhr & G. Pasternak, G. (Eds.), *Analgesics: Neurochemical, Behavioral and Clinical Perspectives* (pp. 289–312). New York: Raven.

Kerlan, R. K. (Ed.). (1991). *Clinics in sports medicine*. Philadelphia: Saunders.

King, A. C., & Arena, J. G. (1984). Behavioral treatment of chronic cluster headache in a geriatric patient. *Biofeedback and Self Regulation, 9*, 201–108.

Kremer, E., Atkinson, J. H., & Ignelzi, R. J. (1981). Measurement of pain: Patient preference does not confound pain measurement. *Pain, 10*, 241–249.

Kwentus, J. A., Harkins, S. W., Lignon, N., & Silverman, J. J. (1985). Current concepts of geriatric pain and its treatment. *Geriatrics, 40*, 48–54, 57.

Lang, E. V., & Hamilton, D. (1994). Anodyne imagery: An alternative to IV sedation in interventional radiology. *AJR, American Journal of Roentgenology, 162*, 1221–1226.

Lehr, J., & Swanson, K. (1990). *Fit, firm & 50*. Chelsea, MI: Lewis.

Linoff, M., & West, C. (1982). Relaxation training systematically combined with music: Treatment of tension headaches in a geriatric patient. *International Journal of Behavioral Geriatrics, 1*, 11–16.

Magni, J., Schifano, F., & DeLeo, D. (1985). Pain as a symptom in elderly depressed patients: Relationship to diagnostic subgroups. *European Archives of Psychiatry and Neurological Sciences, 235,* 143–145.

Maniglia, R., Schwartz, A. B., & Moriber-Katz, S. (1988). Non-steroidal anti-inflammatory nephrotoxicity. *Annals of Clinical and Laboratory Science, 18,* 240–252.

Manton, K. G. (1997). Chronic morbidity and disability in the U.S. elderly populations: Recent trends and population implications. In J. Lomranz & D. I. Mostofsky (Eds.), *Handbook of pain and aging* (pp. 37–68). New York: Plenum.

Masters, J. C., Burish, T. G., Hollon, S. D., & Rimm, D. C. (1987). *Behavior therapy: Techniques and empirical findings* (3rd ed.). San Diego, CA: Harcourt Brace Jovanovich.

McCracken, L. M., Mosley, T. H., Plaud, J. J., Gross, R. T., & Penzien, D. B. (1993, August). *Age, chronic pain and impairment: Results from two clinical samples.* Paper presented at the 7th World Congress on Pain, Paris.

McCullough, P. K. (1991). Geriatric depression: Atypical presentations, hidden meanings. *Geriatrics, 46,* 72–76.

McIntosh, I. B. (1990). Psychological aspects influence the threshold of pain. *Geriatric Medicine, 20,* 37–41.

Meichenbaum, D. H. (1977). *Cognitive-behavior modification.* New York: Plenum.

Melding, P. S. (1995). Psychiatric aspects of chronic pain. In R. Roy (Ed.), *Chronic pain in old age: An integrated psychosocial perspective* (pp. 194–214). Toronto: University of Toronto Press.

Melding, P. S. (1997). Coping with pain in old age. In J. Lomranz & D. I. Mostofsky (Eds.), *Handbook of pain and aging* (pp. 167–184). New York: Plenum.

Melzack, R. (1975). The McGill Pain Questionnaire: Major properties and scoring methods. *Pain, 1,* 277–299.

Melzack, R. (1987). The short-form McGill Pain Questionnaire. *Pain, 30,* 191–197.

Melzack, R., & Katz, J. (1992). The McGill Pain Questionnaire: Appraisal and current status. In D. C. Turk & R. Melzack (Eds.), *Handbook of pain assessment* (pp. 152–168). New York: Guilford.

Meyer, C. L., & Hawley, D. J. (1994). Characteristics of participants in water exercise programs compared to patients in a rheumatic disease clinic. *Arthritis Care and Research, 7,* 85–89.

Middaugh, S. J., Levin, R. B., Kee, W. G., Barchiesi, F. D., & Roberts, J. M. (1988). Chronic pain: Its treatment in geriatric and younger patients. *Archives of Physical Medicine and Rehabilitation, 69,* 1021–1025.

Middaugh, S. J., Woods, S. E., Kee, W. G., Harden, R. N., & Peters, J. R. (1991). Biofeedback-assisted relaxation training for the chronic pain patient. *Biofeedback and Self Regulation, 16,* 361–377.

Moss, M. S., Lawton, M. P., & Glicksman, A. (1991). The role of pain in the last year of life of older persons. *Journal of Gerontology: Psychological Sciences, 46,* P51–57.

Mumford, H. M. (1965). Pain perception threshold and adaptation of normal human teeth. *Archives of Graduate Biology, 10,* 957–968.

Nelson, L., Taylor, F., Adams, M., & Parker, D. E. (1990). Improving pain management for hip fractured elderly. *Orthopaedic Nursing, 9,* 79–82.

Notermans, S. L. H. (1966). Measurement of the pain threshold determined by electrical stimulation and its clinical application. I: Methods and factors possibly influencing the pain threshold. *Neurology, 16,* 1071–1086.

Onghena, P., & Van Houdenhove, B. (1992). Antidepressant-induced analgesia in chronic non-malignant pain: A meta-analysis of 39 placebo-controlled studies. *Pain, 49,* 205–220.

Parmelee, P. A., Katz, I. R., & Lawton, M. P. (1991). The relation of pain to depression among institutionalized aged. *Journal of Gerontology: Psychological Sciences, 46,* P15–21.

Patterson, D. R., Everett, J. J., Burns, G. L., & Marvin, J. A. (1992). Hypnosis for the treatment of burn pain. *Journal of Consulting and Clinical Psychology, 60,* 713–717.

Portenoy, R. K., & Farkash, A. (1988). Practical management of non-malignant pain in the elderly. *Geriatrics, 5,* 29–47.

Portenoy, R. K., Foley, K. M., & Inturrisi, C. E. (1990). The nature of opioid responsiveness and its implications for neuropathic pain: New hypotheses derived from studies of opioid infusions. *Pain, 43,* 273–286.

Procacci, P., Della Corte, M., Zoppi, M., Romano, S., Maresca, M., & Voegelin, M. (1974). Pain threshold measurement in man. In J. J. Bonica, P. Procacci, & C. Pagoni (Eds.), *Recent advances on pain: Pathophysiology and clinical aspects* (pp. 105–147). Springfield, IL: Thomas.

Puder, R. S. (1988). Age analysis of cognitive-behavioural group therapy for chronic pain outpatients. *Psychology and Aging, 3,* 204–207.

Rasmussen, M. J., Hayes, D. L., Vlietstra, R. E., & Thorsteinsson, G. (1988). Can transcutaneous electrical nerve stimulation be safely used in patients with permanent cardiac pacemakers? *Mayo Clinic Proceedings, 63,* 443–445.

Saxon, S. V., & Etten, M. J. (1984). *Psychosocial rehabilitation programs for older adults.* Springfield, IL: Thomas.

Schludermann, E., & Zubek, J. P. (1962). Effect of age on pain sensitivity. *Perceptual and Motor Skills, 14,* 295–301.

Schumacher, G. A., Goodell, H., Hardy, J. D., & Wolff, H. G. (1940). Uniformity of pain threshold in man. *Science, 92,* 110–112.

Schuster, J. M., & Goetz, K. L. (1994). Pain. In C. E. Coffey & J. L. Cummings (Eds.), *Textbook of geriatric neuropsychiatry* (pp. 334–350). Washington, DC: American Psychiatric Press.

Scogin, F., Rickard, H. C., Keith, S., Wilson, J., & McElreath, L. (1992). Progressive and imaginal relaxation training for elderly persons with subjective anxiety. *Psychology and Aging, 7,* 419–424.

Sengstaken, E. A., & King, S. A. (1993). The problems of pain and its detection among geriatric nursing home residents. *Journal of the American Geriatric Society, 41,* 541–4.

Sherman, E. D., & Robillard, E. (1960). Sensitivity to pain in the aged. *Canadian Medical Association Journal, 83,* 944–947.

Sherman, E. D., & Robillard, E. (1964). Sensitivity to pain in relationship to age. *Journal of the American Geriatric Society, 12,* 1037–1044.

Sorkin, B. A., Rudy, T. E., Hanlon, R. B., Turk, D. C., & Stieg, R. L. (1990). Chronic pain in old and young patients: Differences appear less important than similarities. *Journal of Gerontology: Psychological Sciences, 45,* P64–68.

Stern, M. J., Gorman, P. A., & Kaslow, L. (1983). The group counselling v. exercise therapy study: A controlled intervention with subjects following myocardial infarction. *Archives of Internal Medicine, 143,* 1719–1725.

Stewart, R. B., Blashfield, R., Hale, W. E., Moore, M. T., May, F. E., & Marks, R. G. (1991). Correlates of Beck Depression Inventory scores in an ambulatory elderly population: Symptoms, diseases, laboratory values, and medications. *Journal of Family Practice, 32,* 497–502.

Sykes, N. P. (1991). [Letter]. Oral naloxone in opioid associated constipation. *Lancet, 337,* 1475.

Thorsteinsson, G. (1987). Chronic pain: use of TENS in the elderly. *Geriatrics, 42,* 75–82.

Turk, D. C. & Meichenbaum, D. (1994). A cognitive-behavioural approach to pain management. In P. D. Wall & R. Melzack (Eds.), *Textbook of pain* (pp. 1337–1348). Endinburgh: Churchill Livingstone.

Turk, D. C., Okifuji, A., & Scharff, L. (1995). Chronic pain and depression: Role of perceived impact and perceived control in different age cohorts. *Pain, 61,* 93–101.

Van der Does, A. J., & Van Dyck, R., & Spijker, R. E. (1988). Hypnosis and pain in patients with severe burns: A pilot study. *Burns, Including Thermal Injury, 14,* 399–404.

Weinsten, E. J., & Au, P. K. (1991). Use of hypnosis before and during angioplasty. *American Journal of Clinical Hypnosis, 34,* 29–37.

Williams, A. K., & Schulz, R. (1988). Association of pain and physical dependency with depression in physically ill middle-aged and elderly persons. *Physical Therapy, 68,* 1226–1230.

Williamson, G. M., & Schulz, R. (1992). Pain, activity restriction and symptoms of depression among community-residing elderly residents. *Journal of Gerontology: Psychological Sciences, 47,* P367–372.

Williamson, J. (1978). Depression in the elderly. *Age and Aging, 7* (Suppl.), 35–40.

Wisocki, P. A., & Mosher, P. A. (1982). The elderly: An under-studied population in behavioral research. *International Journal of Behavior Geriatrics, 1,* 5–11.

Wisocki, P. A., & Powers, C. B. (1997). Behavioral treatments for pain experienced by older adults. In J. Lomranz & D. I. Mostofsky (Eds.), *Handbook of pain and aging* (pp. 365–382). New York: Plenum.

Woodrow, K. M., Friedman, G. D., Siegalaub, A. B., & Collen, M. F. (1972). Pain tolerance: Differences according to age, sex, and race. *Psychosomatic Medicine, 34*, 548–556.

Yates, P., Dewar, A., & Fentiman, B. (1995). Pain: The view of elderly people living in long-term residential settings. *Journal of Advanced Nursing, 21*, 667–674.

Yehuda, S., & Carasso, R. L. (1997). A brief history of pain perception and pain tolerance in aging. In J. Lomranz & D. I. Mostofsky (Eds.), *Handbook of pain and aging* (pp. 19–35). New York: Plenum.

Zoob, M. (1978). Differentiating the chest pain. *Geriatrics, 33*, 95–101.

CHAPTER 19

The Experience of Bereavement by Older Adults

Patricia A. Wisocki

INTRODUCTION

Bereavement is generally a normal response to loss, an experience shared by all ages and all cultures and even by a number of species (Averill, 1979). It is not an experience unique to the oldest among us, but it probably happens most often and most regularly to them. For example, each year in the United States approximately 800,000 people lose a spouse (Murrell & Himmelfarb, 1989). Most of these people are over age 60. LaRue, Dessonville, and Jarvik (1985) reported that 51% of women and 13.6% of men over the age of 65 have been widowed at least once.

This chapter is organized around four primary areas. First, characteristics of bereavement, with particular emphasis on how older adults (i.e., people over the age of 60) differ in their response to loss from people younger than 60 will be outlined. The literature on this topic is sparse but informative. Second, the evidence for a relationship between bereavement and the physical and mental health of elderly bereaved will be reviewed. The research is extensive on the general topic of bereavement, but relatively little work has been done with the elderly bereaved. Third, evidence for benefits of social support in mitigating the negative effects of the experience of loss for older adults will be presented. And fourth, suggestions for clinical interventions for the elderly when the pain of bereavement becomes too difficult to manage are considered. In addition, several successful treatment strategies are described.

Patricia A. Wisocki • Department of Psychology, University of Massachusetts, Amherst, Massachusetts 01003.

Handbook of Clinical Geropsychology, edited by Michel Hersen and Vincent B. Van Hasselt. Plenum Press, New York, 1998.

CHARACTERISTICS OF BEREAVEMENT

In distinguishing between bereavement, grief, and mourning, Averill (1979) points out that bereavement refers to the real or symbolic loss of a significant object, which may be human or nonhuman, tangible or intangible. He considers grief and mourning to be two distinct aspects of bereavement. Grief is the behavioral face of bereavement, that is, "a set of stereotyped physiological and psychological reactions of biological origin" (p. 341), whereas mourning is the social face, that is, "a conventional pattern of response dictated by the mores and customs of society" (p. 341).

Bereavement is recognized as a process by most theorists, but there is disagreement over whether it proceeds in an ordered sequence of stages, as originally suggested by Lindemann (1944) and later by Kubler-Ross (1970), or has separate components which do not necessarily occur successively or in any particular order (Bowlby, 1980; Bugen, 1977; Parkes, 1972). In stage theories, grief is presumed to pass through a set of normal stages toward resolution. Wortman and Silver (1987) have pointed out that stage theories have been built upon Freud's (1917) concept that grievers must "work through" their losses, and that those who show no grief are abnormal. They do not, however, report evidence indicating that the bereaved who fail to show significant distress are at risk for later pathology. Instead, they note that such individuals may become the target of social criticism for failing to grieve correctly. Most proponents of these theories indicate that bereaved people may not experience all stages and that they may not follow the designated order, but missing a stage or experiencing a stage out of order is often regarded as indicative of pathological grieving.

Theories in which separate components of grieving are postulated include most of the emotional reactions described in the stage theories, but the stages need not occur in a fixed order. The time limits vary per period and the intensity experienced in each period may differ markedly as a function of individual and environmental variables (Bugen, 1977).

Recognizing and accepting the arguments against stage theories, I have nevertheless opted to describe bereavement in stages for the sake of convenience. This description was taken from previous work by Averill and Wisocki (1981) and Wisocki and Averill (1988).

STAGES OF BEREAVEMENT

Stage 1. *Shock*

The bereaved experiences a dazed sense of unreality or numbing that may last several hours or several days, and he or she often reports feeling isolated from the world.

Stage 2. *Protest and Yearning*

The bereaved recognizes the loss, but does not entirely accept it. He or she feels intense pain and longing for the deceased and protests over the fact of loss by means of a variety of "searching" behaviors, including dreams about the dead person, "finding" him or her in familiar places, hallucinations, and so forth. This is also a time of agitation, heightened physiological arousal, and restlessness, sometimes alternating with a feeling of deceleration. The bereaved is preoccupied with memories of the lost person and focuses attention on those aspects of the environment that were associated with past pleasures experienced with the individual. This stage typically lasts for several months.

Stage 3. *Disorganization and Despair*

In this stage the bereaved accepts the fact of the loss and abandons attempts to recover the lost person, but continues to pine for the deceased. The bereaved commonly experiences apathy, withdrawal, loss of energy and despondency, a loss of sexual interest, poor socialization, diminished appetite, sleep disturbances, and other behavioral and somatic problems. The bereaved may experience conflicting emotions and moods, such as despair, hostility, shame, guilt, anger, and irritability. This stage is the most enduring, complex, and difficult phase of the grief process, often lasting a year or more.

Stage 4. *Detachment, Reorganization, and Recovery*

Characteristics of the previous stage are ultimately relieved when the bereaved develops new ways of perceiving and thinking about the world and his or her place in it. A person regains hope and confidence in him or herself and is able to enjoy life again. Most often, this involves establishment of new roles, relationships, and sense of purpose in life. It is not unusual for a person to grieve for several years before a relatively adequate readjustment occurs. Feelings of grief may be triggered continuously by holidays and dates, which mark meaningful events for the bereaved.

GRIEF REACTIONS AMONG OLDER ADULTS

Although there has been little work comparing or differentiating ways older and younger men and women respond to bereavement, several characteristic reactions have been described for older adults. First, the affective experience of grief is more subdued or "flat," and it is often more diffuse and obscured. Although some have suggested that this quality is an indication that older adults are not as pained by their losses as younger adults are, Skelskie (1975) has proposed that such flattened affect may be a sign of inhibited grief or depression, or that it may signal the relinquishing of an interest in life. Burnside (1969) has cautioned that this characteristic pattern may lead to a misdiagnosis of organic brain syndrome. Second, there are more likely to be complaints of a sense of inadequacy, loss of purpose in life, and an unwillingness to "go on" without the deceased. Third, some grief responses may be exaggerated among older adult bereaved individuals, including apathy, self-isolation, and idealization of the deceased (cf. Ball, 1976–1977; Heyman & Gianturco, 1973; Parkes, 1964; Skelskie, 1975; Stern, Williams, & Prados, 1951). Fourth, older bereaved people are more likely to hallucinate (i.e., "see" or "hear") the deceased person (Rees, 1971), a process which has been associated with long happy marriages.

Younger widows have significantly stronger grief reactions than older widows, show greater irritability if the death of a spouse was sudden rather than prolonged, and are more restless (Ball, 1976–1977). Maddison (1968) believed that younger widows were at greater risk for high mortality rates following bereavement than older widows, a finding that was also related to existing financial problems, number of dependent children, preexisting problems with the marriage, multiple crises, problems with the spouse's family, lack of support from family or professionals, and personal problems of the widow herself. Younger bereaved are more likely to have health problems following the loss of a spouse (Maddison & Viola, 1968), higher mortality rates (Kraus & Lilienfeld, 1959), an increase in psychological difficulties (Parkes, 1964), and more sleep disturbances (Gorer, 1965) than older adults.

These descriptions seem to suggest that the older bereaved person is better adjusted to the experience of loss in comparison with the younger bereaved. Not everyone agrees, however. Stern and colleagues (1951) reported that grief reactions of older bereaved in their sample (who were between the ages of 53 and 70) included a greater preponderance of somatic illnesses, such as pain, gastrointestinal problems, and sleep disorders than the younger bereaved. Bettis and Scott (1981) have also stated that these problems are more severe and more long-lasting for the older bereaved person than the younger.

A longitudinal study by Sanders (1981) comparing bereavement outcomes of older and younger widowed individuals determined that under certain conditions the older group of bereaved (i.e., persons over age 65) had more persistent problems in adjustment than the younger group (i.e., people under age 63), compared with matched controls who were not bereaved. Sanders found that duration of bereavement was differentially related to symptomatology and intensity of grief for the two age groups. The younger widowed group responded initially with greater shock, confusion, guilt, and anxiety, but they were able to adjust fairly quickly. The older bereaved initially manifested diminished grief responses, but their reactions became more powerful as time passed, even up to two years after the loss. On the Grief Experience Inventory, the younger bereaved obtained higher scores on the element of guilt, while the older bereaved scored higher on the denial element and on measures of social isolation, depersonalization, death anxiety, and loss of vigor.

Results from the Sanders (1981) study are interesting, in that they point out the painful progression of grief for the older adult and they indicate the importance of taking measures as time passes after a loss. Thus, while preponderance of data suggest that younger bereaved are at higher risk for both physical and mental health problems than older bereaved, the distress and symptomatology experienced by elderly bereaved are, nonetheless, disturbing and often debilitating to their health. Research on the health effects of bereavement are explored in the next section.

EFFECTS OF BEREAVEMENT ON
WELL-BEING OF OLDER ADULTS

Mortality and Morbidity Effects

According to excellent reviews by Stroebe and Stroebe (1987) and Oster-weis, Solomon, and Green (1984), epidemiological evidence from a variety of sources demonstrated an increase in mortality rates for the recently bereaved who experienced spousal loss, although conclusions from the evidence must be drawn carefully because of a number of methodological problems in the various data collection processes described in these studies. These reviews contain detailed critiques of the data and are not repeated here.

In studying widows and widowers of all ages, Helsing, Szklo, and Comstock (1981) have noted increases in deaths from suicide, accidents, cardiovascular disease, and some infectious diseases among widowers and an increase in the risk of death from cirrhosis of the liver among widows. Glick, Weiss, and Parkes (1974) found an increase in hospitalization among the widowed within a year after the loss of a spouse, but only widowers demonstrated significantly more physical health problems. Clayton (1979) reported similar findings in the rate of hospitalization, but only among the young widowed sample. She did not find differences in the number of reported physical problems between those who were married and those who were widowed.

When older adults were specifically studied, however, results were surprising. One might expect older bereaved people to be more vulnerable to the detrimental health effects of bereavement because they initially are more likely to be in poor health. As Stroebe and Stroebe (1987) point out, "the negative health impact of bereavement is generally attributed to the fact that it aggravates or accelerates existing health problems" (p. 185). The bulk of the evidence indicates that it is the younger bereaved who suffer greater health deterioration. For example, Heyman and Gianturco (1973) found a small increase in depressive symptomatology in older widowed women, but no change in health, leisure activities, or anxiety. Norris and Stanley (1987) likewise found no relationship between bereavement and health status, but did find that health status was related to amount of stress in the family prior to occurrence of death and after the death, only if there had been no stress in the family preceding the death. Murrell, Himmelfarb, and Phifer (1988) also reported that, when health status before bereavement was taken into account, there was no relationship between bereavement and self-reported health, nor between bereavement and subsequent death, health problems, or use of medical services by the elderly men and women who participated in their study. Other investigators concur with these findings (Avis, Brambilla, Vass, & McKinlay, 1991; Wolinski & Johnson, 1992). Ferraro (1985) also found that elderly bereaved perceived their health as poorer shortly after loss, but not on a long-term basis.

Thompson, Breckenridge, Gallagher, and Peterson (1984), however, believe that bereavement has more serious health effects on the elderly than these data appear to indicate. They found that, among their sample of 212 widowed adults between the ages of 55 and 83, recently bereaved more often reported a worsening of existing illnesses, development of new illnesses, beginning a new medication, greater use of medication, and poorer health ratings than adults in the control group. There were no differences between groups on number of visits to physicians or hospitalizations. Although recently bereaved men did not report greater morbidity than women in the sample, there were more deaths among them one year after loss of a spouse, and there were more deaths among bereaved than among control group participants. Thompson and colleagues (1984) caution that bereaved men may have underestimated their health problems at the time of the study.

Avis and colleagues (1991) also found that recent bereavement was associated with increased use of prescription medicine; Wolinski and Johnson (1992) reported that it was linked to a greater probability of being placed in a nursing home. Most seriously, Mendes de Leon, Kasl, and Jacobs (1993) provided a weak but positive association between widowhood and mortality in the first 6 months after spousal death for a group of elderly bereaved. This effect was most pronounced for widows between the ages of 65 and 74.

Findings about health consequences of bereavement are complicated by a number of factors pertinent to older adults. We know, for instance, that mortality rates are affected by changes in residence to nursing homes, retirement homes, and institutions (already indicators of poor health), and solitary living (Morse & Wisocki, 1991). Remarriage seems to make a difference in the mortality rates of widowed men, but not of widowed women (Osterweis *et al.*, 1984). Following a death, there are generally marked increases in the consumption of tobacco, alcohol, and drugs (Maddison & Viola, 1968), mostly among people who had used these substances earlier. Emotional stress in response to loss has been implicated in deaths from congestive heart failure (Chambers & Reiser, 1953) and essential hypertension (Wiener, Gerber, Battine, & Arkin, 1975). In a study of death occurrences during stressful times Engel (1961) reported that half his sample of people died immediately after the death of a person close to them and an additional 43% died within sixteen days after the death of someone close. Engel related the majority of these deaths, however, to cardiac arrest in persons with cardiovascular disease, not to bereavement per se.

Another stress factor that may contribute to the bereaved person's health status is related to the demands associated with caring for a relative who is ill, dependent, or dying. Evidence suggests that caregivers worry often about finances and the adequacy of available help; they reduce their participation in social and recreational events; and they frequently experience a great deal of stress in family relationships (e.g. Canton, 1983; Poulshock & Deimling, 1984). As Harlow, Goldberg, and Comstock (1991b) determined, depression scores of a group of elderly men and women prior to widowhood were inversely related to the spouse's health status, indicating perhaps that bereavement begins somewhat before actual death occurs.

It is commonly assumed that opportunity to grieve prior to the loss may ease the impact of the loss and facilitate long-term recovery for the bereaved person. This process, called *anticipatory grief* (Lindemann, 1944), has been examined in a few studies in which suddenness of death was a major variable. Clayton (1979) and Parkes (1972) both found that young widows grieve less and remarry sooner following an anticipated death, as opposed to a sudden death. Lundin (1984) found that sudden death from acute illness was associated with a significant increase in sick days on the part of the bereaved, whereas expected death from chronic illness was not significantly related to the number of sick days.

For the elderly, however, it appears the opposite is true. Gerber, Rusalem, Hannon, Battin, and Arkin (1975) found that elderly widows had a better prognosis if their husbands died suddenly rather than after a lingering illness. Similar results were obtained by Vachon and colleagues (1977), who compared widows of cancer patients with widows of men who suffered from chronic cardiovascular disease. Deaths of the cancer patients were generally anticipated, whereas the deaths of the patients with cardiovascular disease were sudden, although not completely unexpected. One to two months after their loss, 38% of the widows whose husbands had died of cancer reported that they felt worse than they did immediately after the death. Twenty-three percent of the widows of the men who had died of cardiovascular disease reported feeling worse during that same time period, which is a statistically significant difference. Cancer widows were also more likely to feel that they were in poor health following the death of their husbands than the other widows.

Additional evidence is provided by Hill, Thompson, and Gallagher (1988), who found that elderly bereaved women who had anticipated or spontaneously rehearsed for their loss by discussing funeral arrangements, financial security, feelings about being left behind, and prospects for the future if one's spouse died before they did, were more poorly adjusted after their loss, reported significantly more health problems, and tended to show greater levels of depression than those widows who had not engaged in spontaneous rehearsal strategies. These investigators also found no relationship between expectancy of death and the subsequent adjustment to bereavement.

Averill and Wisocki (1981) have offered several reasons why anticipated loss, as compared with sudden loss, should be more debilitating for older adults than for younger adults. The first reason is that death seldom comes as a complete surprise to the elderly. They frequently experience deaths of their friends and family members and receive several reminders of their own vulnerability to mortality. Consequently, some of the value a forewarning might provide to the young may be superfluous to the elderly. Second, anticipation of a threatening event can be a potent source of stress in its own right. Knowing that a spouse will die within a limited time period can add to the stress of bereavement without necessarily conferring compensating benefits. This is especially true if the surviving spouse is suffering from chronic ill health or some other preexisting condition that might be worsened by the stress of caring for a dying partner.

It is important to recognize, however, that caring for a dying partner may also provide purpose and satisfaction to the lives of some elderly. Caregiving may be the primary source of social support for the caregiving partner. Thus, ironically, the third reason why an anticipated bereavement may be particularly difficult for the elderly, is that, with death of a spouse, the caregiving partner loses these positive attributions and affiliations. The fourth reason is related to the third. It is difficult for a person to make personal sacrifices that are often demanded by a dying spouse without experiencing some ambivalence. This is especially true if the spouse's illness has progressed through a series of remissions, increasing risk of premature detachment. An ambivalent relationship prior to death of a partner is frequently cited as an etiological factor in pathological grief (Aldrich, 1974; Parkes, 1972).

Mental Health Effects

Numerous studies of stressful life events and life change events repeatedly confirm loss as a powerful predictor of mental disorder (e.g., Dohrenwend & Dohrenwend, 1974; Rahe, 1979). In an extensive review of the health risks of the bereaved, Stroebe and Stroebe (1987), reported overwhelming support for the idea that bereavement may be a cause of mental illness. Only one study reported dissenting findings. That study was done by Clayton (1979), who studied 109 widowed people and found that both psychiatric consultation and hospitalization were rare following the death of a spouse.

Although the bulk of these studies was conducted with younger adults, it appears that the bereaved older adult is also likely to experience high rates of psychological symptomatology. For example, Richards and McCallum (1979) reported rates of diagnosed depressive disorder or severe psychological distress in 25% to 33% of the elderly bereaved in their sample population within the first year of bereavement. Jacobs, Melson, and Zisook (1987) reported that 10% to 20% of the 800,000 people in the United States who become widows or widowers suffered from severe depression during the first year of bereavement. Carey (1977) not only found that self-reported depression occurred significantly more often among the widowed than among the married, but it was still measurable as long as 13 to 16 months after the loss. In cases where a spouse committed suicide, elderly bereaved were significantly more anxious than their counterparts whose spouses died "natural deaths," but did not differ on other measures of psychological distress; both groups of bereaved elderly demonstrated significantly higher scores on measures of depression and general psychopathology (Farberow, Gallagher, Gilewski, & Thompson, 1987).

Along with depression, the elderly bereaved experience problems with sleep, social support, self-esteem, and impaired functioning (Pasternak *et al.,* 1994).

Progression of bereavement over an extended time has been examined by several researchers and the findings illuminate important aspects about the psychological healing process for elderly bereaved. In a series of studies by Clayton and her colleagues (Bornstein, Clayton, Halikas, Maurice, & Robins, 1973; Clayton, Halikas, & Maurice, 1972; Clayton, Herjanic, Murphy, & Woodruff, 1974), 35% of their sample of older widows and widowers (mean age 61.5) showed signs of depression at 1 month after their losses, 25% at 4 months, and 17% up to a year after the loss. Harlow, Goldberg, and Comstock (1991a) reported similar percentages with their sample of elderly bereaved women. They found that 17.5% of the bereaved showed a higher percentage rate of depressive symptoms after the first year of widowhood. For the majority of the population studied, depressive reactions peaked at 6 months after the loss and returned to baseline levels after the first year, a finding which led them and other researchers (e.g..

Murrell & Himmelfarb, 1989) to conclude that bereavement does not pose a serious threat to mental health among the elderly.

That conclusion was challenged by Mendes De Leon, Kasl, and Jacobs (1994), who, as part of a prospective study, conducted a detailed and extensive examination of the course of depressive symptomatology during the bereavement of 139 elderly widowed men and women between the ages of 65 and 99. They described a 75% increase in depression scores during the first year of bereavement, which returned to prewidowhood levels for most people by the second year after the loss. They did not, however, find this pattern to be true for younger female members of the sample (i.e., those between 65 and 74). For these widows, levels of depressive symptoms did not decline as much after the initial increase and remained elevated long after the first year. In fact, their symptoms persisted into the second and third years following spousal loss. Prevalence rates calculated over the years of the study indicated that 37.5% of older bereaved adults experienced high depressive symptomatology during the first year of bereavement and 16% of the sample were bereaved for more than 1 year. Mendes de Leon and his colleagues concluded from these data that many older bereaved adults, especially those in the lower register of senior citizenship, "experienced clinically significant increases in depressive symptomatology well beyond the normal duration of the grief process, and that many of these indeed are likely to suffer from depressive disorder" (p. 622).

Interestingly in this study, the acutely bereaved reported symptoms of disturbed affect, but not symptoms relating to negative self-appraisal, which the authors proposed may be reflective of the normal manifestation of grief and may provide a useful diagnostic distinction between grief and depression. Indeed, Mendes De Leon and colleagues (1994) compared elderly subjects who had elevated depression scores 1 year after spousal death and nonwidowed elderly subjects who also had high depression scores. They found that the widowed group had levels of negative appraisals that were almost as high as those of the persistently depressed nonwidowed. By contrast, very few of the recently bereaved endorsed the negative appraisal symptoms. These findings led the researchers to conclude that elderly bereaved with persistent elevations of depressive symptomatology after the first year of widowhood may require professional clinical treatment. Information from McHorney and Mor (1988) indicating that bereaved subjects who were classified as depressed increased their contact with physicians, in comparison with the bereaved who were not depressed, lends additional support to this conclusion.

Pasternak and her colleagues (1994) took this notion a step further by identifying a clinically subsyndromal depressed group of elderly bereaved and comparing them with a matched group who were not depressed and a group who were neither depressed nor bereaved. Subjects (average age 68 years) were rated on measures of general functioning, depressive symptoms, sleep disturbances, medical condition, social support, social rhythm stability, and grief intensity every 6 months for 2 years after loss of spouses in the first two groups. Depressed participants consistently demonstrated greater impairments than the other two sets of participants, even after 2 years. They showed continued intense grieving and impaired sleep quality at 18 months after the loss, lower social support, poor self-esteem, and impaired life functioning 1 to 2 years later. Stability of social rhythms was not impaired, however (a finding that the authors suggest may have protected those subsyndromally depressed bereaved from developing more serious forms of depression). All of the bereaved elderly had increased medical problems, as compared with control subjects.

It appears, then, that the elderly bereaved experience multiple psychological problems connected to the grief experience. They are particularly vulnerable to depressive symptomatology, which may persist for several years after the death of a spouse. Depression in cases of bereavement, however, is qualitatively different from chronic clinical depression for elderly men and women. Thus, bereavement does not appear to be a primary etiological factor in most cases of depression in the elderly.

SOCIAL SUPPORT AS A FACTOR IN BEREAVEMENT

In addition to the often painful loss of the person himself or herself, death of a loved one often eliminates an important source of interaction and it may eliminate one's role in society as well. When one's identity has been defined by the relationship to the deceased (e.g., as husband or wife), role loss is a major source of distress and depression in its own right. Such loss may help explain why many elderly bereaved report a sense of meaninglessness and lack of purpose after the death of a spouse, not to mention a sense of social isolation, loneliness, or apathy long after the bereavement process has ended. The survivor may be required to move to a smaller, more manageable residence; children and other relatives may be living at a distance and thus be unable to provide continuing social support; financial resources may be inadequate to sustain a comfortable life style; a person may lack job skills, driving skills, and even self-management skills. For example, many elderly widows have never had experience in managing money and thus are ill prepared to do it. Many elderly widowers have never had experience preparing a meal or maintaining a house, and thus are lacking adequate survival skills.

Perhaps because the social losses are so great, the social network may take on greater importance for people at the time of bereavement. Certainly, results from a number of studies suggest that social factors play a strong role in not only alleviating the stress of the loss (Schwarzer, 1992) but in helping to ameliorate postbereavement depression in the elderly (Norris & Murrell, 1990; Siegel & Kuykendall, 1990).

Bowling (1988–1989) followed 503 widowed elderly for 6 years after loss of their spouses and found that the death rate for widowers over 75 years of age was significantly higher than for the same-aged men in the general population. Multivariate analyses showed that, in addition to being a male over 75 years of age, the most powerful discriminating variables independently associated with mortality were a low happiness rating given by the interviewer, high social class, and having no one to telephone. Bowling suggested that social contact and a happier disposition may have modifying effects on the stress of bereavement and the risk factors associated with subsequent mortality.

From a large epidemiological study, Goldberg, Comstock, and Harlow (1988) interviewed 128 elderly widows (6 months after spousal loss) who had in the original baseline interview reported specifically that they did not need help for an emotional problem and who had completed questionnaires assessing number of people in their social network and quality of the interactions. At the time of the second interview participants were again asked if they needed help with an emotional problem since becoming widowed. Nearly 22% responded affirmatively to the question. In a series of multiple logistic regression analyses, the authors examined the effects of social network variables on the expressed need for help and found that three were significant. First, they found that size of the network was a significant factor in a lack of need for emotional counseling. Widows with networks smaller than 10 people were at greater risk. A similar finding was also reported by Dimond, Lund, and Caserta (1987), who determined that size of the social network, perceived closeness to the members of the network, and the quality of the interaction were significantly related to coping behavior, lower scores on the depression measure, and higher life satisfaction 2 years after spousal loss for 192 elderly bereaved men and women.

The second significant variable from the work of Goldberg and her colleagues (1988) is that number of friends seemed more important than size of one's family. Widows with four or more friends with whom they kept in touch were less likely to feel the need for emotional counseling than those with fewer friends. This finding is similar to the conclusion reached by Arling (1976b), who compared various sources of social support, such as family members, friends, and neighbors on their effect on the morale of elderly widowed. Arling found that contact with friends and neighbors was clearly related to a reduction in loneliness and worry, while contact with family members, especially children, did little to elevate morale.

Goldberg and colleagues' (1988) findings on the value of children to the widow are different from conclusions reached by Arling (1976b). Goldberg and her colleagues found that widows who, at baseline, had reported a very close relationship to their children, were less likely to have a need for help during the bereavement process than were either those widows who had no children or who had a low level of closeness to their children. This finding is also supported by Lopata's (1979) work, in which it was found that the widow's children provided more service and emotional support than her friends. It is possible, however, that participants in Goldberg and colleagues' (1988) study were stronger because they had the security of knowing about the positive quality of their relationship to their children, but that fact may or may not have been related to the importance of developing other relationships with nonfamily members after the loss of the spouse. Indeed, research has consistently shown benefits from friendship networks (cf. review by Ferraro, 1984), whereas research on the family has not shown such benefits and family-based relationships have usually been regarded as providing neutral or even negative effects (cf. review in Mutran & Reitzes, 1984). Results of a number of studies in which family and friends have been compared as sources of support (e.g., Arling, 1976a; Roberto & Scott, 1986) have indicated that support from friends is more important to the widowed.

This finding contradicts common wisdom, which suggests that bereavement demands a pulling together of the family resources; after an initial period of condolence, friends often tend to stay away to allow the bereaved time to share the grief experience within the family. Research findings, however, intimate that a supply of friends is essential in easing the pain of bereavement. Social contacts in various forms, including phone calls, personal visits, and even letters are beneficial for the elderly bereaved.

Lack of a network of social acquaintances may have the same deleterious effect as a lack of good health practices. Those elderly who have lost friends through death or new residential placements, or those who have lost them by exclusive focus on family over a long period of time, or those who never had many friends to begin with, may find it particularly difficult to reenter a social world after the death of a long-time companion.

Worden (1982) feels so strongly about the importance of social support for the bereaved that he has stated that the role of mental health professionals in grief therapy is to provide a substitute for religious and family institutions that have stopped providing necessary support to the bereaved in the culture.

THERAPY FOR THE ELDERLY BEREAVED

Grief is a normal response to loss and not a form of pathology. It is a complex experience, the origins of which may be found in the biological, psychological, and sociocultural history of an individual. Thus, as has been stated elsewhere (Averill & Wisocki, 1981), some of the components of grief, such as protest, search, and depression of activity may reflect biological adaptations, either directly or indirectly. Other components may be the result of psychological factors, such as extinction of habits that have been built up over many years of living with another person. Finally, still other components may reflect social privileges and responsibilities. Any therapeutic regimen that seeks to alleviate the suffering of the bereaved must be sensitive to these historical causes, as well as to the aspects of the current situation that together help determine the nature, severity, and duration of the entire grief experience. It is not the goal of therapy to eliminate grief, but to understand it and alleviate some of its pain.

The various components of grief cannot be attributed to any single cause and thus cannot be alleviated by any single procedure. As has been stated elsewhere (Wisocki & Averill, 1988), goals should be established and intervention procedures should be selected depending on the component reactions that are presenting difficulties. For instance, possible categories of goals may include *physiological concerns,* such as somatic symptoms, insomnia, headaches, compliance to medical regimens, proper nutrition, and self-care activities; *subjective (private) events,* such as devaluative self-statements, disturbing thoughts about taking one's life in order to join the deceased, self-blaming statements about ways one could have kept the deceased alive, and so on; *overt behaviors,* including behavioral excesses commonly occurring during bereavement, such as alcohol consumption or over-medication, compulsions, and avoidance reactions; *interpersonal relationships,* such as reducing isolation, increasing social contacts, assertive behaviors when necessary; and *environmental supports,* which may involve changing environmental structures to support or facilitate therapeutic gains.

Occasionally grieving has pathological aspects. For instance, a person may openly grieve for "too long," a time determined by social custom, but generally meaning more than a year. At times a person seems to devote too much energy and too many resources to celebrating the deceased, such as turning a room in a house into a "shrine" or setting a place at the dining table each day for the deceased person. These prolonged grief experiences are not only troubling in and of themselves, but they may also lead to health-threatening behaviors, such as refusal to eat, withdrawal from companionship, depression, and so forth.

The symptoms of pathological grief have been listed by Wahl (1970) as profound feelings of irrational despair and hopelessness; an inability to accept or deal with feelings of ambivalence toward the deceased person; loss of self-esteem; self-blame for the death; an inability to proffer affection to others; loss of interest in planning for the future; protracted apathy, irritability, or hyperactivity without appropriate affect. This is only a partial list, but it illustrates the commonality of symptoms between normal and pathological grieving. These symptoms become pathological only if they are unduly prolonged or if they are expressed in such a way as to lead to other forms of serious maladaptive behavior.

Worden (1982) believes that pathological grief occurs when four grieving tasks have not been completed: accepting the reality of the loss, experiencing the pain of the loss, adjusting to an environment in which the deceased is not present, and withdrawing emotional energy and reinvesting it in another relationship. The focus in therapy is on the resolution of these tasks, which are achieved by getting the client to talk to the deceased. Methods for accomplishing this goal include role playing, linking objects and photos (i.e., touching special tokens, clothing, pictures, etc. of the deceased as a way of stimulating memories), and the empty-chair technique. Worden also relies heavily on the therapeutic relationship to provide the necessary social support for the bereaved.

Volkan (1975) has developed a short-term model of treatment called "regrief therapy," in which the bereaved undergoes three processes: demarcation, externalization, and reorganization, all designed to separate the bereaved person from the deceased. The person is first encouraged to relive the orginal loss experience by recounting or behaviorally tracing the details of it and abreacting. Confrontation is a technique central to this process and ultimately serves to direct the bereaved's energies toward new objects.

Melges and DeMaso (1980) have developed "grief resolution therapy," based on use of abreactive processes, for removal of elements they feel prevent the resolution of grief.

There are several therapies for pathological bereavement that employ techniques based primarily on behavior therapy. For example, Kleber and Brom (1985) use relaxation, desensitization, and hypnotic imagery to have the bereaved client gradually confront the relevant aspects of his or her loss. They also work with clients in a psychodynamic framework to help them discover and solve intrapsychic conflicts related to loss. Lieberman (1978) has described a similar approach, using systematic desensitization and implosion, a therapy model that he describes as "forced mourning." Ramsay (1977) recommends flooding as the most effective model of therapy because it involves a confrontation with the stimuli associated with the loss and elicits the grief response. In using the flooding procedure, considerable time is devoted to developing details of the client's relationship to the deceased. Guided imagery is also used to have the client re-create the moment of parting to allow expression of unstated thoughts and feelings.

Exposure to stimuli associated with loss is regarded by many as the critical ingredient in overcoming pathological grieving. Research efforts to demonstrate the importance of this factor have produced interesting results. Mawson, Marks, Ramm, and Stern (1981) compared a guided mourning and exposure technique with antiexposure instructions to avoid contact with distressing situations relating to subjects' bereavement. They found that, after 1 month of treatment, subjects in the exposure condition showed less avoidance of bereavement cues and scored better on the Texas Inventory of Grief than the other group. On most other measures, however, the groups improved equally. Sireling, Cohen, and Marks (1988) attempted a replication of this study with an increase in number of subjects and treatment sessions, the addition of more systematic advice, support, and help with relationships, work, and recreational activities, additional affective and cognitive cues, and more assessments. They reported similar results, again favoring the guided mourning and exposure condition.

Specific attempts to provide therapy for bereaved who are elderly have been relatively rare. Probably the most extensive effort directed to alleviation of bereavement-associated pain for the older adult going through a normal grieving process is organized around the use of support groups, such as the widow-to-widow programs and other social networks (cf. Walker, McBride, & Vachon, 1977). These groups exemplify the philosophy that grieving people are helped best by others who have shared the experience. And, as we have seen earlier, the social supportive aspects of group involvement are therapeutic in and of themselves for the older bereaved person.

Gerber, Wiener, Battin, and Arkin (1975) conducted a longitudinal investigation of a sample of elderly bereaved to evaluate the effects of unsolicited crisis intervention on medical outcomes. One hundred sixteen subjects were assigned to a treatment group; 53 were assigned to the nontreatment control group. Subjects in the treatment group were given support for the affective aspects of the grief response, helped to increase their participation in social activities with friends and family members, and helped with practical matters of legal, financial, and household concerns. Interviews were conducted at the homes of the subjects or by telephone. After 6 months intervention was terminated. Evaluations were conducted at 3, 5, 8, and 15 months after the loss. Subjects in the treatment group reported fewer drug prescriptions, fewer consultations with physicians, and fewer experiences of feeling ill. These findings confirmed the health benefits of the therapy and support the incorporation of social and practical elements in an intervention with elderly bereaved.

For the most part, the elderly bereaved seem to benefit from suggestions about restructuring their environment, increasing social contact, and maintaining adaptive behaviors. For specific problems associated with the grieving process, the bereaved might be trained in specific stress-relieving strategies, such as relaxation to assist in sleep induction, self-reinforcement for a more positive attitude, thought stopping about guilt, fears about the future, and so on, and desensitization to avoidance behaviors. Use of such procedures does not mean that the elderly person should not be permitted to express his or her grief openly. All therapeutic models encourage this expression to varying degrees.

As Wisocki and Averill (1988) have pointed out previously, the therapist working with the elderly bereaved should be prepared to extend his or her services in areas which are not strictly psychological in nature. Some of the most serious needs of an elderly client may be economical. The therapist may have to work with the client to establish a budget, open a bank account, pay bills, get a driver's license, and other mundane matters. At the minimum the therapist should be aware of relevant support services available within the client's local community and be able to serve as a catalyst to ensure that the client utilizes those services.

SUMMARY

Bereavement is an experience common to older adults. In many ways, older adults experience bereavement differently from younger adults. These differences are primarily in the intensity of the response to loss, the value of anticipatory grief, and the relationship of bereavement to mortality and morbidity effects. The age groups display similar psychological effects. Severe clinical depression is a particular concern for the bereaved. Among the elderly, however, the quality of negative appraisal frequently associated with clinical depression is often absent, suggesting a possible diagnostic factor indicative of pathological grieving instead of depression.

In this chapter, I addressed these differences and similarities by first, exploring the characteristics of bereavement; second, examining the evidence for the effects of bereavement on the mental and physical health of the elderly bereaved; third, presenting evidence for the benefits of social support in minimizing the negative effects of bereavement; and fourth, describing treatment strategies for the elderly who have difficulty in managing the pain of bereavement.

REFERENCES

Aldrich, C. (1974). Some dynamics of anticipatory grief. In B. Schoenberg, A. Carr, A. Kutscher, D. Peretz, & I. Goldberg (Eds.), *Anticipatory grief* (pp. 3–9). New York: Columbia University Press.

Arling, G. (1976a). The elderly widow and her family, neighbors, and friends. *Journal of Marriage and the Family, 38*, 757–768.

Arling, G. (1976b). Resistance to isolation among elderly widows. *International Journal of Aging and Human Development, 7*, 67–86.

Averill, J. (1979). The functions of grief. In C. Izard (Ed.), *Emotions in personality and psychopathology* (pp. 339–368). New York: Plenum.

Averill, J., & Wisocki, P. (1981). Some observations on behavioral approaches to the treatment of grief among the elderly. In H. Sobel (Ed.), *Behavior therapy in terminal care* (pp. 125–150). Cambridge, MA: Ballinger.

Avis, N., Brambilla, D., Vass, K., & McKinlay, J. (1991). The effect of widowhood on health: A prospective analysis from the Massachusetts Women's Health Study. *Social Science and Medicine, 33*, 1063–1070.

Ball, J. (1976–1977). Widow's grief: The impact of age and mode of death. *Omega, 7,* 307–333.

Bettis, S., & Scott, F. (1981). Bereavement and grief. In C. Eisdorfer (Ed.), *Annual review of gerontology and geriatrics* (pp. 144–159). New York: Springer.

Bornstein, P., Clayton, P., Halikas, J., Maurice, W., & Robbins, E. (1973). The depression of widowhood after thirteen months. *British Journal of Psychiatry, 122,* 561–566.

Bowlby, J. (1980). *Attachment and loss:*Vol. 3. *Loss: Sadness and depression.* New York: Basic Books.

Bowling, A. (1988–1989). Who dies after widow(er)hood? A discriminant analysis. *Omega: Journal of Death and Dying, 19,* 135–153.

Bugen, L. (1977). Human grief: A model for prediction and intervention. *American Journal of Orthopsychiatry, 47,* 196–206.

Burnside, I. (1969). Grief work in the aged patient. *Nursing Forum, 8,* 416–427.

Canton, M. (1983). Strain among caregivers: A study of experience in the United States. *Gerontologist, 23,* 597–604.

Carey, R. (1977). The widowed: A year later. *Journal of Counseling Psychology, 24,* 125–131.

Chambers, W., & Reiser, M. (1953). Emotional stress in the precipitation of congestive heart failure. *Psychosomatic Medicine, 15,* 38–60.

Clayton, P. (1979). The sequelae and nonsequelae of conjugal bereavement. *American Journal of Psychiatry, 136,* 1530–1534.

Clayton, P., Halikas, J., & Maurice, W. (1972). The depression of widowhood. *British Journal of Psychiatry, 1200,* 71–78.

Clayton, P., Herjanic, M., Murphy, G., & Woodruff, R. (1974). Mourning and depression: Their similarities and differences. *Canadian Psychiatric Association Journal, 19,* 309–312.

Dimond, M., Lund, D., & Caserta, M. (1987). The role of social support in the first two years of bereavement in an elderly sample. *Gerontologist, 27,* 599–604.

Dohrenwend, B. S., & Dohrenwend, B. P. (Eds.). (1974). *Stressful life events: Their nature and effects.* New York: Wiley.

Engel, G. (1961). Is grief a disease? *Psychosomatic Medicine, 23,* 18–23.

Farberow, N., Gallagher, D., Gilewski, M., & Thompson, L. (1987). An examination of the early impact of bereavement on psychological distress in survivors of suicide. *Gerontologist, 27,* 592–598.

Ferraro, K. (1984). Widowhood and social participation in later life: Isolation or compensation? *Research on Aging, 6,* 451–468.

Ferraro, K. (1985). The effect of widowhood on the health status of older persons. *International Journal of Aging and Human Development, 21,* 9–25.

Freud, S. (1959). *Mourning and melancholia.* In J. Riviere (Trans.), *Collected papers* (Vol. 4, pp. 152–170). New York: Basic Books. (Original work published 1917)

Gerber, I., Rusalem, R., Hannon, N., Battin, D., & Arkin, A. (1975). Anticipatory grief and aged widows and widowers. *Journal of Gerontology, 30,* 225–229.

Gerber, I., Wiener, A., Battin, D., & Arkin, A. (1975). Brief therapy to the aged bereaved. In B. Schoenberg, I. Gerber, A. Wiener, A. Kutscher, D. Peretz, & A. Carr (Eds.), *Bereavement: Its psychosocial aspects* (pp. 310–333). New York: Columbia University Press.

Glick, I., Weiss, R., & Parkes, C. (1974). *The first year of bereavement.* New York: Wiley.

Goldberg, E., Comstock, G., & Harlow, S. (1988). Emotional problems and widowhood. *Journal of Gerontology: Social Sciences, 43,* S206–208.

Gorer, G. (1965). *Death, grief, and mourning.* London: Crescent.

Harlow, S., Goldberg, I., & Comstock, G. (1991a). A longitudinal study of the prevalence of depressive symptomatology in elderly widowed and married women. *Archives of General Psychiatry, 48,* 1065–1068.

Harlow, S., Goldberg, I., & Comstock, G. (1991b). A longitudinal study of risk factors for depressive symptomatology in elderly widowed and married women. *American Journal of Epidemiology, 134,* 526–538.

Helsing, K., Comstock, G., & Szklo, M. (1982). Causes of death in a widowed population. *American Journal of Epidemiology, 116,* 524–532.

Heyman, D., & Gianturco, D. (1973). Long-term adaptation by the elderly to bereavement. *Journal of Gerontology, 28,* 359–362.

Hill, C. D., Thompson, L., & Gallagher, D. (1988). The role of anticipatory bereavement in older women's adjustment to widowhood. *Gerontologist, 28*, 792–796.

Jacobs, S., Melson, J., & Zisook, S. (1987). Treating depresssion of bereavement with antidepressants: A pilot study. *Psychiatric Clinics of North America, 10*, 501–510.

Kleber, R., & Brom, D. (1985). Psychotherapy and pathological grief controlled outcome study. *Israel Journal of Psychiatry and Related Sciences, 24*, 99–109.

Kraus, A., & Lilienfeld, A. (1959). Some epidemiological aspects of the high mortality rate in the young widowed group. *Journal of Chronic Disease, 10*, 207–217.

Kubler-Ross, E. (1970). *On death and dying*. London: Tavistock.

LaRue, A., Dessonville, D., & Jarvik, L. (1985). Aging and mental disorders. In J. Birren & K. W. Schaie (Eds.), *Handbook of the psychology of aging* (pp. 664–702). New York: Van Nostrand.

Lieberman, S. (1978). Nineteen cases of morbid grief. *British Journal of Psychiatry, 132*, 156–163.

Lindemann, E. (1944). The symptomatology and management of acute grief. *American Journal of Psychiatry, 101*, 141–148.

Lopata, H. (1979). *Women as widows: Support systems*. New York: Elsevier.

Lundin, T. (1984). Morbidity following sudden and unexpected bereavement. *British Journal of Psychiatry, 144*, 84–88.

Maddison, D. (1968). The relevance of conjugal bereavement to preventive psychiatry. *British Journal of Medical Psychology, 41*, 223–233.

Maddison, D., & Viola, A. (1968). The health of widows in the year following bereavement. *Journal of Psychosomatic Research, 12*, 297–306.

Mawson, D., Marks, I., Ramm, E., & Stern, R. (1981). Guided mourning for morbid grief: A controlled study. *British Journal of Psychiatry, 138*, 185–193.

McHorney, C., & Mor, V. (1988). Predictors of bereavement depression and its health services consequences. *Medical Care, 26*, 882–893.

Melges, F., & Demaso, D. (1980). Grief resolution therapy: Reliving, revising, and revisiting. *American Journal of Psychotherapy, 34*, 51–61.

Mendes DeLeon, C., Kasl, S., & Jacobs, S. (1993). Widowhood and mortality risk in a community sample of the elderly: A prospective study. *Journal of Clinical Epidemiology, 46*, 519–527.

Mendes DeLeon, C., Kasl, S., & Jacobs, S. (1994). A prospective study of widowhood and changes in symptoms of depression in a community sample of the elderly. *Psychological Medicine, 24*, 613–624.

Morse, C., & Wisocki, P. (1991). Residential factors in behavioral programming for elderly. In P. Wisocki (Ed.), *Handbook of clinical behavior therapy with the elderly client* (pp. 97–120). New York: Plenum.

Murrell, S., & Himmelfarb, S. (1989). Effects of attachment bereavement and pre-event condition on subsequent depressive symptoms in older adults. *Psychology of Aging, 4*, 166–172.

Murrell, S., Himmelfarb, S., & Phifer, J. (1988). Effects of bereavement/loss and pre-event status on subsequent physical health in older adults. *International Journal of Aging and Human Development, 27*, 89–107.

Mutran, E., & Reitzes, D. (1984). Intergenerational support activities and well-being among the elderly: A convergence of exchange and symbolic interaction perspectives. *American Sociological Review, 49*, 117–130.

Norris, F., & Murrell, S. (1990). Social support, life events, and stress as modifiers of adjustment to bereavement of older adults. *Psychology and Aging, 4*, 150–165.

Norris, F., & Stanley, S. (1987). Older adult family stress and adaptation before and after bereavement. *Journal of Gerontology, 42*, 606–612.

Osterweis, M., Solomon, F., & Green, M. (Eds.). (1984). *Bereavement reactions, consequences, and care*. Washington, DC: National Academy Press.

Parkes, C. (1964). The effects of bereavement on physical and mental health: A study of the case records of widows. *British Medical Journal, 2*, 274–279.

Parkes, C. (1972). *Bereavement: Studies of grief in adult life*. London: Tavistock.

Pasternak, R., Reynolds, C., Miller, M., Frank, E., Fasiczka, A., Prigerson, H., Mazumdar, S., & Kupfer, D. (1994). The symptom profile and two-year course of subsyndromal depression in spousally bereaved elders. *American Journal of Geriatric Psychiatry, 2*, 210–219.

Poulshock, S., & Deimling, G. (1984). Families caring for elders in residence: Issues in the measurement of burden. *Journal of Gerontology, 39,* 230–239.

Rahe, R. (1979). Life change events and mental illness: An overview. *Journal of Human Stress, 5,* 2–10.

Ramsay, R. (1977). Behavioural approaches to bereavement. *Behaviour Research and Therapy, 15,* 131–135.

Rees, W. (1971). The hallucination of widowhood. *British Medical Journal, 4,* 37–41.

Richards, J., & McCallum, J. (1979). Bereavement in the elderly. *New Zealand Medical Journal, 89,* 201–204.

Roberto, K., & Scott, J. (1986). Confronting widowhood. *American Behavioral Scientist, 29,* 497–511.

Sanders, C. (1981). Comparison of younger and older spouses in bereavement outcome. *Omega, 11,* 217–232.

Schwarzer, C. (1992). Bereavement, received social support, and anxiety in the elderly: A longitudinal analysis. *Anxiety Research, 4,* 287–298.

Siegel, J., & Kuykendall, D. (1990). Loss, widowhood, and psychological distress among the elderly. *Journal of Counseling and Clinical Psychology, 58,* 519–524.

Sireling, L., Cohen, D., & Marks, I. (1988). Guided mourning for morbid grief: A controlled replication. *Behavior Therapy, 19,* 121–132.

Skelskie, B. (1975). An exploratory study of grief in old age. *Smith College Studies in Social Work, 45,* 159–182.

Stern, K., Williams, G., & Prados, M. (1951). Grief reactions in later life. *American Journal of Psychiatry, 108,* 289–293.

Stroebe, W., & Stroebe, M. (1987). *Bereavement and health.* Cambridge, England: Cambridge University Press.

Thompson, L., Breckenridge, J., Gallagher, D., & Peterson, J. (1984). Effects of bereavement on self-perceptions of physical health in elderly widows and widowers. *Journal of Gerontology, 39,* 309–314.

Vachon, M., Freedman, K., Formo, A., Rogers, J., Lyall, W., & Freeman, S. (1977). The final illness in cancer: The widow's perspective. *Canadian Medical Association Journal, 177,* 1151–1154.

Volkan, V. (1975). "Re-grief" therapy. In B. Schoenberg, I. Gerber, A. Wiener, A. Kutscher, D. Peretz, & A. Carr (Eds.), *Bereavement: Its psychosocial aspects* (pp. 334–350). New York: Columbia University Press.

Wahl, C. (1970). The differential diagnosis of normal and neurotic grief following bereavement. *Psychosomatics, 11,* 104–106.

Walker, K., MacBride, A., & Vachon, M. (1977). Social support networks and the crises of bereavement. *Social Science and Medicine, 11,* 35–41.

Wiener, A., Gerber, I., Battine, D., & Arkin, A. (1975). The process and phenomenology of bereavement. In B. Schoenberg, I. Berger, A. Wiener, A. Kutchner, D. Peretz, & A. Carr (Eds.), *Bereavement: Its psychsocial aspects* (pp. 53–65). New York: Columbia University Press.

Wisocki, P., & Averill, J. (1988). The challenge of bereavement. In L. Carstensen & B. Edelstein (Eds.), *Handbook of clinical gerontology* (pp. 312–321). New York: Pergamon.

Wolinsky, F., & Johnson, R. (1992). Widowhood, health status, and the use of health services by older adults: A cross-sectional and prospective approach. *Journal of Gerontology: Social Sciences, 47,* 8–16.

Worden, J. (1982). *Grief counseling and grief therapy: A handbook for the mental health practitioner.* New York: Springer.

Wortman, C., & Silver, R. (1987). Coping with irrevocable loss. In G. VandenBos & B. Bryant (Eds.), *Cataclysms, crises, and catastrophies: Psychology in action* (pp. 185–235). Washington, DC: American Psychological Association.

CHAPTER 20

Marriage and Divorce

GARY R. BIRCHLER AND WILLIAM FALS-STEWART

INTRODUCTION

By the year 2000, 13% of the U.S. population will be over 65 years old (Peterson and Bahr, 1989); by 2040 it is estimated that this proportion will reach nearly 25% (Goldberg, 1992). Soon the average American will live up to 25 years *after* raising children to adulthood. A quarter of one's adult life may be spent in retirement. People entering retirement may have to deal with taking care of their aging parents as the number of people over 75 years of age increases (Goldberg, 1992). These significant changes in the demographics of our aging population suggest that families will be composed of more older people and fewer younger people; more divorces and remarriages will require important adjustments between husbands and wives. In particular, there is concern for women in their late 50s and 60s who will be called upon to care for (a) their elderly parents, (b) their adult children, and (c) their spouses (Goldberg, 1992; Peterson and Bahr, 1989). Because women generally outlive their husbands by a decade, it begs the question, "Who will provide for these women?" In this ominous context, marriage, as the persistent and venerable institution that it is, will become more challenged and will be an important resource for the elderly.

On a more positive note, many elderly couples are expected to become more active, more secure financially because they have two incomes, and more healthy and long-lived as a consequence of advances in medical technology. Nevertheless, economic and social support for older adults could become threatened (Neidhardt & Allen, 1993). The need for home health care is expected to grow tremendously (Goldberg, 1992; Peterson & Bahr, 1989). Consequently, there will be increasing pressure on the family to care for older family members, coming at a time when increasing numbers of the elderly from all racial and ethnic groups are living alone by choice or because of lack of alternatives (Lee, 1986; Mindel, 1986).

GARY R. BIRCHLER • Department of Psychiatry, School of Medicine, University of California, San Diego, La Jolla, California 92093-0603.   WILLIAM FALS-STEWART • Department of Psychology, Old Dominion University, Norfolk, Virginia 23529-0267.

Handbook of Clinical Geropsychology, edited by Michel Hersen and Vincent B. Van Hasselt. Plenum Press, New York, 1998.

RECOGNIZED BIASES

Much of the literature in the area of marriage and the elderly has focused on retirement (cf. Szinovasz, Ekerdt, & Vinick, 1992). Relatively little attention has been devoted to a family systems conceptualization of the aging process. Apart from investigations of gender role transitions as a result of retirement, family life cycle theories and research have generally neglected older persons during the *postparental* and *culmination* stages of the marital life cycle (Birchler, 1992; Carter and McGoldrick, 1988). This book is an example of the recent attempts to consolidate and promote the field of geropsychology. We must realize the developmental potential of all generations in the family. To this end, Flori (quoted in Goldberg, 1992) recommends that mental health care providers take a position of *therapeutic realism*, as opposed to *therapeutic pessimism* or *therapeutic idealism*. Examples of therapeutic pessimism include (a) notions that because elderly couples have a limited capacity to change their beliefs, interventions are better devoted to the younger generations, (b) the idea that validating and confirming long-standing patterns of behavior and beliefs is better than expecting changes in them, and (c) beliefs that in treating elderly clients one cannot have much hope for the future; it is preferable to work for acceptance of the inevitable. Such views are not in the best interest of older persons. However, at the other extreme, therapeutic idealism also can miss the mark; practitioners with this bias often minimize age-specific concerns and developmental changes that must be recognized in order to best meet the needs of elderly couples. Seeking a balance between these viewpoints, therapeutic realism accounts for the personal strengths and vulnerabilities of the elderly couple. When understood, validated, and encouraged, the elderly couple has significant potential to become as vibrant, efficient, and competent as their younger counterparts (Wolinsky, 1990).

In this chapter, we will discuss the strengths and vulnerabilities of older couples and review briefly certain better-known aspects of marriage during the postparental and culmination stages of the marital life cycle. The status and implications of divorce and remarriage among the elderly also will be explored. Finally, an approach to working with older adults in the context of conjoint marital therapy will be described.

THE MARITAL RELATIONSHIP
OF OLDER COUPLES

The marital relationships of older couples can best be described by posing and answering a number of relevant questions. Answers to these questions delineate the requisites for viable long-term relationships, illustrate the strengths of older marriages, and highlight vulnerabilities to be identified and treated in therapy. It should be noted that most of the research and the following discussion pertain, in general, either to first marriages or to long-term second or third marriages. The developmental tasks and evolution of relationship dynamics apply most appropriately to two people living together and experiencing an "older marriage," not just older people who become married or remarried. Characteristics of *remarriages* will be discussed later in this chapter.

1. How are older marriages different from younger marriages?

This information is organized according to lifelong changes in marital satisfaction and four important core dimensions or requisites of a longterm intimate
relationship: The *4 Cs* (i.e., Commitment, Caring, Communication, and Conflict
resolution: Birchler & Fals-Stewart, 1994a; Birchler & Schwartz, 1994; Nichols,
1988). As for changes in marital satisfaction over the marital life cycle, reasonable consensus exists that marital satisfaction follows a curvilinear pattern
(Miller, 1976; Rollins & Cannon, 1974; Spanier, Lewis, & Cole, 1975; Troll, 1986).
In order of development, the five stages of the traditional marital life cycle have
been described by Birchler (1992): Newlyweds, Parents Or Not To Be, Mid-life
Adolescence (of the adults), Postparental, and Culmination. Newlyweds are the
happiest, followed by postparental couples (i.e., couples early in retirement).
Couples in the parenting stage or marriages in the midlife adolescence of their
relationship generally are the least satisfied and most conflicted. In particular,
child-rearing and occupational issues seem to trouble many marriages (J. M.
Lewis, 1988; J. M. Lewis, Owen, & Cox, 1988; Nadelson, Polonsky, & Mathews,
1984). Couples experiencing the culmination stage of marital life are nearly as
satisfied as the somewhat younger postparental couples, particularly if they can
retain their health and financial security (Gilford, 1984; Lee, 1988).

Commitment between elder spouses seems to evolve from the passion, independence, and volatility experienced in youth, eventually to attaining a level
of profound loyalty, mutual sharing of activities, a sense of fairness, and a comfortable interdependency in meeting the day-to-day practical challenges of life
(Traupmann & Harfield, 1983; Troll, 1986). *Caring,* including support and understanding, cohesion, affection, and sexual interaction, evolves from physical
attraction and higher intensity emotionality to more stable elements of attachment, mutual caregiving, and, for some, continuing sexual activity emphasizing
warmth and closeness. Sexual activity and marital satisfaction correlate positively (Hammond, 1989), but for many older couples sex is not essential (Troll,
1986). Over time, *Communication* also reaches a more mature form of development. Older couples have a long-term perspective; they are inclined to experience humor, playfulness, and possess good communication skills (Lauer, Lauer,
& Kerr, 1990). Finally, *Conflict resolution* patterns often change from the uneven,
high-conflict, demand-withdraw, or disengaged styles characteristic of younger
marriages to a more passive, consensus-based pattern of low conflict. Even older
distressed marriages tend to have many fewer domestic disagreements (Birchler
& Schafer, 1990; Condie, 1990; Fals-Stewart, Schafer, & Birchler, 1993; Levenson,
Carstensen, & Gottman, 1993, 1994). Cuber and Haroff (1965) found that older
couples were more likely to fit their *passive-congenial* and *devitalized* types of
marriage (compared to the *total, vital,* or *conflict-habituated* types).

2. Is marriage good for older people? Are there gender differences
   in the quality experienced?

A sizable body of research supports the physical and emotional value of being married over being widowed or divorced for both men and women (Goldberg, 1992; Quiroutte & Gold, 1992). Married older people live longer, experience

higher life satisfaction, smoke less, are less depressed, have more financial resources, and have lower rates of institutionalization. However, beyond the *state*
of marriage, and especially for women, it is the *quality* of the marriage that appears to be even more important for individuals' physical and emotional well-
being. More specifically, the positive association between the state of being
married and mental health is stronger for men, whereas marital satisfaction is a
stronger predictor for women's mental health than it is for men's mental health.
In particular, Quirouette and Gold (1992) found that the three variables that best
predicted wives' psychological well-being were (a) husbands' perceptions of the
marriage, (b) husbands' positive well-being, and (c) husbands' physical health.
The authors interpreted these findings from a traditional perspective, suggesting
that because caring for children and the family has been the wives' responsibility, their husbands' satisfaction serves as a powerful determinant of their own
self-esteem. That is, their husbands' perceptions of the quality of the marriage reflect on the wives' levels of competency and thus affect their psychological well-
being. Moreover, with advancing age men tend to become more dependent on
their wives for nurturance, social interaction, and assistance with disabilities,
thus reinforcing wives' caregiver roles. Therefore, when the husbands' senses of
well-being are positive, so are their wives'.

3. What are the basic requisites and developmental tasks associated with a long-term intimate relationship?

It is estimated that only 20% of first marriages will survive to their golden
anniversaries (Brubaker, 1983; Glick & Norton, 1977). What does it take to reach
this amazing milestone? Wynne (1984), suggests that long-term intimate relationships require a mutual commitment to the marriage, attachment and affec-
tional bonding, communication and problem-solving skills (note that these
dimensions are similar to the 4 Cs discussed previously). Cole (1986) has proposed seven developmental tasks or achievements of high-quality long-term
marriages (Cole, 1989) which help partners in older marriages avoid loneliness,
reduce conflict and feel understood: (1) Establish an effective communication
system, (2) be aware of one's own and other's thoughts, feelings, and actions so
one can be responsive to partner's needs, (3) build and maintain a high level of
self-esteem, (4) become comfortable with ambivalence, (5) develop awareness
of one's own and one's partner's sexual needs and desires, (6) be comfortable
with partner's differences and use conflict resolution tools in a creative way,
and (7) develop problem-solving skills to reach mutually agreeable solutions.
Once again, the general emphasis of Cole's analysis is on the 4 Cs.

As energy levels and health change, it is also important for partners in
older couples to (a) establish predictable daily patterns and routines to manage
activities of daily living, such as housing, finances, and social activities, (b)
simplify their lifestyle (i.e., retain fewer material possessions and reduce the
number of routines and responsibilities), (c) develop and maintain healthy
habits regarding sleeping, eating, vitamins, and exercise, (d) shift and balance
workloads based less on traditional gender role responsibilities and more on
ability and cooperation, and (e) develop a plan for long-term financial security.

The final years together are significantly more rewarding if couples develop an effective retirement plan, learn to cope with health limitations and reduced energy levels, and successfully face their own mortality through advance planning (Askham, 1994; Swenson, Eskew, & Kohlhepp, 1981). Finally, family and social relationships can be critical during the culmination stage of the marital life cycle. Not only do spouses need to realize and correct for imbalances in amount of separateness and togetherness, but each partner must make similar adjustments with respect to their children, grandchildren, siblings, and same-generation family and friends.

4. What causes problems for older people in older marriages? What are the areas of vulnerability?

Consensus among gerontologists is that the two greatest threats to older couples are health problems and financial insecurity or poverty (Askham, 1994; Atchley, 1992; Condie, 1989; Hess & Markson, 1986; Quirouette & Gold, 1992). Unfortunately, disability and poverty tend to interact and together they are a significant threat to society as the U.S. population ages. Spousal mental or physical illness has a detrimental effect on both partners' psychological well-being. Major illness also negatively affects marital satisfaction, especially if the couple was experiencing marital distress before the onset of health problems (Quirouette & Gold, 1992). Typically, because wives are more frequently cast in the role of the caregiver, they suffer more or less depending on the level of marital quality. Although high-quality marriages seem to cope fairly well with physical illness, psychiatric illness in the husband significantly affects the psychological well-being of the wife, despite the premorbid level of marital satisfaction. Less is known about how husbands cope with their wives' health problems, but the level of marital satisfaction, for men, seems to be a less significant factor in their mental health.

Financial insecurity and poverty potentially have grave implications for the elderly. Virtually all aspects of their lives can be adversely affected if financial resources are insufficient. The resources include living arrangements (e.g., location and quality of housing, dependence on children or other relatives, space and privacy, need to move), health maintenance (e.g., access to health care, preventive versus remedial care, nutritional aides, illness and institutionalization), and general quality of life options (e.g., travel, material needs and desires, social activities and telecommunications). To the extent that the government reduces economic support in these areas, families will be challenged to compensate—and these changes will affect everyone in our society.

Apart from health and financial difficulties, older couples also are increasingly vulnerable to marital and life dissatisfaction if they have not succeeded in coping with or mastering the developmental tasks just described. Distressed older couples are susceptible to power struggles, high conflict, and isolating avoidance patterns if they have not developed collaborative mutuality in the 4 Cs: Commitment, Caring, Communication, and Conflict resolution. The failure of the partners in the relationship to develop adaptive interactional processes for managing stressful events (Karney & Bradbury, 1995) may lead to a low-quality passive-congenial type of existence at best, or to a lonely and devitalized relationship (Cuber & Haroff, 1965), or it may culminate in separation and divorce (R. A. Lewis & Spanier, 1979).

For ethnic and cultural minorities (e.g., Hispanic and African American families), some recent trends are disturbing. A smaller percentage of members from these groups is getting married, separation and divorce rates are increasing, widowhood is occurring at an alarmingly earlier age, economics are worsening, and traditional familialism and extended family caregiving among these groups are deteriorating. Taken together, it appears that marital satisfaction among elderly cultural minority groups is likely to be lower in the future (Troll, 1986).

Research on other effects of major life events on marital satisfaction have produced mixed findings, with a variety of modifying variables found across studies. For example, departure of children from the home sends many couples into marital distress; yet, in many other cases, this event is liberating and invigorating to the couple (Troll, 1986). Similarly, retirement (discussed next) causes significant problems for some couples, but most adapt gradually and successfully, often with little apparent effect on marital quality (cf. Troll, 1986).

5. What are the effects of retirement on marriage?

As mentioned previously, this is the most researched area and the best-documented aspect of older marriages (Atchley, 1992; Dorfman, 1992; Vinick & Ekerdt, 1992). Accordingly, only the persistent findings are summarized here. First of all, the marital relationship is a central aspect of postparental life; estimates are that 87% of men and 65% of women who retire are married (Atchley, 1992). However, some preretirement expectations do not completely match postretirement experiences. Although men expect and experience more change in retirement than do their wives, husbands tend to overestimate the amount of time they will have for leisure activities (Vinick & Ekerdt, 1992). Wives participate in household activities to a similar extent before and after retirement, but they underestimate how much husbands will actually "help" them. Husbands also have more time for masculine-type household activities (e.g., yardwork, mechanics, woodworking). Interestingly, in one major study (Vinick & Ekerdt,1992), half of the retired couples experienced little or no change in their activities from pre- to postretirement. If planned for adequately, retirement has been found to have relatively little effect on marital satisfaction, especially compared with adverse life events such as declining health, disability, loss of employment, or reduced income.

Retired couples do indicate that they have more time for mutually rewarding activities together, increased communication, and , if required, mutual caregiving. In retirement, marital satisfaction for men tends to increase because there is less competition for their time and interest from nonmarital roles (Lee, 1988). However, a similar effect was not found for wives. Today, if not in the future, most couples approach voluntary retirement with adequate income, a stable relationship, high self-esteem, and good coping skills (Atchley, 1992; Dorfman, 1992).

For some unfortunate older couples, retirement may cause or exacerbate certain problems. Partners' sex-role routines and personal privacy and space may be disrupted. There can be unrealistically high expectations of what will be garnered from the marriage after retirement (e.g., to compensate for years of miscommunication and inattention to the relationship). Increased time together also can cause a conflict over roles; power struggles over dominance in the household can result. Couples who have failed to master the 4 Cs and the other requisite developmental tasks described previously can encounter serious difficulties and disappointments if retirement puts pressure on the marital relationship to provide most of life's satisfactions.

In summary, although partners in elderly couples may become quite interdependent and may even have fewer friends and activities outside of marriage than do their widowed or divorced counterparts, most older couples do adjust rather well to retirement and marital satisfaction is relatively high. However, some couples enter old age continuing a long-standing pattern of marital dissatisfaction, others encounter difficulties as a result of retirement, and still others do well until the relationship is impacted by a significantly adverse life event. In the latter cases, dissolution of the relationship is becoming more frequently employed as a solution to perceived relationship problems among the elderly.

DIVORCE AMONG THE ELDERLY

Surprisingly few studies have explored the relationship between aging and divorce. What little literature exists typically has focused on the impact of divorce on women, primarily because they are at the greatest risk for economic, social, and emotional adjustments after divorce (Hennon, 1983; Morgan, 1992; Uhlenberg, Cooney, & Boyd, 1990). Once again, consider that, overall, the divorce rate for first marriages is about 66% (Castro-Martin & Bumpass, 1989). The remarriage rate is 75% within five years of divorce , and yet 44% of these relationships also end in divorce (Hennon, 1983).

Although rate of divorce decreases as the population ages, divorce after age 40 is not uncommon. For example, in 1985, 23% of divorced women were over age 40, 2% were over age 60 and 1.3% were over age 65 (representing about 10,000 divorces among older persons each year) (Hennon, 1983). Despite the comparatively low divorce rate among elderly couples, there is a concern that divorce rates for older adults are increasing. Divorce has become a more viable and acceptable solution to marital problems throughout our society. From 11% to 18% of women in first marriages after age 40 will obtain a divorce. Of all marriages that survive 15 years, 17% will end in divorce; 11% that last at least 20 years will end in divorce. Divorce feeds on itself. We now expect more from spouses; people are less reluctant and more able financially to engage in serial monogamy. Attesting to this pattern is the high remarriage rate; in the case of the elderly, this is especially true for men. For women, remarriage rates decline sharply with age and are quite low after age 45 (3% remarry in the first year after divorce compared to a 30% remarriage rate for women under 25).

Conservative projections are that less than half of the women born between 1955 and 1959 will be in first marriages at midlife (Uhlenberg *et al.,* 1990). One third of these women will be living outside marriage either in single, divorced, or widowed status. For older women, implications of these increasing divorce and declining remarriage rates are not promising. Research indicates that relative to married, single, or widowed women, divorced females (a) have fewer financial resources, (b) have to work longer than their counterparts, (c) generally suffer more from psychological and self-esteem problems, (d) experience more distress and conflict associated with their families, and (e) experience more disruption in their social contacts and living arrangements (Hennon, 1983; Lee, 1986; Morgan, 1992; Peterson & Bahr, 1989; Uhlenberg *et al.,* 1990). Moreover, consequences for long-term divorced women are almost as severe as for recently divorced older women.

Today's high divorce and remarriage rates among the general population will certainly affect and disrupt family relationships in the years to come. More divorces will cause increased emotional trauma and greater socioeconomic problems. The subsequent increases in second and third marriages surely will complicate extended family relationships. Indeed, the divorce rate among those over 65 years of age is ten times higher for remarriages than it is for first marriages. We believe that following a divorce, men may suffer more than women psychologically because relative to women, older men are more dependent on marriage for intimacy and caregiving. Death rates for divorced males over 65 are 35% higher than for married males; this differential is only 7% for women. However, as just indicated, women are significantly more at risk financially and are more likely to encounter difficulties starting over (Hennon, 1983). Increasing divorce rates, in general, also mean that more older women are likely to have adult children who are divorced. This trend has significant implications for availability of supportive resources for older women. Divorced women in the middle generation are in need of support from their aging parents, who, in turn, are in need of support from their daughters. If the majority of women are divorced and are members of reconstituted families, sources of critical support are complicated and likely to be reduced for both generations. We briefly present some specific information about remarriage among older persons.

REMARRIAGE AMONG THE ELDERLY

Although in the U.S. more than 20% of all marriages are remarriages, relatively little is known about this phenomenon among the elderly (Bowers & Bahr, 1989). We do know that divorced older women (a) tend to be younger than widowed older women, (b) are more likely to be living with children, (c) are less likely to be obligated to a dead spouse, and (d) they are more likely to be in need of economic support. Based on these factors, relative to widowed women, divorced women are more likely to remarry. After age 60, 16% of divorced women remarry, compared to 3% of widowed women (Bowers & Bahr, 1989). A similar pattern is expected among men, but definitive research on this question is not yet available.

Remarriage rates are much lower for women than men because of several factors: (a) There is a sex ratio pool of only two men for every three women at age 65, and this discrepancy increases with age, (b) widows are less inclined to remarry than are widowers, who are more dependent on marriage, and (c) our cultural values dictate that men are able to marry much younger women than vice versa, further improving their selection advantage (Bowers & Bahr, 1989).

The purpose of remarriage seems to be different for older compared to younger couples. Elderly couples are interested primarily in companionship and someone to help in the practical navigation of later life. Accordingly, remarriages among older couples appear to be much more stable than are younger remarriages (53% of women in remarriages before age 50 get divorced compared to only 22% after age 50). The older the age at remarriage, the more stable the relationship seems to be. Interestingly, there appear to be no significant differences in marital satisfaction between younger and older remarried couples. However, some studies suggest that older men are more satisfied with their remarriages than are older women. Again, this finding may be a function of the greater need that men appear to have for marriage and their greater pool of potential partners (Bowers & Bahr, 1989).

MARITAL THERAPY FOR OLDER COUPLES

In comparison with their younger counterparts, the current cohort of elderly couples is more reluctant to request mental health services. If marital difficulties are encountered, they initially tend to seek guidance from their primary care physician or a member of the clergy. Those referred to a marital therapist, often by their adult children, present clinical problems and need therapeutic interventions that are similar to problems and interventions for younger couples (Gatz, Popin, Pino, & VandenBos, 1985). However, there are diagnostic and assessment issues as well as specific methods of facilitating engagement in the therapeutic process that should be considered when treating elderly couples. Let us discuss these three points in more detail.

Presenting Problems

Lauer, Lauer, and Kerr (1990) have described four types of marriage among older persons: (a) long-term maritally satisfied, (b) long-term dissatisfied, (c) short-term pleasurable, and (d) short-term distressed. Satisfied couples do not seek marital therapy; dissatisfied groups are referred for marital treatment. Of the two dissatisfied groups, the short-term dissatisfied are the most likely to seek treatment. They may represent either long-term marriages disrupted by sudden changes or losses that overwhelm one or both spouse's ability to cope, or they may be remarried couples who find themselves in conflict due to any number of adjustment problems or apparent incompatibilities. In any case, these couples tend to be good candidates for marital therapy.

When older couples enter marital therapy, the basic content areas about which they are concerned are similar to the issues presented by younger couples: financial stressors, disputes regarding (adult) children (or grandchildren), conflicts about personality styles and behavioral habits, and perhaps problems regarding sex and affection (Birchler & Fals-Stewart, 1996; Rosenberg, 1989;

Stone, 1987). However, these issues that are found in common with younger couples are very likely to be salient for second or third marriages, where sex, money, relationships with adult children, and rigid personal styles often require mutual adjustment. In remarriages the strong desire for companionship does not obviate the need for accommodation to each partner's families and to each partner's long-standing beliefs, values, and behavior patterns.

In contrast to remarried older couples, partners in long-term marriages usually have resolved many of the marital problems typical of younger couples (Birchler & Schafer, 1990; Fals-Stewart et al, 1993; Rosenberg, 1989). No longer are money management, career conflicts, frequency and variety of sex activities, and disciplining the children the most prominent issues. More likely, a healthy spouse is appearing on behalf of an unhealthy partner; spouses are seeking assistance in adjusting to any of a number of losses in their lives. Careful assessment of these losses and partners' attempts and successes at coping with them are important from both assessment and intervention perspectives. These potential and some inevitable losses include residence; family and friends; financial security; children moving out of the home or away from town; changes in personality, mental status, or physical capabilities; reduced energy or sensory impairments; and diminished self-esteem associated with loss of youth, vocational activities, or role and life expectations (Gafner, 1987; Stone, 1987). Consequently, much of the therapeutic work that can be done is based on a compensatory model of aging, namely, assisting couples to accept the aspects of their losses that cannot be changed, helping them restore aspects lost but restorable, and helping partners to substitute or compensate for losses to the extent possible (Stone, 1987).

Basic Interventions

Most of the basic types of interventions that therapists might use to assist elderly couples with marital problems vary little from contemporary approaches employed with all distressed couples (Birchler & Fals-Stewart, 1996; Gafner, 1987, Stone, 1987). Indeed, we have found cognitive and behavioral approaches to be quite compatible with the treatment needs of older couples. Frequently, treatment goals are expressed in concrete and behavioral terms. Most elderly couples are neither candidates for, nor do they plan on altering their long-standing belief systems. More likely, they simply desire to bring their personal and relationship function in accordance with their long-standing beliefs. In addition, most older couples do not seek insight-oriented or emotionally focused therapy. Despite their proclivity and apparent need to tell stories about their life experiences (Butler, 1974), partners in the couples want to learn expeditiously how to compensate for what they have lost or to reconcile conflicts associated with external stressors or recent remarriages. Accordingly, these couples often prefer a relatively brief, directive, communication and problem-solving oriented therapeutic approach (Stone, 1987). In addition, in a directive role, the therapist may need to be an active mediator and provide more explicit advice than is typically required for younger couples.

The 7 Cs Model

By incorporating the diagnostic and therapy-engagement procedures described in the next section, we have quite successfully used the *7 Cs* model to assess and treat many elderly couples. The model will be only briefly outlined here; the four core dimensions (the 4 Cs) were introduced earlier. The interested reader is referred to Birchler and Fals-Stewart (1994a), and Birchler and Schwartz (1994) for a more extensive discussion of the 7 Cs formulation for the assessment and treatment of marital dysfunction.

In their entirety, the 7 Cs include: *Character features, Contract, Cultural and ethnic factors, Commitment, Caring, Communication,* and *Conflict resolution.* Aspects of the 7 Cs are assessed using a series of behaviorally oriented interviews (Birchler & Schwartz, 1994), a paper-and-pencil Marital Relationship Assessment Battery (Birchler, 1983; Birchler & Fals-Stewart, 1996), and observation of a 10-min sample of marital conflict communication between partners (Basco, Birchler, Kalal, Talbott, & Slater, 1991; Birchler, 1983).

Character features relate to obstructive personality features and the extent of psychopathology present in one or both partners. The continuum of concern ranges from rigid and dominating personality styles, to moderate levels of psychiatric disturbance in one spouse (e.g., depression and anxiety), to presence of major psychiatric disorders in both partners (e.g., both spouses have bipolar depressive disorder; one experiences major depression and the other has a substance abuse problem). The more severe or complex the character features presented by the couple the more likely that individualized treatments will be required either before, concurrent with, or instead of marital therapy (Fals-Stewart, Birchler, Schafer, & Lucente, 1994).

Contract refers to the discrepancy between what partners expect to gain from the marriage and their actual experiences in the relationship. In the absence of good communication and problem-solving skills, unrealistic or divergent partner expectations lead to unrealistic demands, which results in resentments and highly frustrating marital conflict. Some older couples have *implicit* contract problems (i.e., the nature of the conflict is outside their awareness or beyond their present knowledge), others have *explicit* contract problems and frank disagreements (e.g., the husband expects his wife to restrict her time and activities with her adult children and their families and she married him expecting to expand and enjoy access to these families). Most contract problems for older couples in long-term marriages arise as a result of significant life-event changes (e.g., retirement, disability, or other personal growth-related differences between partners). Remarried partners more frequently perceive that they are not getting what they expected from their new partner (e.g., sexual activity, caregiving, help with household chores, financial income, access to or lack of interference from adult children). Treatment includes helping couples identify, clarify, and negotiate and reconcile these various implicit and explicit differences between partners' expectations and experiences.

Cultural and ethnic factors are contextual variables that may affect the marital relationship and the prospects for successful therapy. Family of origin issues are included in this area because certain beliefs, experiences, and cultural traditions from partners' original families may impact the marriage significantly. Potential problems to be addressed include conflict between the spouses concerning racial, ethnic, religious, and socioeconomic class issues. In addition, some couples not only have such conflicts within the marriage, they are struggling against outside interference from family, friends, or society in general. Finally, it is also possible that the therapist comes from a significantly different sociodemographic background (e.g., different race, religion, or significantly younger group than the older couple). In the case of a significant age difference, elderly clients may feel that very young therapists do not have sufficient life experience to understand and be able to treat them; young therapists may feel that they are being treated like the couples' adult children. If any of these age, cultural, or ethnic factors threaten the prospects for successful therapy, then case consultation, case management adjustments (e.g., adding a culturally matched cotherapist to enhance ethnic or racial understanding), or perhaps a referral to another therapist or setting may be required to achieve compatibility. Older couples, especially in circumstances of remarriage, are not immune from the complicating and conflicting effects of cultural and ethnic factors. Any such problems must be addressed and resolved before one can expect a positive outcome from conjoint therapy.

Commitment refers to three interrelated areas: commitment to the marriage (stability), commitment to change (quality), and commitment to the therapeutic process. Of course, it is optimal if both partners have strong personal commitments at all three levels. Unfortunately, entering marital therapy, typically one or both partners fall short in one or more of these three types of commitment. When the assessment process reveals deficiencies in commitment, the underlying issues must be addressed early in therapy. Partners in long-term marriages more likely are committed to stability, but they may need encouragement to commit to quality (i.e., positive change) in the relationship and to the therapy process itself. Older remarried couples frequently have commitment problems in all three areas. Commitment evolves from reliable experience, trust, and expectations for positive relating. Therefore, whatever the therapist can do to join with the clients, to demonstrate competence, to underline credibility for the approach, and to engender hope for future relating contributes to strengthening partners' commitments.

Caring encompasses mutual support and understanding, attachment, cohesion, demonstrations of affection, and sexual interaction. Once again, partners in long-term marriages usually measure up well in this area unless they are challenged by emotional or physical disabilities that have disrupted and damaged the caring bond between partners. Conversely, remarriages are subject to a number of challenges that typically do not confront long-term marriages. Because many older people remarry for companionship and practical interdependency, there may be conflicts regarding the various ways of demonstrating caring. Therapeutic interventions include "Caring Days" (Stuart, 1980), "Love Days" (Weiss & Birchler, 1975), development of both independent and mutually rewarding activities (Birchler, 1983), other exercises to facilitate and enhance the expression of affection (Jacobson & Margolin, 1979), and, if appropriate, sexual relationship enhancement interventions (Gottman, Notarius, Gonso, & Markman, 1976; Heiman, 1986; Stone, 1987).

Communication is a critical skill for older and younger couples alike. Except for the fortunate few golden anniversary couples, many elderly couples who are referred for marital therapy have lost or have never had the opportunity to be fully understood and personally validated. Older men often are inclined to have some difficulty in expressing feelings, while their wives often have more difficulty being assertive. Moreover, as discussed throughout this chapter, these couples usually present under stress while attempting to cope with one or more significant losses. If such losses are profound and emotionally disturbing, even couples with adequate communication skills find themselves in distress and need assistance in identifying, exploring, sharing, and resolving their problems. Remarried older couples frequently need extensive work in developing better communication skills; fortunately, they are often willing and successful participants. Communication skills training (Birchler, 1979; Gottman *et al.,* 1976; Jacobson & Margolin, 1979; Notarius & Markman, 1993) provides a supportive and instructive environment to help motivated couples speak assertively and listen attentively to their mates (for a case study of an older couple, refer to Birchler and Fals-Stewart, 1996).

Conflict resolution refers to three levels of interaction: (a) day-to-day decision making, (b) mutual problem solving of life's problems and relationship issues, and (c) actual conflict management skills needed to resolve overt and covert emotionally charged disputes. Older couples can have certain difficulties at all three levels of conflict resolution. For the most part, long-term marriages are characterized by conflict avoidance and passive responses to marital conflict (Birchler & Fals-Stewart, 1994b). However, the usual caveat applies—if a partner experiences a major mental or physical disability, his or her emotional equilibrium may be disrupted, resulting in an irritable disposition and sometimes culminating in hostility and violence between otherwise compatible partners. As mentioned previously, in such situations, careful medical, psychological, and neuropsychological assessments are indicated to help determine the causes and develop appropriate treatment plans. Alternatively, sometimes short-term remarried partners present for marital therapy and benefit from the standard cognitive-behavioral treatments developed for general problem solving and designed for acute, interpersonal conflict management (Gottman, *et al.,* 1976; Jacobson & Margolin, 1979; Notarius & Markman, 1993).

In summary, the 7 Cs model represents universal dimensions of marital relationships, whether the participants are younger or older in age and regardless of the length of the marriage. Combined with special assessments and engagement-enhancement procedures enumerated in the following sections, interventions based on the 7 Cs and an integrated behavioral couples therapy approach (Christensen, Jacobson, & Babcock, 1995) serve well to help older couples benefit from brief marital treatment experiences.

Special Considerations

There are significant age-related diagnostic issues that are important considerations when working with older couples. Indeed, there is an emerging literature that recommends various therapist attitudes and procedural enhancements that clinicians might well consider. These extra "enhancements" can facilitate both the entry of older couples into therapy and the subsequent effectiveness of therapeutic interventions (Gafner, 1987; Stone, 1987; Wolinsky, 1990).

Diagnostic Issues

Diagnostically, one must be aware of changes in mental and physical functioning that are specifically related to the aging process. Moreover, one should be knowledgeable about the developmental tasks and transitional life events inherent in the postparental and culmination stages of the marital life cycle (Birchler, 1992). Individual spousal changes in mental status, cognitive function, or personality may indicate a variety of problems, including dementia, depression, sensory impairment, malnutrition, misuse of substances (e.g., alcohol, street drugs, medications), drug interactions, and various metabolic conditions. Close collaboration among health care providers may be important in addressing multifaceted problems. Additional areas of assessment that might be particularly relevant to older couples presenting for therapy include lifestyle issues (e.g., eating, drinking, and sleeping habits, recent life disruptions, or a variety of other environmental stressors). In the area of sexuality, it is important to distinguish between normal aging effects on sexual function and sexual dysfunctions that may be unrelated to aging (refer to the chapter on sexuality in this volume). Psychoeducation may be indicated when older partners experience sexual concerns that occur in the normal course of aging; formal sex therapy may be appropriate for other types of sexual dysfunction. The primary determination is how, if at all, the aging process has caused or exacerbated relationship distress.

Engagement Procedures

Special therapy engagement and therapy facilitation techniques recommended for treating elderly couples take into account certain biases, as well as emotional and physical needs that elderly clients may have. Any number of the following enhancements may apply to a given case:

1. Be prepared to counter ageism in both the therapist and in the clients. Do not take the older couple's life experiences, functional status, and potential for change (or the lack thereof) for granted.
2. Assessment and intervention procedures may need to proceed at a slower pace to accommodate trust and credibility issues or to compensate for sensory and energy-level impairments. Older couples may be wary of mental health services and thus seek a greater sense of self-determination. Go slowly, explain interventions carefully, and give clients choices whenever possible.
3. Be flexible in considering the logistics of care. It may be that clients need to be seen in various locations, for varying lengths and total number of sessions, and be accommodated with special seating, lighting, and audio enhancements.
4. Older clients may need more work on trust and attitudes before they can be comfortable with "feeling-talk," conjoint meetings, or certain value-challenging behavioral interventions.

5. Older clients are likely to be suffering from an interaction of physical and psychological maladies, (e.g., memory or sensory impairments causing self-esteem problems, anxiety, depression or irritability).

6. Be aware that older clients often are significantly influenced by important others in their lives (e.g., a family physician, the clergy, well-meaning or interfering family members). These agents of influence need to be taken into account during assessment of the problems and in planning interventions.

7. Finally, despite these considerations, remember that there is no stereotype that fits every elderly couple. Assessments and interventions should be individualized to meet the existing needs in a given case.

THE FUTURE

A review of the existing literature on marriage and divorce in the elderly suggests several areas of concern and questions to be addressed by future research. It should be noted that marriages of people reaching later life in the future may be considerably different from those represented by the present cohort. The prevailing divorce rate, remarriages, changes occurring between the sexes, culturally altered views on marriage itself, and changes in the socioeconomic status of older people—all these factors will significantly impact the life satisfaction of elderly couples and their families (Askham, 1994).

As with other segments of the population, today there exists great heterogeneity among the aged. Many people are in poverty, some are wealthy, while others who are truly needy may be losing support. To reiterate, economic security and good health are the basic prerequisites for successful aging. Sources of socioeconomic support are in transition; more pressure will be brought to bear on the family to provide support for the aged (Quiroutte & Gold, 1992). Family supportive structures prevalent in the past are breaking down. If the current divorce and remarriage rates prevail, it will be even less likely in the future that the elderly will reside with their children (who increasingly are in remarried families themselves).

In the future much more definitive and controlled research is needed in the following areas: adjustment patterns of widows and widowers, alternative family forms in later life, quality of life in later years, gender differences (especially divorce, remarriage, and life satisfaction determinants for males compared to females), social networks and support systems, family characteristics related to a higher quality of late life, more representative samples of the elderly (especially ethnic, racial, and socioeconomic stratifications), spousal variables that predict husbands' well-being, and additional investigations on marital quality and the consequences of divorce and remarriage for the older members of our society.

SUMMARY

Marriage and divorce among the elderly is a population phenomenon in a major transition. Even as the bulk of the U.S. population is aging and is shaping politics, economics and family relationships significantly, over the past several decades the institution of marriage has changed as well. On the one hand, given the prevailing 66% divorce rate, one might conclude that for many, if not the majority, the expectations for what marriage can and should provide to participants frequently are not met. On the other hand, we have not as yet discovered a better model of "permanent" relating, given that the remarriage rate of 75% suggests that most people try marriage again. Unfortunately, although many people attempt marriage a second time, these new relationships will just as likely fail to meet peoples' perceived or actual needs for a marriage. As Stone (1987) so poignantly states it, the older members of our society are not different from us; they *are* us! The perpetuation of marriage and divorce, in serial monogamy style, is resulting in an ever more complex and conflicted society. Children have more and more sets of stepsiblings, stepparents, and stepgrandparents. The future, in this respect, is troublesome.

This chapter is written in an attempt to describe the present status of marriage and divorce among older persons. We need a better understanding of the strengths and developmental accomplishments of long-term marriages, of the promises and pitfalls associated with remarried older couples, and of the various and inevitable challenges that we all will face as the years progress. Such knowledge can only help us to prepare for the future and to help older couples as they seek our assistance in improving the quality of life in their present circumstances. Relationship satisfaction, developmental issues, and gender differences that distinguish older couples' marriages were described along with the requisites for developing and maintaining long-term intimate relationships. In addition, the life events, the biological and relationship transitions that accompany the aging process were contrasted with normal problems and conflicts that may be unrelated to aging, but are known to be difficulties for married couples at all ages. A description of the 7 Cs formulation of marital dysfunction was offered as a conceptual basis for assessment and intervention with older couples. Diagnostic issues related to the clinical presentation of older couples and specific recommendations for facilitating their participation and benefit from marital therapy were discussed. Finally, some implications of present trends for the future of older Americans were presented, along with a number of recommendations for important research investigations that might better prepare us all for our future.

REFERENCES

Askham, J. (1994). Marriage relationships of older people. *Reviews in Clinical Gerontology, 4*, 261–268.

Atchley, R. (1992). Retirement and marital satisfaction. In M. Szinovacz, D. Ekerdt, & B. Vinick (Eds.), *Families and retirement* (pp. 145–158). London: Sage.

Basco, M. A., Birchler, G. R., Kalal, B., Talbott, R., & Slater, M. A. (1991). The clinician rating of adult communication (CRAC): A clinician's guide to the assessment of interpersonal communication skill. *Journal of Clinical Psychology, 47*, 368–380.

Birchler, G. R. (1979). Communications skills in married couples. In A. S. Bellack & M. Hersen (Eds.), *Research and practice in social skills training* (pp. 273–315). New York: Plenum.

Birchler, G. R. (1983). Marital dysfunction. In M. Hersen (Ed.), *Outpatient behavioral therapy: A clinical guide* (pp. 229–269). New York: Grune & Stratton.

Birchler, G. R.(1992). Marriage. In V. B. Van Hasselt & M. Hersen (Eds.), *Handbook of social development: A lifespan perspective* (pp. 397–419). New York: Plenum.

Birchler, G. R., & Fals-Stewart, W. (1994a). Marital dysfunction. In V. S. Ramachandran (Ed.), *Encyclopedia of human behavior* (Vol. 3, pp. 103–113). Orlando, FL: Academic.

Birchler, G. R., & Fals-Stewart, W. (1994b). The Response to Conflict Scale: Psychometric properties. *Assessment, 1*, 335–344.

Birchler, G. R., & Fals-Stewart, W. S. (1996, August). *The Marital Relationship Assessment Battery: A maximal decomposition.* Paper presented at the American Psychological Association annual convention, Toronto, Ontario, Canada.

Birchler, G. R. & Fals-Stewart, W. S. (1996). Marital discord. In M. Hersen & V. B. Van Hasselt (Eds.), *Psychological treatment of older adults: An introductory textbook.* (pp. 315–333). New York: Plenum.

Birchler, G. R., & Schafer, J. (1990, August). *Assessment of older couples entering marital therapy.* Paper presented at the American Psychological Association Convention, Boston.

Birchler, G. R., & Schwartz, L.(1994). Marital dyads. In M. Hersen & S. M. Turner (Eds.), *Diagnostic interviewing* (2nd ed., pp. 277–304). New York: Plenum.

Bowers, I. H., & Bahr, S. J. (1989). Remarriage among the elderly. In S. J. Bahr & E. T. Peterson (Eds.), *Aging and the family* (pp. 85–95). Lexington, MA: Lexington Books.

Brubaker, T. H. (1983). *Family relationships in later life.* Beverly Hills: Sage.

Butler, R. N. (1974). Successful aging and the role of the life review. *Journal of the American Geriatric Society, 22*, 529–535.

Carter, B., & McGoldrick, M. (1988). *The changing family life cycle* (2nd ed.). New York: Gardner.

Castro-Martin, T., & Bumpass, L. (1989). Recent trends in marital disruption. *Demography, 26*, 37–51.

Christensen, A., Jacobson, N. S., & Babcock, J. C. (1995). Integrative behavioral couple therapy. In N. S. Jacobson & A. S. Gurman (Eds.), *Clinical handbook of marital therapy* (2nd ed., pp. 31–64). New York: Guilford.

Cole, C. L. (1986). Developmental tasks affecting the marital relationship in later life. *American Behavioral Scientist, 29* (4), 389–403.

Cole, C. L. (1989). Relationship quality in long-term marriages: A comparison of high-quality and low-quality marriages. In L. Ade-Ridder & C. B. Hennon (Eds.), *Lifestyles of the elderly* (pp. 61–70). Oxford, OH: Human Sciences.

Condie, S. J. (1989). Older married couples. In S. J. Bahr & E. T. Peterson (Eds.), *Aging and the family* (pp.143–158). Lexington, MA: Lexington Books.

Cuber, J., & Haroff, P. (1965). *The significant Americans.* New York: Appleton-Century-Crofts.

Dorfman, L. (1992). Couples in retirement: Division of household work. In M. Szinovacz, D. Ekerdt, & B. Vinick (Eds.), *Families and retirement* (pp. 159–173). London: Sage.

Fals-Stewart, W. S., Schafer, J. C., & Birchler, G. R. (1993). An empirical typology of distressed couples based on the Areas of Change Questionnaire. *Journal of Family Psychology, 7*, 307–321.

Fals-Stewart, W. S., Birchler, G. R., Schafer, J. C., & Lucente, S. (1994). The personality of marital distress: An empirical typology. *Journal of Personality Assessment, 62* (2), 223–241.

Gafner, G. (1987). Engaging the elderly couple in marital therapy. *American Journal of Family Therapy, 15*, 305–315.

Gatz, M., Popin, S. J., Pino, C. O., & VandenBos, G. R. (1985). Psychological interventions with older adults. In J. E. Birren & K. W. Schaie (Eds.), *Handbook of psychology and aging* (3rd ed., pp. 404–425). San Diego, CA: Academic.

Gilford, R. (1984). Contrasts in marital satisfaction throughout old age: An exchange theory analysis. *Journal of Gerontology, 39*, 325–333.

Glick, P. C., & Norton, A. J. (1977). Marrying, divorcing, and living together in the U.S. today. *Population Bulletin, 32*, 1–39.

Goldberg, J. R. (1992). The new frontier: Marriage and family therapy with aging families. *Family Therapy News, 23* (4), 1.

Gottman, J. M., Notarius, C., Gonso, J., & Markman, H. (1976). *A couple's guide to communication.* Champaign, IL: Research Press.

Hammond, D. B. (1989). Love, sex, and marriage in the later years. In E. S. Deichman & R. Kociecki (Eds.), *Working with the elderly* (pp. 255–273). Buffalo, NY: Prometheus Books.

Heiman, J. R. (1986). Treating sexually distressed marital relationships. In N. S. Jacobson & A. G. Gurman (Eds.), *Clinical handbook of marital therapy* (pp. 361–384). New York: Guilford.

Hennon, C. B. (1983). Divorce and the elderly: A neglected area of research. In T. Brubaker (Ed.), *Family relationships in later life* (pp. 149–172). Beverly Hills, CA: Sage.

Hess, B. B.,& Markson, E. W. (1986). *Growing old in America* (3rd ed.). New Brunswick, NJ: Transition Books.

Jacobson, N. S., & Margolin, G. (1979). *Marital therapy: Strategies based on social learning and behavior-exchange principles.* New York: Brunner/Mazel.

Karney, B. R., & Bradbury, T. N. (1995). The longitudinal course of marital quality and stability: A review of theory, method, and research. *Psychological Bulletin, 118,* 3–34.

Lauer, R., Lauer, J., & Kerr, S. (1990). The long-term marriage: Perceptions of stability and satisfaction. *International Journal of Aging and Human Development, 31,* 189–195.

Lee, G. (1986). Marriage and aging. In B. B. Hess & E. W. Markson (Eds.), *Growing old in America* (3rd ed., pp. 361–368). New Brunswick, NJ: Transition Books.

Lee, G. (1988). Marital satisfaction in later life: The effects of non-marital roles. *Journal of Marriage and the Family, 50,* 775–783.

Levenson, R. W., Carstensen, L. L., & Gottman, J. M. (1993). Long-term marriage: Age, gender, and satisfaction. *Psychology and Aging, 8,* 301–313.

Levenson, R. W., Carstensen, L. L., & Gottman, J. M. (1994). Influence of age and gender effect on affect, physiology, and their interrelations. *Journal of Personality and Social Psychology, 67* (1), 56–68.

Lewis, J. M. (1988). The transition to parenthood: II. Stability and change in marital structure. *Family Process, 27,* 149–165.

Lewis, J. M., Owen, M. T., & Cox, M. J. (1988). The transition to parenthood: III. Incorporation of the child into the family. *Family Process, 27,* 411–421.

Lewis, R. A., & Spanier, G. B. (1979). Theorizing about the quality and stability of marriage. In W. R. Burr, R. Hill, F. I. Nye, & I. L. Reiss (Eds.), *Contemporary theories about the family: Research-based theories* (pp. 268–294). New York: Free Press.

Miller, B. C. (1976). A multivariate developmental model of marital satisfaction. *Journal of Marriage and the Family, 38,* 643–657.

Mindel, C. H. (1986). The elderly in minority families. In B. B. Hess & E. W. Markson (Eds.), *Growing old in America* (3rd ed., pp. 369–386). New Brunswick, NJ: Transition Books.

Morgan, L. A. (1992). Marital status and retirement plans. In M. Szinovacz, D. Ekerdt, & B. Vinick (Eds.), *Families and retirement* (pp. 114–126). London: Sage.

Nadelson, C., Polonsky, D. C., & Mathews, M. A. (1984). Marriage as a developmental process. In C. Nadelson & D. C. Polonsky (Eds.), *Marriage and divorce: A contemporary perspective* (pp.127–141). New York: Guilford.

Neidhardt, E. R., & Allen, J. A.(1993). *Family therapy with the elderly.* Newbury Park, CA: Sage.

Nichols, W.C. (1988). *Marital therapy.* New York: Guilford Press.

Notarius, C. I., & Markman, H. (1993). *We can work it out: Making sense of marital conflict.* New York: Putnam's.

Peterson, E. T., & Bahr, S. J. (1989). Epilogue: Prospects for the future. In S. J. Bahr & E. T. Peterson (Eds.), *Aging and the family* (pp. 305–313). Lexington, MA: Lexington Books.

Quirouette, C., & Gold, D. P. (1992). Spousal characteristics as predictors of well-being in older couples. *International Journal of Aging and Human Development, 34* (4), 257–269.

Rollins, B. C., & Cannon, K. L. (1974). Marital satisfaction over the family life cycle: A reevaluation. *Journal of Marriage and the Family, May,* 271–282.

Rosenberg, I. I. (1989). Love and marital problems in the elderly. *University Service News, 3* (2), 3.

Spanier, G., Lewis, R., & Cole, C. (1975). Marital adjustment over the family life cycle: The issue of curvilinearity. *Journal of Marriage and the Family, 37,* 263–276.

Stone, J. D. (1987). Marital and sexual counseling of elderly couples. In G. R. Weeks & L. Hoff (Eds.), *Integrating sex and marital therapy: A clinical guide* (pp. 221–244). New York: Brunner/Mazel.

Stuart, R. B. (1980). *Helping couples change.* New York: Guilford.

Swenson, C. H., Eskew, R. W., & Kohlhepp, K. A. (1981). Stage of family life cycle, ego development, and the marriage relationship. *Journal of Marriage and the Family, 43,* 841–853.

Szinovasz, M., Ekerdt, D. J., & Vinick, B. H. (1992). *Families and retirement.* Beverly Hills, CA: Sage.

Traupmann, J., & Harfield, E. (1983). How important is marital fairness over the lifespan? *International Journal of Aging and Human Development, 17* (2), 89–101.

Troll, L. E. (1986). Marriage. In L. E. Troll (Ed.), *Family issues in current gerontology* (pp. 1–13). New York: Springer.

Uhlenberg, P., Cooney, T., & Boyd, R. (1990). Divorce for women after midlife. *Journal of Gerontology, 45* (1), S3–S11.

Vinick, B., & Ekerdt, D. (1992). Couples view retirement activities: Expectation versus experience. In M. Szinovacz, D. Ekerdt, & B. Vinick (Eds.), *Families and retirement* (pp. 129–144). London: Sage.

Weiss, R. L., & Birchler, G. R. (1975). *Areas of Change Questionnaire.* Unpublished manuscript, University of Oregon, Eugene.

Wolinsky, M. A. (1990). *A heart of wisdom: Marital counseling with older and elderly couples.* New York: Brunner/Mazel.

Wynne, L. C. (1984). The epigenisis of relational systems: A model for understanding family development. *Family Process, 23,* 297–318.

CHAPTER 21

Family Caregiving
Stress, Coping, and Intervention

DOLORES GALLAGHER-THOMPSON, DAVID W. COON,
PATRICIA RIVERA, DAVID POWERS,
AND ANTONETTE M. ZEISS

INTRODUCTION

At present, more than 4 million adults over the age of 65 years receive some type of personal care from family members. This figure is expected to increase as the nation's population of older adults grows to 67.5 million by the year 2050 (U.S. Senate, 1991). In such situations, the care recipient frequently benefits from the physical, emotional, and financial support provided by the family caregiver. However, the personal consequences to the caregiver of fulfilling this responsibility have received much attention in the research literature. This chapter will review the findings from studies with family care providers. We begin with a historical overview of the characteristics of individuals who comprise the majority of caregivers in this country, and review the problems, stresses and hardships they experience. Next, we review theoretical models that have been proposed to explain the process of caregiver distress and its interaction with moderating variables. Then, we examine the various psychologically oriented treatments and forms of intervention currently available, and address issues of their efficacy. Finally, we provide a brief review of the growing literature on special caregiving populations, with particular emphasis on

DOLORES GALLAGHER-THOMPSON • Older Adult Center, Veterans Affairs Health Care System, Palo Alto, California 94304 and Stanford University School of Medicine, Stanford, California.   DAVID W. COON, PATRICIA RIVERA AND DAVID POWERS • Older Adult Center, Veterans Affairs Health Care System, Palo Alto, California 94304.   ANTONETTE M. ZEISS • Training and Program Development, Psychology Service, and Interprofessional Team Training and Development Program, Veterans Affairs Health Care System, Palo Alto, California 94304.

Handbook of Clinical Geropsychology, edited by Michel Hersen and Vincent B. Van Hasselt. Plenum Press, New York, 1998.

the unique needs and concerns of male caregivers and caregivers of various ethnic or minority backgrounds. The chapter closes with recommendations for future research.

FAMILY CAREGIVING IN HISTORICAL PERSPECTIVE

Although public concern for older persons has existed since the founding of this country, their attention and care has largely been a private family matter. In the mid-1800s, individual states began to include family welfare laws in their statutes, outlining a standard of care required of all citizens toward their elderly kin. The Social Security Act of 1930, however, assigned more of the task to public programs and resources, thereby allowing individuals to reduce the level of personal responsibility for care of aged relatives (Schorr, 1980). More recently, demographic, social, and economic pressure have created a shift back toward personal responsibility, and individuals have found themselves in the role of "caregiver" to spouses, elderly parent(s), grandparents, or even friends and neighbors.

Although medical and scientific advances have contributed to increased longevity in this country, it was the increase in births during the 1920s and the postwar "baby boom" that had the greatest impact on aging in this nation. The drop in birthrates in the 1960s contributed to a drastic shift in the proportion of old to young citizens (U.S. Senate, 1991), making it more likely for adult children of today to have living parents and, frequently, grandparents. The increased divorce rate denies older individuals who have not remarried spousal support (a primary source of assistance for frail elders). In divorce situations, more caregiving responsibility may fall on adult children (Cicirelli, 1983), who must struggle to care for two parents who do not live together. Finally, 62% of American women between the ages of 45 and 54 work full-time (U.S. Department of Labor, 1990). This segment of the population is likely to assume the role of family caregiver to an aging parent; the requirements inherent in the dual role of paid employee and unpaid caregiver can contribute to feelings of burden and distress. Moreover, those women who are also mothers shoulder the burden of a third role and may experience even greater stress with these competing demands (Brody, 1990). One might infer that elder abuse or neglect could result from the role overload experienced by these caregivers, but the phenomenon most often seen is the emotional and physical toll paid by family caregivers themselves.

WHO ARE THE INFORMAL CAREGIVERS?

Because the processes of aging and debilitation tend to be gradual, the provision of assistance usually begins with the individual closest in physical proximity to the elder; thus, spouses are natural primary caregivers (Zarit, Birkel, & MaloneBeach, 1989). In situations in which there is no spouse, evidence points to the existence of a hierarchical pattern of responsibility, with primary duties going to the adult female child, then the adult male child, and finally, other family members (Cantor, 1983). A 1982 long-term care survey found that 22% of caregivers sampled were spouses, 30% were children (83% of whom were daughters), and 18% were formal, or paid, caregivers. Indeed, up to three quarters of the caregivers surveyed shared households with a frail elder (R. Stone, Cafferata, & Sangl, 1987), and the majority of unmarried or divorced adult children cited financial hardships as primary reasons for co-residence (Brody, Litvin, Hoffman, & Kleban, 1995; Cutler & Coward, 1992). Other factors that help to determine whether one will accept the responsibility of caregiving include presence of competing role demands, such as employment and marital status, as well as financial status and prior relationship history with the care recipient (Arling & McAuley, 1983; Brody *et al.*, 1996).

Responsibilities associated with caregiving of an elderly individual are numerous and may vary from simple errands which take minutes, to such physically and emotionally challenging tasks as bathing or toileting a confused and frail individual. Although the type of assistance provided depends on the elder's level of disability, caregivers generally provide as-needed assistance in the areas of (1) personal service provision, such as help with instrumental activities of daily living (e.g., balancing the checkbook and supervising medication usage), along with more intimate forms of personal care including dressing, feeding, and bathing, (2) identification of, and linkage to, formal services such as senior day care and transportation, (3) financial support, and (4) emotional support through regular contact, company, and conversation (Horowitz, 1985).

WHAT IS THE PSYCHOLOGICAL IMPACT
OF CAREGIVING

For some individuals, caring for a parent and the sense of reciprocating the nurturance and care once provided by that parent can be very rewarding (Altholz, 1991). National estimates show that approximately 75% of caregivers say caregiving makes them feel useful (U.S. House of Representatives, 1987) and a growing literature suggests that caregiving can lead to personal rewards and satisfaction (Genevay, 1994; Lawton, Moss, Kleban, Glicksman, & Rovine, 1991). For example, people may remain caregivers over an extended period of time for several positive personal outcomes, including the following: caregiving may contribute to self-worth, build self-confidence, and provide companionship (Schulz, Tompkins, & Rau, 1988).

A far greater number of caregivers, however, report negative feelings as a result of the increased responsibility of caring for a disabled or impaired relative. Anger, frustration, and anxiety are common symptoms of caregiver distress and clinical levels of depression in caregivers of Alzheimer's patients have been reported in several studies (reviewed in Schulz, Visintainer, & Williamson, 1990). In addition, use of psychotropic medications among caregivers is higher than that of their noncaregiving counterparts (see also updated review by Schulz, O'Brien, Bookwala, & Fleissner, 1995).

Prevalence of depression among caregivers of impaired elders reported in the caregiving literature ranges from about 20% to more than 80%. However, prevalence rates of clinical diagnoses of depression determined by structured clinical interviews are often noticeably lower than rates derived from self-report inventories that focus on depressive symptoms. Still, caregiving studies incorporating structured clinical interviews, such as the Schedule for Affective Disorders and Schizophrenia (SADS; R. Spitzer & Endicott, 1978), the Diagnostic Interview Schedule (DIS; Robins, Helzer, Croughan, & Ratcliff, 1981), and the Structured Clinical Interview for *DSM-III-R* (SCID; R. L. Spitzer, Williams, Gibbon, & First, 1992) have found significantly higher rates of clinical depression among caregivers compared with the general adult population. For example, in a study of 68 spousal caregivers to individuals with Alzheimer's disease, more than 40% met current criteria for a depressive disorder as measured by the SADS, and another 40% of this sample of caregivers met the same criteria for a time period earlier in their caregiving situation (Coppel, Burton, Becker, & Fiore, 1985). Drinka, Smith and Drinka (1987) found even higher rates of depressive disorders in their study of caregivers for demented patients. Of the 117 caregivers assessed, 83% met *DSM-III* (American Psychiatric Association, 1980) diagnostic criteria for major depression. However, caregivers in this sample provided assistance for patients unable to follow treatment regimens prescribed by specialty clinics. This uniqueness suggests an extra burden for the caregivers, which may have contributed to the high rate of reported depressive disorders.

More recently, Redinbaugh, MacCallum, and Kiecolt-Glaser (1995) investigated recurrent syndromal depression, as identified by Structured Clinical Interview–Nonpatient version (SCID-NP) (Riskind, Beck, Berchick, Brown, & Steer, 1987; Spitzer, Williams, Endicott, & Gibbon, 1987). Syndromal depression in their project included diagnoses of major depression, dysthymia, or depressive disorder not otherwise specified. Among their sample of 103 caregivers for family members with progressive dementia, 53% of these caregivers reported a syndromal depressive disorder at some point over 3 years of caregiving.

Rate of depression seems to remain higher among caregivers than the general population regardless of whether or not they feel they need help for their distress. Gallagher and her colleagues used the SADS to describe their sample of 115 help-seeking caregivers recruited for a psychoeducational intervention (Gallagher, Rose, Rivera, Lovett, & Thompson, 1989). Of these caregivers, 46% were diagnosed with major, minor, or intermittent depressive disorders; an additional 22% of these participants reported some depressive features. As a part of the same study, this team of researchers recruited an additional 58 nonhelp-seeking caregivers from an Alzheimer's disease study, and discovered that 18% of these similarly assessed nonhelp seekers met criteria for depression. More than one third of this nonhelp-seeking group also presented with some depressive symptoms. Even though a larger proportion of help seekers than nonhelp seekers were diagnosed with depression, the proportion of depressed nonhelp-seeking caregivers is still as much as ten times greater than prevalence figures for major depression reported among adults in general (Blazer, Hughes & George, 1987; Koenig & Blazer, 1992).

A more striking picture of the prevalence of depression appears when caregivers are contrasted with comparison groups. Dura, Stukenberg, and Kiecolt-Glaser (1991) administered the SCID to a group of 78 adult children caring for their demented parents and contrasted these results with SCID ratings from a group of 78 comparison subjects of similar age and other demographic characteristics. At time of assessment, 18% of the caregivers presented with clinical depressive disorders versus 0% of the comparison group. Another 26% of these caregivers also met diagnostic criteria for a depressive disorder at some earlier point during the time they provided care, as contrasted with only 4% of the comparison subjects matched on equivalent time periods. These differences between subjects and matched comparison groups hold when subjects are assessed more than once during the course of caregiving. In a study of 69 spousal caregivers and matched noncaregiving adults, 25% of the caregivers as opposed to 0% of the noncaregivers met criteria for a diagnosis of a depressive disorder at an initial assessment point, and 32% of these caregivers and 6% of the comparison subjects met criteria for a depressive disorder at some point during the next 13 months (Kiecolt-Glaser, Dura, Speicher, Trask, & Glaser, 1991).

Similarly, Russo, Vitaliano, Brewer, Katon, and Becker (1995) used another diagnostic interview, the Diagnostic Interview Schedule Version III-R (DIS; Robins *et al.,* 1981), to measure depressive and anxiety disorders among a group of spouse caregivers ($N = 82$) and a group of demographically matched controls. During the time they provided care, 27% of the caregivers met criteria for either a depressive or anxiety disorder and 20% had a major depressive episode. In contrast, only 10% of the noncaregiving controls met criteria for a depressive or anxiety disorder, and only 7% had an established major depressive episode across similar time periods. The current prevalence of major depression in the same group of caregivers ranged from 7.3% at baseline to 9.8% approximately 18 months later, whereas the prevalence rate ranged from 0% to 1.2% among controls. Moreover, caregivers with past psychiatric disorders were found to be twice as likely to have a recurrence or relapse after onset of patient illness as matched controls with previous disorders assessed at comparable time frames.

Standardized self-report inventories, such as the Center for Epidemiologic Studies Depression Scale (CES-D; Radloff, 1977) and the Beck Depression Inventory (BDI; Beck, Rush, Shaw, & Emery, 1979), are also used to assess depression and depressive symptoms in caregivers to elders. Most caregiving studies using the CES-D report means between 14 and 18, with scores of 16 or above indicating that an individual is at risk for clinical depression (e.g. Baumgarten *et al.,* 1992; Pruchno, Kleban, Michaels, & Dempsey, 1990). The average reported CES-D score as well as the proportions of caregivers over the cutoff score of 16 are often well above the typical population means (7.4 to 9.4) and proportions (15% to 20%) described by various epidemiological studies (Futterman, Thompson, Gallagher-Thompson, & Ferris, 1995). For example, Baumgarten and colleagues (1992) using the CES-D with a group of 103 primary caregivers of dementia patients and a group of noncaregiving spouses discovered 38.8% of these caregivers fell above the cutoff score. This is two times the percentage found in the noncaregiving community samples (16.5%). These means and proportions are even higher when caregivers are recruited from either home health service agencies or waiting lists for respite services (e.g., Mohide *et al.,* 1990; Robinson, 1989; Shields, 1992).

Caregiving studies using the Beck Depression Inventory (BDI) have also reported higher means and proportions for caregivers than those found in the general population. For instance, a study that compared caregivers of cognitively versus functionally impaired elders revealed that almost 50% of caregivers to cognitively impaired care receivers and almost 40% of the caregivers to functionally impaired care receivers scored above normal BDI cutoff scores, indicating current depressive symptoms (Gallagher, Wrabetz, Lovett, DelMaestro, & Rose, 1989). Vitaliano, Russo, Young, Teri, and Maiuro (1991) found that 34.2% of spousal caregivers to individuals with Alzheimer's disease scored above the BDI's mild depression cutoff at baseline; this proportion did not change significantly at a 15- to 18-month follow-up assessment. Similarly, Dura and colleagues (1991), in a study of adult children caring for demented parents, determined that mean BDI scores in this group of caregivers were significantly higher than a matched group of noncaregiving controls.

In sum, prevalence rates for depression among caregivers of elders are impressive, whether these rates are determined by structured interview or self-report. Yet, a sizable proportion of caregivers actually do report few depressive symptoms or feelings. Furthermore, a subgroup of these caregivers report very little psychological distress, despite the fact that they complain of caregiver stress and volunteer for various interventions designed to reduce their perceived distress (Zarit, 1990; Zarit, Anthony, & Boutselis, 1987). Variability in prevalence rates reported and the differences in people's experience of the caregiving process has generated a large caregiving literature designed to identify and discuss factors that may contribute to caregiver distress and well-being. Several of these studies have produced mixed results but other findings have been consistently supported by the literature.

Research results from studies exploring the caregiver's relationship to the frail elder imply that both spousal and adult offspring caregivers can experience significant depression. Yet on the whole, intrahousehold caregivers, especially spouses, are more likely to experience distress from extended caregiving than adult offspring caregivers living apart from elders (Baumgarten et al., 1992; George & Gwyther, 1986; Zarit & Whitlatch, 1992). Such level of depression may be further exacerbated by the quality of the caregiver–care receiver relationship prior to the onset of the elder's illness. A high degree of positive attachment between caregiver and patient can presumably contribute significantly to the experience of loss and grief in the altered relationship between patient and caregiver. Alternatively, a low level of attachment, or even a conflicted relationship between caregiver and patient may produce negative affect such as anger and resentment (Robinson, 1989; Schulz & Williamson, 1991). It is possible that caregivers in both scenarios may manifest their negative affect through depressive symptomatology, but further exploration of the caregiver–patient premorbid relationship is warranted.

The caregiving literature overwhelmingly supports the notion that caregiving can adversely affect a caregiver's psychological well-being regardless of the elder's particular illness or disability. Further, many studies suggest that caring for an elder with more frequently occurring problem behaviors places the caregiver at an even higher risk for depression (Baumgarten et al., 1992; Mittelman et al., 1994; Schulz & Williamson, 1991). However, the impact of other patient illness characteristics on caregivers is not as clear. The majority of studies indicate that neither the amount of assistance provided to the elder nor the severity of his or her cognitive impairment is directly explanatory of caregiver depression (e.g., Clipp & George, 1990; Deimling & Bass, 1986; Dura, Stukenberg, & Kiecolt-Glaser, 1990; Dura *et al.,* 1991; Gallagher *et al.,* 1989; Kiecolt-Glaser *et al.,* 1991; Pruchno & Resch, 1989; Russo *et al.,* 1995; Schulz & Williamson, 1991). However, a smaller, but still substantial, group of studies have reported findings supporting these relationships (Baumgarten *et al.,* 1992; Coppel *et al.,* 1985; W. E. Haley, Levine, Brown, Berry, & Hughes, 1987; Russo *et al.,* 1995).

The length of time providing care may contribute to caregiver depression, but the extent and direction of the relationship is uncertain. At first, we might expect that an increasing length of time spent caregiving would wear caregivers down, increase their vulnerability, and exacerbate negative affective states (e.g., Baumgarten *et al.,* 1992: George & Gwyther, 1986), but several studies have not found this to be the case (e.g., Draper, Poulos, Cole, Poulos, & Ehrlich, 1992; Kiecolt-Glaser *et al.,* 1991). In fact, an additional amount of time spent in the caregiving role may actually influence grief and loss processes, including preparation for the frail elder's death, or it may strengthen coping skills and social resources that result in caregiver adaptation (Mullan, 1992; Norris & Murrell, 1987; Pearlin, Mullan, Semple, & Skaff, 1990).

Another cluster of findings supports the contention that being an older Caucasian female (Blazer, 1990; Evans, Copeland, & Dewey, 1991; Mirowsky & Ross, 1990; Williamson & Schulz, 1992) with few economic resources (George, 1983; Mirowsky & Ross, 1990), who is experiencing significant life stressors and who also has few social supports (Dean, Kolody & Wood, 1990; George, 1983; Mirowsky & Ross, 1990; Russell & Cutrona, 1991) increases the risk of developing psychological symptoms of distress. Although there are a few exceptions (see, e.g., Dura *et al.,* 1991; Shields, 1992), caregiving wives and daughters generally report more depression and other psychological distress than comparable husbands and sons (Anthony-Bergstone, Zarit, & Gatz, 1988; Gallagher *et al.,* 1989; Horowitz, 1985; Lieberman & Fisher, 1995; Young & Kahana, 1989). Although our understanding of this gender discrepancy is still unclear, socialization may play a role by permitting women to more freely express their feelings and by promoting different conceptualizations between the sexes of the meaning, roles, and tasks of caregiving (Horowitz, 1985; Miller, 1987; Pruchnol *et al.,* 1990).

Characteristics and qualities of caregivers' social resources may help in managing the situation or help buffer them from negative effects of caregiving. In general, caregiver perceptions of greater amounts of available support, adequacy of social support, and satisfaction with the support received have been reported to be associated with less depression and other negative affective states (Fiore, Coppel, Becker, & Cox, 1986; Mittelman *et al.,* 1994; Oxman, Freeman, Manheimer, & Stukel, 1994). Similarly, particular domains or types of social support, including larger amounts of direct assistance and positive feedback from others as well as higher numbers of self-reported recreational interactions, have also been associated with lower levels of depression. In contrast, two other support characteristics investigated in the literature, namely, a greater need for social support and increased negative interactions with others, appear to be related to more caregiver psychological distress (MaloneBeach & Zarit, 1995; Redinbaugh *et al.,* 1995; Rivera, Rose, Futterman, Lovett, & Gallagher-Thompson, 1991; Thompson, Futterman, Gallagher-Thompson, Rose & Lovett, 1993).

In addition to caregivers' social resources, their psychological resources, including the coping strategies they use to handle the caregiving situation, appear to be related to both the quality and quantity of distress experienced (Coppe *et al.,* 1985; W. E. Haley, Levine, Brown, & Bartolucci, 1987; W. E. Haley, Levine, Brown, Berry, & Hughes, 1987; Pruchno & Resch, 1989). On the one hand, caregivers who use problem-focused coping strategies to reassess situations, seek out alternatives, and take steps to change how stressors are handled seem to experience less depression and more positive caregiver well-being. On the other hand, use of emotion-focused coping strategies that encourage avoidance, escape, and fantasy in response to real and unavoidable caregiver stressors seems to be less effective in reducing depression and other negative affect (Barusch, 1988; W. E. Haley *et al.,* 1987; Pruchno & Resch, 1989; Quayhagen & Quayhagen, 1989; Vitaliano *et al.,* 1991).

In an investigation related to these findings on coping strategies, Hooker, Frazier, and Monahan (1994) addressed the issue of personality and coping style in a study of 50 Alzheimer spousal caregivers. Caregivers scoring high on neuroticism tended to use emotion-focused coping strategies that are associated with depression and increased interpersonal conflict, but those scoring high on extroversion used problem-solving approaches. Because coping strategies are easily taught, it may be useful to identify those caregivers who are at higher risk and provide them with coping skills training in the early stages of their caregiving.

IMPACT OF CAREGIVING ON
PHYSICAL HEALTH

Fengler and Goodrich (1979) have referred to caregivers as "hidden patients," suggesting that caregivers experience significant physical health problems as a result of their exposure to the consistent stress of caregiving. Yet, the research examining caregiving effects on physical health is somewhat limited. Generally, increased emotional distress is often found to be associated with poorer self-reported physical health (Baumgarten *et al.,* 1992; Draper *et al.,* 1992; Mittelman *et al.,* 1994; Schulz *et al.,* 1990; Schulz *et al.,* 1995; Wright *et al.,* 1993). However, we should keep in mind that physical health effects may not become evident until quite some time after caregiving ends (Schulz et al, 1990). In a study comparing the health status of caregivers to noncaregivers, Kiecolt-Glaser and colleagues (1987) found caregivers to have weaker immune responses than noncaregivers. In a recent review of physical health outcome studies of Alzheimer's disease caregivers, Schulz and colleagues (1995) concluded that although caregivers report their health to be worse than that of their noncaregiving peers, the relationships among their perceived health and their actual symptoms, behavior, or use of health care services are tenuous. The studies reviewed did, however, support the relationship between socioeconomic hardship (and its associated stressors such as high perceived stress, low life satisfaction) and negative health outcomes. Finally, these studies evidenced a pattern of health effects specific to caregiving such that caregivers of patients exhibiting cognitive impairments evidenced greater physical health problems, whereas those caring for patients with problem behaviors were more likely to experience psychiatric morbidity.

PSYCHOLOGICALLY ORIENTED INTERVENTIONS FOR TREATMENT OF CAREGIVER DISTRESS

As the previous section has clearly shown, most caregivers experience a considerable amount of psychological distress during their tenure in the caregiving role, with the most prominent negative emotions being depression, frustration or anger, and anxiety. Other feelings, such as guilt, loneliness, fear, and apprehension about the future, have also been reported in some studies. In fact, clinical experience suggests that most caregivers experience a wide range of negative affects over the course of time. In an effort to address these unpleasant mood states, and at the same time encourage caregivers to give and get support from one another, the Alzheimer's disease (AD) support group movement was started over a decade ago. The program was initiated by a woman in Minnesota whose husband had AD and who felt extremely alone in her efforts to give him care. This movement has grown tremendously, so that now there are AD chapters and support groups in most towns and cities throughout the United States, as well as in most countries of the world. The success of the AD movement spawned development of other self-help groups based on type of disability; there are now support groups for caregivers of persons with Parkinson's disease, for those who have suffered multiple strokes (or multiinfarct dementia), or for brain-damaged adults in whom the cause might not be easily determined. However, despite the grassroots success of these groups, few empirical studies have been conducted to evaluate the impact of support group participation on the psychological status of family caregivers. Gonyea (1989), in a review of available literature, found that most participants rated the group experience as helpful, but more objective measures of psychological distress, such as self-report scales for depressive symptoms or frustration tolerance, were rarely used. In addition, there is some evidence that support groups meet the needs of caregivers in terms of gaining knowledge about the particular disease and its likely course over time (Toseland, Rossiter, & Labrecque, 1989). However, there is much less evidence that membership in a support group helps reduce psychological distress and perceived burden, or that caregivers attending support groups gain skills to manage their situations more effectively (Dura *et al.*, 1991; Toseland et al. 1989).

One might argue that support groups serve a valuable function for most caregivers at some stage in the process. However, by themselves, they may not be adequate to help caregivers feel better about themselves or how they are managing, because the focus of support groups is simply on sharing feelings, not on sharing solutions or strategies for improving quality of life. In some instances, support groups may actually be of little value (for example, when the caregiver is in acute distress and needs to know how to deal with his or her strong emotions). Further, as with any intervention, quality of the experience varies greatly according to the personalities of the other participants and the leader (if there is one). Finally, some caregivers are not comfortable expressing themselves in front of a group, no matter how supportive the group tries to be, so that the group venue is likely to be of little benefit. For such caregivers, individual counseling or therapy (depending on the nature and severity of the problem) would be needed.

However, for most caregivers who regularly attend support groups and who do benefit, the time comes when something else seems to be needed so that they can cope more effectively with the stresses and strains of daily caregiving responsibilities and a deteriorating family member. To address these needs, several research groups have focused on the development of psychoeducational programs using specific themes, such as "coping with depression," "coping with frustration," or "coping with stress." Under these rubrics, certain specific skills are taught, usually in a small group or class format, with a relatively small number of participants, to encourage active learning and mastery of cognitive and behavioral coping strategies.

Interventions focused on teaching self-management skills to family caregivers have included such strategies as relaxation training, teaching problem-solving skills, or teaching methods for increasing everyday pleasant events (Greene & Monahan, 1989; W. E. Haley, 1989; Lovett & Gallagher, 1988; Whitlatch, Zarit, & von Eye, 1991). Similar to traditional psychotherapy groups, they are generally small in number: 8 to 10 participants who sign up for a given number of sessions in a closed-end format. Participants are encouraged to share thoughts and feelings and to participate actively through role playing, skill demonstrations, and "homework" opportunities that encourage the practice of new skills outside the group or class setting. In general, those programs that teach a very specific set of skills (such as anger management), rather than a broad array of skills (such as problem solving), report more improvement in terms of reduction in depression and increased well-being in caregivers (Gallagher-Thompson & DeVries, 1994; Lovett & Gallagher, 1988). In general, such short-term, highly focused programs have been effective in reducing caregivers' stress and related negative emotions when levels of distress were high at the outset. Less improvement has been noted among caregivers who were less distressed to begin with, possibly reflecting the fact that the latter had less room for change. Moreover, even when measures of distress did not change significantly over time, caregivers have reported high levels of satisfaction with these interventions (Toseland et al., 1989), along with increased self-efficacy and control over certain aspects of their situation (Steffen, Gallagher-Thompson, Zeiss, & Willis-Shore, 1994).

For those caregivers experiencing more distress, such as those in an episode of major depression or those who are actively abusing or neglecting the elder care receiver, individual counseling or psychotherapy may be indicated. Case reports by Rose and DelMaestro (1990), Kaplan and Gallagher-Thompson (1995), and Dick and Gallagher-Thompson (1995) describe use of methods such as brief psychodynamic therapy or short-term cognitive-behavioral therapy for such individuals; these case studies report excellent results. Few empirical studies have been conducted that evaluate efficacy of psychotherapy with family caregivers, but those that have are encouraging. For example, Gallagher-Thompson and Steffen (1994) found that both brief psychodynamic and brief cognitive-behavioral therapy were effective in significantly reducing clinical levels of depression in a sample of more than 60 family caregivers. Similarly, Toseland and Smith (1990) demonstrated the benefits of individual therapy for caregivers' subjective well-being, particularly for subjects with professional therapists as compared to those meeting with peer counselors.

An individually based behavioral approach trained caregivers in principles and techniques that could be used in the home to manage the troublesome behaviors of their impaired relative more effectively (Pinkston & Linsk, 1984). They taught caregivers to monitor and then change problematic behaviors through reinforcement, cueing, and shaping of more appropriate behaviors (e.g., socialization, dressing, toileting) and reported excellent success with this program. Teri and colleagues have termed this the "A-B-C" approach to behavioral management, referring to the links between antecedent events, behavioral responses, and emotional consequences. They emphasize teaching new behavioral responses and better management of the antecedent events that trigger problematic behaviors, particularly in demented elders (see Teri & Logsdon, 1991; Teri & Uomoto, 1991, for further description of this approach).

Teri and Gallagher (1991) have also described suggested interventions that caregivers could be taught to administer that could be utilized to treat depression in dementia victims. This approach is suggested not only to benefit the care receiver, but is also thought to benefit the caregiver in two ways. First, the caregiver goes through the same activities, designed to dispel depression and create positive mood, as the care receiver; caregivers using this approach have been shown to respond with reduced depression. Second, if the care receiver is less depressed, some tasks of caregiving may be easier, such as getting the patient up and dressed, feeding the patient, and so forth.

Several informative reviews have been published in the past few years that debate the relative efficacy of psychosocial interventions (in general) and psychoeducational interventions (in particular) for improving the psychological function of family caregivers. These reviews include those by Bourgeois, Schulz, Burgio (1996), Gallagher-Thompson (1994b), Knight, Lutzky, and Macofsky-Urban (1993), and Toseland and Rossiter (1989). The reviewers disagree as to which interventions are most effective for reducing caregivers' burden and/or other indices of psychological distress. However, in general, they report that individual psychosocial interventions have been at least "moderately" effective with distressed and depressed caregivers, whereas group interventions had more "modest" effects, with greater variability in responsiveness.

This body of findings suggests that the next generation of caregiver efficacy research should focus on which interventions are most effective for caregivers with certain characteristics (or individual difference variables) at the beginning of treatment as assessed during an intake process. As Snow (1991) has very cogently argued, it is only by carefully studying aptitude by treatment interaction (ATI) effects that we will have an empirical basis for deciding who is most likely to benefit from a given intervention.

Data from a recently completed study by our group confirm the value of this approach. By examining the interaction of anger expression style and type of caregiver class (emphasizing controlling one's depression versus controlling one's frustration), we found that caregivers with more of an "anger-in" style responded significantly better to the controlling depression class, whereas caregivers with more of an "anger out" style benefited considerably more from the controlling frustration class (Gallagher-Thompson, Coon, & Thompson, 1996). Such results encourage further development of models for systematic treatment selection.

Information of this nature can be extremely valuable in assisting program managers to allocate their limited resources to those most in need, at the same time enabling researchers to specify a broad range of services and programs that would be helpful to caregivers who are stressed, but perhaps not seriously distressed. We turn now to what is known currently about the particular needs and most effective approaches with caregivers of different kinds.

ADDRESSING THE UNIQUE NEEDS OF SUBGROUPS OF FAMILY CAREGIVERS

Men in the Caregiving Role

The National Long Term Care Survey, carried out in 1982, until recently was the most recent survey yielding information about different demographic groups of caregivers; it may now be considerably out of date, but it represents a good available source of information. According to that survey, 28% of all caregivers are male (R. Stone *et al.,* 1987). Although several studies have examined differences between male and female caregivers, there is far less research on male caregivers specifically. The results from gender comparison studies may be the reason that male caregiver research is not as advanced as female caregiver research. Studies have consistently shown that men report lower levels of negative feelings, physical symptoms, and burden relative to women (Gallagher, Rose *et al.,* 1989; Young & Kahana, 1989).

A metanalysis of 10 studies of caregiver burden found significantly less burden experienced by men than by women (Miller & Cafasso, 1992), but all reviewed studies used self-report measures of burden. The authors note that the significant gender differences explained only 4% of the variance in caregiver burden (Miller & Cafasso, 1992). It should also be noted that most male primary caregivers are husbands (R. Stone *et al.,* 1987), so that many of the findings discussed here about male caregivers may not apply to male caregivers with other family roles, for example, sons, nephews, sons-in-law, and so forth.

Though some have interpreted these data to indicate that intervention with male caregivers is not as critical as intervention with female caregivers, such a conclusion is probably premature. For example, self-reported levels of depression have been shown to increase in one study of male caregivers over a 2-year period, while female caregivers showed no increase in depression over the same period (Schulz & Williamson, 1991). Also, distress experienced by male caregivers may have been underestimated or misunderstood because of the methods or measuring instruments used to measure distress. Lutzky and Knight (1994) point to previous findings of gender differences in recognizing and reporting emotional states (Notarius & Johnson, 1982; Vinick, 1984) as possible reasons for gender differences in reported caregiver burden. However, Lutzky and Knight (1994) found no gender differences in cardiovascular responsivity (CVR), a physiological, nonself-report measure of stress.

Given these differences between male and female caregivers, it may be that male caregivers have needs different from those of female caregivers in terms of interventions to ameliorate caregiver distress. The experiences of the present authors and anecdotal reports from other therapists who have worked with male caregivers support this contention, but only two research papers to date have examined a psychosocial intervention designed specifically for male caregivers of dementia patients (Davies, Priddy, & Tinklenberg, 1986; Moseley, Davies, & Priddy, 1988).

These two papers are an initial report and follow-up with a support group developed for elderly male caregivers of dementia patients, and address individual case issues as well as general themes. Davies and colleagues (1986) identified several different types of male caregivers, explaining the particular issues they face, and Moseley and colleagues (1988) reported on the status of these caregivers 3 years after the group started. Moseley and colleagues (1988) also discussed several themes that were evident throughout the life of the group. These male caregivers appeared to approach caregiving as "a challenge to be met 'head on' " (p. 733). Their roles changed dramatically, particularly in that they were required to carry out tasks that traditionally fit into their wives' roles. Frustration was overtly discussed more often than sadness, and it took considerably more time for men to become comfortable discussing their emotions in the group relative to the authors' experiences with female caregivers. Finally, the experience of caregiving was not static, but instead was constantly evolving, and the stages of grief described by Kubler-Ross (1969) were evident throughout the process.

The authors made several recommendations for future male caregiver groups, including (1) offering the group as an adjunct to a larger, coeducational information and support activity; (2) keeping the men's group small, with a limited influx of new members; (3) meeting biweekly, rather than weekly, because of caregiving schedule demands; (4) using a low to moderate level of structure; and (5) trying to provide for an exclusively male group "whenever possible" (Moseley *et al.,* 1988, p. 135). The last recommendation is given specifically because of the authors' observations that men are underrepresented and much more passive in mixed-gender groups. No study implementing their suggestions for future male groups has yet been published, although one of the chapters of the national Alzheimer's Association has published a "how-to" manual for leaders who wish to offer men-only support groups; the manual actually contains many of the same observations and suggestions (Keller, 1992).

Unfortunately, no rigorously designed experimental outcome study on the process and results of male caregiving has been published to date, to the authors' best knowledge. Because of this, and because of the limited information currently available on how to best offer services to male caregivers, conclusions about their needs and the types of services that will benefit them must be drawn with caution. Further research is necessary before firm conclusions can be reached about whether treatments that are known to work with women will work as well with men, and whether these treatments are the best way to help male caregivers. We also need further study on similarities and differences between concerns and treatment needs of adult sons versus spouse caregivers, as well as examining how men may function more often than anyone realizes in secondary (rather than primary) caregiving roles. The impact of this on such activities as employment and use of leisure time are two other areas that warrant future investigation.

Ethnic and Cultural Minorities as Family Caregivers

Recently we have seen in this country both a significant increase in immigration of older persons from many different countries and cultures and a definite rise in the life expectancy of racial and ethnic minority elderly, including African Americans, Native Americans, Asian Americans and Pacific Islanders, and persons of Hispanic origins (Jackson, 1988). There are important differences, both between and within these broad racial and ethnic designations, in explanatory models of health and illness. These factors contribute to an extraordinarily complex interaction picture that makes the study of family caregiving patterns in these groups a very challenging (and also rewarding) process.

Kleinman (1980) described eloquently how cultural customs and beliefs about causes and treatments of disease act as strong influences on the kinds of problems that are experienced and the kinds of interventions that are viewed as acceptable. For example, not all cultures experience caregiving as primarily a stressful experience; in such cultures, treatments that focus on the negative aspects of caregiving may not be at all well received. The reader is referred to several studies by Haley and associates focusing on the apparent psychological resilience and positive views about caregiving that have been found among African American caregivers (W. Haley *et al.*, 1995, W. Haley *et al.*, 1996).

Yet on an empirical level, much less is known than should be about the day-to-day caregiving experiences of racial and ethnic minorities as they attempt to support frail elders and maintain them in the home setting. Most of the few available empirical studies have focused on African Americans (cf. the work of Haley and colleagues just noted, along with Dilworth-Anderson & Anderson, 1994; Gonzalez, Gitlin, & Lyons, 1995; Hinrichsen & Ramirez, 1992, for more specific findings). Mexican Americans are currently the fastest growing ethnic group in this country (U.S. Bureau of the Census, 1989). Some research has been completed that focused specifically on the needs of Hispanic families, particularly those caring for a relative with dementia (e.g., Cox & Monk, 1993; Sotomayor & Randolph, 1988), However, virtually no outcome studies have been conducted with any of the major Hispanic subgroups.

Clinical reports by Henderson and Gutierrez-Mayka (1992) and Henderson, Gutierrez Mayka, Garcia, and Boyd (1993) describe in excellent detail how to establish and maintain ethnically sensitive support groups for both the Latino and African American populations of family caregivers in Florida. These writings have encouraged others to think about how best to work with these populations. Recent work (e.g., chapters by Gallagher-Thompson, Talamantes, Ramirez, & Valverde, 1996, and Henderson, 1996) attempts to integrate already published insights with additional clinical experience. Also, several groups of researchers have recently been funded by the National Institute on Aging to undertake more controlled research on the efficacy of several different kinds of psychosocial interventions with several different groups of minority caregivers. This collaborative research program, termed the REACH project, involves six research sites in different parts of the country. It will yield new information about how African American and Hispanic caregivers, in particular, respond to a variety of interventions. Although no published information is yet available from the project, basic descriptive information can be obtained (Ory & Schulz, 1996).

The other major groups, including Asian Americans and Pacific Islanders (e.g., Chinese, Japanese, Korean, Tongan, and Vietnamese Americans), and Native Americans, have been generally overlooked when it comes to caregiving research. In the case of Asian Americans and Pacific Islanders, this may be due in part to language issues that can make it extremely difficult to understand what caregivers and their elders are experiencing and what their needs are. In addition, their cultural customs and values emphasize not complaining about stress within the family, and showing great respect for elders, regardless of their frailties or lack of adequate cognitive function. These values may make it very stigmatizing to seek services and help outside the family for what is essentially regarded as a "family affair" (see Elliott, Di Minno, Lam, & Mei, 1996; Koh & Bell, 1987; McBride & Parreno, 1996; and Tempo & Saito, 1996, for discussion of these issues with particular focus on Chinese, Korean, Filipino, and Japanese American family caregivers, respectively).

Emphasizing the similarities rather than differences among them, Lockery (1991) addressed the role of family and social support among the major racial and ethnic groups just noted. She found several important similarities in perceptions of the roles of family members, including (1) the value placed on intergenerational contact, (2) the tradition of respect toward the elderly, and (3) the clear family obligation for caregiving in the home, rather than in an institutional setting. Lockery points out that these characteristics reflect more "traditional" values, but it is not wise to assume that traditional values are always operative in a given family's situation. Other variables such as immigration status, level of acculturation, degree of family contact, and socialization to the dominant culture and its values will influence these traditions and lead to variations in family members' roles or beliefs. For example, first-generation immigrants are more likely to retain traditional customs or beliefs than are third- or fourth-generation persons, who have become more acculturated to the host country (Landrine & Klonoff, 1992).

The practice of comparing biological subgroups (such as African American and White caregivers) on several variables is becoming more common in caregiver research. However, because race is so interrelated with socioeconomic, educational, and health status, we suggest that its use (as well as the use of these other variables) to explain is limited and can lead to inaccurate conclusions, which may in turn strengthen current stereotypes. For example, some have proposed that minority caregivers experience a double jeopardy due to disadvantages of age and race (Belgrave, Wylie, & Choi, 1993), yet the perception that race always represents a disadvantage may be shortsighted. As noted above, several studies have found that resilience, rather than distress, tends to characterize African American caregivers.

Ethnicity is a concept that refers to cultural lifestyle patterns such as shared language, customs, religion, and values (Fernando, 1991). As a multidimensional construct, it is more difficult to define than race but is more likely to help identify genuine cultural differences in caregiving that are less influenced by socioeconomic status and more by one's beliefs, as related to family and tradition.

Comparisons between ethnic and Anglo caregivers have typically focused on three variables: social support, psychological well-being or burden, and health. Despite the belief that the social support networks of minority caregivers differ from those of Anglos, data have been inconsistent regarding size and frequency of contact (George, 1989; Wood & Parham, 1990). Based on their findings, W. Haley et al. (1996) have suggested that cognitive strategies such as positive appraisal and coping contribute to minority caregivers' abilities to overcome the added hardships imposed by low income and poor health. Others (Gibson, 1982; Wood & Parham, 1990) have suggested that minority caregivers' values and beliefs, along with their life experiences, create a powerful variable which impacts appraisal and coping, so that for many, caregiving is almost automatically less stressful than for Anglo counterparts. Thus, they may not need or want the same kinds of services that have been developed primarily to serve the more well-characterized needs of Anglo caregivers, who are still in the majority in this country. Clearly, future research must be culturally sensitive in the ways it asks about caregiving, and in the types of interventions or services that are proposed to assist minority families with the caregiving process.

A final related point concerns the underutilization of currently existing social and health care services by minority caregivers and their elders. For all the reasons noted here, it should not come as a surprise that caregivers of varied cultural backgrounds do not utilize extant services. For some, this has been a matter of great concern, since their unique needs are apparently not being addressed adequately by the majority culture in its public policy and planning efforts. Henderson and colleagues (1993) theorized that several factors serve to discourage minority use of services such as support groups or clinics. These disincentives include impersonal recruitment and maintenance strategies, inconvenient location of services, and absence of ethnic staff representing the target group. Recommendations include active recruitment strategies that emphasize individual contact via face-to-face interviews and telephone and written follow-up, and an informal, unhurried interpersonal approach which facilitates the development of trust between participants and staff. Additional suggestions have been described by Areán and Gallagher-Thompson (1996). These include active problem solving to handle practical barriers such as transportation difficulties and low literacy levels; use of research funds to defray costs associated with participating in a project over time, such as "sitting" costs for someone to stay with a demented spouse or parent while the caregiver receives services; and staff flexibility around scheduling, so that missed appointments can be made up with a minimum of embarrassment and explanations. These and other recommendations in this section, such as the employment of bilingual and, whenever possible, appropriately bicultural, staff, may seem costly and time-consuming to implement. However, research and practice will continue to lag significantly behind caregivers' needs until such strategies are broadly implemented.

SUMMARY AND FUTURE DIRECTIONS

Research on caregiving and clinical interventions designed to help caregivers have gone through several transformations, as we have reviewed. The field started with a general awareness that caregiving is a stressful responsibility. Research questions in that phase focused on assessing the level of stress and examining the impact of stress on physical and emotional well-being of the caregiver. Other early research examined the behaviors of the demented care receiver as sources of stress. Interventions emphasized support groups, in which caregivers could share information and offer emotional support to each other.

Out of this early work, questions of greater sophistication developed. Caregiving came to be understood as a complex process that could not adequately be captured by notions of level of stress or distress. Instead, researchers began to examine both the rewards and the problems associated with caregiving, and to see how these interacted to create complex emotional and behavioral responses in the caregiving context. Researchers also began to explore caregiving as a longitudinal process, which may be experienced very differently at different points. In this phase, interventions began to shift from simple support groups to more complex psychoeducational models. In both group interventions and individual counseling, an emphasis on understanding and support were maintained, but additional factors were emphasized, such as learning to handle one's own emotional reactions to caregiving, developing skills for maintaining one's own well-being as a caregiver, and developing better problem-solving skills.

Research at the second level produced more information, which led to yet a third phase of caregiver research and intervention. In this latest phase, individual variability in the caregiving experience is being studied even more broadly, with greater sensitivity to racial, ethnic, and other cultural features, as well as to the role of gender of the caregiver: Caregiving is being viewed more in terms of the ongoing, complex relationships between the patient, the caregiver, the broader family or kinship network, and the cultural norms and expectations of a community. In this phase, intervention is being viewed more broadly as well, with sensitivity to how caregiving is defined among different ethnic and cultural groups, and by male as well as female caregivers, and with special attention to factors that influence what skills might be seen as most important for caregivers from different backgrounds.

We applaud these developments in our understanding of the caregiving process and experience. Caregiving for a demented family member can be easy to define at one level, but the complexity and depth of the situation become compelling as research progresses and as our efforts to intervene mature. It would have been hard to predict future directions for research and clinical activity in the beginning, and we should continue to be guided by each wave of research rather than by a pre-set agenda. However, some general ideas about future directions can be suggested.

First, the emphasis on ethnic factors in caregiving needs to continue. To date, only African American and Hispanic caregivers have any appreciable body of research or ongoing initiatives. And each of these groups is complex and multifaceted; rather than pursuing "African American" caregiving, for example, it may be important to recognize issues for subgroups of that general category (e.g., in different parts of the country, caregivers of different socioeconomic status, in matriarchal family structures versus two-parent family structures, for male African American caregivers). At each step, refinements in interventions should keep step with basic research.

At the same time, there is a need to seek underlying principles while examining complexity and diversity. Accumulating facts about different subgroups is an extremely helpful and positive step for many reasons, but part of its value is that it challenges simplistic and culturally biased assumptions about the meaning and experience of caregiving. When basic assumptions are challenged, it becomes possible to search for unifying themes in a more open, less culture-biased way. For example, most caregiver research has started with the assumption that it is important to keep demented patients at home as long as possible, but with a parallel assumption that institutional placement may be necessary and appropriate at certain phases of dementing illness or in certain family situations. One focus of research then becomes the caregiver experiences that might lead to institutional placement of the care receiver. Home caregiving is a widely shared value, but it must be recognized that it is a value and that it flows from particular assumptions about the "best" environment for a demented person, the meaning of "home and family," and so forth. Future research might look at how caregivers try to maintain "optimal" conditions within their own framework, rather than assuming that all caregivers and families share a common perspective or, conversely, simply listing the different strategies observed across different cultural groups.

Finally, the future of caregiving research and intervention will undoubtedly be heavily influenced by the politics of health care provision and financial support for older adults. Caregivers are being expected to carry a heavier and heavier burden as other programs and health care benefits are targeted for cuts in funding. Families receiving all their care in managed care systems, for example, may have very different caregiving experiences from those receiving care in fee-for-service systems. Researchers in this area, as in all areas of health care, must recognize that the pace of change in the next decade will be rapid, and they must stay closely informed about health care policy and take steps as necessary to advocate for caregiving support programs and research funding.

REFERENCES

Altholz, J. A. S. (1991). Caregiving: The emotional rewards and challenges. In C. Nelson-Morrill (Ed.) *The Florida caregiver's handbook* (pp. 7–22). Tallahassee, FL: Healthtrac Books.

American Psychiatric Association. (1980). *Diagnostic and statistical manual of mental disorders* (3rd ed.). Washington, DC: Author.

Anthony-Bergstone, C., Zarit, S. H., & Gatz, M. (1988). Symptoms of psychological distress among caregivers of dementia patients. *Psychology and Aging, 3*, 245–248.

Areán, P. & Gallagher-Thompson, D. (1996). Issues and recommendations for the recruitment and retention of older minorities into clinical research. *Journal of Consulting and Clinical Psychology, 64,* 875–880.

Arling, G., & McAuley, W. (1983). The feasibility of public payments for family caregivers. *Gerontologist, 23,* 300–306.

Barusch, A. (1988). Problems and coping strategies of elderly spouse caregivers. *Gerontologist, 28,* 677–685.

Baumgarten, M., Battista, R. N., Infante-Rivard, C., Hanley, J. A.., Becker, R., & Gauthier, S. (1992). The psychological and physical health of family members caring for an elderly person with dementia. *Journal of Clinical Epidemiology, 45,* 61–70.

Beck, A. T., Rush, J., Shaw, B., & Emery, G. (1979). *Cognitive therapy of depression.* New York: Guilford.

Belgrave, L. L., Wykle, M. L., & Choi, J. M. (1993). Health, double jeopardy and culture: The use of institutionalization by African Americans. *Gerontologist, 33,* 379–385.

Blazer, D. G. (1990). The epidemiology of psychiatric disorders in late life. In E. W. Busse & D. G. Blazer (Eds.), *Geriatric psychiatry* (pp. 235–260). Washington, DC: American Psychiatric Press.

Blazer, D. G. (1994). Geriatric psychiatry. In R. E. Hales, S. C. Yodfsky, & J. A. Talbott (Eds.), *The American Psychiatric Press textbook of psychiatry* (2nd ed., pp. 1405–1421). Washington, DC: American Psychiatric Press.

Blazer, D. G., Hughes, D. C., & George, L. K. (1987). The epidemiology of depression in an elderly community population. *Gerontologist, 27,* 281–287.

Bourgeois, M. S., Schulz, R., & Burgio, L. (1996). Intervention for caregivers of patients with Alzheimer's disease: A review and analysis of content, process, and outcomes. *International Journal of Human Development, 43,* 35–92.

Brody, E. M. (1990). *Women in the middle: Their parent-care years.* New York: Springer.

Brody, E. M., Litvin, S. J., Hoffman, C., & Kleban, M. H. (1995). Marital status of caregiving daughters and co-residence with dependent parents. *Gerontologist, 35,* 75–85.

Cantor, M. H. (1983). Strain among caregivers: A study of experience in the United States. *Gerontologist, 23,* 597–604.

Cicirelli, V. G. (1983). A comparison of helping behavior to elderly parents of adult children with intact and disrupted marriages. *Gerontologist, 23,* 619–625.

Clipp, E. C., & George, L. K. (1990). Caregiver needs and patterns of social support. *Journal of Gerontology: Social Sciences, 45,* S102–S111.

Coppel, D. B., Burton, C., Becker, J., & Fiore, J. (1985). Relationships of cognitions associated with coping reactions to depression in spousal caregivers of Alzheimer's disease patients. *Cognitive Therapy and Research, 9,* 253–266.

Cox, C., & Monk, A. (1993). Hispanic culture and family care of Alzheimer's patients. *Health and Social Work, 18*(2), 92–100.

Cutler, S. J., & Coward, R. T. (1992). Availability of personal transportation in households of elders: Age, gender, and residence differences. *Gerontologist, 32,* 77–81.

Davies, H., Priddy, J. M., & Tinklenberg, J. R. (1986). Support groups for male caregivers of Alzheimer's patients. *Clinical Gerontologist, 5*(3/4), 384–395.

Dean, A., Kolody, B., & Wood, P. (1990). Effects of social support from various sources on depression and elderly *person. Journal of Health and Social Behavior, 2,* 148–161.

Deimling, G. T., & Bass, D. M. (1986). Symptoms of mental impairment among older adults and their effects on family caregivers. *Journal of Gerontology, 41,* 778–784.

Dick, L. P., & Gallagher-Thompson, D. (1995). Cognitive therapy with the core beliefs of a distressed lonely caregiver. *Journal of Cognitive Psychotherapy: An International Quarterly, 9,* 215–227.

Dilworth-Anderson, P., & Anderson, N.B. (1994). Dementia caregiving in blacks: A contextual approach to research. In B. Lebowitz, E. Light, & G. Neiderehe (Eds.), *Mental and physical health of Alzheimer caregivers* (pp. 385–409), New York: Springer.

Draper, B. M., Poulos, C. J., Cole, A. D., Poulos, R. G., & Ehrlich, F. (1992). A comparison of caregivers for elderly stroke and dementia victims. *Journal of the American Geriatrics Society, 35,* 896–901.

Drinka, T. J., Smith, J., & Drinka, P. J. (1987). Correlates of depression and burden for informal caregivers of patients in a geriatrics referral clinic. *Journal of the American Geriatrics Society, 35,* 522–525.

Dura, J. R., Stukenberg, K. W., & Kiecolt-Glaser, J. K. (1990). Chronic stress and depressive disorders in older adults. *Journal of Abnormal Psychology, 99,* 284–290.

Dura, J. R., Stukenberg, K. W., & Kiecolt-Glaser, J. K. (1991). Anxiety and depressive disorders in adult children caring for demented parents. *Psychology and Aging, 6,* 467–473.

Elliott, K. S., Di Minno, M., Lam, D., & Mei, A. (1996). Working with Chinese families in the context of dementia. In G. Yeo & D. Gallagher-Thompson (Eds.), *Ethnicity and the dementias* (pp. 89–102). Washington, DC: Taylor & Francis.

Evans, M. E., Copeland, J. R. M., & Dewey, M. E. (1991). Depression in the elderly in the community: Effect of physical illness and selected social factors. *International Journal of Geriatric Psychiatry, 6,* 787–795.

Fengler, A. P., & Goodrich, N. (1979). Wives of elderly disabled men: The hidden patients. *Gerontologist, 19,* 175–183.

Fernando, S. (1991). *Mental health, race and culture.* Hampshire, England: Macmillan Education.

Fiore, J., Coppel, D. B., Becker, J., & Cox, G. B. (1986). Social support as a multifaceted construct: Examination of important dimensions for adjustment. *American Journal of Community Psychology, 14,* 93–111.

Futterman, A., Thompson, L., Gallagher-Thompson, D., & Fertis, R. (1995). Depression in later life: Epidemiology, assessment, etiology, and treatment In E. E. Beckham & W. R. Leber (Eds.), *Handbook of depression* (2nd ed., pp. 494–525). New York: Guilford.

Gallagher, D., Rose, J., Rivera, P., Lovett, S., & Thompson, L. W. (1989). Prevalence of depression in family caregivers. *Gerontologist, 29,* 449–456.

Gallagher, D., Wrabetz, A., Lovett, S., DelMaestro, S., & Rose, J. (1989). Depression and other negative affects in family caregivers. In E. Light & B. Liebowitz (Eds.), *Alzheimer's disease treatment and family stress: Directions for research* (pp. 218–244). Washington, DC: National Institute of Mental Health.

Gallagher-Thompson, D. (1994a). Clinical intervention strategies for distressed caregivers: Rationale and development of psychoeducational approaches. In E. Light, G. Niederehe, & B. D. Lebowitz (Eds.), *Stress effects on family caregivers of Alzheimer's patients: Research and interventions* (pp. 260–277). New York: Springer.

Gallagher-Thompson, D. (1994b). Direct services and interventions for caregivers: A review of extant programs and a look to the future. In M. H. Cantor (Ed.), *Family caregiving: Agenda for the future* (pp. 102–122). San Francisco: American Society on Aging.

Gallagher-Thompson, D., & DeVries, H. (1994). "Coping with Frustration" classes: Development and preliminary outcomes with women who care for relatives with dementia. *Gerontologist, 34,* 548–552.

Gallagher-Thompson, D., Coon, D., & Thompson, L. W. (1996, November). Anger expression by type of treatment interaction predicts treatment outcomes in family caregivers. Presented at the Gerontological Society of America 49th Annual Scientific Meeting, Washington, DC.

Gallagher-Thompson, D., & Steffen, A. (1994). Comparative effectiveness of cognitive/behavioral and brief psychodynamic psychotherapies for the treatment of depression in family caregivers. *Journal of Consulting and Clinical Psychology, 62,* 543–549.

Gallagher-Thompson, D., Talamantes, M., Ramirez, R., & Valverde, I. (1996). Service delivery issues and recommendations for working with Mexican American family caregivers. In G. Yeo & D. Gallagher-Thompson (Eds.), *Ethnicity and the dementias* (pp. 137–152). Washington, DC: Taylor & Francis.

Genevay, B. (1994). Family issues/family dynamics: A caregiving odyssey to 2001 and beyond. In M. H. Cantor (Ed.), *Family caregiving: Agenda for the future* (pp. 89–101). San Francisco: American Society on Aging.

George, L. K. (1989). Social and economic factors. In E. W. Busse & D. G. Blazer (Eds.). *and Aging, 5,* 277–283.

George, L. K. (1983). *Caregiver well-being. Correlates and relationships with participation in community self-help groups* (Final report to the AARP Andrers Foundation). Durham, NC: Duke University Medical Center.

George, L. K., & Gwyther, L. P. (1984, November). The dynamics of caregiver burden: Changes in caregiver well-being over time. Paper presented at the Annual Scientific Meeting of the Gerontological Society of America, San Antonio, TX.

George, L. K., & Gwyther, L. P. (1986). Caregiver well-being: A multidimensional examination of family caregivers of demented adults. *Gerontologist, 26,* 253–259.

Gibson, R. C. (1982). Blacks in middle and late life: Resources and coping. *Annals of the American Academy of Political and Social Science, 464,* 79–90.

Gonyea, J. G. (1989). Alzheimer's disease support groups: An analysis of their structure, format and perceived benefits. *Social Work in Health Care, 14,* 61–72.

Gonzalez, E., Gitlin, L., & Lyons, K. J. (1995). Review of the literature on African American caregivers of individuals with dementia. *Journal of Cultural Diversity. 2* (2), 40–48.

Gore, S. (1981). Stress-buffering functions of social supports: An appraisal and clarification of research methods. In B. Dohrenwend & B. P. Dohrenwend (Eds.), *Stressful life events and their contexts* (pp. 202–222). New York: Neale Watson Academic.

Greene, V. L., & Monahan, D. J. (1987). The effect of professionally guided caregiver support and education groups on institutionalized care receivers. *Gerontologist, 27,* 716–721.

Greene, V. L., & Monahan, D. J. (1989). The effect of a support and education program on stress and burden among family caregivers to frail elderly persons. *Gerontologist, 29,* 472–480.

Gwyther, L. P. (1990). Letting go: Separation-individuation in a wife of an Alzheimer's patient. *Gerontologist, 30,* 698–702.

Haley, W. E., West, C. A. C, Wadley, V. G., Ford, G. R., White, F. A., Barrett, J. J., Harrell, L. E., & Roth, D. L. (1995). Psychological, social, and health impact of caregiving: A comparison of Black and White dementia family caregivers and noncaregivers. *Psychology and Aging, 10,* 540–552.

Haley, W., Roth, D. L., Coleton, M., Ford, G. R., West, C. A. C., Collins, R. P., & Isobe, T. (1996). Appraisal, coping, and social support as mediators of well-being in Black and White family caregivers of patients with Alzheimer's disease. *Journal of Consulting and Clinical Psychology, 64,* 121–129.

Haley, W. E. (1989). Group intervention for dementia family caregivers: A longitudinal perspective. *Gerontologist, 29,* 481–483.

Haley, W. E., Levine, E. G., Brown, S. L., & Bartolucci, A. A. (1987). Stress, appraisal, coping and social support as predictors of adaptational outcome among dementia caregivers. *Psychology and Aging, 2,* 323–330.

Haley, W. E., Levine, E. G., Brown, S. L., Berry, J. W., & Hughes, G. H. (1987). Psychological, social and health consequences of caring for a relative with senile dementia. *Journal of the American Geriatrics Society, 35,* 405–411.

Henderson, J. N. (1996). Cultural dynamics of dementia in a Cuban and Puerto Rican population in the United States. In G. Yeo & D. Gallagher-Thompson (Eds.), *Ethnicity and the dementias* (pp. 153–166). Washington, DC: Taylor & Francis.

Henderson, J. N., & Gutierrez-Mayka, M. (1992). Ethnocultural themes in caregiving to Alzheimer's disease patients in Hispanic families. *Clinical Gerontologist, 11* (3/4), 59–74.

Henderson, J. N., Gutierrez-Mayka, M., Garcia, J., & Boyd, S. (1993). A model for Alzheimer's disease support group development in African-American and Hispanic populations. *Gerontologist, 33,* 409–414.

Hinrichsen, G. A., & Ramirez, M. (1992). Black and White dementia caregivers: A comparison of their adaptation, adjustment and service utilization. *Gerontologist, 32,* 375–381.

Hooker, K., Frazier, L. D., & Monahan, D. J. (1994). Personality and coping among caregivers of spouses with dementia. *Gerontologist, 34,* 386–392.

Horowitz, A. (1985). Family caregiving to the frail elderly. In M. P. Lawton & C. Maddox (Eds.), *Annual review of gerontology and geriatrics* (Vol. 5, pp. 194–246). New York: Springer.

Jackson, J. S. (1988). Growing old in black America: Research on aging black populations. In J. S. Jackson (Ed.), *The black American elderly: Research on physical and psychosocial health* (pp. 3–16). New York: Springer.

Kaplan, C. P., & Gallagher-Thompson, D. (1995). Treatment of clinical depression in caregivers of spouses with dementia. *Journal of Cognitive Psychotherapy: An International Quarterly, 9,* 35–44.

Keller, J. L. (1992). *Male caregivers' guidebook: Caring for your loved one with Alzheimer's at home.* Des Moines, IA: Alzheimer's Association Des Moines Chapter.

Kiecolt-Glaser, J. K., Glaser, R., Shuttleworth, E. E., Dyer, C. S., Ogrocki, P., & Speicher, C. E. (1987). Chronic stress and immunity in family caregivers of Alzheimer's disease patients. *Psychosomatic Medicine, 49,* 523–535.

Kiecolt-Glaser, J. K., Dura, J. R., Speicher, C. E., Trask, J., & Glaser, R. (1991). Spousal caregivers of dementia victims: Longitudinal changes in immunity and health. *Psychosomatic Medicine, 53,* 345–362.

Kleinman, A. (1980). *Patients and healers in the context of culture.* Berkeley: University of California Press.

Knight, B. G., Lutzky, S. M., & Macofsky-Urban, F. (1993). A meta-analytic review of interventions for caregiver distress: Recommendations for future research. *Gerontologist, 33,* 240–248.

Koenig, H. G., & Blazer, D. G. (1992). Epidemiology of geriatric affective disorders. *Clinics in Geriatric Medicine, 8,* 235–251.

Koh, J. Y., & Bell, W. G. (1987). Korean elders in the United States: Intergenerational relations and living arrangements. *Gerontologist, 27,* 66–71.

Kübler-Ross, E. (1969). *On death and dying.* New York: Macmillan.

Landrine, H., & Klonoff, E. A. (1992). Culture and health-related schemes: A review and proposal for interdisciplinary integration. *Health Psychology, 11,* 267–276.

Lawton, M. P., Moss, M., Kleban, M. H., Glicksman, A., & Rovine, M. (1991). A two-factor model of caregiving appraisal and psychological well-being. *Journal of Gerontology: Psychological Sciences, 46,* P181–P189.

Lieberman, M. A., & Fisher, L. (1995). The impact of chronic illness of the health and well-being of family members. *Gerontologist, 35,* 94–102.

Lockery, S. A. (1991). Family and social supports: Caregiving among racial and ethnic minority elders. *Generations, Fall/Winter,* 58–62.

Lovett, S., & Gallagher, D. (1988). Psychoeducational interventions for family caregivers: Preliminary efficacy data. *Behavior Therapy, 19,* 321–330.

Lutzky, S. M., & Knight, B. G. (1994). Explaining gender differences in caregiver distress: The roles of emotional attentiveness and coping styles. *Psychology and Aging, 9*(4), 513–519.

MaloneBeach, E., & Zarit, S. (1995). Dimensions of social support and social conflict as predictors of caregiver depression. *International Psychogeriatrics, 7,* 25–38.

McBride, M., & Parreno, H. (1996). Filipino American families and caregiving. In G. Yeo & D. Gallagher-Thompson (Eds.), *Ethnicity and the dementias* (pp. 123–135). Washington, DC: Taylor & Francis.

Miller, B. (1987). Gender and control among spouses of the cognitively impaired: A research note. *Gerontologist, 27,* 447–453.

Miller, B., & Cafasso, L. (1992). Gender differences in caregiving: Fact or artifact. *Gerontologist, 32,* 498–507.

Mirowsky, J., & Ross, C. E. (1990). Age and depression. *Journal of Health and Social Behavior, 33,* 187–205.

Mittelman, M., Ferris, S., Shulman, E., Steinberg, G., Mackell, J., & Ambinder, A. (1994). Efficacy of multicomponent individualized treatment to improve the well-being of Alzheimer's caregivers. In E. Light, G. Niederche, & B. D. Lebowitz (Eds.), *Stress effects on family caregivers of Alzheimer's patients: Research and interventions* (pp. 156–184). New York: Springer.

Mohide, E. A., Pringle, D. M., Streiner, D. L., Gilbert, J. R., Muir, G., & Tew, M. (1990). A randomized trial of family caregiver support in the home management of dementia. *Journal of the American Geriatrics Society, 38,* 446–454.

Moseley, P. W., Davies, H. D., & Priddy, J. M. (1988). Support groups for male caregivers of Alzheimer's patients: A follow-up. *Clinical Gerontologist, 7,* 127–136.

Mullan, J. T. (1992). The bereaved caregiver: A prospective study of changes in well-being. *Gerontologist, 32,* 673–683.

National Center for Health Statistics. (1987). Health statistics on older persons, United States. 1986. *Vital and health statistics* (Series 3, No. 25, DHHS Publication No. PHS 87-1409). Washington, DC: U.S. Government Printing Office.

Norris, F., & Murrell, S. (1987). Transitory impact of life-event stress on psychological symptoms in older adults. *Journal of Health and Social Behavior, 28,* 197–211.

Norris, F., & Murrell, S. (1990). Social support, life events, and stress as modifiers of adjustment to bereavement by older adults. *Psychology and Aging, 5,* 429–436.

Notarius, C. I., & Johnson, J. S. (1982). Emotional expression in husbands and wives. *Journal of Marriage and the Family, 44,* 483–489.

Ory, M., & Schulz, R. (1996, November). *Resources for enhancing Alzheimer's caregiver health (REACH). Innovative approaches to AD Caregiving Interventions.* Paper presented at the annual meeting of the Gerontological Society of America, Washington, DC.

Oxman, T., Freeman, D., Manheimer, E., & Stukel, T. (1994). Social support and depression after cardiac surgery in elderly patients. *American Journal of Geriatric Psychiatry, 2*, 309–323.

Pearlin, L. I. (1992). The careers of caregivers. *Gerontologist, 32*, 647.

Pearlin, L. I., Mullan, J. T., Semple, S. J., & Skaff, M. M. (1990). Caregiving and the stress process: An overview of concepts and their measures. *Gerontologist, 30*, 583–595.

Pinkston, E. M., & Linsk, N. L. (1984). Behavioral family intervention with the impaired elderly. *Gerontologist, 24*, 576–583.

Pinkston, E. M., Linsk, N. L, Young, R. N. (1988). Home based behavioral family treatment of the impaired elderly. *Behavior Therapy, 19*, 331–344.

Pruchno, R. A., & Resch, N. L. (1989). Aberrant behaviors and Alzheimer's disease: Mental health effects on spouse caregivers. *Journals of Gerontology: Social Sciences, 44*, S177–S182.

Pruchno, R. A., Kleban, J. E., Michaels, N. P., & Dempsey, N. P. (1990). Mental and physical health of caregiving spouses: Development of a causal model. *Journals of Gerontology: Psychological Sciences, 45* , P192–P199.

Quayhagen, M. P., & Quayhagen, M. (1989). Differential effects of family-based strategies on Alzheimer's disease. *Gerontologist, 29*, 150–155.

Radloff, L. S. (1977). The CES-D scale: A self-report depression scale for research in the general population. *Applied Psychological Measurement, 1*, 382–401.

Redinbaugh, E. M., MacCallum, R. C., & Kiecolt-Glaser, J. K. (1995). Recurrent syndromal depression in caregivers. *Psychology and Aging, 10*, 358–368.

Riskind, J. H., Beck, A. T., Berchick, R. J., Brown, G., & Steer, R. A. (1987). Reliability of DSM-II diagnoses for major depression and generalized anxiety disorder using the structured clinical interview for DSM-II. *Archives of General Psychiatry, 44*, 817–820.

Rivera, P. A., Rose, J., Futterman, A., Lovett, S., & Gallagher-Thompson, D. (1991). Dimensions of perceived social support in clinically depressed and nondepressed female caregivers. *Psychology and Aging, 6*, 232–237.

Robins, L. N., Helzer, J. E., Croughan, J., & Ratcliff, K. S. (1981). National Institute of Mental Health Diagnostic Interview Schedule: Its history, characteristics and validity. *Archives of General Psychiatry, 38*, 381–389.

Robinson, K. M. (1989). Predictors of depression among wife caregivers. *Nursing Research, 38*, 359–363.

Rose, J., & DelMaestro, S. (1990). Separation-individuation conflict as a model for understanding distressed caregivers: Psychodynamic and cognitive case studies. *Gerontologist, 30*, 693–697.

Russell, D. W., & Cutrona, C. E. (1991). Social support, stress, and depressive symptoms among the elderly: Test of a process model. *Psychology and Aging, 6*, 190–201.

Russo, J., Vitaliano, P. P., Brewer, D., Katon, W., & Becker, J. (1995). Psychiatric disorders in spouse caregivers of care-recipients with Alzheimer's disease and matched controls: A diathesis-stress model of psychopathology. *Journal of Abnormal Psychology, 194*, 197–204.

Schorr, A. (1980). *"Thy father and thy mother": A second look at filial responsibility and family policy* (SSA Publication No. 13-11953). Washington, DC: U.S. Department of Health and Human Services.

Schulz, R., & Williamson, G. M. (1991). A 2-year longitudinal study of depression among Alzheimer's caregivers. *Psychology and Aging, 6*, 569–578.

Schulz, R., Tompkins, C. A., Wood, D., & Decker, S. (1987). The social psychology of caregiving: Physical and psychological costs to providing support to the disabled. *Journal of Applied Social Psychology, 17*, 401–428.

Schulz, R., Tompkins, C. A., & Rau, M. T. (1988). A longitudinal study of the psychosocial impact of stroke on primary support persons. *Psychology and Aging, 3*, 131–141.

Schulz, R., Visintainer, P., & Williamson, G. M. (1990). Psychiatric and physical morbidity effects of caregiving. *Journals of Gerontology: Psychological Sciences, 45*, P181–P191.

Schulz, R., O'Brien, A. T., Bookwala, J., & Fleissner, K. (1995). Psychiatric and physical morbidity effects of dementia caregiving: Prevalence, correlates, and causes. *Gerontologist, 35*, 771–791.

Shields, C. G. (1992). Family interaction and caregivers of Alzheimer's disease patients: Correlates of depression. *Family Process, 31*, 19–33.

Snow, R. E. (1991). Aptitude-treatment interaction as a framework for research on individual differences in psychotherapy. *Journal of Consulting and Clinical Psychology, 59*, 205–216.

Sotomayor, M., & Randolph, S. (1988). A preliminary review of caregiving issues and the Hispanic family. In M. Sotomayor & H. Curiel (Eds.), *Hispanic elderly: A cultural signature* (pp. 137–160). Edinburg, TX: Pan American University Press.

Spitzer, R., & Endicott, J. (1978). Research diagnostic criteria: Rationale and reliability. *Archives of General Psychiatry, 35,* 773–782.

Spitzer, R. L., Williams, J. B., Endicott, J., & Gibbon, M. (1987). *Structured clinical interview for DSM-II-R disorders—Nonpatient version (SCID-NP).* New York: New York State Psychiatric Institute, Biometrics Research Department.

Spitzer, R. L., Williams, J. B., Gibbon, M., & Furst, M. B. (1992). The structured clinical interview for DSM-III-R (SCID). I: History, rationale, and description. *Archives of General Psychiatry, 49,* 624–629.

Steffen, A. M., Gallagher-Thompson, D., Zeiss, A. M., & Willis-Shore, J. (1994, August). *Self-efficacy for caregiving: Psychoeducational interventions with dementia family caregivers.* Paper presented at the American Psychological Association, Los Angeles.

Stone, R., Cafferata, G. L., & Sangl, J. (1987). Caregivers of the frail elderly: A national profile. *Gerontologist, 27,* 616–626.

Tempo, P., & Saito, A. (1996). Techniques of working with Japanese American families. In G. Yeo & D. Gallagher-Thompson (Eds.), *Ethnicity and the dementias* (pp. 109–122). Washington, DC: Taylor & Francis.

Teri, L., & Gallagher, D. G. (1991). Cognitive-behavioral interventions for treatment of depression in Alzheimer's patients. *Gerontologist, 21,* 413–416.

Teri, L., & Logsdon, R. (1991). Identifying pleasant activities for individuals with Alzheimer's disease: The Pleasant Events Schedule-AD. *Gerontologist, 21,* 124–127.

Teri, L., & Uomoto, J. (1991). Reducing excess disability in dementia patients: Training caregivers to manage patient depression. *Clinical Gerontologist,* 49–63.

Thompson, E., Futterman, A., Gallagher-Thompson, D., Rose, J., & Lovett, S. (1993). Social support and caregiving burden in family caregivers of frail elders. *Journal of Gerontology: Social Sciences, 48,* S245–S254.

Toseland, R. W., & Rossiter, C. M. (1989). Group interventions to support family caregivers: A review and analysis. *Gerontologist, 29,* 438–448.

Toseland, R. W., & Smith, G. C. (1990). Effectiveness of individual counseling by professional and peer helpers for family caregivers of the elderly. *Psychology and Aging, 5,* 256–263.

Toseland, R. W., Rossiter, C. M., & Labrecque, M. D. (1989). The effectiveness of peer-led and professionally led groups to support family caregivers. *Gerontologist, 29,* 465–471.

U.S. Bureau of the Census. (1989). "Projections of the populations of the United States, by age, sex, and race: 1988 to 2080," by Gregory Spencer. *Current Population Reports* Series P-25, No. 1018.

U.S. Department of Labor, Bureau of Labor Statistics. (1990). *Employment and earning, 37* (1). Washington, DC: U.S. Government Printing Office.

U.S. House of Representatives Select Committee on Aging. (1987). *Exploding the myth: Caregiving in America* (Committee Publication No. 99-1611). Washington, DC: U.S. Government Printing Office.

U.S. Senate Special Committee on Aging, the American Association of Retired Persons, the Federal Council on the Aging, and the U.S. Administration on Aging. (1991). *Aging America: Trends and projections.* (Publication No. (FCoA) 91-28001). Washington, DC: U.S. Department of Health and Human Services. Washington, DC.

Vinick, B. H. (1984). Elderly men as caretakers of wives. *Journal of Geriatric Psychiatry, 17,* 61–68.

Vitaliano, P. P., Russo, J., Young, H. M., Teri, L., & Maiuro, R. D. (1991). Predictors of burden in spouse caregivers of individuals with Alzheimer's disease. *Psychology and Aging, 6,,* 392–402.

Whitlatch, C. J., Zarit, S. H., & von Eye, A. (1991). Efficacy of interventions with caregivers: A reanalysis. *Gerontologist, 31,* 9–14.

Williamson, G. M., & Schulz, R. (1992). Physical illness and symptoms of depression among elderly outpatients. *Psychology and Aging, 7,* 343–351.

Wood, J. B., & Parham, F. A. (1990). Coping with perceived burden: Ethnic and cultural issues in Alzheimer family caregiving. *Journal of Applied Gerontology, 9,* 325–339.

Wright, L., Clipp, E., & George, L. (1993). Health consequences of caregiver stress. *Medicine, Exercise, Nutrition, and Health, 2,* 181–195.

Young, R. F., & Kahana, E. (1989). Specifying caregiver outcomes: Gender and relationship aspects of caregiver strain. *Gerontologist, 29,* 660–666.

Zarit, S. H. (1990). Interventions with frail elders and their families: Are they effective and shy? In M. A. P. Stephens, J. H. Crowther, S. E. Hobfoll, & D. L. Tennebaum (Eds.), *Stress and coping in later life families* (pp. 241–265). Washington, DC: Hemisphere.

Zarit, S. H., & Whitlatch, C. J. (1992). Institutional placement: Phases of the transition. *Gerontologist, 32,* 665–672.

Zarit, S. H., Anthony, C. R., & Boutselis, M. (1987). Interventions with caregivers of dementia patients: Comparison of two approaches. *Psychology and Aging, 2,* 225–232.

Zarit, S. H., Birkel, R. C., & MaloneBeach, E. (1989). Spouses as caregivers: Stresses and interventions. In M. Z. Goldstein (Ed.), *Family involvement in the treatment of the frail elderly.* Washington, DC: American Psychiatric Association.

Zeiss, A., & Lewinsohn, P. (1986). Adapting behavioral treatment for depression to meet the needs of the elderly. *Clinical Psychologist, 39,* 98–100.

CHAPTER 22

Prevention

Peter V. Rabins

INTRODUCTION AND DEFINITIONS

Prevention is the ultimate goal of the health professional. However, prevention in the mental health field has had a checkered career. Broad promises have not been backed up with results and prospective trials have been few and far between (Wilson, Simpson, & McCaughey, 1983).

Prevention

Prevention is defined as the avoidance or diminution of ill health and its sequelae. Three levels of prevention have been defined. *Primary prevention* is the total avoidance of a condition. Childhood vaccination and water fluoridation are two examples of successful primary prevention. *Secondary prevention* is defined as the prompt recognition of a disorder and initiation of appropriate treatment. Here the goal is to minimize acute morbidity and eliminate its sequelae. The identification and treatment of individuals who have had sexual contact with a person with syphilis is an example. *Tertiary prevention* is the provision of maximal treatment that minimizes the long-term sequelae of chronic illness. Tertiary prevention is appropriate for conditions such as personality disorder, schizophrenia, manic depression, and dementia.

A task force of the Institute of Medicine (IOM) (Mrazek & Haggerty, 1994) has suggested a modification of this categorization for the mental health fields. The three stages it identified are treatment, management, and maintenance.

Both sets of definitions have inherent difficulties. For example, it is often not clear whether an action is secondary or tertiary prevention. On the other hand, the IOM categorization does not recognize that complete avoidance is the ultimate goal of prevention.

Peter V. Rabins • Department of Psychiatry and Behavioral Sciences, Johns Hopkins University School of Medicine, Baltimore, Maryland 21287-7279.

Handbook of Clinical Geropsychology, edited by Michel Hersen and Vincent B. Van Hasselt. Plenum Press, New York, 1998.

The interest in the prevention of emotional disorder is not new. For example, eminent American psychiatrist Adolf Meyer (1915) stated the following: "Where, then, shall we attack the problem of prevention? By reinforcing the existing helps, the hospitals, the dispensaries, the special agencies; by adapting the schools to the needs of the pupils; by facing pointedly the problems of alcoholism and syphilis; but above all, by starting a quiet work of community-organization, building up manageable district units, and by inspiring a constructive atmosphere among people who can know and understand people each other and who have common needs" (p. 557). Meyer also suggested that efforts be made to counsel families of persons with major mental illness and cautioned against raising hopes unrealistically. These suggestions remain appropriate 80 years later.

Risk Factors

One important approach to developing prevention strategies is the identification of risk factors. Three measurements have been developed to convey the degree of risk. Both the *odds ratio* and the *relative risk* measure the strength of the relationship between single risk factors and a disorder or disease. Each is defined as the ratio of incident (new) cases in persons with the risk factor to the number of cases in persons without the risk factor. The two measures differ in the sources of data used to calculate them. The odds ratio is based on data from cohort or case control studies, whereas relative risks are calculated on data from population-based samples. The third measure, *attributable risk,* refers to the percentage of cases of a disorder caused by a specific risk factor. It differs from the odds ratio and relative risk because its value depends on the prevalence (frequency) of the risk factor in the population.

Clinical Logics

A final set of definitions important to prevention are two models of clinical logic. *Categorical* or *dichotomous* logic is used when a condition is either present or absent. Examples from medicine are a broken bone or a heart attack. Schizophrenia, bipolar disorder, and dementia are mental health examples. This approach dates back to the 17th-century writings of the British physician Sydenham, who suggested that clusters of signs and symptoms can be found among many patients and that these clusters are similar across cultures and eras. This approach is sometimes referred to as the disease or "medical" model because it assumes an underlying biological abnormality.

A second type of clinical logic is labeled *continuous* or *dimensional.* It is used for human characteristics that are universal and distributed in the population in a Gaussian (so-called bell curve or normal) fashion. Personality, grief, and reaction to stress are examples of characteristics for which this logic is used. This method dates back to the ancient Greeks, who believed that an imbalance of "humors" caused behavior problems and illness. Almost 150 years ago the statisticians Gauss and Galton developed many of the statistics we use today to measure dimensional features. In this form of logic, disorder is attributed to an individual's differing in degree or amount (for example, 2 standard deviations) from the norm. Medical examples include blood pressure and height. Whereas categorical abnormalities and categorical disorders are either present or absent, dimensional attributes are present in all people but vary among individuals by amount.

Prevention Strategies

There are two approaches to prevention. The *population-based* or *universal* strategy aims at preventing disorder by focusing on as many members of a population as possible (for example, lowering salt and cholesterol intake in the population so as to lower rates of heart attack and stroke). The *high risk* strategy intervenes with those at greatest risk (e.g., treating all individuals whose blood pressure is above 160/90 mm hg) with a goal of preventing morbidity in these high-risk individuals. The choice of strategy depends on the prevalence of the disorder in the population (high prevalence favors the population-focused; low prevalence increases the benefit of a high-risk strategy), the clinical logic used (categorical logic favors a high-risk strategy; dimensional logic favors the population-based approach), the morbidity of the condition (prevention for low-morbidity disorders can be justified only if they are common), and a scientific understanding of what the risk factors are (based in part on relative and attributable risks). Table 22-1 illustrates these issues.

One important aspect of the dimensional as opposed to categorical disorders is that prevention in dimensional conditions is most effectively accomplished by changing the population *distribution* of a trait or behavior; that is, by changing the position of as many people as possible toward a "more desirable" point on the Gaussian curve. Because there are so many more people who score in this "normal" range for a trait that confers risk than people who score in the abnormal range, more cases of disorder are prevented among people in the "normal" range than in the categorically abnormal range. For example, individuals with a systolic blood pressure above 160 mm Hg are at highest risk of stroke and heart attack. Treating this group for "hypertension," that is, treating this group as having a categorical abnormality, decreases the number of strokes and heart attacks that occur in the population. This is an example of the high-risk categorical model. However, lowering the blood pressure of *everyone* whose blood pressure is in the "normal" range (120–160) actually prevents a *greater number* of strokes and heart attack, because the number of individuals

Table 22-1. Targets and Models of Prevention

	Targeted	Universal
Focus	individual	population
Model	individual health	public health
Prevalence	low	high
Logic	dichotomous	continuous

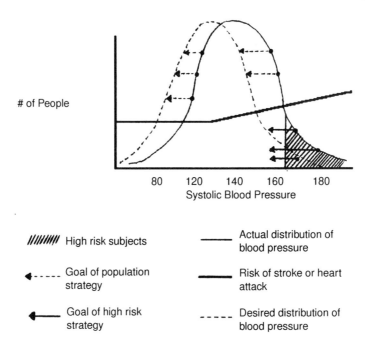

# of People

80   120   140   160   180
Systolic Blood Pressure

////// High risk subjects

—— Actual distribution of blood pressure

◄----- Goal of population strategy

—— Risk of stroke or heart attack

◄—— Goal of high risk strategy

----- Desired distribution of blood pressure

Figure 22-1. Schematic of blood pressure treatment using population and high risk strategies.

in this group is much greater than in the group with blood pressure greater than 160 and because the linkage between blood pressure and stroke is present in this "normal" range. Figure 22-1 illustrates this schematically.

These principles have significant implications for prevention in the mental health field. If linkages between psychological morbidity and specific personality traits, coping styles, living arrangements, socioeconomic conditions, and common life events (all factors that are distributed in the population in a graded fashion) are identified, then changing how all individuals behave would be the most effective way to diminish the prevalence of psychological morbidity in the community at large. On the other hand, individuals at risk for low-prevalence, high-morbidity diseases (e.g., schizophrenia, manic-depression, HIV infection) or at high risk for psychological morbidity because they are in certain work settings, disasters, caregiving situations, or have certain medical illnesses (that is, conditions for which the categorical mode of logic is most appropriate) will be helped best by a high-risk strategy.

PREVENTION OF MENTAL DISORDER AMONG OLDER ADULTS

The Epidemiologic Catchment Area study examined approximately 20,000 Americans during the early 1980s to provide data on the prevalence of mental disorder in the United States (Robins & Regier, 1991). Figure 22-2 compares prevalence among persons 60 years old and older with younger individuals. Several points are notable:

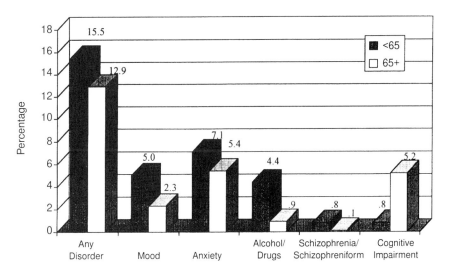

Figure 22-2. One-month prevalence of psychiatric disorders by age. ECA Wave I Data.

First, total prevalence of disorder among the elderly is high. One fifth of older adults suffer from some form of mental disorder. Second, disorders vary greatly in their prevalence. Anxiety disorder and cognitive disorder are several times more prevalent among the elderly than mood disorder, substance abuse disorder, or schizophrenia. Finally, and perhaps most importantly, all disorders other than cognitive impairment are *less* prevalent in the elderly than in the young.

However, these data reflect the categorical logic of the *Diagnostic and Statistical Manual of Mental Disorders* (American Psychiatric Association, 1994), the formal nomenclature proposed by the American Psychiatric Association. If one takes a dimensional approach and examines the rates of symptoms, a different picture emerges. For example, symptoms of depression become more prevalent in the elderly. Studies that explain why the elderly have more symptoms and less disorder are sorely needed. Also needed are studies to identify who among older adults are at highest risk and whether strategies aimed at lowering risk are efficacious.

Data that demonstrate effective prevention in the elderly are sparse. One way to decide which strategy for prevention might be most appropriate to study is to understand prevalence of psychological and psychiatric morbidity in the population. The following sections review what is known about categories of mental disorder and about the dimensions of distress and predispositions.

PREVENTION OF CATEGORICAL DISORDERS

Dementia

The dementias provide several examples of successful prevention. Indeed, some of the greatest advances in prevention have occurred among the dementias. At the beginning of the 20th century, neurosyphilis accounted for 15% of persons hospitalized for mental illness in the United States. Although tertiary syphilis (syphilis involving the nervous system) still occurs, it is now rare. This has occurred because of effective secondary prevention that depends on the prompt tracing of people who have had sexual contact with an infected individual and on the use of antibiotics. Surprisingly, the rate of syphilis has not declined dramatically between 1920 and 1990 as can be seen in Figure 22-3. The success in prevention has been the avoidance of long-term sequelae (tertiary syphilis) by secondary prevention.

An example of effective primary prevention in dementia is that of pellagra. This was a common cause of mental illness (including dementia) in the United States at the beginning of the century. The discovery that pellagra is caused by vitamin B_6 deficiency led to food fortification with B vitamins. This has almost totally eradicated this disease. This is an example of a low-prevalence disorder prevented by a population strategy (education and vitamin fortification) that was practical because it was inexpensive and easy to administer.

Prevalence of vascular dementia (dementia due to blood vessel disease) varies geographically. The dramatic decline in the rate of stroke and heart attack that has occurred in the United States over the past 20 years and more recently in other areas of the world suggests that primary prevention of this form of dementia is a possibility and that vascular dementia *might* decline in incidence. As discussed earlier, changes in behavior (eating better and exercising more) are likely responsible for the decline (primary prevention) in stroke. There is also weak evidence of secondary prevention. Meyer (1986) demonstrated that individuals with a single stroke who were treated with aspirin and followed for $2^1/_2$ years had better cognition than a placebo-treated comparison group. The treated group also experienced better blood brain flow (as measured by brain scan). This study suggests the possibility that daily low-dose aspirin might prevent stroke and, therefore, dementia.

These three examples illustrate several aspects of prevention. Neurosyphilis prevention occurred because a biological treatment, penicillin, be-

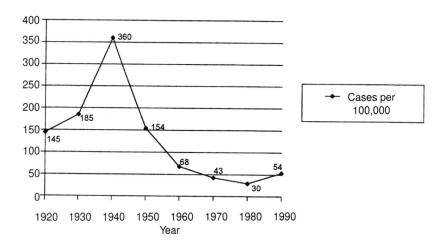

Figure 22-3. Reported cases of syphillis

came available and provided a reason for identifying and promptly treating those infected with the syphilis spirochete. That is, an ill group (the category) could be treated promptly (secondary prevention). The population-based intervention, encouraging safe-sex practices such as condom use, was not a major factor, as primary infection rates did not decline before the introduction of penicillin in the 1940s. The successful prevention of pellagra, on the other hand, resulted from a universal intervention (vitamin B fortification, school breakfast and lunch programs and improved socioeconomic circumstances).

Vascular dementia prevention requires multiple strategies. Primary prevention with both a high-risk strategy (treating high blood pressure and diabetes aggressively) and population strategy (lowering fat and salt intake and increasing physical activity) coupled with secondary prevention (drugs [aspirin and anticoagulants] and surgery [coronary bypass surgery and endarterectomies]) will be most successful because the risk factors are dimensional, common, and responsive to a number of different treatments.

Alzheimer's disease (AD) is by far the most common cause of dementia. There are no proven prevention strategies at present but there are several tantalizing leads. Head trauma has been confirmed as a risk factor with a relative risk between 1.5 and 2. Prevention strategies that decrease head injury due to accidents and boxing could decrease the incidence of AD. Several genetic causes (four have been identified thus far) and genetic modifiers (the APOE-E4 gene) have been identified. If diet or medication could block or delay the undesirable actions of these genes most individuals would die before ever developing the disease. Low education may be another risk factor for AD. If this proves to be the case then improved early-life education could be an important primary prevention strategy.

Preliminary research suggests that estrogens and nonsteroidal anti-inflammatory medicines (e.g., ibuprofen) might decrease the risk of developing AD. Because many of the epidemiologic studies demonstrating these effects did not control for education and social class, their validity is not yet established. It will be important to determine whether the adverse effects of these drugs might outweigh whatever protection they provide. Another controversial preventive factor is activity level. Several studies show that people who maintain activity are less likely to develop AD; however, it seems most plausible that diminished activity is the earliest sign of dementia rather than that inactivity causes dementia.

Delirium

Delirium is a cognitive disorder in which people are unable to perform cognitive tasks at their usual level and are also inattentive and drowsy. It is common among older persons who are hospitalized, in whom prevalence ranges from 20% to 35% and incidence (that is, the development of delirium during the hospitalization) is approximately 10% to 15%. Having a dementia is the highest risk factor (relative risk is approximately 5). The dementia is not causative but is a predisposing factor. Strategies that identify individuals at high risk (low cognitive score, older age, weight, more medications, history of alcoholism) and then carefully monitor them might prevent delirium (primary prevention) or allow earlier recognition and more prompt treatment (secondary prevention).

Mood Disorder

There is no evidence that mood disorder can be primarily prevented. However, research shows that injury to the left anterior quadrant of the brain due to stroke greatly increases the risk of developing major depression following stroke (Robinson, Kubos, Starr, Rao, & Price, 1984). A trial of antidepressants or psychotherapy or both in persons with a new stroke in this area of the brain would be intriguing, but this study has not been carried out yet.

Secondary prevention of mood disorder is possible, on the other hand. Earlier recognition of depression through better training for clinicians and the use of self-administered screening questionnaires are secondary preventive strategies. One study (German, Shapiro, & Skinner, 1985) demonstrated that providing the scores from screening questionnaires to clinicians improved the treatment of elderly individuals.

Suicide is a behavior with several causes. Rates in the United States are highest in older persons and have increased more among persons 80 years old or older than in any other groups (MMWR, 1996). Approximately 60% of suicides in older adults are due to depression and another 30% occur in individuals with substance abuse disorder (Conwell, Olsen, Caine, & Flannery. 1991). Studies in both the United States and Great Britain suggest that most persons who commit suicide have seen a medical practitioner several weeks prior to the suicide attempt. These data suggest that primary prevention of suicide is best accomplished by earlier and more effective recognition of both depression and substance abuse (a secondary prevention high-risk strategy). This will require improved clinician training (to recognize disorders and to assess for suicidal ideation) that is best provided by mental health practitioners.

Depression and manic-depression (unipolar and bipolar mood disorder) are frequently recurrent. Frequency of relapse can be decreased by psychotherapy and medication (tertiary prevention).

PREVENTION OF DIMENSIONAL DISORDERS

Overview

The relationships among personality, coping strategies, life change, and "stress" are complex. Studies have not shown that "prophylactic" interventions such as preretirement or stress management training have demonstrable preventive benefits (although these certainly appear to benefit some individuals), nor has prevention been shown to prevent prolonged grief reactions. In one well-designed community-based trial, individuals randomized to group treatment after the death of a loved one were not less symptomatic than individuals who did not receive treatment (Vachon, Lyall, & Rogers, 1980).

On the other hand, caregivers of persons with chronic illnesses have demonstrated decreased emotional distress with treatment. To date, 9 of 11 controlled trials of interventions that target caregivers of persons with dementia have proven effective in improving caregiver mood and morale (Rabins, 1996). Interventions that provide caregivers with emotional support are more effective than those that offer only educational information. The combination of emotional support and education is most effective. Two studies have shown that nursing home placement can be delayed by caregiver interventions. These trials have generally studied caregivers of individuals attending memory assessment centers, day treatment centers, or similar facilities. Therefore, it is possible that the study participants may have been "high-risk" individuals. Nevertheless, there is good evidence to support secondary preventive efficacy for support groups of the chronically ill.

An intriguing set of experiments carried out in the United States by Rodin and colleagues (Rodin, 1986; Rodin & McAvay, 1992) suggests that "giving control" to older individuals can improve their psychological well-being. In one study implemented in a nursing home, individuals who were allowed to tend to plants and make decisions regarding them fared better emotionally than those who did not. Although these studies have been carried out in narrowly defined populations and have relied on interventions and responses that may be culturally specific, the results show the important impact that environmental design can have on behavior and mood and suggest that environments that maximize the choice of older persons can prevent demoralization and inactivity.

Degree of memory decline associated with usual aging varies widely (Schaie, 1994). Providing instruction on memory enhancement strategies may lessen the amount of decline (Schaie, 1994).

Substance Abuse Disorder

Alcohol abuse remains a problem in late life although many studies suggest that prevalence of alcohol use and abuse declines in late life. Several studies suggest that this is due to the declining health of some individuals. Alcohol abuse makes up the bulk of substance abuse disorders in the elderly now but it is quite likely that as younger cohorts grow old the abuse of narcotics, stimulants, hallucinogens, and other drugs will increase.

Although some individuals, particularly women, first develop alcohol problems in mid or late life, substance abuse usually begins early in life. Thus, primary prevention efforts aimed at young individuals will likely be the most effective way of preventing late-life substance abuse disorder. Further research is needed to demonstrate effectiveness of currently available treatments in the elderly. Clearly, however, because many individuals do not respond to these therapies, more effective treatments are needed. It is not known whether older adults respond better to some types of therapy than to others.

SUMMARY

Most categorical mental disorders are uncommon and their genesis is multifactorial. Therefore, population-based primary preventive strategies for diseases such as manic-depression and schizophrenia are unlikely to be developed in the near future. On the other hand, dimensional and behavioral disorders, such as age-associated memory changes, sadness, distress due to caregiving, substance abuse, and obesity are common enough that population-based strategies could be effective.

Secondary preventive strategies for individuals and groups of individuals at high risk for vascular dementia, delirium, and suicidal behavior are effective, as are tertiary preventive strategies that improve long-term care of persons with mood disorder, schizophrenic disorders, substance abuse disorder, anxiety disorder, and behavioral symptoms accompanying dementia, and the emotional, educational, and social support of caregivers. As Meyer warned 80 years ago, it is important that we neither oversell nor trivialize prevention. Well-designed research is our best hope for developing interventions that can prevent mental morbidity and identify those at risk.

REFERENCES

American Psychiatric Association. (1994). *Diagnostic and statistical manual of mental disorders* (4th ed.). Washington, DC: Author.

Conwell, Y., Olsen, L., Caine, E. D., & Flannery, C. (1991). Suicide in late life: Psychological autopsy findings. *International Psychogeriatrics, 3,* 59–66.

German, P. S., Shapiro, S., & Skinner, E. A (1985). Mental health of the elderly: Use of health and mental health services. *Journal of the American Geriatics Society, 33,* 246–252.

Meyer, A. (1915). Where should we attack the problem of prevention of mental defects and mental disease? *Survey, 34,* 557–560.

Meyer, J. S., Judd, B. J., & Tawaklna, T. (1986) Improved cognition after control of risk factors for multi infarct dementia. *Journal of the American Medical Association, 256,* 2203–2209.

Mrazek, P. J., & Haggerty, R. J. (Eds.). (1994). *Reducing risks for mental disorders: Frontiers for preventive intervention research.* Washington, DC: National Academy Press. Institute of Medicine.

Morbidity and Mortality Weekly Report [MMWR]. (1996). Suicide among older persons—United States, 1980–1992. *MMWR, 45,* 3–6.

Rabins, P. V. (1996). Caring for persons with dementing illnesses: A current perspective. In L. Heston (Ed.), *Progress in Alzheimer's disease and similar conditions* (pp. 277–289). Washington, DC: American Psychiatric Press.

Robins, L. E. & Regier, D. A. (Eds.). (1991). *Psychiatric disorders in America.* New York: Free Press.

Robinson, R. G., Kubos, K. L., Starr, L. B., Rao, K., & Price, T. R. (1984). Mood disorders in stroke patients: Importance of location of lesions. *Brain, 107,* 81–93.

Rodin, J. (1986). Aging and health: Effects of the sense of control. *Science, 233,* 1271–1276.

Rodin, J., & McAvay, G. (1992). Determinants of change in perceived health in a longitudinal study of older adults. *Journals of Gerontology, 47,* 373–384.

Schaie, K. W. (1994). The course of adult intellectual development. *American Psychologist, 49,* 304–313.

Vachon, M. L. S., Lyall, W. A. L., Rogers, J, et al. (1980). A controlled study of self-help intervention for widows. *American Journal of Psychiatry, 137,* 1380–1384.

Wilson, L. B., Simpson, S., & McCaughey, K. (1983). The status of preventive care for the aged: A meta-analysis. In S. Simpson, L. B. Wilson, J. Hermalin, & R. Hess (Eds.), *Aging and prevention* (pp. 23–38). New York: Haworth.

CHAPTER 23

Minority Issues

Sherrill L. Sellers, James S. Jackson, and Cheryl Burns Hardison

INTRODUCTION

This chapter addresses the influence of cultural and ethnic factors on health among minority group older persons. Because of the existence of more extensive national data (Stanford & Du Bois, 1992), we focus primarily on Hispanic American, African American, and American Indian elderly. We realize that these three groups do not capture the full diversity of material, social, and life experiences among the vast array of minority elderly groups (J. S. Jackson, Albright, et al., 1995). They are, however, a sizable subset of the rapidly growing population of minority older adults. We are unable in the space allotted for this chapter to examine the complicated heterogeneity among even these three groups. Thus, we direct our attention primarily to common factors that may increase risk of, or enhance resilience to, poor physical health and mental health outcomes. Specifically, we examine the meaning and significance of minority group status to physical and psychological health and suggest that a culturally sensitive theoretical framework for research and interventions with ethnic minority older persons must attend to (1) sociohistorical context, (2) significance of minority group status, and (3) cultural reality of life among ethnic and racial minorities. These three recommendations evolve from assuming a life-course perspective on aging. A life-course perspective considers the unfolding of lives through time (J. S. Jackson & Sellers, 1997). This perspective is particularly important for considering the lives of ethnic minority older persons in whom experiences in adolescence and early adulthood, as well as cohort and period events, influence health trajectories, health behaviors, and attitudes toward health professionals (Riley, 1996).

Sherrill L. Sellers, James S. Jackson, and Cheryl Burns Hardison • Program for Research on Black Americans, Institute for Social Research, University of Michigan, Ann Arbor, Michigan 48106-1248.

Handbook of Clinical Geropsychology, edited by Michel Hersen and Vincent B. Van Hasselt. Plenum Press, New York, 1998.

The chapter is divided into four sections. In the first section, we briefly describe some of the major demographic characteristics of the three cultural groups. In the second, we present recent data on the physical and mental health status of these elderly. In the third section, we address caregiving. The objective of this section is to frame the discussion of caregiving in a ethnic and cultural context, furthering the development of culturally sensitive care for minority elderly (J. S. Jackson, Burns, & Gibson, 1992). We conclude with specific recommendations for researchers, policymakers, and health care providers.

ELDERLY ETHNIC MINORITIES IN THE
UNITED STATES—DEMOGRAPHICS

Anticipating the primary recommendations, we suggest the need for more research and services grounded in a sociohistorical context. The health status of American Indian older people provides an important illustration. McCabe and Cueller (1994) suggest that American Indian elderly live in worse material conditions than those of majority group older persons in the United States. Thus, some of the problems associated with older age affect American Indian older adults at an earlier chronological age than majority elders and earlier than some better-off minority group older persons. Specifically, Manson and Callaway (1988) found that a 50-year-old American Indian confronts the health challenges of a 65-year-old White American. Hence, the central concepts of gerontology, age, aging, elderly, must include individual biography, diversity within and between ethnic group members, and sociohistorical context (Riley, 1996).

Several terms have been used to describe racial and ethnic groups. Some focus on a group's relationship with others; other terms focus on language, region of origin, and dietary habits. The concepts of culture, race, and ethnic group are prominent in the study of ethnic minority aging. Yet, there is considerable conceptual confusion over the use of these terms. We use the term *ethnic minority elderly* to convey age, ethnicity, and sociohistorical status. We begin with a conceptualization of minority and majority. The *majority* or dominant group is defined as the group that has power and uses it to control social institutions and processes for its own benefit (Blauner, 1972). A *minority* group is defined as a group that is distinguishable on the basis of skin color, language, culture, religion, or other observable characteristics (Wirth, 1945). Minority groups have less power than the majority group; they control fewer resources and have unequal access to social rewards (King & Williams, 1995). Often a distinguishing feature of a minority group is its *culture.* We adopt the definition offered by Swidler (1986), who defines culture as a symbolic vehicle of meaning, including beliefs and rituals as well as informal practices such as language and activities of daily life. In other words, culture refers to the ways of living that people devise to meet biological and psychosocial needs. These ways of living are passed down through the generations, but may vary over time and across regions. Culture is not independent; rather, it develops from the social environment in which individuals are embedded. What is most salient for our purpose is the recognition that individuals' culture will influence their definition of illness, perceptions of symptoms, and health behaviors (Levine & Gaw, 1995;

Snow, 1983). *Ethnicity* refers to connectedness based on shared norms and values. It is often used interchangeably with race. However, ethnicity and race technically have very different meanings. We prefer the term ethnicity, primarily because it focuses attention on social and historical context, rather than questionable genetic and biological differences. We refer to those individuals over age 65 as *ethnic minority elderly*. The term, although not lyrical, aims to convey both ethnic and sociohistorical status. In addition, we use the terms Black, rather than African American, and American Indian rather than Native American, to be consistent with census reports.

Four groups have been identified as ethnic minorities: Blacks, Hispanic Americans, Asian Americans, and American Indians (including American Indians, Eskimos, and Aleuts). It is estimated that by the year 2030, of the people 65 years and older, 15% will be members of these four ethnic groups. And, by the year 2050, ethnic minority elderly will comprise 21% of the total U.S. population (J. Angel & Hogan, 1994). This chapter presents demographic and epidemiologic data for Blacks, Hispanic Americans, and American Indians.[1] Blacks comprise 12% of the total U.S. population and nearly 11% of this population is over the age of 60. Projections indicate that by the year 2000, elderly Blacks will comprise about 8.5% of the total U.S. population age 65 and over and by 2040, 12.5% of that population (Ruiz, 1995).

Hispanic Americans comprise about 8% of the total U.S. population and are relatively youthful (median age 25.9 compared with 32.5 for total U.S. population); consequently, the proportion of Hispanic elderly is certain to increase. Projections suggests that from the years 2000 to 2050, the Hispanic elderly population will more than quadruple. That is, in the year 2000, Hispanics are expected to comprise 4.9% of the elderly; by 2050 this number is expected to increase to 11.7% of all elderly (Garcia, 1991). American Indians comprise about 1% of the total U.S. population (U.S. Bureau of the Census, 1990), with some 6% being over the age of 65. Compared to other ethnic minority elderly, much less is known about elderly American Indians. However, trends and projections suggest that the elderly among these groups will also increase. According to the 1990 census, there are nearly 2 million American Indians in the United States. Of this group, only 108,000 are over the age of 65. However, this number represents an increase of nearly 70% since 1980. There are expected to be 276,000 65 years of age and older by 2020 and 467,000 by 2030 (McCabe & Cueller, 1994). Although these projections indicate an increase in ethnic minority elderly, problems related to the census undercount may actually underestimate the increases (J. Angel & Hogan, 1994).

Considerable heterogeneity exists between and among these ethnic minority groups. For example, in 1989, 48% of the approximately 1 million Hispanic elderly were of Mexican descent. Cuban (18%), Puerto Rican (11%), Central and South American (8.4%), and "Other Hispanic" (15%) comprise the

---

[1]We have excluded Asian Americans from detailed discussion because of the relative dearth of national estimates on this population, as compared with the other three groups. For an excellent review of the health status of Asian Americans see the Stanford Geriatric Center Paper Series.

remaining groups (J. Angel & Hogan, 1994). Factors such as urbanicity, acculturation, education, and socioeconomic status make generalization across groups tenuous. For example, in 1987, 91% of the elderly Hispanic population resided in urban areas, compared with 83% of Black elderly, 72% of White elderly, and 54% of American Indian elderly (John, 1994; Villa, Cuellar, Gamel, &Yeo, 1993).

Nevertheless, commonalities among the ethnic minority elderly also exist. Poverty, gender-related issues, and household living arrangements are particularly salient examples. Specific income and poverty rates vary, but the pattern is similar across ethnic minority elderly. In 1990, about 10% of all White elderly lived in poverty. Also in 1990, median income for Hispanic elderly was $7,060 (somewhat above the poverty line), while slightly more than 20% of Hispanic elderly had incomes below the poverty line. Similar data for Black elderly indicated that more than 30% of this population was below the poverty level (Ruiz, 1995). American Indians had similar income and poverty patterns, with incomes slightly higher than those of elderly Blacks, but slightly less than those of Hispanic elderly (McCabe & Cuellar, 1994). For American Indian elders the poverty level varied by urbanicity. Those residing in urban areas had lower poverty rates (25%) compared with their rural counterparts (39%) (Baker & Lightfoot, 1995).

Gender is also an important risk factor for poverty among ethnic minority elderly. Women comprise 58% of the elderly population, but nearly 74% of the elderly poor are women (Taeuber, 1992). Poverty is particularly high among black American elderly women; for those 75 years of age and older, poverty rates are 2.5 times that of majority women (43.9% compared with 17.3%) (Ruiz, 1995). Further, because of differences in longevity and mortality in general, elderly women outnumber elderly men (Herzog, 1989). In 1990, for individuals between the ages of 65 and 74, the gender ratio was 71 Black men to 100 Black women. For Hispanic elderly, the ratio for Puerto Rican elderly was 1 to 1; for Mexican American elderly the ratio was 91 men to 100 women (J. Angel & Hogan, 1994). The gender ratio for American Indian elderly closely resembles that of black elderly with 77 men to 100 women at ages 65 to 74; the ratio declines to 59 to 100 after age 85 (McCabe & Cuellar, 1994). Given these statistics, we believe that it is essential for researchers, policy makers, and program providers to incorporate considerations of the intersection of ethnicity and gender into their theorizing, policies, and programs related to ethnic minority elderly.

Household living arrangements illustrate the similarities and differences among ethnic minority elderly. The most common household arrangement among ethnic minority elderly is to live with a spouse. Black elderly, however, do not follow this pattern, in part because of higher rates of marital disruption throughout the life course. Approximately 30% of Black elderly live alone, a pattern similar to that of majority elderly (J. Angel & Hogan, 1994). Most ethnic minority elderly live in multigenerational families. Lopez and Aguilera (1991) found that more than 75% of Hispanic elderly lived with other family members compared with 67% of White elderly and 63% of Black elderly. In a study that examined factors that influenced community living arrangements of unmarried White and minority elderly, Black and Hispanic elderly were less likely to live alone, regardless of health status (R. Angel, Angel, & Himes,

1992). R. Angel and colleagues (1992) also found that old age, low levels of education and income, and having more children contributed to elderly living with others rather than alone.

PHYSICAL HEALTH

Demographic projections suggest that the proportion of ethnic minority elderly will increase in the coming decades. These elderly are more likely to be female, to live with family members, and to be of lower socioeconomic status. Such factors in turn influence the physical and mental health status of ethnic minority elderly. This section selectively reviews the physical health status of ethnic minority elderly. The specific health topics include mortality rates, chronic illness conditions (e.g., arthritis, diabetes, hypertension), and leading causes of mortality (e.g., diseases of the heart, cancer, stroke).

One of the more important differences between ethnic minority elderly and their majority counterparts is their longevity. In 1995, the life expectancy at birth was 73.8 years for White males and 80 years for White females, compared with 64.5 years for Black males and 74.3 years for Black females. Hispanic men and women have life expectancy rates comparable to majority elderly, 74.9 years for men and 82.2 years for women. For American Indians the life expectancy at birth is 71.5 years for males and 80.2 years for females (U.S. Bureau of the Census, 1996). (*Authors' note:* We conservatively report the middle assumption figures.)

Based on age-specific mortality rates, it appears that a mortality crossover occurs at some point between the ages of 65 and 85 for Blacks, Hispanic Americans, and American Indians. This crossover indicates that ethnic minority elderly who live to reach these ages will live, on average, longer than their majority counterparts. Blacks, for example, are at greater risk of dying at every age, until after the age of 75, when their life expectancy becomes greater than that of Whites (Richardson, 1990). For American Indians the crossover occurs after age 65 (John, 1994). Several scholars have attempted to explain the mortality crossover phenomenon genetically, as an artifact of age misreporting, or as an environmental-biological interaction related to successive mortality sweeps in different age groups among vulnerable minority populations (e.g., Gibson & Jackson, 1992; J. J. Jackson, 1985; Manton, Poss & Wing, 1979). The empirical evidence in support of these speculations is surprisingly limited. For Blacks, in the past few decades the age at which the crossover occurs has increased, suggesting largely socially contextualized, rather than mainly genetic, causes (Richardson, 1990).

With the exception of some Asian American groups, ethnic minority elderly generally have poorer health status when compared with Americans of European descent. Coupled with the fact that almost 85% of those aged 65 or greater report at least one chronic condition, it is clear that ethnic minority elderly are at risk for chronic conditions. The most common chronic conditions include arthritis, hypertension, and diabetes (Herzog, 1989). For example, approximately 50% of the Black elderly population report having some form of arthritis (Cohen & Van Nostrand, 1995).

Rates of hypertension are highest among Blacks, followed by Hispanics, American Indians, and then White Americans (Villa *et al.,* 1993). Among Black elderly, hypertension affects almost 37% of males and 64% of females (Richardson, 1990). Research by Sherman James and colleagues (James, Hartnett, & Kalsbeek, 1983; James, Strogatz, Wing, & Ramsey, 1987) suggests an important cultural component in the high prevalence of hypertension among Blacks. James and colleagues suggest that Blacks' sheer determination even in the face of overwhelming odds (John Henryism) may be a risk factor for hypertension. Other researchers have highlighted the impact of racism and discrimination (J. S. Jackson *et al.,* 1996).

Compared with majority elderly, there is a greater prevalence and incidence of noninsulin-dependent diabetes among ethnic minority elderly. Blacks over the age of 65 have almost three times the incidence of diabetes compared with majority elderly (Richardson, 1990). Prevalence of diabetes in Mexican and Puerto Rican populations is almost double that of Whites, and this prevalence increases with age. Diabetes is the fifth leading cause of death among American Indians (Indian Health Service, 1991). Diabetes is also a contributing factor in other diseases and health complications including blindness, stroke, heart disease, and kidney failure (John, 1994).

Richardson (1990) notes, "essentially blacks die of the same diseases as whites (diseases of the heart, cancer, and cerebrovascular diseases), but at an earlier age . . ." (p. 5). Among Hispanic Americans, mortality rates for specific causes vary by national origin. Using 1980 census data, Rosenwaike (1987) found that Puerto Rican-born males had the highest rates of death from heart disease, compared with Cuban-born and Mexican-born. For Hispanic women, those who were Cuban-born had the lowest rates, while Puerto Rican-born women had the highest rates (Rosenwaike, 1987). John (1994) reported that according to the Indian Health Service, the leading causes of mortality among American Indian elderly were heart diseases, malignant neoplasms (cancer), cerebrovascular diseases (stroke), pneumonia, diabetes, and accidents.

The leading cause of death for all older adults is cardiovascular disease. Villa and colleagues (1993) noted that although cardiovascular mortality is declining, the decline has been less dramatic for Hispanic elderly and is still the leading cause of death. During 1985–1987, more than 35% of American Indian elderly died from diseases of the heart (John, 1994). John (1994) reported that heart disease was also the leading cause of death among American Indians aged 45 to 64.

Cancer rates vary by ethnic group and type of cancer. According to the Office of Minority Health Resource Center (1988), Black males have the greatest likelihood of dying from cancer, compared with all other groups. Villa and colleagues (1993) reported that compared with the total older U.S. population, Hispanic elderly had decreased risk of breast cancer and increased risk of liver, pancreatic, stomach and cervical cancers. Cervical cancer among Hispanic women more than 65 years of age was particularly high. Villa and colleagues (1993) speculated that this increase may be, in part, one effect of the lower likelihood of older Hispanic women to have Pap tests. The investigators suggest that this lesser likelihood reflects a cultural emphasis on personal privacy. Among American Indian elderly, cancer is the seconding leading cause of death, accounting for 17.5% of all deaths during 1985–1987 (John, 1994). Lung cancer is particularly problematic and is associated with the prevalence of smoking.

Among Black and American Indian elderly, cerebrovascular disease is the third leading cause of death (Richardson, 1990; John, 1994). Compared with other Hispanic groups, Rosenwaike (1987) found that Mexican-born elderly had the highest rate of cerebrovascular disease mortality; Cuban-born elderly had the lowest rate. He speculated that these differences may be attributed to migrant selection and within-group lifestyle differences. Specifically, compared with more recent immigrants of Hispanic origin, pre-1980 immigrants from Cuba were a select group from the higher social classes (Rosenwaike, 1987).

Debates surrounding genetic versus social factors are particularly prominent with regard to the pattern of mortality among ethnic minority elderly. The high prevalence of diabetes and hypertension suggests the possibility of genetic causes. However, there is also a clear link between these illnesses and sociocultural factors, such as diet and exercise. Further, obesity is a leading risk factor for a number of poor health outcomes, including diabetes, hypertension, and coronary heart disease, and is particularly prevalent among ethnic minority elderly women (Richardson, 1990). Yet, there is very little research on cultural attitudes toward obesity. Such research is essential. To be successful, efforts to reduce morbidity and mortality among ethnic minority elderly must consider cultural factors such as food preferences and sedentary lifestyles, as well as structural factors such as limited financial resources and racial discrimination.

MENTAL HEALTH

Mental health is, in part, a cultural construction, and is subject to considerable interpretation and speculations regarding its origins, illness prevention strategies, and treatment options. Mental health research is currently dominated by a disease model and clinically based studies (Vega & Rumbaut, 1991). This emphasis is particularly problematic for research on minority mental health in general, and ethnic minority elderly in particular. Ethnic minority elderly may associate mental health with mental illness and are likely to view mental illness as something of which to be ashamed (Baker & Lightfoot, 1995). They may be less likely to seek assistance (J. S. Jackson & Wolford, 1992). As Wykle and Kaskel (1991) add, underutilization of mental health resources may reflect differences in cultural attitudes. Ethnic minority elderly are less likely than majority elderly to mention mental or emotional problems during physician visits. In addition, mental health problems may be masked or confounded by physical health issues. Kasl and Berkman (1981) suggest that compared with the situation in younger individuals, physical and mental health may be more closely related among the elderly. Further, some research has reported major health problems and depression to be highly associated (Brown, Ahmed, Gary, & Milburn, 1995; Stanford & Du Bois, 1992). In their community study of Black adults, Brown and colleagues (1995) found that among those reporting depression, 75% indicated having major physical health problems.

Miranda (1991) estimated that 15% to 25% of all older persons have some form of mental health problem, either dementing diseases or major mental disorder. This figure skyrockets to an estimated 70% to 90% for those older adults in institutional settings (Knight, Santos, Teri, & Lawton, 1995). For ethnic minority elderly, specific rates of mental illness vary by disorder (Stanford & Du Bois, 1992). This section presents several mental health outcomes including subjective well-being and selected serious mental disorders.

Well-being may be considered a positive measure of mental health (Lebowitz & Niederehe, 1992). Although there are a number of measures of well-being, life satisfaction tends to be the one most frequently used (George, 1993). In general, life satisfaction appears to be slightly higher among older persons than among younger people (Rodgers, 1982). Research indicates that level of life satisfaction varied among ethnic minority elderly. In a recent analysis using data from the National Survey of Black Americans, J. S. Jackson and Neighbors (1996) found an increase in life satisfaction over a 13-year period, despite decreases in economic and social resources, across all age groups. They also found a trend toward older age group members' reporting greater satisfaction compared with their younger counterparts. In contrast, Andrews, Lynos, and Rowland (1992) reported that less than half (48%) of older Hispanics were very satisfied with their lives, compared with 62% of the general population of U.S. elderly. In a small study of elderly American Indians, Johnson and colleagues (1986) found a high level of life satisfaction (about 64%). They also found that objective measures of life satisfaction were less predictive of mental health than subjective measures. Older American Indians were more likely to equate life satisfaction with not feeling lonely and good hearing and vision. The authors speculate that this finding may reflect cultural differences between majority and American Indian elderly.

Among all older persons, aside from dementing conditions, affective disorders are one of the most common psychiatric problems (Lebowitz & Niederehe, 1992). Rabins (1992), using ECA data, estimated that nearly 6% of all elderly met the criteria for an anxiety disorder. Prevalence rates for symptoms of anxiety are even higher. Prevalence of depressive disorders are estimated at between 1% to 2% for all older persons. As with anxiety, rates of depressive symptoms are estimated at 20% for older adults. Interestingly, in general, ethnic minority elderly tend to have rates of diagnosed depression that are comparable to their White counterparts, but report higher rates of depressive symptoms (Brown *et al.*, 1995). In fact, symptoms of depression are the most common psychological symptoms reported by black elderly (Turnbull & Mui, 1995). Several researchers have found high rates of depressive symptoms among Hispanic elderly (Markides & Krause, 1986; Stanford & Du Bois, 1992). In a small study of Hispanic elderly, Lopez-Aqueres, Keep, Plopper, Staples, and Brummel-Smith (1984) found that 26% of the Hispanic elderly had major depression or dysphoria. Surprisingly, Markides and Krause (1986) found that high levels of association with children actually increased depressive symptoms among Hispanic elderly. In one of the few studies that examined the mental health of American Indians, Manson, Shore, and Bloom (1985) found that, for all age groups, depression was the most frequently diagnosed problem.

The most common cause of severe cognitive impairment in old age is Alzheimer's disease (Herzog, 1989). Its incidence for those more than 65 years of age is estimated at 10.3% (Evans, Funkenstein, & Albert, 1989). Prevalence of

Alzheimer's has been assumed to be the same for majority and minority elderly (between 5% and 10%), yet, we know very little about the incidence, prevalence, or course of Alzheimer's disease among ethnic minority elderly (Stanford & Du Bois, 1992).

The interrelationship between physical and mental health is very complex and research in this area is plagued by problems of confounding measures and cross-sectional designs (Herzog, 1989). For example, research indicates that members of ethnic minority groups disproportionately "somatize" psychological problems. That is, these individuals manifest psychological problems as physical symptoms. Yet, several symptom checklists used to ascertain the presence of mental health problems are designed to rule out physical health problems. This may result in the underreporting of mental health problems among minority groups (Vega & Rumbaut, 1991). Depressive symptoms provide a striking illustration. As mentioned previously, ethnic minority elderly tend to have higher rates of depressive symptoms. Depressive symptoms include factors such as low self-esteem, dysphoric mood, loss of energy, and difficulty concentrating. The same symptoms are associated with physical ailments. Diagnoses may be directed toward physical conditions when in fact psychological treatment is needed.

Mental and physical health, culture, and sociohistorical context converge when the relationship between health and stress is examined. For example, ethnic minority elderly may reside in areas that place them at increased risk of crime. Experiences with mugging, purse-snatching, and witnessing violence may increase anxiety. Chronic anxiety may be associated with stress-related illness. Further, these factors influence the level and type of exercise and activities available to elderly in their living environments. Although considerable research has described an association between stress and health, we know very little about the relationships between stress and health among ethnic minority elderly. In addition, we have very limited knowledge of how stress changes over the life course. Consider an African American male aged 15; he is considered violent, dangerous, and a threat to others. Now age this individual 50 years. Society now considers him to be less of a threat. We do not know the impact of this racialized stress; that is, whether the individual has become accustomed to alienation, whether the stress has increased vulnerability to other stressors, or whether racial and age discrimination interact in such a way as to actually buffer their individual effects.

For ethnic minorities in general, and ethnic minority elderly in particular, strategies for coping with stress often take religious form (Dressler, 1991). Prayer may be an appropriate strategy for some health concerns, but may need to be supplemented with other interventions (Chatters & Taylor, 1989). Physicians, social workers, and other health care specialists may need to be aware of the cultural context in which symptoms are described and understood (Gaines, 1992). Further, relative to their majority counterparts, mental health service use among ethnic minorities is low. Wykle and Kasel (1991) suggest that these differences may be a reflection of cultural attitude about mental health and mental health services and treatments. Padgett (1995) notes that despite emphasis by mental health researchers on a stress and coping approach to understanding mental health among ethnic minorities, few researchers have applied the stress paradigm to ethnic minority elderly (J. S. Jackson, Antonucci & Gibson, 1995; Padgett, 1995).

Finally, considerations of the mental health of ethnic minority elderly must also address the relationship between culture, etnicity, and misdiagnosis (Adebimpe, 1981; Jeste, Naimark, Halpain, & Lindamer, 1995; Neighbors, 1984; Wade, 1993). Additional research is needed to identify those factors, be they structural or individual, that affect diagnosis (Littlewood, 1992). It is clear, however, that for ethnic minority groups, culture, ethnicity, and social context influence symptom manifestation, intervention strategies, and treatment outcomes.

INFORMAL AND FORMAL CAREGIVING

In the previous sections we described indicators of the physical and mental health status of ethnic minority elderly. This section examines current trends in caregiving. Differences in caregiving patterns between ethnic minority and White majority are attributed either to cultural or socioeconomic causes. Lockery (1991) contends that family history and lifestyle differences among minority groups influence attitudes and expectations of caregiving. Although there are overlapping similarities, minority families also differ by such factors as availability of family and friends, amount of contact with support networks, conditions of immigration, length of residence in the United States, socialization processes, socioeconomic status (Lockery, 1991), levels of acculturation and assimilation (Henderson, Guiterrez-Mayka, & Garcia, 1993), and fertility and family living arrangements (R. Angel *et al.,* 1992). Hence, the widely varying findings in the literature on the differences in helping patterns between majority and ethnic minority elderly may reflect the complexity of within- and between-group differences (Lockery, 1991).

Historically, informal caregiving among family and friends has played a major role in the care and support of ethnic elderly (J. S. Jackson, Albright, *et al.,* 1995). Culture plays an important role in the provision of social support, living arrangements, and other aspects of caregiving. Worobey and Angel (1990) found that Blacks, Whites, and Hispanics differed in their pattern of living arrangements after experiencing a disabling event. Whites tended to enter nursing homes, Blacks continued to live in their predisability situation, and Hispanic elderly lived with family.

There is a growing trend in research on informal support systems among ethnic minority elderly to challenge assumptions about the existence, as well as benefits, of the extended family. Existence of widespread, extensive, and effective family support among ethnic minorities cannot be taken for granted (White-Means & Thornton, 1990). For example, in a study of Mexican Americans, Markides, Boldt, and Ray (1986) found that elderly Mexican Americans were not more likely to be cared for by their family network than elderly majority Americans. The authors interpreted this finding by suggesting that environmental stressors, such as language and low economic status, interfere with cultural and family support networks that ordinarily would be provided to aging Hispanics.

Furthermore, it is commonly surmised that large extended minority families provide sufficient intergenerational support for their members. However,

Lockery (1991) maintains that the notion of available intergenerational support is built on a number of erroneous assumptions. In particular, this research assumes that most minority families care for their members (Lockery, 1991; Morrison, 1995). Further, researchers who adopt an uncritical view of the extended family often consider evidence of nonformal service use as understandable and acceptable.

Caregivers of ethnic minority elderly require additional research. One assumption about these caregivers is that they do not use various support groups or services because they are either self-reliant or already receiving support from others. In fact, methods used by service organizations to attract caregivers in the general population have been unsuccessful with minority communities. One common explanation is lack of trust and familiarity with staffs of organizations providing such services. For example, minority caregivers seldom attend support group meetings for those caring for victims of Alzheimer's disease (Levine & Lawler, 1991). In addition to addressing emotional strains, support groups provide valuable information for caregivers. Since minority caregivers do not attend these meetings, they may be ill prepared for legal and financial uncertainties often inherent in caring for the elderly (Levine & Lawler, 1991).

Social work practitioners and researchers are beginning to address the underutilization of services by minority caregivers. One study examined efforts to involve the Black church and clergy in disseminating knowledge about Alzheimer's disease and caregivers' support services (Chadiha, Morrow-Howell, Darkwa, & MicGillick, 1994). Only when training sessions were incorporated into previously scheduled meetings were ministers and laypersons willing to participate. The authors caution that severity of other social problems may take away from the clergy members' ability to give attention to Alzheimer's disease (Chadiha *et al.,* 1994). Further, even though African American social workers were used as recruiters for the study, their outsider status may have affected the participation of ministers and laypersons in the program. Likewise, the use of culturally sensitive approaches, such as high levels of personal contact and multiple referral sources, along with perseverance, is crucial for recruiting minority caregivers into support groups (Henderson *et al.,* 1993; Chadiha *et al.,* 1994).

SUMMARY AND RECOMMENDATIONS

In this chapter we have discussed the meaning and significance of aging and minority group status in considering physical and psychological health. Although there are few well-developed frameworks, it is clear that a culturally sensitive theoretical framework for research and interventions with ethnic minority elderly must attend to sociohistorical content, significance of minority group status, and the cultural reality of ethnic minorities.

Our recommendations are organized with these three principles in mind. Consideration of sociohistorical context suggests concerns about longevity and cohort differences (Riley, 1996). One of the most important changes in human history is our increasing longevity. Through the early part of this century the life expectancy for adult males hovered around 40 years of age. Changes in health care, medical technology, decreased infant mortality, and decreased adult morbidity and mortality have lengthened the life span to 74 years for White males. Life expectancy for Blacks has improved dramatically. An African American woman born in 1900 had a life expectancy of 33.5 years. A Black woman born in 1985 may expect to live 75.3 years. For Black men, the figures are 32.5 and 65.3 years (Griffith & Baker, 1995). Yet, it is important to remember that these changes are in our recent history. Longevity has far-reaching implications for family patterns, service provision, and social policy. Equally important, given that increased longevity is a rather recent historical phenomenon, society is just beginning to create the sociocultural frameworks from which to understand and negotiate longer life.

In his classic essay on cohort and social change, Ryder (1965) defined a cohort in terms of its aggregate biography. Future cohorts of ethnic minority elderly will be both similar to and different from previous cohorts (Baker, 1994). Experience with racial discrimination provides a striking illustration. Blacks who are now 75 were probably born in the rural South, experienced childhood poverty, and were middle-aged during the civil rights movement. Contrast this to Blacks born in 1975, who will be 75 in the year 2050. These individuals in all likelihood were born in an urban setting, raised in diverse neighborhoods, and benefited from the opening up of opportunities. We can only speculate about the effects of a changing racial system on the health and well-being of ethnic minorities. This is clearly a fruitful area of research.

Minority group status has important implications for the well-being of ethnic elderly. It is in this area that the intersection of individual, group, and social and material context comes to the fore. Two examples illustrate the importance of considering both the individual and minority group status. The first example is that of a retired African American male of average weight, whose blood pressure during a routine physical examination appears to be slightly elevated. Is he a candidate for medication? It is possible, particularly when one considers the high prevalence of hypertension among African Americans. However, it is also possible that the individual finds doctor visits extremely stressful, hence the elevated blood pressure. Health care providers must learn to balance group indicators with individual biography. A second example involves the financial hardships that disproportionately affect ethnic minority elderly. The financial status of ethnic minority elderly has improved, but lags far behind that of their White counterparts (Chen, 1995). Although individuals may prepare for aging, large numbers of ethnic minority elderly are employed in areas that do not include adequate retirement benefits. These older persons depend mainly on Social Security. New cohorts of ethnic minority elderly may have opportunities to "plan for retirement." Yet, it is also possible that they too will be trapped in employment settings that preclude setting aside monies for later life.

Consideration of the cultural reality of life among ethnic minority elderly leads to a number of recommendations. Researchers and practitioners will need to consider the cultural resources available to these elderly. Cultural resources, such as the Black church, are important points of intervention among African American elderly (Griffith & Baker, 1995). A second resource, having pride in the ability to endure adversity, may reflect cultural belief systems that act as an important buffer for individuals and groups of ethnic minority elderly. A third resource may come through intergenerational relations. Griffith and Baker (1995) speculated that lower rates of suicide among African American elderly in part may be related to their important roles in the family (J. S. Jackson, Antonucci, & Gibson, 1995). They noted that suicide rates among ethnic elderly may be rising, perhaps indicating increasing stressors (J. S. Jackson, Antonucci, & Gibson, 1995). Related to these increasing stressors, as noted in the discussion of caregiving, ethnic minority families are under growing pressures (economic as well as social) and may be compromised in their ability to care for elderly. The threat to elderly may take the form of exploitation, neglect, or abuse. Unfortunately, there is limited research on the factors associated with elder abuse among ethnic minorities. With the increases in longevity and aging of the baby boom cohort, research in this area is essential.

No discussion of minority group aging would be complete without consideration of Riley's (1992) concept of structural lag, defined as the mismatch between social opportunities and individual aging. For ethnic minority elderly, the mismatch may be particularly severe, such that past and current contextual influences overwhelm factors that are attributable to aging-related processes. Old age cannot be divorced from earlier stages of life and nowhere is this clearer than among ethnic minority elderly. Among several groups of ethnic minority elderly, most have experienced economic difficulties, inadequate health care, and the stress of discrimination.

Another consideration is a cultural understanding of health, illness, and disease (Gaines, 1992; Padgett, 1995). Health and mental health services must reach out to older minority adults. This outreach should involve multiple community locations, from primary health centers to churches to the homes of older adults (J. S. Jackson, Albright, et al., 1995). These services must be sensitive to the lifestyles, cultural preferences, behaviors, attitudes, and values of ethnic racial minorities (J. S. Jackson et al., 1992), as well as barriers to service use. Language may be the most pressing barrier to providing accurate diagnosis and appropriate intervention strategies for ethnic minority elderly. Researchers have found that, among Blacks, stress is often discussed in a religious idiom, as "trials and tribulations" (Dressler, 1991). For nonnative speakers of English, the language barrier is even more problematic. Specifically, a number of ethnic minority elderly may be unable to speak or read English (Browne & Broderick, 1994). For ethnic minority elderly, inability to articulate symptoms in a manner prescribed by the dominant culture may result in misdiagnoses. Efforts to increase service use by ethnic minority elderly will need to employ creative strategies for informing and serving these populations. Using skilled interpreters as a standard practice is one strategy for developing culturally sensitive services. However, caution must be exercised. Interpreters mediate between the clinician and the patient; an untrained interpreter could create a number of problems, including misdiagnosis. Nevertheless, judicious use of interpreters, nontraditional service settings (e.g., the church), and creative outreach and recruitment strategies are approaches that move beyond standard efforts to more effectively influence the health and well-being of ethnic minority elderly.

Finally, the heterogeneity within and between ethnic minority elderly must be explored further (J. S. Jackson, Antonucci, & Gibson, 1995). Research on American Indians and Asian American elderly is especially sparse (Stanford &

Du Bois, 1992). Similarly, our knowledge of the incidence and prevalence of such important issues as elder abuse is nearly nonexistent among ethnic minority elderly. Further, gender differences within groups requires more study (Brown, Milburn, & Gary, 1992). As we have argued elsewhere, gender, socioeconomic, and ethnic minority status cannot be divorced from one another in fruitfully studying the lives of ethnic minority elderly (Gibson & Jackson, 1992).

The growth in the number of ethnic minority elderly over the next 50 to 75 years will place increasing burdens on family, other informal supports, and formal delivery of material and social services. Close examination of cultural factors, minority group determined life experiences, and the organization of formal systems of care will be required in order to provide effective services to the largest growing segment of the new elderly population. The belief that these considerations are of secondary importance to the effective organization and delivery of physical and mental geriatric health care will no longer be possible.

REFERENCES

Adebimpe, V. (1981). Overview: White norms and psychiatric diagnosis of black patients. *American Journal of Psychiatry, 138,* 279–285.

Andrews, J., Lynos, B., & Rowland, D. (1992). Life satisfaction and peace of mind: A comparative analysis of elderly Hispanic and other elderly Americans. *Clinical Gerontologist, 11,* 21–42.

Angel, J., & Hogan, D. (1994). The demography of minority aging populations. In J. S. Jackson, J. Albright, T. P. Miles, M. R. Miranda, C. Nunez, E. P. Stanford, B. W. K. Yee, D. L. Yee, & G. Yeo (Eds.), *Minority elderly: Five goals toward building a public policy base* (2nd ed., pp. 9–12). Washington, DC: Gerontological Society of America.

Angel, R., Angel, J., & Himes., C. (1992). Minority group status, health transitions, and community living arrangements among the elderly. *Research on Aging, 14,* 496–521.

Baker, F. M. (1994). Psychiatric treatment of older African Americans. *Hospital and Community Psychiatry, 45*(1), 32–37.

Baker, F. M., & Lightfoot, O. (1995). Psychiatric care of ethnic elderly. In A. Gaw (Ed.), *Culture, ethnicity, and mental illness* (pp. 517–552). Washington, DC: American Psychiatric Press.

Blauner, R. (1972). *Racial oppression in America.* New York: Harper & Row.

Brown, D. R., Milburn, N. G, & Gary, L. E. (1992). Symptoms of depression among older African-Americans: An analysis of gender differences. *Gerontologist, 32* (6), 789–795.

Brown, D. R., Ahmed, F., Gary, L. E., & Milburn, N. G. (1995). Major depression in a community sample of African Americans. *American Journal of Psychiatry, 152* (3), 373–378.

Browne, C., & Broaderick, A. (1994). Asian and Pacific island elderly: Issues for social work practice and education. *Social Work, 39,* 252–259.

Chadiha, L., Morrow-Howell, N., Darkwa, O., & MicGillick, J. (1994). Targeting the black church and clergy for disseminating knowledge about Alzheimer's disease and caregivers's support services. *American Journal of Alzheimer's Care and Related Disorders and Research, 9,* 17–20.

Chatters, L. M., & Taylor, R. J. (1989). Age differences in religious participation among black adults. *Journal of Gerontology: Social Sciences, 44,* S183–S189.

Chen, Y. P. (1995). Improving the economic security of minority persons as they enter old age. In J. S. Jackson, J. Albright, T. Miles, M. Miranda, C. Nunez, E. Stanford, B. Yee, D. Yee, & G. Yeo (Eds.), *Minority elders: Five goals toward building a public policy* (2nd ed., pp. 22–31). Washington, DC: Gerontological Society of America.

Cohen, R. A., & Van Nostrand, J. F. (1995). *Trends in the health of older Americans: United States, 1994.* Washington, DC: National Center for Health Statistics.

Dressler, W. (1991). *Stress and adaptation in the context of culture: Depression in a southern black community.* New York: State University of New York Press.

Evans, D., Funkenstein, H., & Albert, M. (1989). Prevalence of Alzhemier's disease in a community population of older persons higher than previously reported. *Journal of the American Medical Association, 262*, 2251–2556.

Gaines, A. D. (1992). From DSM-I to II-R; Voices of self, mastery and the other: A cultural constructivist reading of U.S. psychiatric classification. *Social Science and Medicine, 35* (1), 3–24.

Garcia, A. (1991). The changing demographic face of Hispanics in the United States. In M. Sotomayor (Ed.), *Empowering Hispanic families: A critical issue for the '90's.* (pp. 21–38). Milwaukee, WI: Family Service America.

George, L. (1993). Economic status and subjective well-being: A review of the literature and an agenda for future research. In N. Culter, D. Gregg, & M. P. Lawton (Eds.), *Aging, money and life satisfaction* (pp. 69–99). New York: Springer.

Gibson, R. C., & Jackson, J. S. (1992). The black oldest old: Health, functioning and informal support. In R. M. Suzman, D. P. Willis, & K. G. Manton (Eds.), *The oldest old* (pp. 321–340). New York: Oxford University Press.

Griffith, E., & Baker, F. M. (1995). Psychiatric care of African Americans. In A. Gaw (Ed.), *Culture, ethnicity, and mental illness* (pp. 147–173). Washington, DC: American Psychiatric Press.

Henderson, J., Guiterrez-Mayka, M., & Garcia, J. (1993). A model of Alzheimer's disease support group development in African-American and Hispanic populations. *Gerontologist, 33*, 409–414.

Herzog, R. (1989). Physical and mental health in older women: Selected research issues and data sources. In A. R. Herzog, K. Holden, & M. Seltzer (Eds.), *Health and economic status of older women* (pp. 35–91). Amityville, NY: Baywood.

Indian Health Service. (1991). *Trends in Indian health.* U.S. Department of Health and Human Services, Public Health Services. Washington, DC: U.S. Government Printing Office.

Jackson, J. J. (1985). Race, national origin, ethnicity, and aging. In R. B. Binstock & E. Shanas (Eds.), *Handbook of aging and the social sciences* (pp. 264–303). New York: Van Nostrand Reinhold.

Jackson, J. S., & Neighbors, W. (1996). Changes in African American resources and mental health 1979 to 1992. In H. Neighbors & J. Jackson (Eds), *Mental health in Black America* (pp. 189–212). Thousand Oaks, CA: Sage.

Jackson, J. S., & Sellers, S. L. (1997). Psychological, social, and cultural perspectives on minority health in adolescence: A life-course framework. In D. Wilson, J. Rodrigue, & W. Taylor (Eds.), *Health-promoting and health-compromising behaviors among minority adolescents* (pp. 29–54). Washington, DC: American Psychological Association.

Jackson, J. S., & Wolford, M. L. (1992). Changes from 1979 to 1987 in mental health status and help-seeking among African Americans. *Journal of Geriatric Psychiatry, 25*, 15–67.

Jackson, J. S., Burns, C., & Gibson, R. (1992). An overview of geriatric care in ethnic and racial minority groups. In E. Calkins, P. J. Davis, A. B. Ford, & P. R. Katz (Eds.), *Practice of Geriatrics* (2nd ed., pp. 57–64). Philadelphia: Harcourt Brace Jovanovich.

Jackson, J. S., Albright, J., Miles, T. P., Miranda, M. R., Nunez, C., Stanford, E. P., Yee, B. W. K., Yee, D. L., & Yeo, G. (Eds.). (1995). *Minority elderly: Five goals toward building a public policy base* (2nd ed.). Washington, DC: Gerontological Society of America.

Jackson, J. S., Antonucci, T. C., & Gibson, R. C. (1995). Ethnic and cultural factors in research on aging and mental health: A life-course perspective. In D. K. Padgett (Ed.), *Handbook on ethnicity, aging and mental health* (pp. 22–46). New York: Greenwood/Praeger.

Jackson, J. S., Brown, T., Williams, D., Torres, M., Sellers, S., & Brown, K. (1996). Perceptions and experiences of racism and the physical and mental health status of African Americans: A thirteen-year national panel study. *Ethnicity and Disease, 6*, 132–147.

James, S., Hartnett, S., & Kalsbeek, W. (1983). John Henryism and blood pressure differences among black men. *Journal of Behavioral Medicine, 6*, 259–278.

James, S., Strogatz, D., Wing, S., & Ramsey, D. (1987). Socioeconomic status, John Henryism, and hypertension in blacks and whites. *American Journal of Epidemiology, 126*, 664–673.

Jeste, D. V., Naimark, D., Halpain, M. C., & Lindamer, L. A. (1995). Strengths and limitations of research on late-life psychoses. In M. Gatz (Ed.), *Emerging issues in mental health* (pp. 72–96). Washington, DC: American Psychological Association.

John, R. (1994). The state of research on American Indian elders' health, income security, and social support networks. In J. S. Jackson, J. Albright, T. Miles, M. Miranda, C. Nunez, E. Stanford, B.

Yee, D. Yee, & G. Yeo (Eds.), *Minority elders: Five goals toward building a public policy base* (2nd ed., pp. 46–58). Washington, DC: Gerontological Society of America.

Johnson, F., Cook, E., Foxall, M., Kelleher, E., Kentopp, E., & Mannlein, E. (1986). Life satisfaction of the elderly American Indian. *International Journal of Nursing Studies, 23*(3), 265–273.

Kasl, S., & Berkman, L. (1981). Some psychosocial influences on the health status of the elderly: The perspective of social epidemiology. In J. L. McGaugh & S. B. Kiesler (Eds.), *Aging, biology and behavior* (pp. 345–385). New York: Academic.

King, G., & Williams, D. (1995). Race and health: A multidimensional approach to African-American health. In C. Benjamin, I. Amick, S. Levin, A. R. Tarlov, & D. C. Walsh (Eds.), *Society and Health* (pp. 93–130). New York: Oxford University Press.

Knight, B., Santos, J., Teri, L., & Lawton, M. P. (1995). Introduction: The development of training in clinical geropsychology. In B. Knight, L. Teri, P. Wohlford, & J. Santos (Eds.), *Mental health services for older adults* (pp. 1–8). Washington, DC: American Psychological Association.

Lebowitz, B. D., & Niederehe, G. (1992). Concepts and issues in mental health and aging. In J. E. Birren, R. B. Sloane, & G. D. Cohen (Eds.), *Handbook of mental health and aging* (2nd ed., pp. 3–26). New York: Academic.

Levine, J., & Lawlor, B. (1991). Family counseling and legal issues in Alzheimer's disease. *Psychiatric Clinics of North America, 14,* 385–396.

Levine, R., & Gaw, A. (1995). Culture-bound syndrones. *Culture Psychiatry, 18*(3), 523–536.

Littlewood, R. (1992). Psychiatric diagnosis and racial bias: Empirical and interpretative approaches. *Social Science & Medicine, 34,* 141–149.

Lockery, S. (1991). Family and social support: Caregiving among racial and ethnic minority elderly. *Generations, 15,* 58–62.

Lopez, C., & Aguilera, E. (1991). *On the sidelines: Hispanic elderly and the continuum of care.* Washington, DC: National Council of La Raza.

Lopez-Aqueres, A., Keep, B., Plopper, M., Staples, F., & Brummel-Smith, K. (1984). Health needs of the Hispanic elderly. *Journal of the American Geriatric Society, 32,* 191–198.

Manson, S., & Callaway, D. (1988). Health and aging among American Indians. Issues and challenges for the biobehavioral sciences. In S. M. Mason & N. Dinges (Eds.), *Health and behavior: A research agenda for American Indians* (pp. 160–210). Denver: University of Colorado Health Sciences Center.

Manson, S., Shore, J., & Bloom, J. (1985). The depressive experience in American Indian communities: A challenge for psychiatric theory and diagnosis. In A. Kleinman & Y. Good (Eds.), *Culture and depression* (pp. 331–368). Berkeley, CA: University of California Press.

Manton, K., Poss, S., & Wing, S. (1979). The black/white mortality crossover: Investigation from the perspective of the components of aging. *Gerontologist, 19,* 291–300.

Markides, K., & Krause, N. (1986). Older Mexican Americans. *Generations, 10,* 31–34.

Markides, K., Boldt, J., & Ray, L. (1986). Sources of helping and intergenerational solidarity: A three generation study of Mexican Americans. *Journals of Gerontology, 41,* 506–511.

McCabe, M., & Cuellar, J. (1994). *Aging and health: American Indian/Alaska native elderly* (2nd ed.). Working Paper Series No. 6. Palo Alto, CA: Stanford Geriatric Education Center.

Miranda, M. (1991). Mental health services and the Hispanic elderly. In M. Sotomayor (Ed.), *Empowering Hispanic families: A critical issue for the '90s.* (141–154). Milwaukee, WI: Family Service America.

Morrison, B. (1995). A research and policy agenda on predictors of institutional placement among minority elderly. *Journal of Gerontological Social Work, 24,* 17–28.

Neighbors, H. (1984). The distribution of psychiatric morbidity in African Americans: A review and suggestions for research. *Community Mental Health Journal. 20,* 5–18.

Office of Minority Health Resource Center. (1988). Closing the gap: Cancer and minorities. Office of Minority Health, Public Health Service. Washington, DC: U.S. Department of Health and Human Services.

Padgett, D. (1995). Concluding remarks and suggestions for research and service delivery. In D. Padgett (Ed.), *Handbook on ethnicity, aging, and mental health* (pp. 304–319). Westport, CT: Greenwood.

Rabins, P. (1992). Prevention of mental disorder in the elderly: Current perspectives and future prospectus. *Journal of the American Geriatrics Society, 40,* 727–733.

Richardson, J. (1990). *Aging and health: Black American elderly*. Stanford, CA: Stanford Geriatric Education Center Working Paper Series No 4. Ethnogeriatic Reviews.

Riley, M. (1992). Aging in the twenty-first century. In N. Culter, D. Gregg, & M. P. Lawton (Eds.), *Aging, money and life satisfaction* (pp. 23–36). New York: Springer.

Riley, M. (1996). Age stratification. In J. E. Birren (Ed.), *Encyclopedia of gerontology: Age, aging and the aged* (pp. 81–92). New York: Academic.

Rodgers, W. (1982). Trends in reported happiness within demographically defined subgroups, 1957–78. *Social Forces, 60,* 826–842.

Rosenwaike, I. (1987). Mortality differentials among persons born in Cuba, Mexico, and Puerto Rico residing in the United States, 1979–1981. *American Journal of Public Health, 77,* 603–606.

Ruiz, D. (1995). Profile of ethnic elderly. In D. Padgett (Ed.), *Handbook on ethnicity, aging, and mental health* (pp. 3–21). Westport, CT: Greenwood.

Ryder, N. (1965). The cohort as a concept in the study of social change. *American Sociological Review, 30,* 843–861.

Snow, L. F. (1983). Traditional health beliefs and practices among lower class black Americans. *Western Journal of Medicine, 139*(6), 820–828.

Stanford, E. P., & Du Bois, B. C. (1992). Gender and ethnicity patterns. In J. E. Birren, R. B. Sloane, & G. D. Cohen (Eds.), *Handbook of mental health and aging* (2nd ed., pp. 99–117). New York: Academic.

Swidler, A. (1986). Culture in action: Symbols and strategies. *American Sociological Review, 51,* 273–286.

Taeuber, C. (1992). *Income and poverty trends for the elderly.* Population Division, Bureau of the Census, U.S. Department of Commerce. Washington, DC: U.S. Government Printing Office.

Turnbull, J., & Mui, A. (1995). Mental health status and needs of black and white elderly: Differences in depression. In D. Padgett (Ed.), *Handbook on ethnicity, aging, and mental health* (pp. 73–98). Westport, CT: Greenwood.

U.S. Bureau of the Census. (1990). *Population estimates by age, sex, race, and Hispanic origin: 1980 to 1988.* Current population reports. (Series P-25, No. 1045). Washington, DC: U.S. Government Printing Office.

U.S. Bureau of the Census. (1996). *Population projections of the United States by age, sex, race, and Hispanic origin: 1995 to 2050.* Current population reports. (Series P-25, No. 1130). Washington, DC: U.S. Government Printing Office.

Vega, W., & Rumbaut, R. (1991). Ethnic minorities and mental health. *Annual Review of Sociology, 17,* 351–383.

Villa, M., Cuellar, J., Gamel, N., & Yeo, G. (1993). *Aging and health: Hispanic American elderly* (2nd ed.) SGEC Working Paper Series Number 5 Ethnogeratic Reviews. Stanford, CA: Stanford Geriatric Education Centers.

Wade, J. (1993). Institutional racism: An analysis of the mental health system. *American Journal of Psychiatry, 127,* 329–355.

White-Means, S. I., & Thornton, M. C. (1990). Ethic differences in the production of informal home health care. *Gerontologist, 30* (6), 758–768.

Wirth, L. (1945). The problem of minority groups. In R. Linton (Ed.), *The science of man in the world crisis* (pp. 99–117). New York: Columbia University Press.

Worobey, J., & Angel, R. (1990). Functional capacity and living arrangements of unmarried elderly persons. *Journal of Gerontology: Social Sciences, 45,* 95–101.

Wykle, M., & Kaskel, B. (1991). Increasing the longevity of minority older adults through improved health status. In J. S. Jackson, J. Albright, T. Miles, M. Miranda, C. Nunez, E. Stanford, B. Yee, D. Yee, & G. Yeo (Eds.), *Minority elders: Five goals toward building a public policy base* (2nd ed., pp. 32–39). Washington, DC: Gerontological Society of America.

CHAPTER 24

Physical Activity

WARREN W. TRYON

INTRODUCTION

There are at least five reasons for geropsychologists to be interested in physical activity. The first reason is that activity is a prominent life-span developmental *personality* variable. We will see that stable individual activity differences begin prenatally, are universally recognized as a major dimension of infant temperament, comprise a facet of introversion which is recognized as an important personality trait by all investigators, and remain stable throughout adult life. The ability to ambulate and lead an active life assumes greater importance with advanced age. Perception of health in oneself and others is directly proportional to physical activity. *Active lifestyle,* therefore, constitutes an important individual difference for geropsychologists.

A second reason for geropsychologists to be interested in physical activity is its connection with *physical health.* Evidence is reviewed that exercise promotes both physical and mental health in older people as well as middle-aged or young adults. Older people benefit proportionally, but to a lesser absolute degree, than younger people, but it is never too late to assume a more active life style. Active lifestyle is directly related to physical health.

A third reason for geropsychological interest in activity is that exercise appears to improve *mental health* and *cognitive functioning.* Activity seems to reduce depression, which is quite frequent among older people given loss of job through retirement, loss of friends and relatives through death, and a clearer recognition of the limits of their life span. Exercise also seems to improve cognition, perhaps through better blood flow. Chronic diseases, such as lung disease, arthritis, heart disease, and other ailments, reduce activity and alter previously established individual activity differences. Physical disease and injury modify preexisting personality differences. These factors alter the activity distributions with age.

WARREN W. TRYON • Department of Psychology, Fordham University, Bronx, New York 10458-5198.

Handbook of Clinical Geropsychology, edited by Michel Hersen and Vincent B. Van Hasselt. Plenum Press, New York, 1998.

A fourth reason for geropsychologists to be interested in physical activity is that *sleep* disorders are directly proportional to age and because sleep can be productively studied via actigraphy. The Sleep-Onset Spectrum (SOS) is described to properly understand the perspective actigraphy provides regarding sleep. Validation of wrist actigraphy for sleep assessment is addressed and applications to sleep disorders experienced by the elderly are considered.

A fifth reason for geropsychologists to be interested in physical activity is to better understand developmental changes in *circadian rhythm*. Our biological clocks deteriorate over time and some disorders of aging can be understood in these terms. Core body temperature defines the strongest circadian rhythm; activity level is the second most prominent circadian rhythm. Actigraphy makes it easy to obtain high-quality activity data every minute of the day and night for up to 22 consecutive days from people under natural conditions. Data collection can continue by downloading and reinitializing the actigraphs.

PERSONALITY

Activity is a prominent life-span developmental personality variable from before birth, through infancy and childhood, into adulthood and old age.

Prenatal

Activity is arguably the first personality variable to form stable individual differences. Eaton and Saudino (1992) review 14 studies validating maternal fetal counts. Maternal counts tend to underestimate instrument detectable fetal movements. However, correlations between maternal and instrumented recorded counts ranged from .32 to .99; six articles reported correlations of .97 to .99. Eaton and Saudino (1992) studied daily fetal movement counts obtained once per week from 7 A.M. until 11 P.M. from 46 women with normal pregnancies. Significant and substantial between-fetus differences ($F(45, 495) = 174.33$, $p < .0001$) were found. Individual stability, calculated as a generalizability coefficient and interpreted as a reliability coefficient, based on recordings for 1 week was found to be .93.

Infancy

Goldsmith and colleagues (1987) considered four approaches to temperament and concluded that all theorists agree that activity level and emotionality are valid, primary, and replicable dimensions of temperament. Zuckerman (1991, pp. 7–8) reported that activity is one of nine defining features of temperament. Activity consistently emerges as an important variable in Zuckerman's (1991) discussion of genetic influences during infancy and early childhood (pp. 111–116). For example, by age 9, activity is among the temperament facets with the highest heritability ratios. Kagan and Snidman (1991) also consider motor activity to be an important aspect of infant temperament.

Adulthood

The index of Zuckerman's (1991) book identifies 43 of 428 pages (10%) wherein the importance of activity to an understanding of the psychobiology of personality is discussed. Buss and Plomin (1984) consider activity to be one of the "Big 3" personality factors. Zuckerman (1991, pp. 28–29) identifies activity as one of five primary personality factors. Costa and McCrae (1992) conclude that activity develops into a facet of Extraversion in the Five Factor Model of personality. They characterize the activity (E4) Extraversion facet as follows: "A high Activity score is seen in rapid tempo and vigorous movement, in a sense of energy, and in a need to keep busy. Active people lead fast-paced lives. Low scorers are more leisurely and relaxed in tempo, although they are not necessarily sluggish or lazy" (p. 17).

Old Age

The five personality factors, including the activity facet, remain stable throughout adulthood into old age (Costa & McCrae, 1980, 1994) where the activity factor assumes greater prominence as *activity lifestyle* (Hultsch, Hammer, & Small, 1993). Activity impairment is an important aspect of disability and is therefore of increasing importance throughout late life. Insofar as inactivity is unhealthy, death selects out inactive people thereby skewing the activity distribution to the right. Disease counters this trend by reducing activity level in the more active people who survive thereby skewing the activity distribution to the left. The relative effects of these two processes are presently unknown. Consequently, we do not know how their joint effect alters activity distributions in the elderly. Disease mediated inactivity probably has a negative effect on one's psychological state. Inactivity is, to this extent, a causal antecedent of depression in the elderly and consequently an important mental health concern.

ACTIVITY AND DISABILITY

Hypokinetic Disease

Kraus and Raab (1961) coined the term "hypokinetic disease" to describe a spectrum of physical and mental disorder induced by inactivity. It is interesting that disabilities normally associated with aging can be partially produced in young healthy persons by protracted inactivity. Bortz (1982) discovered important parallels between normal aging and inactivity regarding the cardiovascular system, blood components, body composition, metabolic and regulatory functions, and the nervous system.

Motor control decreases with age and these changes are most noticeable on more demanding tests (Joseph & Roth, 1988; Wallace, Krauter, & Campbell, 1980). Joseph and Roth (1993) summarized experimental evidence indicating that motor performance deteriorates primarily as the result of impaired dopaminergic function due to striatal dopamine receptor loss. Receptor density increase in rats has been achieved through the administration of estrogen or prolactin.

Active Life Style

General

O'Brien and Vertinsky (1991) point out that women outlive their male counterparts but often these extra years of life entail chronic illness and disability. These authors indicate that "... evidence is rapidly accumulating that physical mobility is a critical survival need for the elderly" (p. 348). "Indeed, about 50% of what we currently accept as aging is now understood to be *hypokinesia,* a disease of 'disuse,' the degeneration and functional loss of muscle and bone tissue" (p. 348, emphasis added). The long-term benefits of exercise on health are both broad and substantial.

Active life expectancy (ALE) refers to the years before disability alters one's functional status (see Manton, Stallard, & Liu, 1993). ALE is an important determinant of the health and service needs of persons over 65 years of age. Mobility is recognized as an essential component of self-care. Guralnik and Simonsick (1993) report that "the assessment of functional status and disability is now widely employed by those caring for older patients and those studying the health problems of older populations" (p. 3). Disability regarding activities of daily living increases rapidly after age 65. Guralnik and Simonsick (1993) report that 22% of women and 15% of men over age 65 are sufficiently disabled that they either need help to live at home or are institutionalized. By age 75, the sex difference in disability is pronounced; and at age 85, 62% of women and 46% of men need help to live at home or are in a nursing home. Woollacott (1993) observes that many older adults lose the ability to ambulate outside their home because they cannot maintain their balance on uneven surfaces and in moving vehicles such as a bus or train. Frail elderly nursing home residents are frequently very inactive.

Siu and colleagues (1993) underscored the need to measure functioning in the very old and concluded that most measures were developed on middle-aged and young-old persons. Their objective was to develop a measure of functioning in old-old persons. Manton and colleagues (1993) observed that single ALE estimates cannot address individual disability effects over time nor can they reflect intervention effects. Multiple measurements are required for these purposes. Actigraphy, discussed in the next section, is especially suited for longitudinal activity measurement. Gerety and colleagues (1993) complained that existing assessment devices are insensitive to individual differences. Accordingly, they embarked on creating a more suitable Physical Disability Index (PDI). Their goals were to detect individual differences and changes in functioning over time. They wanted to avoid ceiling and floor effects and sought to reduce reporting bias. They chose tasks to measure strength, range of motion, balance, mobility, and fine motor activities and administered this test battery to 259 nursing home residents aged 60 to 98 (mean 78.3 years). Time for completion ranged from 46 to 83 min (mean 60 min).

Actigraphy

Technological advances provide gerontologists with instruments that can quantify activity. Tryon (1985, 1991) reviewed instruments for measuring activity. Tryon and Williams (1996) introduced a new fully proportional actigraph capable of quantifying 128 levels of activity, averaging the results over user-selectable, often 1-min, epochs, and storing the result in memory 24 hours per day for 22 consecutive days before filling memory. Measurements can be made every second if desired with the consequence that memory fills up 60 times faster than when using 1-minute recording epochs. Even faster recording rates are now possible. Ambulatory Monitoring Inc. (Ardsley, NY) and Computer Science and Applications, Inc. (Shalimar, FL) offer rapid sampling actigraphs capable of making ten readings per second (10 Hz).

Actigraphy solves the problems of (1) sensitivity to individual differences and (2) avoidance of floor and ceiling effects for two types of behavioral samples. First, one can attach an actigraph to the subject while they perform prescribed movements such as the standardized assessments mentioned earlier. For example, Rosnow and Breslau (1966) assessed walking up and down stairs to the second floor and walking a half mile. Less demanding tests include walking across the room (Guralnik & Simonsick, 1993) and walking an 8-foot course (Guralnik *et al.*, 1994). Such tests could be better quantified by attaching an actigraph to the waist, wrist, and/or ankle. Measuring behavior on a 128-point scale 10 times each second and recording the average each second means that 60 data points are obtained each minute. These large data sets ensure that (1) individual differences will arise and (2) no subject will get all zeros (floor effect) or all values of 128 (ceiling effect).

The second type of behavioral sample is a 24-hour sample of the subject's natural behavior for 7, 14, or 21 days. The longer the sample the more repeatable each subject's mean value, the clearer individual differences will become. Some subjects will undoubtedly be more variable than others. Because the standard error of the mean equals the standard deviation of the sample divided by the square root of the sample size, more certainty can be obtained for a more variable subject by collecting more data points through extending the observation period. Hence, statistical significance can be found for even small individual differences. Floor effects cannot occur because everyone moves to some degree over a 1- or 2-week period. It is impossible for a person to wear an activity monitor for this period of time without recording any activity. Ceiling effects also cannot occur because even young healthy people cannot continuously emit the maximum activity detectable by modern actigraphs 24 hours a day for 7, 14, or 21 consecutive days.

Beyond the question of behavioral sample size is sample representativeness. If the person's routine is about the same each day, then a 1-week behavioral sample constitutes seven replications of a representative day. This conclusion assumes that the 7 chosen days are representative of days in general for that subject. If the person works or volunteers on Mondays and Wednesdays in the same setting, then a 1-week sample contains only 2 volunteer days but 5 nonvolunteer days. Then there is the question of whether weekend days are comparable to weekdays. From the perspective of representativeness, a 2-week sample is reasonably small. Brief behavioral samples taken during standardized testing may not be representative; the generalizability of such results may thus be questionable. This is not to say that activity measurements taken during standard conditions do not generalize; rather, the burden of proof is on the investigator who wishes to so generalize. Consequently, standard test results should be compared with 2-week, or longer, samples to demonstrate generalizability.

The site of attachment is also important. Waist activity primarily reflects ambulation. Since a person's center of gravity is near the waist, movement of this site is among the most energy-intensive movements we typically make. Wrist movement also occurs during ambulation, except when carrying something, but it also reflects purposive activities while seated. Wrist activity clearly discriminates sleep from wake (Tryon, 1991, 1996). The ankle is a third possible site of attachment but is the least preferred because the jarring associated with footfalls can produce artificially large readings. The investigator selects one or more sites of attachment depending upon the objective.

It is possible to combine the standardized test and naturalistic behavioral sample approaches by instructing or prompting subjects to perform specified activities at prescribed times each day. Seven to 14 repeated measurements would result if the required exercises were performed just once each day for 1 or 2 weeks. Two or three times this many measurements could be obtained if subjects were instructed to repeat these behaviors two or three times each day.

Activity assessments taken at yearly or monthly intervals would enable one to calculate inverse growth (decline) curves thereby quantifying the rate at which activity decreases over time. This approach is the reverse of what the pediatrician does when placing infants on a growth curve to anticipate adult stature and weight.

A potential limitation of obtaining 24-hour activity levels is that they quantify habitual activity rather than the person's capacity for activity. It must always be the case that the person is capable of being as active as they have been measured to be. Therefore, habitual activity establishes a lower bound on activity capacity. Evaluation of an upper limit can be accomplished by motivating the person to increase or maximize activity during a test period. However, habitual activity level may be more important to psychological and physical health than maximum ability to be active.

Actigraphy provides a noninvasive and cost-effective technology for obtaining extended activity lifestyle measurements. Gathering data about self-reported activity is an inexpensive alternative. However, Sidney and Shephard (1977) reported substantial discrepancies between self-reported and measured activity. This is to be expected for several reasons. People are largely unaware of their activity level because their attention is focused on what they are doing rather than on the mechanics of how they are doing it. Second, devices can quantify physical forces more accurately and consistently than can humans. However, people are better at judging quality of activity such as whether their activity was productive or symptomatic behavior such as pacing or restlessness.

PHYSICAL HEALTH

Activity relates to health in two reciprocal ways. First, activity appears to reduce the risk of death by disease and seems to promote physical health. Elderly people evaluate their own health, and the health of others, in terms of activity (Burnside, 1978; Gueldner & Spradley, 1988) with more active persons perceived as healthier. Second, disease and depression reduce activity and actigraphy can be used to quantify this change.

The important role activity plays in maintaining health is clarified through forced inactivity. Kraus and Raab's (1961) concept of "hypokinetic disease" is important here. It is interesting that disabilities normally associated with aging can be partially produced in young healthy persons by protracted inactivity. Palmore (1970) suggested that exercise is the health practice most strongly associated with longevity in the elderly.

Exercise Reduces Disease Risk

Activity has beneficial effects for those with coronary artery disease (Oberman, 1985; Paffenbarger & Hyde, 1984; K. E. Powell, Thompson, Caspersen, & Kendrick, 1987; Salonen, Puska, & Tuomilehto, 1982), obesity (Colvin & Olson, 1983; Hoiberg, Bernard, Watten & Caine, 1984; Marston & Criss, 1984; Westover & Lanyon, 1990), colon cancer (Slattery, Schumacher, Smith, West, & Abd-Elghany, 1988), and all-cause mortality in both young (Blair *et al.*, 1989; Bouchard, Shepard, Stephens, Sutton, & McPherson, 1990; Fox, Naughton, & Haskell, 1971), middle-aged (Leon, Connett, Jacobs, & Rauramaa, 1987; Morris *et al.*, 1973; Morris, Everitt, Pollard, Chave, & Semmence, 1980), and older adults (Blumenthal, *et al.*, 1989; Cunningham, Rechnitzer, Howard, & Donner, 1987; A. C. King, Taylor, Haskell, & DeBusk, 1989). Blair and colleagues (1989) reported that the decline in death rates with increased levels of fitness is most pronounced in older persons.

Magnus, Matroos, and Strackee (1979) reported a significant negative association between sustained light physical exercise, mainly walking, cycling, or gardening, and acute coronary events. Of the 473 subjects, 220 walked, cycled, or gardened less than 4 hours per week. Smoking was reported to weaken the benefits of exercise. Redwood, Rosing, and Epstein (1972) reported that light physical exercise, such as walking, lowers blood pressure. Slattery, Jacobs, and Nichaman (1989) analyzed 17- to 20-year mortality data on 3,043 subjects and reported that small increases in activity confer substantial protection against death by coronary disease. Expending just 250 Kcal per week through exercise was sufficient to gain benefit. This level of activity corresponds to just 10 min per day of light activity such as walking on a flat surface at 3 mph. In sum, a small amount of activity taken consistently is healthier than being entirely sedentary. Many older people are able to engage in activity at such a nonaerobic activity level.

Paffenbarger, Hyde, Wing, and Steinmetz (1984) reported that the rate of all-cause mortality per 10,000 man-years of observation among 16,936 Harvard alumni between 1962 and 1978 was 84.8 for those expending less than 500 calories through exercise per week, 66.0 for those expending 500 to 1,999 calories per week, and 52.1 for those expending 2,000 or more calories per week ($p < .001$). The mortality rates for total cardiovascular diseases associated with the three exercise levels are 39.5, 30.8, and 21.4 ($p < .001$). The rates for death from respiratory disease across the three exercise levels are 6.0, 3.2, and 1.5 ($p < .001$). The rates for death from all cancers are 25.7, 19.2, and 19.0 ($p < .026$). The benefits of exercise also extend to mental health: The rates for death by suicide are 5.1, 3.2, and 2.9 ($p < .049$). As a control condition, death by accidental means was unrelated to exercise. The three rates were 3.6, 3.9, and 3.0 ($p < .147$). The 2,000-calorie-per-week activity expenditure reduces to just 286 calories per day, which is within the capacity of many people. Similar results are presented by Paffenbarger, Wing, and Hyde (1978). It is not difficult to expend 500 calories per day through activity.

Paffenbarger, Hyde, Wing, and Hsieh (1986) further reported on the 16,936 Harvard alumni sample and revealed that walking 9 or more versus 3 miles per week reduced the risk of death by 21%. Persons expending 3,500 calories per week had an all-cause mortality rate half that of those expending less than 500 calories per week. Expending 2,000 calories or more per week reduced all-cause death risk 28% below those expending less than 500 calories per week.

Energy expenditure can be measured by a waist-worn accelerometer-based device retailed under the name Caltrac [TM] (Muscle Dynamics, 201000 Hamilton Avenue, Torrance, CA 90502) (Tryon, 1991a, p. 49). The author has worn this device for 610 days and finds that his daily energy expenditure due to activity ranges from 173 to 1,116 Kcal with many values in the 500 Kcal range, 645 Kcal being the midrange value. This results in a minimum of $173 \times 7 = 1,211$ Kcal per week and more likely $500 \times 7 = 3,500$ Kcal per week. Caltrac also calculates estimated basal and total calories expended.

Exercise Promotes Physical Health

It has been suggested that the deterioration of the central nervous system with age is partly the result of chronic mild hypoxia (Gibson & Peterson, 1982) due to atherosclerosis (Bierman, 1978; Mintz & Mankovsky, 1971) and inactive life styles (deVries, 1983). Fox and colleagues (1971) conclude that exercise may improve the quality of life as much or more than it may extend life.

Ades, Waldmann, and Gillespie (1995) demonstrated that elderly people can benefit from physical conditioning. They compared spontaneous recovery to formal reconditioning in 23 postcoronary bypass surgery patients and 23 control subjects. The mean age was 68 years for both groups. The training protocol was for 3 hours of activity per week for 3 months. Only the experimental groups displayed evidence of conditioning such as lowered heart rate.

Glucose tolerance deteriorates with aging (Davidson, 1979). The normal decline of activity and increase in adiposity with age adversely affect glucose metabolism. Endurance exercise has clearly been shown to reduce insulin in young people (D.S. King *et al.*, 1988; LeBlanc, Nadeau, Richard, & Tremblay, 1981) and in master athletes (Rogers, King, Hagberg, Ehsani, & Holloszy, 1990;

Seals *et al.*, 1984). Although these studies have demonstrated reduced plasma insulin in response to an oral glucose challenge, the more definitive hyperglycemic clamp procedure was not used. Kirwan, Kohrt, Wojta, Bourey, and Holloszy (1993) used this improved procedure to evaluate the effects of endurance exercise training on 12 subjects (5 men, 7 women) aged 60 to 70 years and a young normally active control group of 7 men and 5 women 23 to 26 years old. Exercise primarily entailed walking and running on an indoor track or treadmill supplemented with stationary cycling and rowing for 45 minutes, plus warm-up and cool-down, 4 days per week for 9 months. Results indicated a significant decline in plasma insulin concentration.

Uncertainty remains over the proper intensity of activity. Minor, Hewett, Webel, Anderson, and Ray (1989) noted that lower-intensity exercise programs may result in improved day-to-day functioning of patients with rheumatoid arthritis and osteoarthritis in the absence of substantial increases in maximal oxygen uptake. However, Paffenbarger and Hale (1975) studied coronary mortality among 6,351 men aged 35 to 74 years over a 22-year period or until age 75. They report that repeated *bursts* of high energy activity protects against coronary mortality. Data were analyzed in terms of Kcal per minute without reference to duration. Perhaps relatively short periods of exertion can have substantial health benefits.

Haskell (1985) observed that the general guidelines for prescribing exercise are based more on what is required to improve physical conditioning than what is necessary to prevent disease or extend longevity. Previous investigators have assumed that exercise requirements are the same for both criteria but this may not be the case. A plausible explanation is that it is easier for investigators to demonstrate improved physical conditioning than it is to demonstrate disease prevention or longevity increases. Hence, investigators choose to demonstrate the effects of exercise on physical performance. It is possible that frequent participation in low-intensity exercise has both psychological and physical benefits.

Life Extension

Goodrick (1980) reported that exercised male rats outlived their nonexercised controls by 19.3%. Exercised female rats outlived their non exercised controls by 11%. Holloszy, Smith, Vining, and Adams (1985) reported that exercised males rats outlived unexercised controls by 11.8%. Holloszy and Schechtman (1991) placed this figure at 9.6%. One problem with these studies is that exercised male rats do not increase caloric intake to compensate for exercise and therefore resemble calorie restricted animals; calorie restriction has been known since 1935 to increase life span (Holloszy, 1993). Female rats increase food intake to compensate for energy expended through activity. Therefore, Holloszy (1993) compared 60 exercised female rats with 64 sedentary controls. Exercise increased average life expectancy by about 9%. This effect was observed for every subject except for the first and last to die. The first exercised animal and first nonexercised animal to die had the same life span. The same was true for the last animal to die in both groups. They died at the same age. Hence, no increase in maximum longevity was observed. At every other rank ordered position, the exercised animal lived longer than the nonexercised animal. Consequently, exercise produces a very consistent effect.

Paffenbarger and colleagues (1986) reported that the number of years human life was extended through activity depended on the age at which subjects entered their study. Subjects entering between the ages of 35 and 39 lived 2.51 years longer if they expended 2,000 or more calories through exercise each week than if they expended less than 500 calories per week. This longevity increase reduced to 0.42 years for those who entered the study between the ages of 75 and 79. On average, activity promoted longevity for all subjects by 2.15 years. Harvard alumni are not typical of the U.S. population. Their age-specific death rates are roughly half those for White males in the United States. This fact makes the present results conservative. Samples with higher death rates may benefit considerably more through activity increases than did this healthier Harvard sample.

Quantify Recovery

Major surgery such as coronary artery bypass or hip replacement reduces activity to zero during the operation. Minor movements return during recovery as the effects of anesthesia wear off. Nursing efforts are focused toward facilitating self-care and ambulation which entail wrist and waist activity. Implementation of the Prospective Payment System (PPS) in 1984 has motivated hospital planners to identify patients who can safely be discharged early (Ensberg, Paletta, Galecki, Dacko, & Fries, 1993). Activity growth curves can be used to quantify recovery. Time to achieve preoperative activity can be predicted if baseline activity measurements are taken prior to surgery either in preparation for surgery or as part of a routine physical examination.

EXERCISE IMPROVES MENTAL HEALTH

Exercise Reduces Depression

Simons, McGowan, Epstein, Kupfer, and Robertson (1985) critically evaluated the following seven studies. Greist and colleagues (1979) divided 24 men and women aged 18 to 30 years into a running, time-limited psychotherapy and time-unlimited psychotherapy for 10 to 12 weeks. Graphic presentation of Symptom Checklist (SCL-90) results suggested significant and equivalent reductions in depression for subjects in all three groups which makes exercise as effective as psychotherapy. Greist (1984) divided 60 depressed subjects into an exercise group, relaxation group, or group therapy. After 12 weeks, SCL-90 scores again were significantly, but equally, reduced for all three groups. Doyne, Chambless, and Beutler (1983) demonstrated the antidepressive effects of exercise for 4 women using a single subject research design. Doyne, Chambless, and Beutler (1983) divided 41 women with minor depression into an 8-week exercise group and a control group. Significant reductions in Beck Depression Inventory (BDI) scores and Hamilton Rating Scale for Depression scores occurred for subjects in the exercise but not the control groups. McCann and Holmes (1984) divided 43 college women into exercise, relaxation training, and no treatment groups. BDI scores reduced significantly more for the exercisers than the other two groups. Fremont and Craighead (1984) divided 49 mildly to moderately depressed men and women aged 19 to 62 years into three groups: running, cognitive therapy, and running plus cognitive therapy for 10 weeks. Exercise was as effective as cognitive therapy and their combination in reducing depression.

Martinsen (1984) studied 49 hospitalized depressed men and women aged 17 to 60 years. All subjects received individual psychotherapy and occupational therapy. Twenty-four subjects also received exercise training. After 9 weeks, patients receiving exercise had significantly lower BDI scores than did control subjects. Unfortunately for our purposes, the oldest subject in the above-mentioned studies was 62. The antidepressive effects of exercise in the elderly remain to be demonstrated. However, Folkins and Sime (1981) evaluated theory and research relating physical fitness training to psychological variables in both normal and clinical populations and some of the reviewed studies entailed geriatric samples that evidenced improvement. Yet, Fillingim and Blumenthal (1993) reviewed studies regarding mood and neuropsychological test effects of aerobic exercise on elderly subjects and concluded that results have been inconsistent. Recommendations to improve future research include developing tests that are more sensitive to the effects of exercise.

The following biological mechanism makes it likely that running and other repetitive exercises are antidepressive for persons of all ages. B. L. Jacobs (1994) and B. L. Jacobs and Fornal (1993) reported laboratory evidence from cats showing that repetitive activity patterns release serotonin from the Raphe nuclei in the brainstem. Increasing availability of serotonin by decreasing reuptake is the way some of the more modern antidepressant medications work. Therefore, there is a known physical basis that explains how repetitive activity like running can reduce depression. This finding gives new meaning to the term *psychopharmacology*. Normally the term refers to the psychological and behavioral effects of medications. Here we suggest that repetitive activity can release additional serotonin. One can self-stimulate with serotonin by running and other repetitive behaviors such as calisthenics. This finding suggests that compulsive behaviors, including compulsive activity by anorectics, may be reinforced by the antidepressive effects of additional serotonin release.

Running is a less viable option for older than younger persons for at least two reasons. First, knee and foot problems sufficient to contraindicate running become increasingly common with age. Second, cerebellar dysfunction leading to instability increases with age. It is well known that balance is impaired with advancing age (Woollacott, 1993). As a result, risk of injury from falling increases with age. However, the fact that running appears to have its antidepressive effects through repetitive motor actions, central pattern generated activities, means that less strenuous repetitive activities may also have antidepressing characteristics. Rapidly pedaling an exercycle set to a low or moderate energy consumption level is one possibility. Movement classes emphasizing repetitive actions may be another. These movements can be performed in a pool to further reduce joint stress.

Exercise Reduces Anxiety

Exercise has been shown to reduce anxiety (Petruzzello, Landers, Hatfield, Kubitz, & Salazar, 1991) and increase perceptions of personal efficacy (Mc-Auley, Courneya, & Lettunich, 1991). McAuley (1992) reported that although self-efficacy was predictive of adherence to the early stages of an organized exercise program, previous participation was the best predictor of later adherence to an exercise program. However, 4 months after the end of an exercise program, self-efficacy was the best predictor of continued exercise (McAuley, 1993). McAuley, Lox, and Duncan (1993) conducted a 9-month follow-up study of a 5-month structured walking program with 44 (53.5%) of the 82 subjects completing the program (26 women, 18 men). Results revealed that adherence efficacy significantly predicted exercise maintenance ($r(42) = .43$, $p < .001$) and that program attendance significantly predicted efficacy ($r(42) = .42$, $p < .01$). Program attendance was associated with a lower percentage of fat ($r(42) = -.47$, $p < .001$), and a lower percentage of fat was associated with higher rate of oxygen uptake (VO_2 max) ($r(42) = -.46$, $p < .001$).

EXERCISE IMPROVES COGNITION

Clarkson-Smith and Hartley (1989) hypothesized that high-exercise persons would exceed low-exercise persons in cognition, reaction time, working memory, and reasoning ability but not vocabulary. They tested their hypothesis by interviewing and examining 300 men and women aged 55 to 91. Group assignment was made on the basis of an extensive interview covering estimated kilo calories expended per week and the number of hours per week engaging in strenuous (above 0.1 Kcal/min/kg of body weight) exercise. The high-exercise subjects expended at least 3,100 Kcal per week while the low-exercise subjects expended less than 1,900 Kcal per week. Results showed that the high-exercise group was more physically fit than the low-exercise group; they had a significantly higher vital capacity and significantly lower heart rate. Significant differences favoring the high-exercise group were found on all three reasoning tests, two of three working memory tests, and all three reaction time tests after controlling for age, education, and vocabulary scores. A small but significant difference in vocabulary favoring the high-exercise group emerged. The authors cautioned that uncontrolled differences in diet or other unmeasured variables could potentially explain the results. The decision to be active is probably correlated with several other lifestyle changes. However, it is easier to quantify activity level than other lifestyle changes. If activity level can be used as proxy for a set of health-related behaviors then high-quality activity measurements can be used to evaluate health status.

Dustman and colleagues (1984) examined the impact of 4 months of aerobic exercise training on the neuropsychological function of three groups of subjects. The aerobic exercise group consisted of nine men and four women aged 55 to 68 years. These subjects exercised at 70% to 80% of their maximum age-adjusted heart rate for individually determined periods of time that became longer over 4 months of training. An exercise control group of nine men and six women aged 55 to 70 years participated in strength and flexibility exercises. A nonexercise control group of nine men and six women aged 51 to 70 years was tested and retested. Results revealed significant improvement for the aerobic exercise but not the other two groups on the Critical Flicker Fusion, Digit Symbol, Simple Reaction Time, and Stroop Interference and Total Times.

Gerontologists are interested in separating the effects of normal aging from disease in elderly patients. This distinction is complicated by the putative relationship between activity lifestyle and cognitive performance. Hultsch and colleagues (1993) examined the relationships between self-reported activity lifestyle and cognition in 484 community-dwelling adults (293 women, 191 men) aged 55 to 86 years. Testing was completed in three 2-hour sessions. Results indicated that the Active Life Style correlated $r(482) = -.22$, $p < .001$ with semantic processing time, $r(482) = -.27$, $p < .001$ with comprehension time, $r(482) = .14$, $p < .01$ with working memory, $r(482) = .13$, $p < .01$ with vocabulary, $r(482) = .21$, $p < .001$ with verbal fluency, $r(482) = 26$, $p < .001$ with world knowledge, $r(482) = .18$, $p < .001$ with word recall, and $r(482) = .23$, $p < .001$ with text recall. Active lifestyle was also significantly correlated with education ($r(482) = .21$, $p < .001$), gender ($r(482) = .33$, $p < .001$; men more active than women), and age ($r(482) = -.20$, $p < .001$; older persons less active than younger persons). The authors conclude that "Active Life Style is a more powerful predictor of cognitive performance for the older subjects than for the middle-aged subjects" (p. P8). Effect size is illustrated by noting that adding Active Life Style to predictor equations increases explainable variance from 15% to 48%.

Stones and Kozma (1989) investigated the effects of exercise on Symbol Digit coding performance (given symbols, subjects had to identify digits) in 40 younger (mean age = 21.2 years) and 40 older (mean age = 62.9 years) as a function of energy expenditure. Subjects expending less than 1.5 Kcal/kg/day were classified as sedentary; subjects expending more than this amount were classified as nonsedentary (Stephens, Craig, & Ferris, 1986). The significant exercise effect favored older subjects. Older exercisers completed the task, on average, in 203.9 ($SD = 41.0$) seconds versus 242.3 ($SD = 63.0$) seconds for non exercisers. Younger exercisers ($M = 148.1$, $SD = 22.6$) were essentially equal to non-exercisers ($M = 145.9$, $SD = 19.6$).

Hill, Storandt, and Malley (1993) compared the cognitive performance of 87 sedentary subjects receiving 9 to 12 months of exercise with 34 matched controls aged 60 to 73 years. The experimental group tested the same at posttest on the Wechsler Memory Scale Logical Memory but control subjects tested significantly lower. The authors concluded that exercise may slow down the effects of aging on memory.

R. R. Powell (1974) studied the effects of 12 weeks of exercise on the cognitive performance of 13 male and 17 female geriatric mental patients (mean age = 69.3 yrs). Significant differences on the Progressive Matrices Test and the Wechsler Memory Scale were reported but not for the Memory-for-Designs test.

EXERCISE ADHERENCE

Dishman (1990) reported that approximately 50% of participants in supervised exercise programs drop out. Dishman (1991) critically reviewed 56 studies designed to increase or maintain exercise. He observed that most studies have not used direct measures of physical activity or fitness and therefore he questioned the validity of the findings. Self-report evidence indicates that all published behavioral and cognitive behavioral interventions produce statistically significant and clinically meaningful activity increases. Follow-up data beyond 3 months are generally unavailable.

Knapp (1988) presents a seven-point method for reducing relapse. Situations that place the person at risk for relapse are identified. Plans are made to avoid or cope with these high-risk situations. Expectancies of positive outcome are adjusted to place the consequences of not exercising in proper perspective. Alternative plans are made for vacationing and when other disruptions of normal routine are encountered. Preparation is made for the tendency to completely give up when a brief relapse occurs. The pleasure obtained from exercise is optimized. Self-defeating dialogues and images pertaining to not exercising and in favor of inactivity are blocked.

NOCTURNAL ACTIVITY

Activity assessment is normally associated with diurnal behavior but nocturnal activity is of special importance for the elderly. Inactivity is the norm during the hours that others are asleep. Short low-intensity activity episodes are not generally disruptive of other persons' sleep. However, pacing and other forms of hyperactivity are common in patients with Alzheimer's disease (AD) (Reisberg et al., 1987; Teri, Larsen, & Reifler, 1988; Winograd & Jarvik, 1986). Some demented patients walk constantly and find it difficult to remain seated if unrestrained. Although this behavior may be tolerable during the day, it is quite intolerable during the night and is an important contributing cause of caregiver burnout leading to institutionalization of the care receiver (Reisberg et al., 1987; Sanford, 1975).

SLEEP

Sleep is predominantly defined and studied in EEG terms by polysomnographers. However, Rechtschaffen (1994), a leading contributor to this field, insists that "physiological measures derive their value as indicators of sleep from their correlations with the behavioral criteria, not from any intrinsic ontological or explanatory superiority" (p. 5). He further concludes that "any scientific definition of sleep that ignores the behaviors by which sleep is generally known unnecessarily violates common understanding and invites confusion" (p. 4). Alternative methods primarily entail sleep logs and actigraphy.

Sleep logs are easy to request. However, awareness decreases over the sleep-onset period thereby depriving subjects of the cognitive resources needed to discriminate when sleep begins. The perception of sleep onset may largely be a function of auditory threshold increases blocking out normal sounds. Awakenings during the night may entail only partial consciousness. It is, therefore, not surprising that self-reports do not agree well with objective sleep indices. Carskadon and colleagues (1976) compared self-reports of sleep with polysomnography on 122 subjects over a total of 368 nights. They reported that most subjects underestimated the time slept and the number of arousals from sleep, and overestimated the time required to fall asleep.

Activity also has been used to study sleep (Tryon 1991, pp. 149–195). Some studies use bed or mattress stabilimeters to monitor motility (Kleitman, 1963, pp. 81–91; Svanborg, Larsson, Carlsson-Nordlander, & Pirskanen, 1990; Webb, 1968, pp. 11–13). Other studies determine sleep onset using active (Birell, 1983; Bonato & Ogilvie, 1989; Espie, Lindsay & Espie, 1989; Granada & Hammack, 1961; Kelley & Lichstein, 1980; Sack, Blood, Percy, & Pen, 1995; Stickgold & Hobson, 1994; Thoman, Acebo, & Lamm, 1993) or passive (Franklin, 1981; Perry & Goldwater, 1987; Viens, De Koninck, Van den Bergen, Audet, & Christ, 1988) behaviors. Actigraphy employs primarily wrist-worn computerized devices to quantify and record activity at user-specified epochs, often 1-min intervals. Tryon (1991, pp. 149–195; 1996) reviewed studies validating sleep scoring based on actigraphy. Sadeh, Hauri, Kripke, and Lavie (1995) recently reviewed the actigraphy literature and concluded that "Actigraphy provides a cost-effective method for longitudinal, natural assessment of sleep-wake patterns" (p. 300). The Standards of Practice Committee (1995) of the American Sleep Disorders Association has recently issued guidelines for the clinical use of actigraphy in evaluating and diagnosing sleep disorders on the basis of Sadeh and colleagues' (1995) review.

The wrist is the preferred site of attachment because it is more active than the waist during sleep (J. J. van Hilten, Middelkoop, Kuiper, Kramer, & Roos, 1993). Comparisons of left and right wrists have found the left wrist more active than the right (Webster, Messin, Mullaney, & Kripke, 1982), the right wrist more active than the left (Sadeh, Sharkey, & Carskadon, 1994), or both wrists equally active (J. J. van Hilten, Middelkoop, et al., 1993). Recording activity every 30 seconds, J. J. van Hilten, Middelkoop, et al. (1993) reported that when data for the dominant wrist were submitted to the sleep-wake scoring algorithm developed for the nondominant wrist, and vice versa, agreement rates ranged from 93% to 99% across all 36 subjects.

Sleep-Onset Spectrum

The one point of consistent disagreement between wrist actigraphy and PSG pertains to determination of sleep-onset latency (SOL). Some poor sleepers can lie awake quietly for about an hour prior to the onset of EEG defined Stage 1 Sleep. Wrist actigraphy identifies sleep onset much earlier. This discrepancy in SOL is fully understandable once one realizes that sleep onset is not a discrete event but entails a sequence of physiological changes over an interval of time that Ogilvie and Wilkinson (1988) and Ogilvie and Harsh (1994) refer to as the sleep-onset period (SOP). Tryon (1991) prefers the term Sleep Onset Spectrum (SOS) because it emphasizes that an orderly and predictable transitional sequence of events characterize the sleep-onset process. EEG Stage 1 sleep onset was validated using the behavioral "gold standard" that people drop handheld objects when they go to sleep because muscle tone decreases prior to EEG-defined sleeponset (cf. Blake, Gerard, & Kleitman, 1939; Perry & Goldwater,

1987; Snyder & Scott, 1972). The validational criteria for EEG Stage 1 sleep are *behavioral* and can be used to correct wrist actigraphic SOL estimates. Ogilvie, Wilkinson, and Allison (1989) instructed subjects to keep a 90-gram handheld "deadman" switch closed while awake. Decreased muscle tone associated with EEG Stage 1 sleep-onset reduced the subject's grip sufficiently to allow the switch to open.

The ability to study sleep behaviorally under natural conditions is a most welcome addition to geropsychology because sleep problems increase dramatically as a result of normal and pathological aging (Bliwise, 1994b). To be able to study sleep noninvasively under natural conditions rather than in a sleep laboratory with an array of sensors attached to the head, eye, ear, nose, chest, and legs is especially important for elderly subjects whose sleep is more easily disturbed than that of younger subjects. Wrist actigraphy affords an opportunity to better evaluate sleep variability because sleep can be studied for weeks at a time if desired. The expense of a sleep laboratory typically restricts investigations to two nights with the first night's data being discarded because of well-known first-night artifact. Van Hilten, Braat, and colleagues (1993) reported no first-night effect associated with home wrist actigraphy. The scientific advantages of wrist actigraphy for the longitudinal study of sleep and its variability extend to subjects of all ages.

Sleep and Aging

Bliwise (1993, 1994a, 1994b) reviewed changes in sleep due to normal aging and dementia. Bliwise (1994b) defined normal sleep in the aged as what occurs in persons over the age of 60 years. I confine myself to behavioral indices. Aging is associated with increased nocturnal awakenings. Sleep onset is delayed in older persons; this delay explains why they consume the preponderance of sleep medications. Elderly women are greater users of sleep medications than are elderly men reflecting their more troubled sleep. Disease and chronic illness compromise the sleep of elderly people. Excessive bedrest disrupts the sleep-wake schedule of even young people. Curtailment of daytime napping can improve nighttime sleep. Some elderly people fear dying in their sleep and are therefore afraid to go to sleep. This fear is not unfounded as people tend to be born and to die at night (Kryger, Roth, & Carskadon, 1994). Women may experience more rapid sleep deterioration than men; this implies greater dysregulation of sleep-wake cycles in women than in men. Breathing abnormalities increase with age up to at least 60 years of age. These problems can further compromise sleep. Forty-five percent of independently living persons over the age of 65 experience periodic leg movements (PLMs) during sleep, which can cause awakening.

Tune (1968) obtained sleep charts from 240 subjects for 8 weeks. Twenty men and 20 women represented six different age ranges from the 20s to the 70s. The total sleep times for these age groups decreased slightly over the first four age groups, increased slightly from age 60 to 70, and then decreased slightly after age 70.

Middelkoop and Kerkhof (1990) obtained nondominant wrist actigraphy over two consecutive days from 14 older (mean age = 71 years; 5 women, 9 men) and 21 younger (mean age = 24 years; 12 women, 9 men) subjects. All subjects were reportedly good sleepers. The only significant finding was that older subjects slept longer (mean = 489 min, SD = 44 min) than younger subjects (mean = 455 min, SD = 50 min) subjects.

Van Hilten, Braat, and colleagues (1993) used wrist actigraphy to evaluate the sleep of 99 healthy subjects (43 men, 56 women) aged 50 to 98 years over 6 successive nights sleeping in their own beds. The only significant sex effect was that women had more periods of immobility, defined as 1-min epochs of zero activity, than men. Sleep indices were consistent over all 6 nights. No first-night effect was observed like that associated with sleep laboratory study. Hence, no adaptation period seems required. No significant age differences were reported.

Kripke, Ancoli-Israel, Klauber, and Wingard (1995) reported data on 355 adults aged 40 to 64 years who underwent 3 nights of home pulse oximetry and wrist actigraphy (Actillume (tm)) recording. They found breathing disordered sleep in 5.6% of Whites (n = 285), 15.9% of Hispanics (n = 44), and 16.7% of Blacks (n = 12).

Kuo and colleagues (1995) obtained 6 nights of polysomnography from 22 women aged 59 to 79 years (mean = 68.1), and 8 men aged 63 to 78 years (mean = 70.1). They reported significantly more movement time for men than women due to a higher prevalence of sleep apnea and Periodic Limb Movements in Sleep (PLMS), a movement disorder that disrupts sleep.

Thoman and colleagues (1993) stated that polysomnography is more problematic with older than younger persons because their sleep is more fragile and more easily disrupted by attached electrodes (cf. Bliwise, 1994a). Hence, they developed a Home Monitoring System (HMS) consisting of a thin pressure-sensitive mattress pad capable of measuring respiration and voluntary movements. Four nights of motility records for 40 women aged 65 to 94 years (mean = 77.6) were scored in 30-s epochs for Time-in-Bed, Sleep Latency, Sleep Period, Sleep, Total Sleep Time, Longest Sustained Sleep Period, Wake After Sleep Onset, Frequency of Waking, Respiratory Disturbance Index, and Periodic Leg Movements while subjects slept in their own beds. No "first night" effect was found for any variable. Reliability estimates ranged from .70 to .80. No significant correlations with age emerged for any variable.

Sleep Disorders

Tryon (1991, pp. 149–195, 1996, 1997) has reviewed the applicability of actigraphy to sleep disorders in general. The following material is focused on the elderly.

Insomnia and Sleep Quality

Moran, Thompson, and Nies (1988) reviewed sleep disorders associated with aging. Sleep latency, the time taken to fall asleep, remained constant but sleep quality deteriorated with increasing age. Sleep quality deteriorates because the number of awakenings after sleep onset increase and the duration of these awakenings increase with age, resulting in less satisfying sleep. Seriously fragmented sleep is a sign of delirium in the elderly.

Pollak, Perlick, Linsner, Wenston, and Hsieh (1990) surveyed 1,855 community residents aged 65 to 98 years (mean = 75.4) and reinterviewed them at 6-month intervals over the next 3.5 years. During this time 309 respondents were placed in nursing homes. Difficulty falling asleep and maintaining sleep, and waking too early was significantly associated (χ^2 (3, $N = 736$) = 10.22, $p < .017$) with nursing home placement.

Pollak, Ford, McGuire, Vaisman, and Zendell (1995) obtained 9 consecutive days of nondominant-wrist actigraphy from 52 elder-caregivers and the persons they were giving care to. The caregivers were younger (mean age = 63.5 years) than the elders they cared for (mean age = 78.4 years), but predominantly female in both cases (54% female caregivers, 57% female elders). Results indicated that the caregivers were more active during the day than the elders but less active at night. Increased nocturnal activity on the part of elders probably reflects their impaired sleep.

Most age-related changes in sleep and estimates of sleep disorders in the elderly, such as those just mentioned, have been obtained from clinical populations (Pollak, Perlick, & Linsner, 1992). These results may not generalize to elderly persons who do not seek treatment for their sleep problems. Therefore, Pollak et al. (1992) interviewed 1,856 elderly residents residing in the Bronx, NY (cf. Pollak, Perlick, & Lisner 1986; Pollak et al., 1990) and selected 31 insomniacs and 23 age- and gender-matched control subjects to wear a wrist actigraph (PMS-8, Vitalog, Inc.) and keep a sleep diary for 14 consecutive nights. Results revealed equivalent 24-hour activity levels with significantly different patterns. However, when data above a specified threshold were analyzed, insomniacs were found to be significantly less active than controls. Imposing the threshold was equivalent to restricting data analysis from about 8:30 A.M. to almost 10:00 P.M. Insomniacs were found to be less active than controls during these times of the day. From about 2:00 A.M. until 8:00 A.M. insomniacs became up to twice as active as control subjects. The combined effect is that insomnia is associated with a difference between activity lows and highs that is smaller than that in normal control subjects. This represents a blunting of the circadian cycle.

Apnea

Svanborg and colleagues (1990) used a static-charge-sensitive bed (SCSB) to monitor respiration and ear oximetry to monitor oxygen saturation in an effort to detect obstructive sleep apnea (OSAS) in 77 patients aged 17 to 68 years (mean = 49 years) suspected of having obstructive sleep apnea syndrome. Obstructive apneas leave a special SCSB signature. Concurrent oxygen reduction confirms that breathing halted or was significantly impaired when this signature occurred. Control subjects were 17 healthy nonhabitually snoring men and women aged 15 to 58 years (mean = 36 years). Concurrent polysomnography was used as the criterion measure. Results indicated that 55 of the 77 subjects had OSAS. The SCSB plus oximetry detected all subjects with apnea: 100% sensitivity. Seven additional false-positive cases were identified for a specificity of 67%. Hence, recording behavioral movements during sleep caused by variations in respiration, along with ear oximetry, offer a cost-effective method of screening for OSAS.

Restless Legs

Flemming, Clark, Wood, and Ramirez (1994) demonstrated that leg actigraphy can reliably detect polysomnography-defined PLMS. They initially validated leg actigraphy using 39 subjects (18 men, 21 women; mean age 45.0 years) for whom 2 nights of data were collected as part of a larger polysomnography PLMS study. Using 60-s recording epochs, they reported that activity counts of 30 or more following four epochs of less than 30 counts were associated with arousal. They reported that ankle actigraphy correctly identified 87.7% of PSG-defined PLMS with a false-negative rate of 3.1% and a false-positive rate of 9.2%. The authors cross-validated their findings on 65 subjects (24 men, 41 women) of mean age 46.2 years for whom 1 night of data were available resulting in 89.7% correct identification with false-negative and false-positive rates of 2.6% and 7.7%, respectively.

Massie, Daniels, and Juszynski (1995) used Flemming and colleagues, (1994) ankle actigraphy methodology to measure PLMS in 14 healthy adults (7 men, 7 women) aged 23 to 56 years (mean = 35.2) for 3 consecutive nights while subjects slept in their own beds. No "first night" effect was found. The authors reported that 65.6% of all leg movements were below the 30-count threshold associated with arousal indicating that about one third of leg movements produced arousal.

Trenkwalder and colleagues (1995) evaluated restless legs syndrome using actigraphy and polysomnography in 32 White men and women aged 29 to 73 years. Actigraphic data revealed a time course similar to that of polysomnography in measuring response to L-dopa treatment.

Kazenwadel and colleagues (1995) described a new actigraphic method for detecting PLMs using high-resolution, high-speed recording. An accelerometer placed on the top of the foot is connected to a recording unit that digitizes the amplitude of movements on a 0 to 253 scale and integrates and records movement over each tenth of a second (10 Hz). Blocking the data into half-second epochs, the authors were able to accurately monitor PLMs in 30 subjects aged 29 to 74 years as validated by standard electromyography.

Arthritis

Lavie, Epstein, and colleagues (1992) investigated the effect of rheumatoid arthritis (RA) on sleep using 4 consecutive nights of 1-min epoch wrist activity. The experimental group consisted of 13 women (mean age = 55.8 years) outpatients diagnosed as having active classical or definite RA. Twelve healthy women (mean age = 54.6 years) served as normal controls. A third group of 9 women (mean age = 35.5 years) with chronic back pain were also studied. The results revealed that the sleep of patients with RA was clearly more fragmented than that of normal controls. The sleep of persons with chronic back pain was also more fragmented than the sleep of control subjects but not as severely fragmented as patients with RA. After controlling for age, significant between-group differences were obtained for sleep duration, sleep efficiency, mean activity level, and longest interval of continuous sleep. The clinical variable most closely associated with actigraphic recordings was degree of evening pain which was significantly correlated with activity during sleep ($r(11) = .62$, $p <$ .03), with sleep efficiency ($r(11) = -.66$, $p < .03$), and with percentage of epochs of zero activity ($r(11) = -.66$, $p < .01$). Pain during sleep was significantly correlated with the percentage of epochs of zero activity ($r(11) = -.68$, $p < .01$).

Parkinson's Disease

Van Hilten and colleagues (1994) used 6 successive nights of wrist actigraphy to evaluate the sleep of 89 nondepressive patients (50 men, 34 women) with ideopathic Parkinson's disease (PD) and 83 age-matched (mean = 66.7 years) healthy controls (38 men, 45 women). Results revealed that patients with PD had a significantly higher activity level than controls. Those PD patients with sleep complaints had a significantly higher movement index defined as the number of 1-min epochs with more than zero activity counts. The mean immobility index, number of epochs of zero activity, did not differentiate the two groups. Activity level ($r(81)= .458$, $p < .001$) was significantly correlated with levodopa use. In the 34 subjects not receiving levodopa, activity level was significantly correlated with disease severity ($r(32)= .510$, $p < .002$). Resting tremor did not influence the activity readings taken during sleep because tremor disappears during sleep.

CIRCADIAN RHYTHMS

The previous sections have focused either on daytime or nighttime activity. This section is comprehensive in that it is concerned with 24-hour activity samples. Modern actigraphy makes collecting these data very simple. Tryon and Williams (1996) describe a small, lightweight device capable of recording data every minute of the day and night for 22 days before memory is filled. Downloading and reprogramming takes just a few minutes and enables another data collection cycle. This process can be repeated indefinitely to obtain very comprehensive rest(sleep)-wake data. The subject need only wear the device. Noncompliance is easily detected by a flat line where minimal movement should be present.

Most biological functions are not constant but vary throughout the day and night (Kryger *et al.*, 1994). Temperature and activity are the two most frequently studied indices of circadian regulation in the laboratory. More research has been conducted on activity than on temperature because it is easier to continuously measure revolutions of a rodent activity wheel than it is to obtain rectal temperatures at fixed intervals. Small computerized wrist- and waist-worn actigraphs methodologically extend the activity literature to humans.

Circadian rhythms are poorly developed at birth but become much better defined during the first month or two of life (Weinert, Sitka, Minors, & Waterhouse, 1994). The newborn infant sleeps much of the time. A transition period of sleep and wake during some part of every hour is followed by consolidating sleep into a single period and wake into another period resulting in the normal sleep-wake circadian cycle by the end of the first year of life (Sadeh, 1994). Psychological circadian rhythms for subjective activation, mood, and performance efficiency also develop (Monk, 1994). Sleep remains consolidated into a single period in healthy adults. Normal aging fractionates nocturnal sleep by interspersing periods of wakefulness (Bliwise, 1993, 1994b). Napping during the day further fractionates the circadian rhythm.

The biological clock seems to be located in the suprachiasmatic nuclei (SCN) of the anterior hypothalamus (Bliwise, 1994b; Harrington, Rusak, & Mistleberger, 1994; Kryger *et al.*, 1994). Mistleberger and Rusak (1994) indicated that the human biological sleep-wake clock has a natural period of about 25 hours. This means that people naturally go to sleep about an hour later each day if isolated from all temporal cues, called *zeitgebers,* that entrain the circadian rhythm to a 24-hour solar cycle. Light is a powerful zeitgeber and can be used to phase shift circadian rhythms (Mistleberger & Rusak, 1994). Feeding animals once per day causes activity to peak at feeding time (Mistleberger & Rusak, 1994). Ablating the SCN in the rat produces ultradian sleep-wake cycles with a periodicity of 3 to 4 hours (Harrington *et al.*, 1994). The human SCN decreases in size with age especially beyond 80 years of age (Bliwise, 1994b).

Aging Effects

The effects of aging on circadian rhythm were studied by Lieberman, Wurtman, and Teicher (1989) using wrist actigraphy in 17 men aged 65 to 94 years (mean = 71.4 years) and 23 women aged 65 to 85 years (mean = 74.6 years). All were in good health and not institutionalized. A young comparison group consisted of 15 men aged 21 to 35 years (mean = 27.7 years) and 14 women aged 19 to 31 years (mean = 24.5 years). Activity was measured over 15-min epochs for 3 full days while subjects temporarily resided at the MIT Clinical Research Center to control for living conditions. A wide range of recreational opportunities were available. The results revealed that a consolidated sleep-wake circadian cycle extended into old age, the primary difference being that older persons were more active in the early morning than the young subjects. However, young men were as active as older men by midmorning and were more active by evening. Young women were less active than older women except during the evening, when they were slightly more active. Women were significantly less active than men. The most prominent effect of age was to move the time of peak activity from 1513 hours to 1326 hours. This temporal adjustment is referred to as a phase advance.

Renfrew, Pettigrew, and Rapoport (1987) used nondominant wrist actigraphy to study the circadian rhythm of 43 men aged 21 to 83 years (mean = 51.9 years) for 9 consecutive days. Three age groups were constructed. Subjects aged 21 to 39 years were classified as young ($n = 13$); those 40 to 59 years were classified as middle-aged ($n = 12$); and those 60 to 83 years old were classified as old ($n = 18$). Circadian amplitude refers to the difference between periods of highest and lowest activity. The stability of the circadian cycle is thought to be directly proportional to its amplitude (Van Gool & Mirmiran, 1986; Wever, 1979). Results revealed that the young subjects were least active at night and most active during the day (i.e., they demonstrated the greatest difference between low and high activity periods: they had the greatest circadian amplitude).

The middle-aged subjects were more active during the night and less active during the day than the other two groups. They had the smallest difference between low and high activity and therefore the lowest circadian amplitude. The old group was intermediate between the young and middle-aged subjects. Comparing just the old and the young, it was found that older subjects were more active at night and less active during the day than young subjects on both weekdays and weekends. The younger subjects began their active phase approximately 1 hour later on the weekends than during the weekdays. Older subjects kept the same schedule throughout the week.

The circadian cycle remains largely intact until late life, when it begins to fragment. Sleep problems during the night produce daytime sleepiness which leads to napping, thereby breaking the consolidated sleep-wake cycle into two or more sleep-wake cycles per day. D. Jacobs, Ancoli-Israel, Parker, and Kripke (1989) used wrist actigraphy to study the sleep-activity patterns of 19 elderly nursing home residents aged 71 to 99 years (mean = 84.4 years) for a single 24-hour period using 1-min recording epochs. Results indicated an average of 11.73 hours of sleep ($SD = 3.59$ hr). Sleep was distributed, on average, over every one of the 24 hours. The mean number of minutes asleep was approximately 15 or more of each hour. Conversely, there was no hour during which subjects were awake all of the time. Only 6 of the 19 subjects experienced even a single hour of consolidated sleep and only 3 subjects experienced 2 hours of consolidated sleep. The circadian sleep-wake cycle for these residents resembles that of the neonate and probably increases confusion regarding date and time of day. Some part of this deterioration is undoubtedly due to the effects of aging on the biological clock, SCN of the hypothalamus.

However, Witting, Kwa, Eikelenboom, Mirmiran, and Swaab (1990) used actigraphs to monitored rest-activity cycles in 13 elderly subjects (2 men, 11 women, aged 71 to 85 years), and 6 young control subjects (4 men, 2 women, aged 29 to 55 years) using wrist actigraphy for 90 to 168 hours. They reported that the rest-activity cycle of the two groups was comparable. Low statistical power may well be responsible for the lack of significant differences.

Dementia

Van Someren, Mirmiran, and Swaab (1993) conclude that deterioration of the biological clock results in a dampened circadian rhythm thereby causing several age-related problems with sleep and wakefulness. Aharon-Peretz and colleagues (1991) used actigraphs to compare the circadian rhythms of 10 patients with multi-infarct dementia (mean age = 75.6), 15 patients with Alzheimer's dementia (mean age = 72.8), and 11 age-matched healthy volunteers (mean age = 69.0) for 8 consecutive days. Analysis of variance revealed that Alzheimer and control subjects were not significantly different on any variables. However, multi-infarct dementia subjects were significantly and substantially more active and had lower sleep efficiency (minutes asleep/minutes in bed) than Alzheimer's or control subjects.

Fishbein, Ferris, and Reisberg (1995) reported a progressive circadian rhythm decline in patients with Alzheimer's dementia (AD). They used wrist actigraphy to monitor the sleep-wake cycles of 15 reliably diagnosed patients with AD (mild to severe) and 6 healthy age-matched controls for 12 consecutive days. Spectral analysis revealed that four activity cycles per 24 hours characterized the behavior of the healthy control subjects with little nocturnal activity. Five to eight activity cycles characterized the AD patients. Hence, dementia appears to increase the number of activity cycles per day. Moreover, these cycles were phase shifted to an earlier clock time. A progressive increase in nocturnal activity was observed as dementia severity increased from mild to severe. Sanford (1975) identified night wandering as an important factor leading to the institutionalization of elderly dependents.

Depression

Raoux and colleagues (1994) used 24-hour nondominant wrist actigraphy to evaluate 26 depressed inpatients before and after 4 weeks of chemotherapy. Pretreatment included two 24-hour periods before drug treatment began. Posttreatment included the final three 24-hour periods prior to discharge. Activity level improved markedly at posttreatment. No difference was found between morning and afternoon activity. Circadian amplitude increased significantly as a result of treatment, largely because of increased diurnal activity.

Sleep

Bliwise (1994a) indicated that very few studies of sleep in well-documented cases of AD exist. Lower sleep efficiency and greater frequency of arousal and awakening seemed to occur in demented compared to control subjects. The effect size appeared to closely parallel the degree of dementia.

Differential diagnosis of dementia and depression is challenging but actigraphy may be informative in this regard. Bliwise (1994a) reported that depressed subjects experienced greater sleep disturbances than did demented subjects. Nocturnal actigraphy may be able to discriminate depressed from demented subjects on the basis of the degree of sleep disruption. The main confusion on the basis of sleep data alone would be between severely demented and depressed subjects but a differential diagnosis is relatively easy in these cases using other information. The important contribution of sleep data is that they may help distinguish depression from mild dementia.

Pollak and colleagues (1995) obtained 9 consecutive days of wrist actigraphy using 30-s recording epochs on 17 demented and 52 nondemented elders and their respective caregivers. The rest-activity cycles of the demented subjects were phase shifted more than 4 hours earlier than for the nondemented subjects. The rest-activity cycle for the caregivers living with the demented subjects was phase shifted approximately 3 hours earlier than for the caregivers living with the nondemented subjects. Given that normal aging tends to phase advance the circadian cycle (Lieberman *et al.*, 1989; Renfrew *et al.*, 1987), dementia appears to emulate advanced aging.

Witting and colleagues (1990) monitored rest-activity cycles in 12 Alzheimer's disease patients (2 men, 10 women, aged 71 to 86 years), 13 elderly control subjects (2 men, 11 women, aged 71 to 85 years), and 6 young control subjects (4 men, 2 women, aged 29 to 55 years) using wrist actigraphy for 90 to 168 hours. They reported that the rest-activity cycle of the demented subjects was disturbed in direct proportion to the severity of the dementia.

Dementia is associated with personality changes including agitated behaviors (Eisendorfer *et al.*, 1992) and sleep-wake disorders (Reisberg *et al.*, 1987; Teri *et al.*, 1988; Winograd & Jarvik, 1986). These behaviors are an important contributing cause of caregiver burnout leading to institutionalization of the care receiver (Reisberg, *et al.*, 1987).

Satlin and colleagues (1991) studied the locomotor activity of 11 demented men and 8 demented women, aged 59 to 92 years (mean = 72.6 years). Eight of 19 subjects were clinically defined as "pacers." Eight healthy volunteers (5 men, 3 women) aged 67 to 75 years served as control subjects. Activity was measured using 5-min epochs over 48 to 72 hours with waist (vest)-worn actigraphs (Ambulatory Monitoring, Inc., Ardsley, NY). The results showed that pacers were 66% more active than controls whereas the remaining demented subjects were 39% less active than control subjects. Pacers' nocturnal activity was approximately four times greater than that of control subjects. This finding is similar to that reported by Teicher and colleagues (1988) for depressed geriatric patients.

The stability of the circadian cycle is thought to be directly proportional to its amplitude (Van Gool & Mirmiran, 1986; Wever, 1979). The authors evaluated circadian strength by dividing the circadian amplitude by the daily average (mesor). Although pacers had a 22% lower relative amplitude than controls, this difference was not statistically significant because of the small sample size. The acrophase, time of maximum activity, was delayed, occurring later in the day, by 126 min, 2 hr and 10 min, (3:14 P.M.) relative to control subjects (1.08 P.M.).

Ancoli-Israel, Klauber, Butters, Parker, and Kripke (1991) used wrist actigraphy and Respitrace/Medilog respiration recordings in 152 women and 83 men residing in a skilled nursing facility to show that dementia and sleep apnea are related. All residents with severe sleep apnea were also found to be severely demented. Apnea disrupts sleep and deprives one of oxygen which may exacerbate the symptoms of dementia.

Lavie, Aharon-Peretz, and colleagues (1992) compared the sleep of 10 normal controls (6 women, 4 men) aged 71.37 years on average with 10 patients (2 women, 8 men) with multi-infarct dementia of average age 76.03 years, and 12 patients (9 women, 3 men) of average age 75.06 years using four periods of 5 to 7 days of wrist actigraphy. The results indicated that only the multi-infarct dementia group showed evidence of disturbed sleep. The authors noted that the Alzheimer's patients suffered only mild dementia and that sleep disruption may occur only as dementia worsens.

Sundowning

Psychopathology disturbs normal circadian rhythm. Switches from depression to mania can drastically shorten or eliminate the sleep period at the point of transition and dramatically increase activity level (Bunney *et al.*, 1977; Tryon, 1991, pp. 65–82). Tryon (1997) discusses the role of activity in *DSM-IV* disorders. Some patients with Alzheimer's disease evidence "sundowning." This is a syndrome of confusion and agitation occurring in the late afternoon and early evening (Evans, 1987). Bliwise (1994a) reports that the most difficult part of sundowning for the caregiver is that the patient is active and noisy at night when the caretaker is trying to sleep. Sundowning is, therefore, one of the most common causes of institutionalization of demented geriatric patients.

The fact that sundowning symptoms occur at approximately the same time each day led Satlin, Volicer, Ross, Herz, and Campbell (1992) to conclude that they reflected a circadian disorder. Accordingly, the authors sought to alleviate the behavioral and sleep disturbances of patients with Alzheimer's disease using properly timed bright light. Subjects were 10 inpatients (9 men, 1 woman) aged 70.1 years on average. Most began yelling or pacing between 2 and 4 P.M. Most patients had sleep disorders and frequently napped during the day. Activity was measured with a waist (vest)-worn actigraph for 48 hours during the first and third week of the study. From 7 to 9 P.M. during the intervening week, subjects received 2 hours of bright (1500 to 2000 lux) light while seated in a geri-chair. Clinical ratings of sleep and wakefulness improved (decreased) significantly from 6.2 pretreatment to 3.0 during treatment to 2.3 posttreatment. The percentage of total daily (24-hour) activity occurring between 1:00 P.M. and 7:00 A.M. decreased significantly during treatment from 18.4% to 11.6% but then increased to 17.1% after treatment ended, indicating that light has a temporary effect on nocturnal activity. The severity of sundowning correlated $r(8) = .74$, $p < .01$ with the relative rest-activity amplitude calculated as the difference between peak and average activity. The degree of improvement was significantly correlated with initial sundowning score ($r(8) = .65$, $p < .01$) during treatment and during posttreatment ($r(8) = .77$, $p < .004$). The authors report that two Japanese studies also indicate that bright light is an effective treatment for Alzheimer's disease and multi-infarct dementia. Czeisler and colleagues (1986) report that properly timed bright light can phase shift the circadian cycle and augment its amplitude.

Teicher and colleagues (1988) used actigraphs to measure activity levels and circadian rhythms for 48 to 64 hours in eight hospitalized geriatric unipolar depressed patients and eight healthy elderly controls in a similar environment. The peak activity of depressed patients was at 3:54 P.M. versus 1:51 P.M. for control subjects ($t(14) = 4.67$, $p < .001$). The nearly 4:00 P.M. time of peak activity for depressed patients suggests that they could be mistakenly diagnosed as sundowning.

CONCLUSIONS/SUMMARY

Geropsychologists have at least five reasons for interest in physical activity. A conclusion is associated with each of these reasons.

1. Activity is a truly life-span developmental personality variable. Stable individual differences in activity level begin prenatally. All theorists and investigators recognize activity level as a primary dimension of infant temperament. Such unanimous theoretical agreement and such consistent empirical support is extremely rare in psychology. Activity level appears to reduce to a

facet of Introversion/Extroversion in adulthood primarily because it is represented by so few items on adult personality inventories. It is a well-known psychometric fact that reducing the number of items pertaining to a construct generally reduces the prominence of that construct in factor analyses. Ability to ambulate and choice of an active lifestyle assume ever greater importance as an individual difference or personality factor with increasing age. Chronic physical illness moderates the expression of personality factors with increasing age. We therefore conclude that it is appropriate for geropsychologists to examine the roots of activity differences in the elderly by obtaining naturalistic activity measurements from younger cohorts.

2. Evidence was reviewed associating activity level and physical health. The term "hypokinetic disease" coined by Kraus and Raab (1961) merits additional consideration at this time given that our population is rapidly aging and that the annual cost of medical care for many of us increases as we reach old age. O'Brien and Vertinsky's (1991) estimation that about 50% of what we currently accept as aging results from hypokinesis indicates that aging can be reduced in clinically meaningful ways. People of all ages benefit from avoiding a sedentary lifestyle. The largest risk reduction of death from all causes occurs when one moves out of the least activity category thereby demonstrating the value of even modest activity increases. We therefore conclude that it would be useful for geropsychologists to further investigate the health risks and benefits associated with objectively measured activity levels in elderly persons.

Another important contribution of actigraphy to behavioral medicine is that it may be used to quantify recovery from illness or surgery. Surgical patients have nearly zero activity levels immediately after surgery and are able to ambulate and care for themselves to a degree at discharge. Convalescence is normally associated with further activity increases. We therefore conclude that the rate and extent of return to preoperative activity level can be used as an objective marker of recovery from surgery and important illness.

3. Evidence was reviewed showing that activity apparently improves mental health by reducing depression and anxiety. Evidence was reviewed demonstrating that activity improves cognitive functioning, perhaps through increased blood flow. The paucity of research in this area leads us to conclude that it is appropriate for geropsychologists to further investigate the mental health benefits associated with increased activity in the elderly.

4. Nocturnal wandering while caretakers attempt to sleep is a major reason for institutionalization of the care receiver. Actigraphy can objectively document the extent to which nocturnal wandering occurs. Sleep disorders become increasingly common with advanced age. The possibility of longitudinal studies of sleep in the person's own home through wrist actigraphy offers geropsychologists new opportunities to learn more about normal sleep and developmental changes in sleep across the life span. The Sleep-Onset Spectrum (SOS) was described and the gradual and continuous process of going to sleep was emphasized. Poor sleepers seem to take longer to complete the sleep-onset process and older persons appear to become poorer sleepers. Contributions of actigraphy in the assessment of sleep disorders was reviewed. Hence, we conclude that geropsychologists have a clear interest in learning more about the similarities and differences of the sleep-onset process in older healthy persons compared to younger poor sleepers and in

using actigraphy to obtain the necessary longitudinal and naturalistic behavioral samples.

5. Advanced age is associated with deterioration in our biological clocks thereby producing changes in our circadian rhythm. Dementia exacerbates this deterioration. Uniform agreement exists that activity level is the second most prominent index of circadian rhythm. Core body temperature is the indicator of choice but is much more difficult to obtain over days, weeks, and months than actigraphic data which can now be provided every minute of the day and night for 22 consecutive days prior to downloading the data and beginning again. We therefore conclude that geropsychologists can advance our understanding of circadian rhythms by obtaining 2-week or longer activity records from elderly persons as they live in their natural environment.

6. Activity as a theoretical construct has long been of interest to psychologists. Empirical methods of obtaining activity data have largely been confined to self-report via questionnaire, diary, or log. These data have questionable reliability and validity primarily because they are limited by memory and compliance factors and subjects' willingness to be honest with themselves and with others. Moreover, people cannot be expected to quantify physical forces as accurately as instruments can. The technology of actigraphy has matured considerably (cf. Tryon & Williams, 1996) and now is technically feasible and cost effective. We therefore conclude that future investigators should use some type of instrument when investigating activity.

REFERENCES

Ades, P. A., Waldmann, M. L., & Gillespie, C. (1995). A controlled trial of exercise training in older coronary patients. *Journal of Gerontology: Medical Sciences, 50A,* M7–M11.

Aharon-Peretz, J., Masiah, A., Pillar, T., Epstein, R., Tzischinsky, O., & Lavie, P. (1991). Sleep-wake cycles in multi-infarct dementia and dementia of the Alzheimer type. *Neurology, 41,* 1616–1619.

Ancoli-Israel, S., Klauber, M. R., Butters, N., Parker, L., & Kripke, D. F. (1991). Dementia in institutionalized elderly: Relation to sleep apnea. *Journal of the American Geriatric Society, 39,* 258–263.

Bierman, E. L. (1978). Atherosclerosis and aging. *Federal Proceedings, 37,* 2832–2836.

Birrell, P. C. (1983). Behavioral, subjective, and electroencephalographic indices of sleep onset latency and sleep duration. *Journal of Behavioral Assessment, 5,* 179–190.

Blair, S. N., Kohl, H. W., Paffenbarger, R. S., Jr., Clark, D. G., Cooper, K. H., & Gibbons, L. W. (1989). Physical fitness and all-cause mortality: A prospective study of healthy men and women. *Journal of the American Medical Association, 262,* 2395–2401.

Blake, H., Gerard, R. W., & Kleitman, N. (1939). Factors influencing brain potentials during sleep. *Journal of Neurophysiology, 2,* 48–60.

Bliwise, D. L. (1993). Sleep in normal aging and dementia. *Sleep, 16,* 40–81.

Bliwise, D. L. (1994a). Dementia. In M. H. Kryger, T. Roth, & W. C. Dement (Eds.), *Principles and practice of sleep medicine* (2nd ed., pp. 790–800). Philadelphia: W. B. Saunders.

Bliwise, D. L. (1994b). Normal Aging. In M. H. Kryger, T. Roth, & W. C. Dement (Eds.), *Principles and practice of sleep medicine* (2nd ed., pp. 26–39). Philadelphia: W. B. Saunders.

Blumenthal, J. A., Emery, C. F., Madden, D. J., George, L. K., Coleman, R. E., Riddle, M. W., McKee, D. C., & Williams, R. S. (1989). Cardiovascular and behavioral effects of aerobic exercise training in healthy older men and women. *Journal of Gerontology: Medical Sciences, 44,* M147–M157.

Bonato, R. A., & Ogilvie, R. D. (1989). A home evaluation of a behavioral response measure of sleep/wakefulness. *Perceptual and Motor Skills, 68,* 87–96.

Bortz W. M., II. (1982). Disuse and aging. *Journal of the American Medical Association, 248,* 1203–1208.

Bouchard, C., Shepard, R. J., Stephens, T., Sutton, J. R., & McPherson, B. D. (1990). *Exercise, fitness and health.* Champaign, IL: Human Kinetics.

Bunney, W. E., Jr., Wehr, T. R., Gillin, J. C., Post, R. M., Goodwin, F. K., & van Kammen, D. P. (1977). The switch process in manic-depressive psychosis. *Annals of Internal Medicine, 87,* 319–335.

Burnside, I. M. (1978). *Working with the elderly.* North Scituate, MA: Duxbury.

Buss, A. H. & Plomin, R. (1984). *Temperament: Early developing personality traits.* Hillsdale, N.J.: Erlbaum.

Carskadon, M. A., Dement, W. C., Mitler, M. M., Guilleminault, C., Zarcone, V. P., & Spiegel, R. (1976). Self-reports versus sleep laboratory findings in 122 drug-free subjects with complaints of chronic insomnia. *American Journal of Psychiatry, 133,* 1382–1388.

Clarkson-Smith, L., & Hartley, A. A. (1989). Relationships between physical exercise and cognitive abilities in older adults. *Psychology and Aging, 4,* 183–189.

Colvin, R. H., & Olson, S. B. (1983). A descriptive analysis of men and women who have lost significant weight and are highly successful at maintaining the loss. *Addictive Behaviors, 8,* 287–295.

Costa, P. T., Jr. & McCrae, R. R. (1980). Still stable after all these years: Personality as a key to some issues in adulthood and old age. In. P. B. Baltes & O. G. Brim (Eds.), *Life-span development and behavior* (pp. 65–102). New York: Academic.

Costa, P. T., Jr. & McCrae, R. R. (1992). *Revised NEO Personality Inventory (NEO PI-R) and NEO Five-Factor Inventory (NEO-FFI): Professional manual.* Odessa, FL: Psychological Assessment Resources.

Costa, P. T., Jr., & McCrae, R. R. (1994). Stability and change in personality from adolescence through adulthood. In C. F. Halverson, Jr., G. A. Kohnstamm, & R. P. Martin (Eds.), *The developing structure of temperament and personality from infancy to adulthood* (pp. 139–150). Hillsdale, NJ: Erlbaum.

Cunningham, D. A., Rechnitzer, P. A., Howard, J. H., & Donner, A. P. (1987). Exercise training of men at retirement: A clinical trial. *Journals of Gerontology, 42,* 17–23.

Czeisler, C. A., Allan, J. S., Strogatz, S. H., Ronda, J. M., Sanchez, R., Rios, C. D., Freitag, W. O., Richardson, G. S., & Kronauer, R. E. (1986). Bright light resets the human circadian pacemaker independent of the timing of the sleep-wake cycle. *Science, 233,* 667–671.

Davidson, M. B. (1979). The effect of aging on carbohydrate metabolism: A review of the English literature and a practical approach to the diagnosis of diabetes mellitus in the elderly. *Metabolism, 28,* 688–705.

deVries, H. A. (1983). Physiology of exercise and aging. In D. S. Woodruff & J. E. Birren (Eds.), *Aging* (2nd ed., pp. 285–304). New York: Van Nostrand.

Dishman, R. K. (1990). Determinants of participation in physical activity. In C. Bouchard, R. J., Shephard, T. Stephens, J. R. Sutton, & B. D. McPherson (Eds.), *Exercise, fitness and health* (pp. 75–102). Champaign, IL: Human Kinetics.

Dishman, R. K. (1991). Increasing and maintaining exercise and physical activity. *Behavior Therapy, 22,* 345–378.

Doyne, E. J., Chambless, D. L., & Beutler, L. E. (1983). Aerobic exercise as a treatment for depression in women. *Behavior Therapy, 14,* 434–440.

Dustman, R. E., Ruhling, R. O., Russell, E. M., Shearer, D. E., Bonekat, H. W., Shigeoka, J. W., Wood, J. S., & Bradford, D. C. (1984). Aerobic exercise training and improved neuropsychological function of older individuals. *Neurobiology of Aging, 5,* 35–42.

Eaton, W. O., & Saudino, K. J. (1992). Prenatal activity level as a temperament dimension? Individual differences and developmental functions in fetal movement. *Infant Behavior and Development, 15,* 57–70.

Eisendorfer, C., Cohen, D., Paveza, G. J., Ashford, J. W., Luchins, D. J., Gorelick, P. B., Hirschman, R. S., Freels, S. A., Levy, P. S., Semla, T. P., & Shaw, H. A. (1992). An empirical evaluation of the Global Deterioration Scale for staging Alzheimer's disease. *American Journal of Psychiatry, 140,* 190–194.

Ensberg, M. D., Paletta, M. J., Galecki, A. T., Dacko, C. L., & Fries, B. E. (1993). identifying elderly patients for early discharge after hospitalization for hip fracture. *Journal of Gerontology: Medical Sciences, 48,* M187–M195.

Espie, C. A., Lindsay, W. R., & Espie, L. C. (1989). Use of the sleep assessment device (Kelley and Lichstein, 1980) to validate insomniacs' self-report of sleep pattern. *Journal of Psychopathology and Behavioral Assessment, 11,* 71–79.

Evans, L. K. (1987). Sundown syndrome in institutionalized elderly. *Journal of the American Geriatric Society, 35,* 101–108.

Fillingim, R. B., & Blumenthal, J. A. (1993). Psychological effects of exercise among the elderly. In P. Seraganian (Ed.), *Exercise psychology: The influence of physical exercise on psychological processes* (pp. 237–253). New York: Wiley.

Fishbein, W., Ferris, S., & Reisberg, B. (1995). Progressive circadian rhythm decline in Alzheimer's disease. *Sleep Research, 24,* 519.

Fleming, J., Clark, C., Wood, C., & Ramirez, C. (1994). Leg actigraphy reliably detects Periodic Limb Movements during sleep. *Sleep Research, 23,* 437.

Folkins, C. H., & Sime, W. E. (1981). Physical fitness training and mental health. *American Psychologist, 36,* 373–389.

Fox S. M., III, Naughton, J. P., & Haskell, W. L. (1971). Physical activity and the prevention of coronary heart disease. *Annals of Clinical Research, 3,* 404–432.

Franklin, J. (1981). The measurement of sleep onset latency in insomnia. *Behaviour Research and Therapy, 19,* 547–549.

Fremont, J., & Craighead, L. W. (1984). *Aerobic exercise and cognitive therapy for mild/moderate depression.* Presented at the Association for Advancement of Behavior Therapy, Philadelphia.

Gerety, M. B., Mulrow, C. D., Tuley, M. R., Hazuda, H. P., Lichtenstein, M. J., Bohannon, R., Katen, D. N., O'Neil, M. G., & Gorton, A. (1993). Development and validation of a physical performance instrument for the functionally impaired elderly: The physical disability index (PDI). *Journal of Gerontology: Medical Sciences, 48,* M33–M38.

Gibson, G. E., & Peterson, C. (1982). Biochemical and behavioral parallels in aging and hypoxia. In E. Giacobini, G. Filogamo, G. Giacobini, & A. Vernadakis (Eds.), *The aging brain: Cellular and molecular mechanisms of aging in the nervous system* (pp. 107–122). New York: Raven.

Goldsmith, H. H., Buss, A. H., Plomin, R., Rothbart, M. K., Thomas, A., Chess, S., Hinde, R. A., & McCall, R. B. (1987). Roundtable: What is temperament? Four approaches. *Child Development, 58,* 505–529.

Goodrick, C. L. (1980). Effects of long-term voluntary wheel exercise on male and female Wistar rats. *Gerontology, 26,* 22–33.

Granada, A. M., & Hammack, J. T. (1961). Operant behavior during sleep. *Science, 133,* 1485–1486.

Greist, J. H. (1984). Exercise in the treatment of depression. *Coping with mental stress: The potential and limits of exercise intervention.* Washington, DC: NIMH Workshop.

Greist, J. H., Klein, M. H., Eischens, R. R., Faris, J., Gurman, A. S., & Morgan, W. P. (1979). Running as treatment for depression. *Comprehensive Psychiatry, 20,* 41–54.

Gueldner, S. H., & Spradley, J. (1988). Outdoor walking lowers fatigue. *Journal of Gerontological Nursing, 14,* 6–12.

Guralnik, J. M., & Simonsick, E. M. (1993). Physical disability in older Americans. *Journals of Gerontology, 48,* 3–10.

Guralnik, J. M., Simonsick, E. M., Ferrucci, L., Glynn, R. J., Berkman, L. F., Blazer, D. G., Scherr, P. A., & Wallace, R. B. (1994). A short physical performance battery assessing lower extremity function: Association with self-reported disability and prediction of mortality and nursing home admission. *Journal of Gerontology: Medical Sciences, 49,* M85–M94.

Harrington, M. E., Rusak, B., & Mistleberger, R. E. (1994). Anatomy and physiology of the mammalian circadian system. In M. H. Kryger, T. Roth, & W. C. Dement (Eds.), *Principles and practice of sleep medicine* (2nd ed., pp. 286–300). Philadelphia: Saunders.

Haskell, W. L. (1985). Physical activity and health: Need to define the required stimulus. *American Journal of Cardiology, 55,* 4D–9D.

Hill, R. D., Storandt, M., & Malley, M. (1993). The impact of long-term exercise training on psychological function in older adults. *Journal of Gerontology: Psychological Sciences, 48,* P12–P17.

Hoiberg, A., Bernard, S., Watten, R. H., & Caine, C. (1984). Correlates of weight loss in treatment and at follow-up. *International Journal of Obesity, 8,* 457–465.

Holloszy, J. O. (1993). Exercise increases average longevity of female rats despite increased food intake and no growth retardation. *Journal of Gerontology: Biological Sciences, 48,* B97–B100.

Holloszy, J. O., & Schechtman, K. B. (1991). Interaction between exercise and food restriction: Effects on longevity of male rats. *Journal of Applied Physiology, 70,* 1529–1535.

Holloszy, J. O., Smith, E. K., Vining, M., & Adams, S. A. (1985). Effect of voluntary exercise on longevity of rats. *Journal of Applied Physiology, 59,* 826–831.

Hultsch, D. F., Hammer, M., & Small, B. J. (1993). Age differences in cognitive performance in later life: Relationships to self-reported health and activity life style. *Journal of Gerontology: Psychological Sciences, 48,* P1–P11.

Jacobs, B. L. (1994). Serotonin, motor activity and depression-related disorders. *American Scientist, 82,* 456–463.

Jacobs, B. L., & Fornal, C. A. (1993). 5-HT and motor control: A hypothesis. *Trends in Neuroscience, 16,* 346–352.

Jacobs, D., Ancoli-Israel, S., Parker, L., & Kripke, D. F. (1989). Twenty-four-hour sleep-wake patterns in a nursing home population. *Psychology and Aging, 4,* 352–356.

Joseph, J. A., & Roth, G. S. (1988). Upregulation of striatal dopamine receptors and improvement of motor performance in senescence. In J. A. Joseph (Ed.), *Central determinants of age-related declines in motor function. Annals of the New York Academy of Science, 15,* 355–362.

Joseph, J. A., & Roth, G. S. (1993). Hormonal regulation of motor behavior in senescence. *Journals of Gerontology, 48* (Special Issue), 51–55.

Kagan, J., & Snidman, N. (1991). Temperamental factors in human development. *American Psychologist, 46,* 856–862.

Kazenwadel, J., Pollmächer, T., Trenkwalder, C., Oertel, W. H., Kohnen, R., Künzel, M., & Krüger, H.-P. (1995). New actigraphic assessment method for periodic leg movements (PLM). *Sleep, 18,* 689–697.

Kelley, J. E., & Lichstein, K. L. (1980). A sleep assessment device. *Behavioral Assessment, 2,* 135–146.

King, A. C., Taylor, C. B., Haskell, W. L., & DeBusk, R. F. (1989). Influence of regular aerobic exercise on psychological health: A randomized, controlled trial of healthy middle-aged adults. *Health Psychology, 8,* 305–324.

King, D. S., Dalsky, G. P., Clutter, W. E., Young, D. A., Staten, M. A., Cryer, P. E., & Holloszy, J. O. (1988). Effects of exercise and lack of exercise on insulin secretion. *American Journal of Physiology, 254,* E537–E542.

Kirwan, J. P., Kohrt, W. M., Wojta, D. M., Bourey, R. E., & Holloszy, J. O. (1993). Endurance exercise training reduces glucose-stimulated insulin levels in 60- to 70-year-old men and women. *Journal of Gerontology: Medical Sciences, 48,* M84–M90.

Kleitman, N. (1963). *Sleep and wakefulness.* Chicago: University of Chicago Press.

Knapp, D. N. (1988). Behavioral management techniques and exercise promotion. In R. K. Dishman (Ed.), *Exercise adherence: Its impact on public health* (pp. 203–235). Champaign, IL: Human Kinetics.

Kraus, H., & Raab, W. (1961). *Hypokinetic disease.* Springfield, IL: Thomas.

Kripke, D. F., Ancoli-Israel, S., Klauber, M. R., & Wingard, D. L. (1995). U.S. population estimate for disordered sleep breathing: High rates in minorities. *Sleep Research, 24,* 268.

Kryger, M. H., Roth, T., & Carskadon, M. (1994). circadian rhythms in humans: An overview. In M. H. Kryger, T. Roth, & W. C. Dement (Eds.), *Principles and practice of sleep medicine* (2nd ed., pp. 301–308). Philadelphia: Saunders.

Kuo, T. F., Bootzin, R. R., Bell, I. R., Wyatt, J. K., Rider, S. P., & Anthony, J. L. (1995). Normative sleep characteristics in the elderly: A six-night PSG study. *Sleep Research 24,* 125.

Lavie, P., Aharon-Peretz, J., Klein, F., Gruner, F., Epstein, R., Tzischinsky, O., & Herer, P. (1992). Sleep quality in geriatric depressed patients: Comparison with elderly demented patients and normal controls and the effects of Moclobemide. *Dementia, 3,* 360–366.

Lavie, P., Epstein, R., Tzischinsky, O., Gilad, D., Nahir, M., Lorber, M., & Scharf, Y. (1992). Actigraphic measurements of sleep in rheumatoid arthritis: Comparison of patients with low back pain and healthy controls. *Journal of Rheumatology, 19,* 362–365.

LeBlanc, J., Nadeau, A., Richard, D., & Tremblay, A. (1981). Studies on the sparing effect of exercise on insulin requirements in human subjects. *Metabolism, 30,* 1119–1124.

Leon, A. S., Connett, J., Jacobs, D. R., Jr., & Rauramaa, R. (1987). Leisure-time physical activity levels and risk of coronary heart disease and death. *Journal of the American Medical Association, 258,* 2388–2395.

Lieberman, H. R., Wurtman, J. J., & Teicher, M. H. (1989). Circadian rhythms of activity in healthy young and elderly humans. *Neurobiology of Aging, 10,* 259–265.

Magnus, K., Matroos, A., & Strackee, J. (1979). Walking, cycling, or gardening, with or without seasonal interruption, in relation to acute coronary events. *American Journal of Epidemiology, 110,* 724–733.

Manton, K. G., Stallard, E., & Liu, K. (1993). Forecasts of active life expectancy: Policy and fiscal implications. *Journals of Gerontology, 48* (Special Issue), 11–26.

Marston, A. R., & Criss, J. (1984). Maintenance of successful weight loss: Incidence and prediction. *International Journal of Obesity, 8,* 435–439.

Martinsen, E. W. (1984). Interaction of exercise and medication in the psychiatric patient. *Coping with mental stress: The potential and limits of exercise intervention.* Washington, DC: NIMH Workshop.

Massie, C., Daniels, R., & Juszynski, G. (1995). Leg actigraphy: Preliminary normative data. *Sleep Research, 24,* 284.

McAuley, E. (1992). The role of efficacy cognitions in the prediction of exercise behavior in middle-aged adults. *Journal of Behavioral Medicine, 15,* 65–88.

McAuley, E. (1993). Self-efficacy and the maintenance of exercise participation in older adults. *Journal of Behavioral Medicine, 16,* 103–113.

McAuley, E., Courneya, K. S., & Lettunich, J. (1991). Effects of acute and long-term exercise on self-efficacy responses in sedentary, middle-aged males and females. *Gerontologist, 31,* 534–542.

McAuley, E., Lox, C., & Duncan, T. E. (1993). Long-term maintenance of exercise, self-efficacy, and physiological change in older adults. *Journal of Gerontology: Psychological Sciences, 48,* P218–P224.

McCann, I. L., & Holmes, D. S. (1984). Influence of aerobic exercise on depression. *Journal of Personality and Social Psychology, 46,* 1142–1147.

Middlekoop, H. A. M., & Kerkhof, G. A. (1990). Nocturnal wrist motor activity and subjective sleep quality in young and elderly subjects. *Journal of Interdisciplinary Cycle Research, 21,* 218–219.

Minor, M. A., Hewett, J. E., Webel, R. R., Anderson, S. K., & Ray, D. R. (1989). Efficacy of physical conditioning exercise in patients with rheumatoid arthritis and osteoarthritis. *Arthritis and Rheumatism, 32,* 1396–1405.

Mintz, A. Y., & Mankovsky, N. B. (1971). Changes in the nervous system during cerebral atherosclerosis and aging. *Geriatrics, 26,* 134–144.

Mistleberger, R. E., & Rusak, B. (1994). Circadian rhythms in mammals: Formal properties and environmental influences. In M. H. Kryger, T. Roth, & W. C. Dement (Eds.), *Principles and practice of sleep medicine* (2nd ed., pp. 277–285). Philadelphia: Saunders.

Monk, T. H. (1994). Circadian rhythms in subjective activation, mood, and performance efficiency. In M. H. Kryger, T. Roth, & W. C. Dement (Eds.), *Principles and practice of sleep medicine* (2nd ed., pp. 321–330). Philadelphia: Saunders.

Moran, M. G., Thompson, T. L., & Nies, A. S. (1988). Sleep disorders in the elderly. *American Journal of Psychiatry, 145,* 1369–1378.

Morris, J. N., Chave, S. P. W., Adam, C., Sirey, C., Epstein, L., & Sheehan, D. J. (1973). Vigorous exercise in leisure-time and the incidence of coronary heart-disease. *Lancet, 1,* 333–339.

Morris, J. N., Everitt, M. G., Pollard, R., Chave, S. P. W., & Semmence, A. M. (1980). Vigorous exercise in leisure-time: Protection against coronary heart disease. *Lancet, 2,* 1207–1210.

Oberman, A. (1985). Exercise and the primary prevention of cardiovascular disease. *American Journal of Cardiology, 55,* 10D–20D.

O'Brien, S. J., & Vertinsky, P. A. (1991). Unfit survivors: Exercise as a resource for aging women. *Gerontologist, 31,* 347–357.

Ogilvie, R. D., & Harsh, J. R. (1994). *Sleep onset: Normal and abnormal processes.* Washington, DC: American Psychological Association.

Ogilvie, R. D., & Wilkinson, R. T. (1988). Behavioral versus EEG-based monitoring of all-night sleep-wake patterns. *Sleep, 11,* 139–155.

Ogilvie, R. D., Wilkinson, R. T., & Allison, S. (1989). The detection of sleep onset: Behavioral, physiological, and subjective convergence. *Sleep, 12,* 458–474.

Paffenbarger, R. S., Jr. & Hale, W. E. (1975). Work activity and coronary heart mortality. *New England Journal of Medicine, 292,* 545–550.

Paffenbarger, R. S., Jr., & Hyde, R. T. (1984). Exercise in the prevention of coronary heart disease. *Preventive Medicine, 13,* 3–22.

Paffenbarger, R. S., Jr., Wing, A. L., & Hyde, R. T. (1978). Physical activity as an index of heart attack risk in college alumni. *American Journal of Epidemiology, 108,* 161–175.

Paffenbarger, R. S., Jr., Hyde, R. T., Wing, A. L., & Steinmetz, C. H. (1984). A natural history of athleticism and cardiovascular health. *Journal of the American Medical Association, 252,* 491–495.

Paffenbarger, R. S., Jr., Hyde, R. T., Wing, A. L., & Hsieh, C. C. (1986). Physical activity, all-cause mortality, and longevity of college alumni. *New England Journal of Medicine, 314,* 605–613.

Palmore, E. (1970). Health practices and illness among the aged. *Gerontologist, 10,* 313–316.

Perry, T. J., & Goldwater, B. C. (1987). A passive behavioral measure of sleep onset in high-alpha and low-alpha subjects. *Psychophysiology, 24,* 657–665.

Petruzzello, S. J., Landers, D. M., Hatfield, B. D., Kubitz, K. A., & Salazar, W. (1991). A meta-analysis on the anxiety-reducing effects of acute and chronic exercise. *Sports Medicine, 11,* 143–182.

Pollak, C. P., Perlick, D., & Linsner, J. P. (1986). Sleep in the elderly: Survey of an urban community. *Sleep Research, 15,* 54.

Pollak, C. P., Perlick, D., Linsner, J. P., Wenston, J., & Hsieh, F. (1990). Sleep problems in the community elderly as predictors of death and nursing home placement. *Journal of Community Health, 15,* 123–135.

Pollak, C. P., Perlick, D., & Linsner, J. P. (1992). Daily sleep reports and circadian rest-activity cycles of elderly community residents with insomnia. *Biological Psychiatry, 32,* 1019–1027.

Pollak, C. P., Ford, T., McGuire, P. J., Vaisman, S., & Zendell, S. (1995). Motor activity of community elders and their caregivers. *Sleep Research, 24,* 536.

Powell, K. E., Thompson, P. D., Caspersen, C. J., & Kendrick, J. S. (1987). Physical activity and the incidence of coronary heart disease. *Annual Review of Public Health, 8,* 253–287.

Powell, R. R. (1974). Psychological effects of exercise therapy upon institutionalized geriatric mental patients. *Journals of Gerontology, 29,* 157–161.

Raoux, N., Benoit, O., Dantchev, N., Denise, P., Franc, B., Allilaire, J. F., & Widlocher, D. (1994). Circadian pattern of motor activity in major depressed patients undergoing antidepressant therapy: Relationship between actigraphic measures and clinical course. *Psychiatry Research, 52,* 85–98.

Rechtschaffen, A. (1994). Sleep onset: Conceptual issues. In R. D. Ogilvie & J. R. Harsh (Eds.), *Sleep onset: Normal and abnormal processes* (pp. 3–17). Washington, DC: American Psychological Association.

Redwood, D. R., Rosing, D. R., & Epstein, S. E. (1972). Circulatory and symptomatic effects of physical training in patients with coronary artery diseases and angina pectoris. *New England Journal of Medicine, 286,* 959–965.

Reisberg, B., Borenstein, J., Salob, S. P., Ferris, S. H., Frannsen, E., & Georgotas, A. (1987). Behavioral symptoms in Alzheimer's disease: Phenomenology and treatment. *Journal of Clinical Psychiatry, 48,* 9–15.

Renfrew, J. W., Pettigrew, K. D., & Rapoport, S. I. (1987). Motor activity and sleep duration as a function of age in healthy men. *Physiology and Behavior, 41,* 627–634.

Rogers, M. A., King, D. S., Hagberg, J. M., Ehsani, A. A., & Holloszy, J. O. (1990). Effect of 10 days of inactivity on glucose tolerance in master athletes. *Journal of Applied Physiology, 68,* 1833–1837.

Rosnow, I., & Breslau, N. (1966). A Guttman health scale for the aged. *Journals of Gerontology, 21,* 556–559.

Sack, R. L., Blood, M. L., Percy, D. L., & Pen, J. C. (1995). A comparison of sleep onset latency measured by PSG, actigraphy and behavioral response. *Sleep Research, 24,* 540.

Sadeh, A. (1994). Assessment of intervention for infant night waking: Parental reports and activity-based home monitoring. *Journal of Consulting and Clinical Psychology, 62,* 63–68.

Sadeh, A., Sharkey, K., & Carskadon, M. A. (1994). Activity-based sleep-wake identification: An empirical test of methodological issues. *Sleep, 17,* 201–207.

Sadeh, A., Hauri, P. J., Kripke, D. F., & Lavie, P. (1995). The role of actigraphy in the evaluation of sleep disorders. *Sleep, 18,* 288–302.

Salonen, J. T., Puska, P., & Tuomilehto, J. (1982). Physical activity and risk of myocardial infarction, cerebral stroke and death: A Longitudinal study in eastern Finland. *American Journal of Epidemiology, 115,* 526–537.

Sanford, J. R. A. (1975). Tolerance of debility in elderly dependents by supporters at home: Its significance for hospital practice. *British Medical Journal, 23,* 471–473.

Satlin, A., Teicher, M. H., Lieberman, H. R., Baldessarini, R. J., Volicer, L., & Rheaume, Y. (1991). Circadian locomotor activity in Alzheimer's disease. *Neuropsychopharmacology, 5,* 115–126.

Satlin, A., Volicer, L., Ross, V., Herz, L., & Campbell, S. (1992). Bright light treatment of behavioral and sleep disturbances in patients with Alzheimer's disease. *American Journal of Psychiatry, 149,* 1028–1032.

Seals, D. R., Hagberg, J. M., Allen, W. K., Hurley, B. F., Dalsky, G. P., Ehsani, A. A., & Holloszy, J. O. (1984). Glucose tolerance in young and older athletes and sedentary men. *Journal of Applied Physiology, 56,* 1521–1525.

Sidney, K. H., & Shephard, R. J. (1977). Activity patterns of elderly men and women. *Journals of Gerontology, 32,* 25–32.

Simons, A. D., McGowan, C. R., Epstein, L. H., Kupfer, D. J., & Robertson, R. J. (1985). Exercise as a treatment for depression: An update. *Clinical Psychology Review, 5,* 553–568.

Siu, A. L., Hays, R. D., Ouslander, J. G., Osterwell, D., Valdez, R. B., Krynski, M., & Gross, A. (1993). Measuring functioning and health in the very old. *Journal of Gerontology: Medical Sciences, 48,* M10–M14.

Slattery, M. L., Schumacher, M. C., Smith, K. R., West, D. W., & Abd-Elghany, N. (1988). Physical activity, diet, and risk of colon cancer in Utah. *American Journal of Epidemiology, 128,* 989–999.

Slattery, M. L., Jacobs, D. R., Jr., & Nichaman, M. Z. (1989). Leisure time physical activity and coronary heart disease death: The US railroad study. *Circulation, 79,* 304–311.

Snyder, F., & Scott, J. (1972). The psychology of sleep. In N. S. Greenfield & R. A. Sternback (Eds.), *Handbook of psychophysiology* (pp. 645–708). Toronto, Ontario, Canada: Holt, Rinehart and Winston.

Standards of Practice Committee. (1995). Practice parameters for the use of actigraphy in the clinical assessment of sleep disorders. *Sleep, 18,* 285–287.

Stephens, T., Craig, C. L., & Ferris, B. F. (1986). Adult physical fitness in Canada: Findings from the Canada Fitness Survey 1. *Canadian Journal of Public Health, 77,* 285–290.

Stickgold, R., & Hobson, J. A. (1994). Home monitoring of sleep onset and sleep-onset mentation using the Nightcap (tm). In R. D. Ogilvie & J. R. Harsh (Eds.), *Sleep onset: normal and abnormal processes* (pp. 141–160). Washington, DC: American Psychological Association.

Stones, M. J., & Kozma, A. (1989). Age, exercise, and coding performance. *Psychology and Aging, 4,* 190–194.

Svanborg, E., Larsson, H., Carlsson-Nordlander, B., & Pirskanen, R. (1990). A limited diagnostic investigation for obstructive sleep apnea syndrome. *Chest, 98,* 1341–1345.

Teicher, M. H., Lawrence, J. M., Barber, N. I., Finklestein, S. P., Lieberman, H. R., & Baldessarini, R. J. (1988). Increased activity and phase delay in circadian motility rhythms in geriatric depression. *Archives of General Psychiatry, 45,* 913–917.

Teri, L., Larsen, E. B., & Reifler, B. V. (1988). Behavioral disturbance in dementia of Alzheimer's type. *Journal of the American Geriatric Society, 36,* 1–6.

Thoman, E. B., Acebo, C., & Lamm, S. (1993). Stability and instability of sleep in older persons recorded in the home. *Sleep, 16,* 578–585.

Trenkwalder, C., Stiasny, K., Pollmächer, T., Wetter, Th., Schwarz, J., Kohnen, R., Kazenwadel, J., Krüger, H. P., Ramm, S., Kunzel, M., & Oertel, W. H. (1995). L-dopa therapy of uremic and ideopathic restless legs syndrome: A double-blind, crossover trial. *Sleep, 18,* 681–688.

Tryon, W. W. (1985). The measurement of human activity. In W. W. Tryon (Ed.), *Behavioral assessment in behavioral medicine* (pp. 200–256). New York: Springer.

Tryon, W. W. (1993). The role of motor excess and instrumented activity measurement in Attention-Deficit Hyperactivity Disorder. *Behavior Modification, 17,* 371–406.

Tryon, W. W. (1996). Nocturnal activity and sleep assessment. *Clinical Psychology Review, 16,* 197–213.

Tryon, W. W. (1997). Motor Activity and *DSM-IV.* In S. M. Turner & M. Hersen (Eds.), *Adult psychopathology and diagnosis* (3rd ed., pp.547–577). New York: Wiley.

Tryon, W. W., & Williams, R. (1996). Fully proportional actigraphy: A new instrument. *Behavior Research Methods Instruments & Computers, 28,* 392–403.

Tune, G. S., (1968). Sleep and wakefulness in normal human adults. *British Medical Journal, 2,* 269–271.

Van Gool, W. A., & Mirmiran, M. (1986). Aging and circadian rhythms. *Progress in Brain Research, 70,* 255–277.

van Hilten, B., Hoff, J. I., Huub, A. M., Middelkoop, M. A., van der Velde, E. A., Kerkhof, G. A., Wauquier, A., Kamphuisen, H. A. C., & Roos, R. A. C. (1994). Sleep disruption in Parkinson's disease. *Archives of Neurology, 51,* 922–928.

van Hilten, J. J., Braat, E. A. M., van der Velde, E. A., Middelkoop, H. A. M., Kerhof, G. A., & Kamphuisen, H. A. C. (1993). Ambulatory activity monitoring during sleep: An evaluation of internight and intrasubject variability in healthy persons aged 50–98 years. *Sleep, 16,* 146–150.

van Hilten, J. J., Middelkoop, H. A. M., Kuiper, S. I. R., Kramer, C. G. S., & Roos, R. A. C. (1993). Where to record motor activity: An evaluation of commonly used sites of placement for activity monitors. *Electroencephalography and Clinical Neurophysiology, 89,* 359–362.

van Someren, E. J. W., Mirmiran, M., & Swaab, D. F. (1993). Non-pharmacological treatment of sleep and wake disturbances in aging and Alzheimer's disease: Chronobiological perspectives. *behavioral Brain Research, 57,* 235–253.

Viens, M., De Koninck, J., Van den Bergen, R., Audet, R., & Christ, G. (1988). A refined switch-activated time monitor for the measurement of sleep-onset latency. *Behaviour Research and Therapy, 26,* 271–273.

Wallace, J. E., Krauter, E., & Campbell, E. (1980). Motor and reflexive behavior in the aging rat. *Journals of Gerontology, 35,* 364–370.

Webb, W. B. (1968). *Sleep: An experimental approach.* New York: Macmillan.

Webster, J. B., Messin, S., Mullaney, D. J., & Kripke, D. F. (1982). Transducer design and placement for activity recording. *Medical & Biological Engineering & Computing, 20,* 741–744.

Weinert, D., Sitka, U., Minors, D. S., & Waterhouse, J. M. (1994). The development of circadian rhythmicity in neonates. *Early Human Development, 36,* 117–126.

Westover, S. A., & Lanyon, R. I. (1990). The maintenance of weight loss after behavioral treatment. *Behavior Modification, 14,* 123–137.

Wever, R. A. (1979). *The circadian system of man: Results of experiments under temporal isolation.* New York: Springer-Verlag.

Winograd, C. H., & Jarvik, L. F. (1986). Physician management of the demented patient. *Journal of the American Geriatric Society, 34,* 295–308.

Witting, W., Kwa, I. H., Eikelenboom, P., Mirmiran, M., & Swaab, D. F. (1990). Alterations in the circadian rest-activity rhythm in aging and Alzheimer's disease. *Biological Psychiatry, 27,* 563–572.

Woollacott, M. H. (1993). Age-related changes in posture and movement. *Journals of Gerontology, 48* (Special Issue), 56–60.

Zuckerman, M. (1991). *Psychobiology of personality.* Cambridge, England: Cambridge University Press.

CHAPTER 25

Approaches to Diagnosis and Treatment of Elder Abuse and Neglect

RONALD D. ADELMAN, HENNA SIDDIQUI,
AND NANCY FOLDI

INTRODUCTION

A 1991 congressional report estimated that each year 1.5 to 2 million older people are physically injured, psychologically mistreated, financially exploited, or neglected by family members (U.S. Congress, House Select Committee on Aging, 1991). Because much of this abuse and neglect occurs between spouses, this phenomenon must be viewed in the context of domestic violence, and much of it constitutes criminal offenses.

Elder abuse and neglect has been called a silent epidemic. Often, the elderly victim is reluctant to divulge mistreatment due to overwhelming feelings of shame and fear. It is highly probable that many older victims are never discovered. Indeed, some estimate that only 1 in 14 elder abuse or neglect cases is actually reported to a public agency (*American Medical Association Diagnostic and Treatment Guidelines on Elder Abuse and Neglect*, 1992). Given the present incidence of mistreatment and the projected growth of the older population, it is crucial that health care providers for the elderly learn to recognize and intervene on behalf of victimized older people. However, it must be recognized that the information base about abuse and neglect of older persons is limited. More research is needed to better understand the causes of elder mistreatment, tactics to

RONALD D. ADELMAN • Division of Geriatrics and Gerontology, New York Hospital–Cornell Medical Center, New York, New York 10021.   HENNA SIDDIQUI • Division of Geriatrics, Winthrop–University Hospital, Mineola, New York 11501,   NANCY FOLDI • Division of Neurology, Winthrop–University Hospital, Mineola, New York 11501.

Handbook of Clinical Geropsychology, edited by Michel Hersen and Vincent B. Van Hasselt. Plenum Press, New York, 1998.

prevent this problem, and ways to successfully intervene. The goals of this chapter are to define family-mediated elder abuse and neglect, to discuss approaches to detection and assessment, and to outline possible strategies for intervention.

EPIDEMIOLOGY

The epidemiology of elder mistreatment has been better understood since the results of a 1986 survey conducted by the Family Research Laboratory at the University of New Hampshire (Pillemer & Finkelhor, 1988). Two thousand twenty randomly selected elderly people living in the Boston metropolitan area were interviewed and 32 of every 1,000 people 65 years of age and older reported being mistreated. *Abuse* was defined as physical abuse, which included hitting, slapping, and pushing; *neglect* involved depriving a person of something needed for daily living; and *chronic verbal aggression* included verbal threats and insults. Because this survey did not include financial exploitation and other forms of elder mistreatment, the 3.2% incidence underestimates the problem

The Family Research Laboratory investigators discovered that most abuse is committed by one spouse against another; 65% of abuse cases were between spouses, whereas only 23% involved an adult child abusing a parent. Of note was that elderly husbands were abused twice as often as elderly wives. It is not known whether the abuse perpetrated by wives was a form of retaliation. Also, the survey found that elderly wives are more seriously injured by their husbands than elderly husbands are by their wives.

Recently, the Women's Initiative of the American Association of Retired Persons categorized family-mediated elder abuse and neglect as follows: (l) early-onset spousal and partner abuse and neglect continuing into later life, (2) late-onset spousal and partner abuse and neglect during later life, and (3) abuse and neglect by adult children and other relatives (Adelman & Breckman, 1995).

Another important finding from the University of New Hampshire study was that the abusers usually were dependent on the person they abused, for example, an adult child dependent for housing and economic support. Close proximity of living arrangements of victim and abuser was noted to be a significant risk factor for the occurrence of abuse and neglect; elderly individuals living alone were less likely to experience abuse. The survey also demonstrated that mistreatment occurred across all economic levels, religions, and age groups among the elderly.

DEFINITIONS

There are three main forms of elder mistreatment: physical, psychological, and financial. Physical abuse and neglect includes striking, shoving, beating, restraining, or feeding improperly. Sexual assault is also included under this subheading. Psychological abuse and neglect may manifest in threatening remarks, insults, commands, or ignoring the older individual. This form of abuse and neglect causes emotional stress for an older person. Ageist behavior in the form of infantilism, whereby the older person is treated as a child, also constitutes a form of psychological mistreatment. Financial abuse and neglect includes the misuse or exploitation of or inattention to an older person's possessions or funds. Conning, pressuring an older individual to distribute assets, or irresponsibly managing the victim's money comprise financial mistreatment. It is important to realize that usually several types of abuse co-occur. For example, if an elderly woman is being physically abused by her alcoholic son, she is likely to be experiencing psychological mistreatment as well (Breckman & Adelman, 1988).

THEORIES OF CAUSATION

There are four main theories of causation for elder abuse and neglect. More research needs to be done to properly substantiate these suggested etiologies. The theories include (1) psychopathology of the abuser; (2) stress; (3) transgenerational violence; and (4) dependency (Pillemer, 1986)

Psychopathology of the Abuser

The disproportionate numbers of abusers with serious psychiatric conditions and drug and alcohol problems is the basis for this etiologic theory (Wolf & Pillemer, 1989). Health professionals working in psychiatric institutions should become aware of elder abuse and neglect. When an adult child has a psychiatric illness requiring hospitalization, the patient may often be discharged to the parents' home. Patients who are not violent while institutionalized can be violent at home. Careful scrutiny for the potential for domestic violence must be part of every discharge plan. Therefore, appropriate provisions for follow-up are essential if prevention of elder mistreatment is a priority.

Stress

Death in the family, financial stresses, the responsibilities of caregiving, and other tensions can create anger and frustration that some individuals express through acts of violence (Strauss, Gelles, & Steinmetz, 1980). One study investigated family violence with Alzheimer's disease patients and found that 5.4% of caregivers in the study were violent to the patients. The variables most associated with violence were caregiver depression and living arrangements (Paveza, Cohen, Isdorfer, & Freels, 1992).

Transgenerational Violence

This etiologic concept theorizes that violent behavior is a learned method of expressing anger and frustration (Wolf & Pillemer, 1989). This theory postulates that when children are treated with violence, they develop the same patterns of behavior from direct observation.

Dependency

This theory postulates that when family members are dependent on an older relative for housing, finances, emotional support, and other needs, the dependent family member may become resentful and then be predisposed to abusive or neglectful behavior (Hwalek, Sengstock, & Lawrence, 1984; Pillemer & Finkelhor, 1988; Wolf, Godkin, & Pillemer, 1984). This theory also implies that older individuals who are cognitively or functionally dependent on their families for care are at increased risk for abuse and neglect.

These four unproven etiologic theories should be conceptualized as potential risk factors for elder abuse and neglect. Systematically inquiring about the issues incorporated in these theories is useful to the health professional seeking to detect and evaluate this form of domestic violence.

DETECTION

There are many factors that make detection of elder abuse and neglect difficult. These factors can be divided into two basic types: the barriers of detection caused by issues of the health care professional and the barriers that are secondary to issues of the victim or the abuser. These barriers are discussed in the following sections.

Aiding in Detection: Training of Health Care Professionals

It is incumbent on the community of health care professionals to be able to detect abuse in the elderly. To facilitate this, every clinical setting should have a protocol for detecting elder mistreatment. At the Mount Sinai/Victim Services Agency Elder Abuse Project, geriatricians-in-training were trained in such detection (Ansell & Breckman, 1988).

Interview Rules

When interviewing an older patient, particularly an individual accompanied by a relative, it is crucial to spend some time with the older person alone. This provides opportunity not only to detect mistreatment, but also to provide a forum in which to establish rapport with the identified individual. The interview (and when appropriate the physical examination) should be performed completely separately from an accompanying relative who is suspected of mistreatment (Quinn & Tomita, 1986). Barriers to detection are numerous, but when a victim does not even have the opportunity for confidential interaction, affinity with the health provider will be difficult to develop. Without a trusting relationship between health professional and older victim, mistreatment most likely will go undetected.

Questions to Ask

As health care professionals are rarely trained in detection, it is helpful to have available concrete questions that can be used. In the program at the Mount Sinai Medical School/Victim Services Agency Elderly Abuse Project from New York City, geriatriciains-in-training were instructed to direct some of these questions to patients:

- Has anyone at home ever hurt you?
- Has anyone ever touched you without your consent?
- Has anyone ever made you do things you didn't wish to do?
- Has anyone taken anything that was yours without asking?
- Has anyone ever scolded or threatened you?
- Have you ever signed any documents that you didn't understand?
- Are you afraid of anyone at home?
- Has anyone ever failed to help you take care of yourself when you needed help?

These questions can be utilized by psychologists, nurses, social workers, and physicians (Ansell & Breckman, 1988).

Detection of Physical Abuse

Physical abuse and neglect can be manifested by unexplained injuries or evidence inconsistent with medical findings. For example, if an x-ray reveals multiple fractures of different ages and this evidence does not fit the clinical past and present history provided, the clinician should be suspicious of underlying mistreatment. Signs may include fractures, welts, lacerations, burns, and bruises. Suspicion of sexual abuse must be considered when any of the following is noted: torn or bloody underclothing; difficulty in walking or sitting; discomfort, itching or bruising in the genital area; or unexplained venereal disease or genital infections. Additional signs or symptoms of physical mistreatment include dehydration, malnutrition, hypothermia or hyperthermia, poor hygiene in a dependent older patient, inadequate or inappropriate clothing, and lack of supportive devices such as eyeglasses, hearing aids, or dentures. Unexpected or unexplained deterioration in an older person's health should also be evaluated. The presence of decubitus ulcers or signs of mismedication also require investigation.

Health care personnel must investigate the specifics of each injury and not misattribute conditions because of incomplete history taking or ageist stereotyping. For example, the health professional should assess each new fracture. A relative accompanying an older patient with a fracture may attribute the problem to a fall caused by poor balance. Although falls are common in the aging population, the injury needs to be carefully assessed and the possibility of abuse must be considered.

Observations

Certain types of behavioral observations by the health professional are helpful in the detection of elder mistreatment. The professional should consider possible elder abuse and neglect when any of the following instances are observed (Breckman & Adelman, 1988):

- the patient appears fearful of a family member;
- the patient appears reluctant to respond when questioned;
- the patient and family member have conflicting stories as to how an event occurred;
- the health professional observes the family member to be hostile, angry, or impatient with the elderly individual;
- the family member is overly concerned about costs for necessary items for the older individual (e.g., radiology tests, hearing aid);
- the family member tries to prevent the health professional from interacting with the older individual privately;
- the family member prevents or resists necessary services from coming into the home (e.g., visiting nurse, physical therapy).

Aiding in Detection: Barriers of Victims and Abusers

Although personnel in mental health and medical settings need training, it is equally important to highlight situations in which the abuser and victim present with specific features that should raise suspicion.

Factors in the Victim

Several aspects of the victim make it difficult to detect abuse or neglect. Clearly, the victim may feel shame and not be able to disclose mistreatment. Fear of retaliation may be another impediment. Another formidable barrier to detection is the lack of awareness about this phenomenon on the part of older people: victims may be unable to report abuse or neglect because they are not aware that what they are experiencing qualifies as mistreatment.

Factors in the Abuser

The abuser also plays a role in creating barriers to detection. Certain risk factors, however, should raise suspicion.

Deterring Contact.   Naturally, the abuser may deter the possibility of having the victim come into contact with health care professionals or friends. The older individual may be newly isolated in that he or she does not have opportunities to be with other people or pursue desired activities. This may also take the form of preventing the victim from seeing health professionals (e.g., missed or delayed appointments). The abuser also may prevent any one health professional from seeing the whole picture (consider the pattern of physician or hospital "hopping"). For example, an abuser who is responsible for multiple fractures can probably avoid seeing the same physician or emergency room to conceal a pattern of behavior that would indicate mistreatment.

The perpetrator also holds a certain authority over and can instill fear in the victim, affecting the presentation to the outside world. This may take the form of the victim's not revealing information for fear of retaliation from the abuser, thus not disclosing events.

Other Risk Factors of the Abuser.   Certain psychological or physical or environmental risk factors of the abuser should raise suspicion. For example, there may be a family member with a history of mental illness or a drug or alcohol problem; or there may be a history of violence in the family; the patient or family member may be dependent on the other for housing, finances, or emotional support; or there may be stress in the family (e.g., loss of job, death of a significant other).

ASSESSMENT

Once there is suspicion of elder abuse or neglect, a careful assessment of the victim's situation must be made. This evaluation needs to be extensive and to include both medical and psychosocial parameters.

Victim Access

The first component to assess is the access the provider will have to the victim. The abuser usually limits the victim's exposure to the outside world and often refuses to allow a professional to visit the home. Abusers closely monitor the victim's contact with the outside world to prevent disclosure of mistreatment. Often, the health professional is the only individual to whom the victim has access which underscores the importance of health providers' recognizing this form of domestic violence. In general, the key to access is persistence and tenacity on the part of the health professional. At times, health professionals need to become quite ingenious to gain access to the isolated victim.

Abuse Pattern

Mistreatment often increases in severity and frequency over time. If the pattern of abuse has escalated, and the older victim is being severely abused, the victim may be in serious danger.

Assessment of Emergency

The health provider must decide whether emergency intervention needs to be taken. Professionals in the aging network may not be knowledgeable about the seriousness of domestic violence and its criminal context. A victim's life may be in jeopardy; therefore, careful scrutiny of the victim's safety is a critical component of assessment. An outlook that emphasizes that mistreatment is derived primarily from caregiver stress undermines a domestic violence perspective and the seriousness of elder abuse and neglect.

Intentionality

It is imperative to learn whether the abuse is intentional. For example, determining that a relative intended to cause harm by mismedicating an older individual (versus nondeliberate mismedication occurring from an improper understanding of the physician's orders) has significant implications for the approach toward intervention.

Who Is Abusing?

The assessment should also attempt to determine who is inflicting the abuse. There may be more than one perpetrator and an accurate assessment is crucial in order to determine appropriate interventions. For example, it must be ascertained whether the suspected abuser is a family member.

Assessing the Interpersonal Dynamic Situation

Dependency profiles of both the victim and the abuser need to be determined. Is the victim dependent on the abuser or is the abuser the dependent one? External stresses, such as unemployment, retirement, and the death of someone close, are considered potential risk factors for elder mistreatment.

It is important to ascertain whether the victim perceives the seriousness of the problem or denies the presence of abuse and neglect. The victim's awareness of the mistreatment and whether the victim is in denial or recognizes the problem will ultimately determine the types of intervention options available to the victim at his or her present stage of awareness.

Cognitive, Psychological, and Physical Level of the Abused

The assessment must determine whether the victim is cognitively impaired. Typically, this will involve a neuropsychological evaluation of the victim that will be used to determine the level of comprehension or appreciation of the situation. That is, does the victim appreciate the risks of staying in an abusive situation? Is the victim competent to access help, follow a safety plan, and escape if abuse recurs? Similarly, any active psychological symptoms secondary to Axis I or Axis II diagnoses (e.g., psychosis, depression, or significant stressors) need to be assessed. Their contributions can significantly affect the victim's ability to follow any future recommendations. The victim's medical status is also important to determine: Is there a medical condition or mobility problem that will require special management? For example, if the patient is wheelchair-bound, this may limit the use of certain shelters that are not set up for the nonambulatory.

Resources

The victim's resources need to be determined. What financial resources does the patient have? Does the victim own his or her residence? What emotional support is available to the victim? Are there concerned family and friends who are willing to help the victim?

INTERVENTION

Intervention can be planned only after a thorough assessment has been conducted. After assessment, the health professional will understand the severity of maltreatment, the victim's insight into the abuse, the victim's cognitive capabilities, the victim's resources, and community resources (Breckman & Adelman, 1988). Intervention can then occur in several areas: safety, treatment of the victim, treatment of cause of mistreatment, and criminal and legal steps. These are discussed in the sections below.

Safety

Immediate action must take place if the assessment reveals that the victim is in danger. Information about previous interventions is crucial. For example, if previous court orders of protection were not successful, it is essential to determine why, so that the same failed approach is avoided. Provision of emergency supports is an integral part of intervention. If an older victim is endangered, providing respite housing or help in getting immediate medical attention may be the first line of action.

Treatment of the Victim

It is essential to determine the victim's *awareness* of the mistreatment. Breckman's model (Breckman & Adelman, 1988) is a useful tool with which to understand the victim's state of mind concerning elder mistreatment. Breckman categorizes victims according to the following stages: denial, recognition, or rebuilding. Although Breckman's model acknowledges that a victim's stage of awareness can fluctuate, it is important that the worker plan interventions that are appropriate for the victim's level of awareness; otherwise, the intervention is likely to fail. For example, if an older victim is still in a stage of reluctant admission about her adult son who is perpetrating violence, it is unlikely that she will proceed with a court order of protection against him.

Another essential part of intervention is the provision of *psychological* treatment. If physical or financial mistreatment is occurring the older individual must also be experiencing psychological victimization. Individual counseling or psychotherapy is necessary for the victim to begin to rebuild self-esteem and recover from the effects of victimization. Victims of elder mistreatment have found that participation in a victims' support group is beneficial. In addition, elder abuse victims are often depressed. Among the elderly, depression can manifest with cognitive changes that are reversible with appropriate treatment. Therefore, a careful mental health assessment is paramount in a comprehensive intervention strategy. Naturally, counseling the elder abuse victim should be viewed as a long-term endeavor; the mental health professional should anticipate progress in incremental steps, rather than in rapid advances with short-term resolution.

Some older victims are reluctant to report mistreatment because they fear the only option available to them is admission to a nursing home. Interventions that are successful in eliminating the source of violence will allow the older victim to reclaim his or her home. When this is not possible, exploring alternative living arrangements is another intervention possibility. Adult homes, life-care communities, and senior housing are possible options.

Providing *educational* information is a major focus of intervention. Education includes teaching victims about abuse and neglect and teaching them that options do exist. It also includes teaching victims to devise safety plans to follow if they are endangered.

Nonemergent medical assistance is also crucial. Mistreatment victims often have been neglected medically and after detection of mistreatment these needs must be addressed.

Treatment of Causes

Assistance that addresses causes of elder abuse and neglect is a third line of intervention. For example, referral to drug or alcohol rehabilitation can be offered to addicted abusers and respite services or home care support can be arranged for stressed caregivers. Psychotherapeutic work with the abuser (e.g., support groups for caregivers) may also be indicated as a vehicle to keep an alliance with those who may still be involved in the victim's care. It is important to recognize that abusers usually do not abuse continuously, and between episodes they may display fairly normal behavior. Unless there are persons who can fill the void in the life of the victim if the abuser is removed, it may be extremely difficult for the older victim to forgo contact with the abuser.

Legal and Criminal Issues

Health professionals must become familiar with their state laws. If mandatory reporting is not required, the health professional can present options to the mentally competent victim who can then decide how to proceed. When a victim is cognitively impaired, most decisions are better made by an interdisciplinary team. Decisions need to be made with full awareness of the severity of the violence, the lifestyle choice history of the individual, and the legal ramifications. Protective service laws govern intervention and reporting for incompetent victims; thus again, health professionals need to be familiar with these state laws. When a victim is ready to embark on a legal route, providing legal aid is an essential part of intervention. If a victim is going to obtain an order of protection through family or criminal court, advocacy for the older victim through the criminal justice system is indispensable.

REFERENCES

Adelman, R., & Breckman, R. (1995). Elder abuse and neglect. In *The Merck manual of geriatrics* (2nd ed., pp. 1408–1416). Whitehouse Station, NJ: Merck.

American Medical Association diagnostic and treatment guidelines on elder abuse and neglect. (1992). Chicago: American Medical Association.

Ansell, P., & Breckman, R. (1988). *Assessment of elder mistreatment: Issues and considerations. Elder mistreatment guidelines for health care profession: Detection, assessment and intervention.* New York: Mount Sinai/Victim Services Agency's Elder Abuse Project.

Breckman, R. S., & Adelman, R. D. (1988). *Strategies for helping victims of elder mistreatment.* Newbury Park, CA: Sage.

Hwalek, M., Sengstock, M., & Lawrence R. (1984, November). *Assessing the probability of abuse of the elderly.* Paper presented at the annual meeting of the Gerontological Society of America, San Antonio, TX.

Paveza, G., Cohen, D., Eisdorfer, C., & Freels, S. (1992). Severe family violence and Alzheimer's disease: Prevalence and risk factors. *Gerontologist, 32* (4), 493–497.

Pillemer, K. (1986). Risk factors in elder abuse: Results from a case-control study. In K. Pillemer & R. Wolf (Eds.), *Elder abuse: conflict in the family* (pp. 236–266). Dover, MA: Auburn House.

Pillemer, K., & Finkelhor, D. (1988). The prevalence of elder abuse: A random sample survey. *Gerontologist, 28,* 51–57.

Quinn, M., & Tomita, S. (1986). Elder abuse and neglect. New York: Springer.

Strauss, M., Gelles, R., & Steinmetz, S. (1980). *Behind closed doors: Violence in the family.* Garden City, NY: Anchor/Doubleday.

U.S. Congress, House Select Committee on Aging. (1991). *Elder abuse: What can be done?* Washington, DC: U.S. Government Printing Office.

Wolf, R., & Pillemer, K. (1989). *Helping elderly victims: the reality of elder abuse.* New York: Columbia University Press.

Wolf, R., Godkin, M., & Pillemer, K. A. (1984). *Elder abuse and neglect: Report from the model projects.* Worcester: University of Massachusetts Medical Center, University Center on Aging.

Index